South University Library
Richmond Campus
2151 Old Brick Road
Glen Allen, Va 23060

Handbooks in Health, Work, and Disability

For further volumes:
http://www.springer.com/series/8766

Robert J. Gatchel · Izabela Z. Schultz
Editors

Handbook of Occupational Health and Wellness

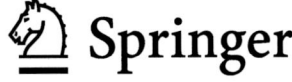

Editors
Robert J. Gatchel
Department of Psychology
The University of Texas at Arlington
Arlington, TX, USA

Izabela Z. Schultz
Department of Educational and
 Counseling Psychology
The University of British Columbia
Vancouver, BC, Canada

ISBN 978-1-4614-4838-9 (hardcover) ISBN 978-1-4614-4839-6 (eBook)
ISBN 978-1-4899-7635-2 (softcover)
DOI 10.1007/978-1-4614-4839-6
Springer New York Heidelberg Dordrecht London

Library of Congress Control Number: 2012952680

© Springer Science+Business Media New York 2012, First softcover printing 2015
This work is subject to copyright. All rights are reserved by the Publisher, whether the whole or part of the material is concerned, specifically the rights of translation, reprinting, reuse of illustrations, recitation, broadcasting, reproduction on microfilms or in any other physical way, and transmission or information storage and retrieval, electronic adaptation, computer software, or by similar or dissimilar methodology now known or hereafter developed. Exempted from this legal reservation are brief excerpts in connection with reviews or scholarly analysis or material supplied specifically for the purpose of being entered and executed on a computer system, for exclusive use by the purchaser of the work. Duplication of this publication or parts thereof is permitted only under the provisions of the Copyright Law of the Publisher's location, in its current version, and permission for use must always be obtained from Springer. Permissions for use may be obtained through RightsLink at the Copyright Clearance Center. Violations are liable to prosecution under the respective Copyright Law.
The use of general descriptive names, registered names, trademarks, service marks, etc. in this publication does not imply, even in the absence of a specific statement, that such names are exempt from the relevant protective laws and regulations and therefore free for general use.
While the advice and information in this book are believed to be true and accurate at the date of publication, neither the authors nor the editors nor the publisher can accept any legal responsibility for any errors or omissions that may be made. The publisher makes no warranty, express or implied, with respect to the material contained herein.

Printed on acid-free paper

Springer is part of Springer Science+Business Media (www.springer.com)

Dedicated to the memory of Dr. Andy Baum, my best friend and colleague of over 30 years

—Robert J. Gatchel

Preface

This *Handbook* integrates the growing clinical research evidence related to the emerging transdisciplinary field of occupational health and wellness. This expanding field is especially important because of the growing costs, including social and economic, and those associated with human suffering. Indeed, numerous statistics have found a clear relationship between health status and risks in the workplace on one hand, and financial and productivity losses on the other. With these challenges in mind, it is not at all surprising that new models and occupational intervention approaches are being developed to address the wide range of issues in this field. Moreover, the recent national and international unrest caused by unemployment and political uncertainties, the rampant distrust of government and big business, and the problems associated with rising health care costs all add up to continuing changes that will have to be taken into account in future developments in this field.

The *Handbook* will be of great interest to physicians, psychologists, occupational therapists, vocational rehabilitators, labor relations and human-resource professionals, employee and family assistance counselors, disability case managers, supervisors/employers, as well as researchers and academicians alike. As delineated in the table of contents, there is a wide array of important topics, ranging from current conceptual approaches to health and wellness in the workplace, to common problems in the workplace such as presenteeism/abstenteeism, to common illnesses and job-related burnout, to prevention and intervention methods. The book consists of five major parts. *Part I*, "Introduction and Overview," provides an overview and critical evaluation of the emerging conceptual models that are currently driving the clinical research and practice in the field. This serves as the initial platform from which to better understand the subsequent topics to be discussed. *Part II*, "Major Symptoms and Disorders in the Workplace," exposes the reader to the types of critical occupational health risks that have been well documented, as well as the financial and productivity losses associated with them. In *Part III*, "Evaluation of Occupational Causes and Risks to Workers' Health," a comprehensive evaluation of these risks and causes of such occupational health threats is offered. This leads to Part IV, "Prevention and Intervention Methods," which delineates techniques to prevent or intervene with these potential occupational health issues. Finally, Part V, "Research, Evaluation, Diversity and Practice," addresses epidemiology, program evaluation, cultural considerations, and future directions.

All contributors to the *Handbook* were asked to provide a balance among theoretical models, current best-practice guidelines, and evidence-based documentation of such models and guidelines. The contributors were carefully selected for their unique knowledge, as well as their ability to meaningfully present this information in a comprehensive manner. At first blush, this may appear to be a quite diverse array of topics to cover in one book. However, we made it our mission to provide the most comprehensive coverage of the field to date. Even we were pleasantly surprised by the convergence of models, issues, and clinical research that resulted across the 26 chapters, albeit in a different light. Each chapter added a unique thread to the overall fabric of the present *Handbook*, making it a comprehensive overview of the field of occupational health and wellness. At the same time, the unique contributions of constructs such as stress, wellness, support, adaptive/maladaptive behaviors, and group and individual differences are represented across this overall fabric.

We would like to acknowledge the authors for their valuable state-of-the-art contributions and for making this *Handbook* come to fruition in a timely manner. We also especially thank Janice Stern of Springer, who supported the vision of this *Handbook* series and encouraged us during our journey. In addition, we are indebted to Pedro Cortes at The University of Texas at Arlington for his technical contributions to the development of the *Handbook*.

Arlington, TX, USA　　　　　　　　　　　　　　　　　　　　Robert J. Gatchel
Vancouver, BC, Canada　　　　　　　　　　　　　　　　　　Izabela Z. Schultz

Contents

Part I Introduction and Overview

1 **Conceptual Approaches to Occupational Health and Wellness: An Overview**... 3
Robert J. Gatchel and Nancy D. Kishino

2 **Theories of Psychological Stress at Work** 23
Philip J. Dewe, Michael P. O'Driscoll, and Cary L. Cooper

3 **The Growth of Occupational Health Psychology** 39
Heather Graham, Krista J. Howard, and Angela Liegey Dougall

Part II Major Symptoms and Disorders in the Workplace

4 **Work-Related Musculoskeletal Disorders and Pain** 63
Ann Marie Hernandez and Alan L. Peterson

5 **Cardiovascular Disease and the Workplace** 87
Alexandra L. Terrill and John P. Garofalo

6 **Challenges Related to Mental Health in the Workplace** 105
Carolyn S. Dewa, Marc Corbière, Marie-José Durand, and Jennifer Hensel

7 **Cancer Survivors and Work**... 131
Michal C. Moskowitz, Briana L. Todd, and Michael Feuerstein

8 **The Problem of Absenteeism and Presenteeism in the Workplace** 151
Krista J. Howard, Jeffrey T. Howard, and Alessa F. Smyth

9 **Occupational Burnout** 181
Cindy A. McGeary and Donald D. McGeary

10 **Self-medication and Illicit Drug Use in the Workplace** 201
Fong Chan, Ebonee Johnson, Emma K. Hiatt, Chih Chin Chou, and Elizabeth da Silva Cardoso

11 Beyond the Playground: Bullying in the Workplace and Its Relation to Mental and Physical Health Outcomes ... 219
Madeline Rex-Lear, Jennifer M. Knack, and Lauri A. Jensen-Campbell

Part III Evaluation of Occupational Causes and Risks to Workers' Health

12 Promoting Mental Health Within Workplaces ... 243
Bonnie Kirsh and Rebecca Gewurtz

13 Workplace Injury and Illness, Safety Engineering, Economics and Social Capital ... 267
Henry P. Cole

14 The Role of Work Schedules in Occupational Health and Safety ... 297
Jeanne M. Geiger-Brown, Clark J. Lee, and Alison M. Trinkoff

15 Work–Family Balance Issues and Work–Leave Policies ... 323
Rosalind. B. King, Georgia Karuntzos, Lynne M. Casper, Phyllis Moen, Kelly D. Davis, Lisa Berkman, Mary Durham, and Ellen Ernst Kossek

16 Workers' Compensation and Its Potential for Perpetuation of Disability ... 341
Michael E. Schatman

Part IV Prevention and Intervention Methods

17 Health and Wellness Promotion in the Workplace ... 365
William S. Shaw, Silje E. Reme, and Cécile R.L. Boot

18 Stress Reduction Programmes for the Workplace ... 383
Tores Theorell

19 Primary and Secondary Prevention of Illness in the Workplace ... 405
Brian R. Theodore

20 Organizational Aspects of Work Accommodation and Retention in Mental Health ... 423
Izabela Z. Schultz, Terry Krupa, E. Sally Rogers, and Alanna Winter

21 Employee Assistance Programs: Evidence and Current Trends ... 441
Mark Attridge

Part V Research, Evaluation, Diversity and Practice

22 Epidemiological Methods for Determining Potential Occupational Health and Illness Issues 471
J. Mark Melhorn, Charles N. Brooks, and Shirley Seaman

23 Program Evaluation of Prevention and Intervention Methods 495
Richard C. Robinson, John P. Garofalo, and Pamela Behnk

24 Gender and Cultural Considerations in the Workplace 513
Nicolette Lopez, Hollie Pellosmaa, and Pablo Mora

25 Addressing Occupational Workplace Issues "In Action": An Ongoing Study of Nursing Academic Program Directors 535
Ronda Mintz-Binder

26 Occupational Health and Wellness: Current Status and Future Directions 549
Robert J. Gatchel

Index 565

Contributors

Mark Attridge, Ph.D., M.A. Attridge Consulting, Inc., Minneapolis, MN, USA

Pamela Behnk University of Kansas School of Medicine, North Kansas, Witchita, KS

Lisa Berkman, Ph.D. Department of Society, Human Development and Health, Harvard University, Cambridge, MA, USA

Cécile R.L. Boot, Ph.D. VU University Medical Center, EMGO Institute for Health and Care Research, Amsterdam, The Netherlands

Charles N. Brooks Bellevue, WA, USA

Elizabeth da Silva Cardoso, Ph.D. Department of Educational Foundations and Counseling Programs, Hunter College, City University of New York, New York, NY, USA

Lynne M. Casper, Ph.D. Department of Sociology, University of Southern California, Los Angeles, CA, USA

Fong Chan, Ph.D. Department of Rehabilitation Psychology and Special Education, University of Wisconsin—Madison, Madison, WI, USA

Chih Chin Chou, Ph.D. Department of Disability and Psychoeducational Studies, University of Arizona, Tucson, AZ, USA

Henry P. Cole, Ed.D. Department of Psychology, University of Kentucky College of Public Health, Lexington, KY, USA

Cary L. Cooper, C.B.E. Management School Office, Lancaster University Management School, Lancaster University, Lancaster, UK

Marc Corbière, Ph.D. Department Centre for Action in Work Disability Prevention and Rehabilitation, University of Sherbrooke, Longueuil, Longueuil, QC, Canada

Kelly D. Davis, Ph.D. Department of Human Development and Family Studies, Penn State University, University Park, PA, USA

François Desmeules, P.T., Ph.D. Axe de recherche clinique—Unité de recherche en orthopédie, Centre de recherche de l'Hôpital Maisonneuve-

Rosemont (CRHMR), School of Rehabilitation, University of Montreal & Maisonneuve-Rosemont Hospital Research Center (CRHMR), Montréal, QC, Canada

Carolyn S. Dewa, M.P.H., Ph.D. Centre for Research on Employment and Workplace Health, Centre for Addiction and Mental Health, Toronto, ON, Canada

Department of Psychiatry, University of Toronto, Toronto, ON, Canada

Philip J. Dewe, Ph.D. Department of Organizational Psychology, Birkbeck, University of London, London, UK

Angela Liegey Dougall, Ph.D. Department of Psychology, The University of Texas at Arlington, Arlington, TX, USA

Marie-José Durand, Ph.D. Department Faculty of Medicine and Health Sciences, University of Sherbrooke, Longueuil, Longueuil, QC, Canada

Mary Durham, Ph.D. The Center for Health Research, Kaiser Permanente, Center for Health Research, Portland, OR, USA

Michael Feuerstein, Ph.D., M.P.H. Department of Medical and Clinical Psychology and Preventive Medicine and Biometrics, Uniformed Services University of the Health Sciences, Bethesda, MD, USA

John P. Garofalo, Ph.D. Department of Psychology, Washington State University Vancouver, Vancouver, WA, USA

Robert J. Gatchel, Ph.D., A.B.P.P. Department of Psychology, The University of Texas at Arlington, Arlington, TX, USA

Jeanne M. Geiger-Brown, Ph.D., R.N. Department of Family and Community health, University of Maryland School of Nursing, Baltimore, MD, USA

Rebecca Gewurtz, Ph.D. Department School of Rehabilitation, McMaster University, Hamilton, ON, Canada

Heather Graham, Ph.D. Department of Psychology, University of Texas at Arlington, Arlington, TX, USA

Jennifer Hensel, M.D. Department of Psychiatry, University of Toronto, Toronto, ON, Canada

Ann Marie Hernandez, Ph.D. Department of Psychiatry, University of Texas Health Sciences Center at San Antonio, San Antonio, TX, USA

Department of Psychiatry—Mail Code 7792, University of Texas Health Sciences Center at San Antonio, San Antonio, TX, USA

Emma K. Hiatt, Ph.D. Department of Rehabilitation Psychology and Special Education, University of Wisconsin—Madison, Madison, WI, USA

Jeffrey T. Howard, M.A. Department of Demography, The University of Texas—San Antonio, San Antonio, TX, USA

Krista J. Howard, Ph.D. Department of Psychology, Texas State University—San Marcos, San Marcos, TX, USA

Lauri A. Jensen-Campbell, Ph.D. Department of Psychology, University of Texas at Arlington, Arlington, TX, USA

Ebonee Johnson, Ph.D. Department of Rehabilitation Psychology and Special Education, University of Wisconsin—Madison, Madison, WI, USA

Georgia Karuntzos, Ph.D. RTI International, Research Triangle Park, NC, USA

Rosalind B. King, Ph.D. Eunice Kennedy Shriver National Institute of Child Health and Human Development, National Institutes of Health, Bethesda, MD, USA

Bonnie Kirsh, Ph.D. Department of Occupational Science and Occupational Therapy, University of Toronto, Toronto, ON, Canada

Nancy D. Kishino, O.T.R., C.V.E. West Coast Spine Restoration Center, Riverside, CA, USA

Jennifer M. Knack, Ph.D. Department of Psychology, Clarkson University, Potsdam, NY, USA

Ellen Ernst Kossek, Ph.D. School of Human Resources and labor Relations, Michigan State University, East Lansing, MI, USA

Purdue University Krannert School of Management & Susan Bulkeley Butler Leadership Center, West Lafayette, Indiana West Lafayette, IN, USA

Terry Krupa, Ph.D. Department School of Rehabilitation Therapy, Queen's University, Kingston, ON, Canada

Clark J. Lee, J.D. Center for Health and Homeland Security, University of Maryland, Baltimore, MD, USA

Nicolette Lopez, Ph.D. Department of Psychology, University of Texas at Arlington, Arlington, TX, USA

Cindy A. McGeary, Ph.D. Department of Psychology, University of Texas at Arlington, Arlington, TX, USA

Donald D. McGeary, Ph.D., A.B.P.P. Department of Psychiatry, The University of Texas health Science Center San Antonio, San Antonio, TX, USA

J. Mark Melhorn, M.D. The Hand Center, Wichita, KS, USA

Ronda Mintz-Binder, D.N.P., R.N., C.N.E. Department of Nursing, College of Nursing, The University of Texas at Arlington, Arlington, TX, USA

Phyllis Moen, Ph.D. Department of Sociology, University of Minnesota, Minneapolis, MN, USA

Pablo Mora, Ph.D. Department of Psychology, University of Texas at Arlington, Arlington, TX, USA

Michal C. Moskowitz, B.A. Department of Medical and Clinical Psychology and Preventive Medicine and Biometrics, Uniformed Services University of the Health Sciences, Bethesda, MD, USA

Michael P. O'Driscoll, Ph.D. Department of Psychology, University of Waikato, Hamilton, New Zealand

Hollie Pellosmaa, M.HuServ. Department of Psychology, University of Texas at Arlington, Arlington, TX, USA

Kadija Perreault, P.T., M.Sc., Ph.D. Laval University & Centre for Interdisciplinary Research in Rehabilitation and Social Integration, Quebec City, QC, Canada

Alan L. Peterson, Ph.D., A.B.P.P. Department of Psychiatry, University of Texas Health Sciences Center at San Antonio, San Antonio, TX, USA

Department of Psychiatry—Mail Code 7792, University of Texas Health Sciences Center at San Antonio, San Antonio, TX, USA

Silje E. Reme, Ph.D. Harvard School of Public Health and Liberty Mutual Research Institute for Safety, Hopkinton, MA, USA

Madeline Rex-Lear, Ph.D. Department of Psychology, University of Texas at Arlington, Arlington, TX, USA

Richard C. Robinson, Ph.D. The University of Texas Southwestern Medical Center at Dallas, Dallas, Texas, USA

E. Sally Rogers, Sc.D. Department—Center for Psychiatric Rehabilitation, Boston University, Boston, MA, USA

Jean-Sébastien Roy, P.T., Ph.D. Laval University & Centre for Interdisciplinary Research in Rehabilitation and Social Integration (CIRRIS), Quebec City, QC, Canada

Michael E. Schatman, Ph.D., C.P.E. Schatman-Robinson Pain Psychology Associates, Foundation for Ethics in Pain Care, Bellevue, WA, USA

Izabela Z. Schultz, Ph.D. Department of Educational and Counselling Psychology, and Special Education, The University of British Columbia, Vancouver, BC, Canada

Shirley Seaman The Hand Center, Whichita, KS, USA

William S. Shaw, Ph.D. Liberty Mutual Research Institute for Safety, Hopkinton, MA, USA

Alessa F. Smyth, M.A. Department of Psychology, Texas State University—San Marcos, San Marcos, TX, USA

Alexandra L. Terrill, Ph.D. Department of Psychology, Washington State University Vancouver, Vancouver, WA, USA

Brian R. Theodore, Ph.D. Department of Anesthesiology and Pain Medicine, University of Washington, Seattle, WA, USA

Tores Theorell, M.D., Ph.D. Karolinska Institutet and Stockholm University, Stockholm, Sweden

Briana L. Todd, M.S. Department of Medical and Clinical Psychology, Uniformed Services University of the Health Sciences, Bethesda, MD, USA

Alison M. Trinkoff, Sc.D., R.N., F.A.A.N. Department of Family and Community Health, University of Maryland School of Nursing, Baltimore, MD, USA

Alanna Winter BC Women's Hospital & Health Centre, Vancouver, BC, Canada

Part I
Introduction and Overview

Conceptual Approaches to Occupational Health and Wellness: An Overview

Robert J. Gatchel and Nancy D. Kishino

As will be discussed in this chapter, there is an ever-growing body of clinical research evidence related to the field of occupational health and wellness. Part of this is due to the fact that we are in the midst of rapid global economic growth, with the attendant complex international and financial systems that produce an array of potentially significant problems, such as environmental and occupational hazards/diseases, worker safety and compensation issues, as well as psychosocial stress. The increase in clinical research in these areas has also produced numerous conceptual models/approaches to try to account for phenomena such as stress–illness relationships, individual differences in resiliency and productivity, and cross-cultural factors that affect occupational health and wellness. We will introduce the reader to some of these models in this chapter. Before doing so, a brief historical overview of events that have led to the development of this ever-expanding field will be provided.

Historical Overview

Occupational Compensation Issues

In modern western industrial countries, there has been a long history of attempts to deal with health issues associated with the work environment. Indeed, with the start of the industrial revolution, the financial issues of compensation for negligent accidental injuries in the workplace became significant. As succinctly reviewed by Anderson (1991), the first actual successful personal work injury case of this type in the English High Court dated back to 1836. In such cases, it was important to provide proof of negligence in the actual workplace, but the litigation was not valid if there was so-called contributory negligence on the part of the worker, or if the actual accident was caused by "ordinary risks" in the workplace. However, the following year, the English courts accepted the "fellow-servant" doctrine, which stated that an employer was not responsible for negligence on the part of another employee or

---

R.J. Gatchel, Ph.D., ABPP (✉)
Department of Psychology, The University of Texas at Arlington, Arlington, TX, USA
e-mail: gatchel@uta.edu

N.D. Kishino, OTR, CVE
West Coast Spine Restoration Center, 6177 River Crest Dr. #A, Riverside, CA 92507, USA
e-mail: nancykishino@msn.com

Table 1.1 Health insurance history in the USA

Post World War II—US employer-based health insurance
Medicare and Medicaid—1965
HMO Act—1973
Federal Health Insurance, Patient Protection and Affordable Care Act—2010

"fellow-servant." Of course, this was the expected "push back" from employers who were used to using workers and then simply replacing them with new workers without the need to pay any compensation. Indeed, this perspective was captured in the writings of individuals such as Engel's (*The Condition of the Working Class in England*, 1845) and Marx (*Das Kapital*, 1867) who portrayed the terrible ways in which industrial-revolution capitalism exploited workers, which produced alienation of workers when treated simply as commodities in the growing capitalistic system (Engels, 1845; Marx, 1867).

The next step, though, toward modern compensation laws was the English "Fatal Accident Act," which required some financial compensation to the family of a person killed by an accident at the workplace. Moreover, at about this same point in time, German law decreed that railroad companies were responsible for any accidents that occurred on the new Berlin–Potsdam Railroad. As Anderson (1991) goes on to note:

> Parallel development in Germany and England during the 1880s resulted in more comprehensive insurance laws. Bismarck introduced a comprehensive social insurance system in Germany, which included workers' compensation, and compulsory insurance was introduced in England through the Employers Liability Act (1880). Up until this time, fault had to be proven by the injured worker. This was abolished in England by the Workman's Compensation Act (1887), which, by 1911 covered all workers and not only those injured in accidents but also those with industrial diseases and sickness as well. (pp. 531–532)

In Europe, this industrial liability became part of a social security and welfare system, as well as the working conditions. For example, by 1992, every nation in the European Union was required to adapt, into their own national legislative mandate, that employers were responsible for evaluating all major occupational risk factors that may negatively affect employee health and safety. However, in the USA, the acceptance of employer responsibility was initially developed as a separate, no-fault system. It was not until 1908 that the Federal Employees Compensation Act was passed and, in 1914, the California Industrial Accident Act was subsequently passed. Unlike a federal disability system that existed in Europe, employers in the USA were sold private insurance coverage with the promise of immunity from liability suits on behalf of an employee. After World War II, such US employer-based health insurance became common. Thus, private insurance companies, such as Liberty Mutual Insurance Co., were developed as the "middle man" between employees and the State in workers' compensation cases. The State bought this private insurance from such companies, which then would protect the States by making any liability claims the responsibility of private insurance carriers such as Liberty Mutual. Each State was free to purchase their own workers' compensation insurance policies for workers of that State. Because of this, the workers' compensation insurance requirements will be quite different from State to State. By 1949, separate workers' compensation systems existed in all States. Moreover, as noted in Table 1.1, in 1954, the Social Security Disability Act was passed by Congress, which created a "second major layer of disability compensation" administered by the Federal government. Thus, in terms of actual physical injuries caused in the workplace, workers started to become more protected by compensation systems, although there were many vagaries across the different systems that could make it either easier or more difficult to obtain palpable benefits across workers and across different States. Subsequently, Medicare and Medicaid were introduced in 1965. The Health Management Organization (HMO) Act was passed in 1973 which opened up managed care networks in the private sector. Most recently, the federal health care plan was passed in 2010, which is still encountering a great deal of resistance. Finally, we would be

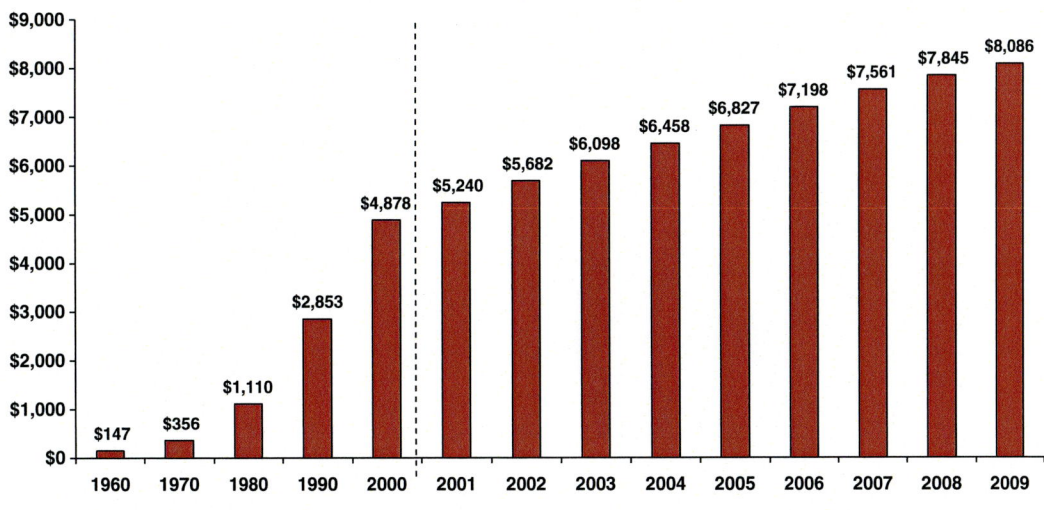

Fig. 1.1 Notes: Personal health-care expenditures are spending for health care services, excluding administration and net cost of insurance, public health activity, research, and structures and equipment. Out-of-pocket health insurance premiums paid by individuals are not included in Consumer Out-of-Pocket; they are counted as part of Private Health Insurance. Medicaid spending for the State Children's Health Insurance Program (which began in 1998) is included in Other Government Programs, not in Medicaid. Source: Kaiser Family Foundation calculations using NHE data from Centers for Medicare and Medicaid Services, Office of the Actuary, National Health Statistics Group, at http://www.cms.hhs.gov/NationalHealthExpendData/. *Source*: National health expenditures per capita 1960–2009

remiss if not to mention the fact that, over the years in the USA, the national expenditures for health care have increased dramatically (see Fig. 1.1). There has also been a shift in who is responsible for these health-care expenditures (Fig. 1.2).

"Unhealthy" Work Environments

Another area of occupational health concerns started to occur with the great advances in science during the nineteenth century. This marked the era where "better life through better chemistry" became the mantra. A broad range of chemical and biological neurotoxins, such as lead, mercury, organic solvents, and asbestos fibers, were introduced into the workplace. For example, an Ohio inventor named Thomas Midgley Jr. developed an interest in the industrial applications of chemistry. As reviewed by Bryson (2003), while working for the General Motors Research Corp., Midgley investigated a new compound called *tetraethyl lead*, and discovered that it could significantly reduce the degenerative condition known as "engine knock" in automobiles. Because of its success, it became a routine additive to gasoline. Unfortunately, lead is a neurotoxin, and too much exposure to it can significantly damage the central nervous system, and cause associated symptoms such as blindness, insomnia, kidney failure, and cancer. Indeed, once production of leaded gasoline started, many of the workers involved in this production started to develop significant neurological symptoms associated

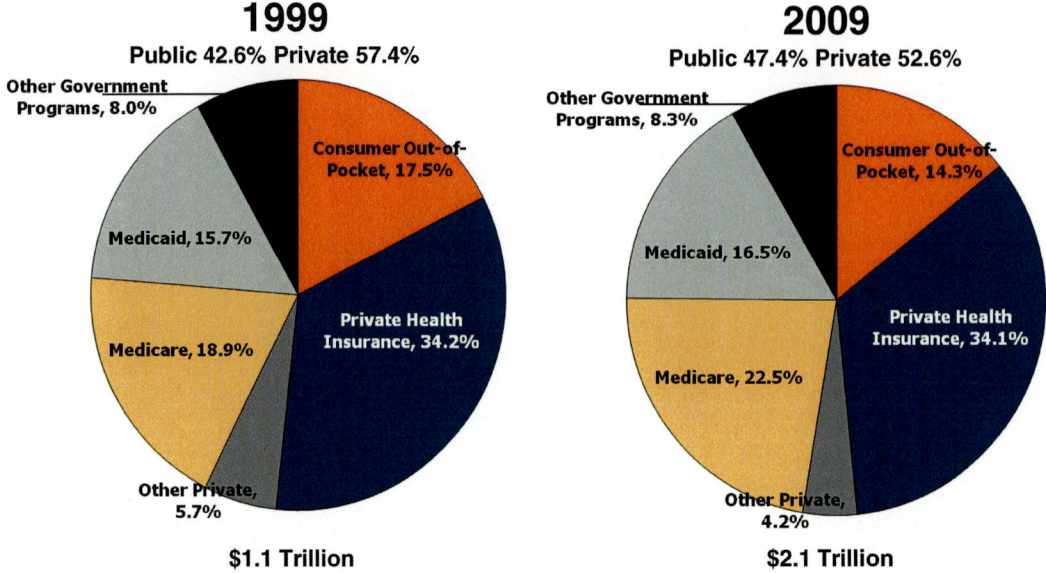

Fig. 1.2 Source: US health-care expenditures by source of payment, 1999 and 2009. Centers for Medicare and Medicaid Services, Office of the Actuary, National Health Statistics Group, at http://www.cms.hhs.gov/NationalHealthExpendData/

with over-exposure, such as neurological disorders highlighted by staggered gait and confused faculties indicative of lead poisoning. However, because of the great deal of money being produced by this lead additive (indeed, three of America's largest corporations—General Motors, DuPont, and Standard Oil—formed a joint enterprise called the Ethyl Gasoline Corp.), there was a major corporation/political denial of these adverse symptoms on workers. It was not until it became known that leaded gas engine exhaust became a major environmental threat to the atmosphere that the Clean Air Act of 1970 was finally passed which eliminated the sale of all leaded gasoline in the USA in 1986. Subsequently, it was immediately found that lead levels in the blood of Americans fell by 80 %. Lead was also subsequently removed from indoor paints and other products. However, unfortunately, the amount of lead in the atmosphere continues to grow even today due to mining, smelting, and other industrial activities in the USA, as well as in the rest of the World. Moreover, because of the great amount of economic pressure to maintain/increase industrial growth with new scientific discoveries for which no health hazards are *currently* known, it is often the case that problematic symptoms and diseases must first occur before there is any federally backed pressure to curtail such processes. For example, this may currently be the case in the widespread use of plastics, which are produced from by-products of the refining of oil and natural gas (producing *polyethylenes* that are carcinogen risks). However, the "proof of burden" rests on the workers/general population to empirically demonstrate, in a scientifically acceptable manner, a "cause–effect" relationship between a certain newly isolated neurotoxin and negative health consequences. This, unfortunately, can take many years if not decades to demonstrate. Of course, the Environmental Protection Agency has been developed to help monitor this, but often there may be political pressure by large multi-national companies to "overlook" premature assumed illness consequences.

Medicolegal Issues and Occupational Injuries

In other chapters of this Handbook, various issues related to occupational injuries will be reviewed. Of course, whenever there is an occupational accident or injury, there are usually medicolegal issues that ensue. Because of this, it is important to become aware of such issues and how they have been evaluated in the past and present. Howard, Kishino, Johnston, Worzer, and Gatchel (2010) have recently provided an overview of this topic in the context of pain-related injuries. However, the major issues are generalizable to other work-related injuries, issues such as losses and gains, malingering, and "litigation neurosis." These will be reviewed next.

Losses and Gains

The development and perpetuation of work-related disability can be attributed to both losses and gains following an occupational injury (Worzer, Kishino, & Gatchel, 2009). Losses and gains at the most basic level are quite relatively easy to identify. For example, once an injury occurs, a primary loss may be reflected by the loss of employment; a primary gain could be seen as the alleviation of guilt/conflict manifested in physical symptoms (Dersh, Polatin, Leeman, & Gatchel, 2009). In marked contrast, secondary losses and gains are consequential to the initial incident. Following a traumatic event (such as an occupational injury), for example, there is often a downward spiral of occurrences that may exacerbate the chronic injury-produced condition. Some examples of these secondary losses can include: financial loss; loss of social relationships at work; loss of respect from family and friends; loss of community approval, and guilt over disability (Dersh, Gatchel, & Kishino, 2005). The culmination of these losses can perpetuate the chronic occupational injury. Similarly, secondary gains have been found to maintain the disability as well. While earlier definitions of secondary gain were associated with the support one received from others following a traumatic event (Freud, 1917), subsequent renditions of the term secondary gain have been attributed to the gain of financial rewards related to disability (Finneson, 1976).

While secondary gain is often deemed as a form of reinforcement for disability behaviors, Worzer et al. (2009) distinguish the two concepts, such that reinforcement relates to external factors (such as monetary gain), whereas secondary gain relates to internal factors (such as the motivation to seek monetary gain). In point of fact, secondary gains have long been viewed as a main motivator that contributes to malingering in chronic disability populations (Fishbain, 1994; Worzer et al.).

Malingering

The term malingering has developed a negative connotation, in that a person is considered to be intentionally projecting exaggerated physical or and/or psychosocial symptoms for the purpose of gaining external rewards (American Psychiatric Association, 2000). While these rewards often include obtaining financial compensation, the act of malingering is also noted in the avoidance of activities, such as military duty or employment, or in obtaining drugs. According to the DSM-IV, at least two of the following four criteria must be met for a diagnosis of malingering:
- Referred by an attorney in order to obtain compensation for an injury or illness.
- No objective findings supporting the claimed disability.
- The lack of cooperation with therapeutic interventions or diagnostic evaluations.
- Antisocial personality disorder, with a history of behaviors such as violence, impulsive behavior, lack of regard for safety, failure to maintain work, and stealing.

However, there has been criticism of the DSM-IV's criteria as being moralistic and lacking in empirical validity. Rogers (1997), for example, regards the above criteria to be quite lacking in that, by meeting just two of the four components, only two-thirds of the individuals were found to be properly diagnosed. Furthermore, he identified that, for every malingerer correctly diagnosed, four other individuals are misclassified. Obviously, this reflects an unacceptably higher false-positive rate.

One particular area which has received extensive attention in terms of malingering is whiplash injuries, usually occurring after a motor vehicle collision. Such collisions often produce injuries to the neck or other body regions, and subsequent persistent pain and disability. Over the years, accumulated evidence suggested that such injuries involved not only a medical issue but were also influenced by external, non-injury psychosocial factors (Schrader et al., 1996). In fact, some have suggested that patients involved in litigation, or seeking legal representation for the whiplash injury, often must repeatedly "prove" their illness as real (Hadler, 1996; Harder, Veilleux, & Suissa, 1998). This, in turn, causes the individual to overly focus on his/her symptoms, with the resultant skewing of the perception of the magnitude of their pain, suffering, and disability. This, unfortunately, can promote delayed recovery from the injuries. The same pattern can emerge in patients with occupational injury disabilities.

Are all individuals with occupational disabilities and motor vehicle injuries malingerers? According to Dersh and colleagues (2009), the general assumption from the medicolegal perspective is that there is a high potential for malingering in workers' compensation populations based on the prevalence of secondary gains. However, most researchers have failed to show a strong relationship between malingering and general workers' compensation disability. Simply because secondary gains are present do not imply that the individual is a malingerer (Fishbain, Rosomoff, Cutler, & Rosomoff, 1995). In fact, true malingering is sometimes considered to be connected to sociopathy, such that there is a history of "deviant or maladaptive behaviors," whereas most individuals injured on the job show little to no psychopathology prior to the incident (Dersh et al., 2009).

An alternative model of malingering put forth by Rogers (1997) describes malingering as an adaptation, such that people will assess their specific goals and then utilize malingering as a method to obtain those goals. According to this model, the act of malingering is only associated with the attainment of the specific goals and not with any other social realms. While these malingerers are seen to participate in all opportunities to exhibit and validate their disability, they will tend to be non-compliant in the actual treatment program. Non-malingerers, however, should be expected to show difficulties with all facets of their lives.

Through a review of the literature on malingering and disability, Fishbain et al., (1999) identified that the proportion of chronic pain patients who are probable malingerers ranged between 1.25 and 10.4 %, whereas Mittenberg, Patton, Canyock, and Condit (2002) estimated the base rate for probable malingering and symptom exaggeration for individuals with workers' compensation disability to reach 32 %. Within a workers' compensation population reporting "stress" injuries, Sumanti, Brauer Boone, Savodnik, and Gorsuch (2006) concluded that between 9 and 29 % of the cohort exhibited non-credible psychiatric symptoms, and 8 % showed non-credible cognitive deficiencies.

Fishbain and colleagues proposed that the degree of malingering for patients may be better understood when evaluated on different levels, such that some individuals can be regarded more as "true" malingerers, while others fall into a "partial" range. The distinction between these levels depends on the actual health condition of the individual. A true malingerer will have no health or disability ailments and will falsify the health assessments to appear to be ill; whereas a partial malingerer, who has some form of disability, will be more likely to exaggerate the symptoms (Fishbain, 1999).

"Compensation Neurosis" and "Litigation Neurosis"

In the medicolegal context, the terms Compensation Neurosis and Litigation Neurosis refer to the amplification of physical and psychosocial symptoms, whether conscious or unconscious, when faced with secondary gains (Fishbain et al., 1995; Robinson, Rondinelli, Scheer, & Weinstein, 1997). In fact, compensation neurosis was first introduced in the 1880s as part of industrial accident litigation (Margoshes & Webster, 2000). It was thought that people who had work-related disability would exaggerate their somatic complaints due to the fact that they suffered from psychiatric disorders (such as depression and neurosis). However, once they received a "curative" financial settlement, they were then able to return-to-work. Recent studies, though, have refuted this concept (Margoshes & Webster, 2000). Some earlier research has shown that, when comparing individuals with similar disabilities, those with occupational injuries have been found to demonstrate poorer treatment outcomes as compared to those whose injuries are not related to workers' compensation (Rainville, Sobel, Hartigan, & Wright, 1997; Robinson et al., 1997). In contrast, research has also shown that chronic pain patients who may be identified as having "litigation neurosis" showed no physical improvement following a resolution of their disability claims (Bellamy, 1997; Fishbain et al., 1995). Bellamy (1997) cites several theories as to why the "malingerer" would continue to feign symptoms after the disability case is settled. One theory states that the continuation of disability may be a form of punishment toward the entity (e.g., the "non-caring Company") that caused the injury. A second theory proposes that recovering from the disability would be seen as admission to fraud, and the chronic disability-case patient may feel the need to defend his/her disability for fear of the loss of benefits. In a more comprehensive approach to defining compensation neurosis, because the system provides financial rewards for illness and injury, the physician is often seen as the "gatekeeper" to the disability benefits. Therefore, the chronic disability patient feels the need to exaggerate his/her symptoms when being challenged or re-examined (Bellamy, 1997).

Malingering and Workers' Compensation

While the incidence rate of true malingering has been identified to be fairly low, oftentimes the employers and insurance providers make assumptions regarding the nature or severity of the injury and the intent of the injured employee. By doing so, the practitioner or insurance provider may develop a certain bias toward individuals with occupational injuries. Patients with chronic occupational injuries tend to display increased disability, which is often noted as limited function. Functional disability is affected by not only the physical condition, but also can be exacerbated by cognitive and psychosocial factors (such as fear of re-injury). Through the recognition and resolution of barriers that impede recovery, patients with chronic occupational musculoskeletal injuries, for example, are better able to regain function and resume normal activities, thus lessening disability behaviors (McIntosh, Melles, & Hall, 1995). Similar to the effects of psychosocial distress, disability behaviors have often been thought to hinder recovery for individuals with chronic occupational injuries. The term disability behavior relates to the individual's sickness role based on the perception of a benefit associated with the injury (Gatchel, 2004). It is possible for these disability behaviors to be interpreted as malingering. And if so, the consequence of limiting or withholding treatment can result in additional distress and further exacerbate disability behaviors, thus perpetuating the malingering assumption (Margoshes & Webster, 2000).

As noted by Margoshes and Webster (2000), the current and more enlightened approach to this issue of malingering is the biopsychosocial model (a model we will emphasize later in this present chapter). They go on to point out that one should respond to a patient's illness, behaviors, and possible malingering by providing appropriate treatment and rehabilitation. As they highlight:

> … models looking at disability exaggeration were unable to predict poor outcomes for chronic low back pain patients in a multidisciplinary treatment program. This may be because the program studied provided counseling that addressed those factors that led to disability exaggeration, including "fear of re-injury, overly protective spouses, physician warnings against painful activity, anxiety, depression, and other personality features"… It is therefore recommended that rehabilitation programs include counseling to address these factors. (p. 58)

The Assessment of Malingering

Finally, while it is hypothesized that many chronic disability patients may exhibit malingering tendencies, the detection of malingering can be difficult to validate. Rogers, Harrell, and Liff (1993) put forth the following clinical evaluation strategies that can be used to detect malingering:
- *The floor effect strategy*: Individuals identified as malingering will score in ranges that even individuals with grave impairments would not score.
- *The performance curve strategy*: Individuals identified as malingering will score poorly on all responses, whereas an honest responder will score positively on the easier questions and poorly on the more difficult questions.
- *The magnitude of error strategy*: Individuals identified as malingering will exhibit a pattern of grossly incorrect answers as compared to incorrect answers that are a close approximation of the correct answers.
- *The symptom validity testing strategy*: Individuals identified as malingering will exhibit performances in the below-chance ranges based on simple binomial probability calculations for large numbers of trials.
- *The Atypical Presentation Strategy*: Individuals identified as malingering will exhibit cognitive ability deficiencies that do not mirror those of individuals with true cognitive impairment.
- *The violation of learning principles strategy*: Individuals identified as malingering will exhibit poor results on basic learning and memory tests that deviate from normal levels.

Several other assessment methods have also been developed and utilized in an attempt to detect malingering. Scoring patterns on the *Minnesota Multiphasic Personality Inventory-2* (MMPI-2; Butcher, Dahlstrom, Graham, Tellegen, & Kaemmer, 1989) have been shown to suggest malingering, specifically with respect to elevations of the F scale (Greene, 1997). The *Structured Interview of Reported Symptoms* (SIRS) was designed to directly parallel Roger's detection strategies (Rogers, Bagby & Dickens, 1992). Other assessments that have been used to detect malingering include basic IQ testing and neuropsychological testing (Conroy & Kwartner, 2006). Most recently, a Special Issue on Malingering and its assessment was published in *Psychological Injury and Law* [March, 2011, *4* (1)]. However, a strong word of caution should be raised here. From a medicolegal standpoint, the presence of secondary gain (e.g., financial reward) following an occupational injury can provide an individual with the motivation to "malinger" or to exaggerate physical and psychological symptoms. However, the prevalence of true malingering in chronic disability populations has been shown to be fairly low (Howard, Kishino, Johnston, Worzer, & Gatchel, 2010). The main quandary is in knowing the best method to assess potential malingering. Several strategies have been developed for such assessment, such as those just mentioned. However, it is the contention of many that it is more clinically feasible and valid to move away from the overly subjective and perjorative term "malingering" in the occupational pain and disability evaluation. Instead, replace that subjective construct method with a more comprehensive biopsychosocial-based approach to identify barriers to recovery that may significantly affect patient effort/responses on objective performance tests, as well as consistency in reporting certain symptoms or deficits. This biopsychosocial approach would be more clinically effective in determining possible pain and resulting disability.

A careful and comprehensive evaluation is quite warranted in order to prevent patients from taking advantage of the medical, insurance, and legal systems. As Hadler (1996) has noted: "If you have to prove you are ill, you can never get well…" (p. 2397). Thus, there may be external pressure on patients to prove they are really ill. This should be kept in mind when evaluating patients. Also, the misdiagnosis of an individual as a "malingerer" can inappropriately drop patients from their deserved medical benefits. Such assessment data are greatly needed in order to "tailor" the most effective biopsychosocial treatment program to the unique needs of specific patients. For individuals with occupational injuries, if malingering goes undetected, then those individuals are able to take advantage of the medical, insurance, and legal systems. However, if malingering is misdiagnosed, then individuals with true disability can be erroneously dropped from their deserved benefits.

Occupational Stress

Another important area of occupational health and illness that has become more recently recognized is occupational stress. Indeed, stress is ubiquitous in the workplace. Many jobs involve pressure to complete increasing amounts of work, and these pressures can contribute to social overload and stress (Baum, Gatchel, & Krantz, 1997). Much of this research in the area of occupational stress and health started in the 1990s, with attempts to determine which occupations were most stressful, or which characteristics of particular occupations were causes of elevated risks of coronary heart disease (Karasek & Theorell, 1990). Indeed, it was found that several broad types of working conditions had been associated with coronary heart disease risk (Baum et al., 1997). These include the psychological demands of the job, autonomy on the job (e.g., how much input workers have in making decisions), and satisfaction on the jobsite. Job demands refer to job conditions that tax or interfere with the workers' performance abilities, such as workload and work responsibilities. The level of job autonomy refers to the ability of the workers to control the speed, nature, and conditions of work. Job satisfaction includes gratification of the workers' needs and aspirations derived from employment. It has been found that low levels of control over one's job, as well as excess of workload, seem to be a particular important combination in heightening job-related stress. Karasek and Theorell (1990) have proposed that conditions of high work demands, combined with few opportunities to control the job situation (e.g., slow decisional latitude), are associated with increase coronary heart disease risk. The conditions of high demand and low control are called *high strain* situations. Indeed, the Karasek "job demand/control" hypothesis has been tested in several populations, and has been shown to predict cardiovascular disease or mortality in studies of male Swedish workers and studies of men and women in the USA (Karasek & Theorell; Karasek et al., 1988; Schnall et al., 1990). In a later chapter in this Handbook, Theorell provides a more thorough review of these above studies.

Another interesting study of occupational stress and coronary heart disease among women also illustrates how job conditions may contribute to coronary disease. Work and family demands and one's control over these situations appear to be important buffers of stress. For example, it has been found that working women (that is, women who had been employed outside the home for more than one half of their adult lives) were compared to housewives and with men. Results revealed that working women in general were not at a significantly higher risk of subsequent coronary heart disease than housewives. However, it was found that the following were more likely to develop coronary heart disease: clerical workers, who perhaps have low job control; working women with children, who have high family demands; and women whose bosses were unsupportive (Baum et al., 1997). Interestingly, the likelihood of coronary heart disease increases linearly with the number of children for working women. Relatedly, in a recent and more thorough review of the literature, Terrill, Garofalo, Soliday, and Craft (2012) have proposed a more comprehensive model for why coronary heart disease is a leading cause of mortality in adult women, particularly working mothers (they also provide a more detailed review of this in a later chapter in the present Handbook). They suggest it is due to a confluence of factors. Among them are the following:

- The multiple roles that potentially place conflicting demands resulting in increased stress (such as responsibilities of childcare, housework, their paid employment, and financial worries).
- Biological pathways such as estrogen-related factors, sympathetic nervous system reactivity, and allostatic load.

As will be discussed, it is now almost universally accepted that there is a relationship between work-related stress and ill health. There are now active occupationally-based programs developed for work–stress prevention. Indeed, as noted below:

> The nature of work is changing at whirlwind speed. Perhaps now more than ever before, job stress poses a threat to the health of workers and, in turn, to the health of the organization.
> National Institute of Occupational Safety and Health (NIOSH)

Indeed, beginning in the 1990s, NIOSH has played a major role in the USA in further promoting the importance of occupational health and safety standards. It is mandated by federal law to conduct research on the types of working conditions that may be hazardous to the mental and/or physical health of workers, as well as to disseminate this research in order to prevent future workplace injuries/illnesses. Other countries have similar research institutes, such as: the Institute for Psychological Factors and Health, part of the Karolinska Institute in Sweden; the Finnish Institute of Occupational Health; and the Institute of Work, Health and Organizations (I-WHO), at the University of Nottingham in the UK.

The Nature of Stress

Because the construct of stress underlies many of the topics in this Handbook, it will be worthwhile to review important issues related to the nature of stress here at the outset. This has been previously reviewed in greater detail by Gatchel and Baum (2009). Stress is a complex process, which leads to a broad-based series of changes across the entire organism. Most clinical researchers agree that stress is initiated and regulated by the central nervous system (CNS), which provides information about the environment and the periphery, and then interprets and acts on this information. The CNS consists of the brain and spinal cord, and connects to peripheral nerves that relay sensory information and executes directions to and from the brain. Part of this process is appraisal, a neurally based interpretation of afferent stimuli in the context of beliefs and perceptions of resources and other conditions. Depending on the nature of this process, the CNS issues commands to the body, either to maintain ongoing activity or to modify it to deal with the object of this appraisal. Thus, one can view the brain as "taking in" information about the environment, as well as the state of the rest of the body and, if this appraisal yields the "conclusion" that prevailing conditions may threaten harm, loss or excessive demand, stress responses are then produced.

It should be noted that all the basic principles of this appraisal process are not yet known, but research has indicated that two neuroendocrine systems are the primary underlying instigators of integrated stress responses. For example, upon recognition of threat or demand, the sympathetic nervous system (SNS) and the hypothalamic–pituitary–adrenocortical (HPA) axis will respond, and then accomplish a number of basic and excitatory functions. The SNS innervates most regions of the body, descending from the hypothalamus and extending to most organ systems and tissues throughout the body. Activation of the SNS results in increased physiological reactivity (such as heart rate, blood pressure, respiration, and other functions) that distributes nutrients to the body. Changes in hemodynamic responses then result in greater blood flow, delivering oxygen and glucose to the cells and organs of the body. Increased respiration increases oxygen available, and other changes liberate energy into easily transportable form. This permits stronger, faster responses. At the same time, SNS activity modifies the distribution of blood to specific parts of the body, whereby constriction of some blood vessels causes reduction of blood flow to the gut, skin and reproductive systems, and selective dilation of other blood vessels, resulting in increased muscle tone, strength, and performance. SNS activation as a consequence of perceived threat or demand produces an aroused, alert and strengthened organism in preparation for coping (e.g., the well-known "fight or flight" reflex).

Of course, the initial arousal of the SNS is a function of the nervous system, but neural stimulation of the SNS is relatively short-lived and may not be sufficiently intense to evoke the required strong responses. Therefore, to some extent, prolonged and more intense responses are associated with endocrine system release of epinephrine from the adrenal medullae and norepinephrine from both the adrenal medullae and from neurons in the SNS. The release of these hormones into circulation have the same effects as SNS arousal accomplished by direct neural stimulation, but take longer to "clear" the system, and may produce a more intense response. The release of epinephrine, for example, stimulates the same heart and respiratory changes that accompany neural stimulation of the SNS, but the different mechanisms that convey these effects (e.g., receptor binding vs. synaptic transmission) alter the strength and persistence of responding. Some effects of SNS arousal appear to be exclusive to endocrine responses but, for the most part, these neuroendocrine responses work together. The HPA axis is different and, although it is also an integrated neuroendocrine response originating in the hypothalamus, it unfolds in different ways and accomplishes different things. For example, activity in this system is initiated by release of corticotrophin-releasing hormone (CRH) in the brain, which stimulates the pituitary to produce adrenocorticotropic hormone (ACTH), which then travels to the adrenals and stimulates release of corticosteroids from the adrenal cortex. In humans, these glucocorticoids are primarily cortisol, a hormone that has important anti-inflammatory and metabolic effects. Stress appraisals are believed to be associated with CRH release, and the arousal of the HPA has been considered another principal driver of the overall stress response.

These two above systems work together in order to provide redundant coverage of some survival functions and complementary coverage of others. The SNS and HPA differ in how responsive they are. For example, the SNS causes measurable changes in circulating sympathetic hormones and increased cardiac and respiratory function, almost immediately after stimulation. However, the HPA axis is more "sluggish," and can take up to 20–30 min to show responses after stimulation (Dickerson & Kemeny, 2004). Moreover, the effects of SNS activation can dissipate as rapidly as they appeared, while HPA responses are more long-lived. Both are catabolic in nature, in that they break down energy stores, and also increase capture and transport of oxygen and distribution of glucose to areas of the body. Each has a number of important targets and functions, some of which overlap with stress. Together, they provide the regulatory basis for the energizing effects of stress.

Stress and Health

The above systems, and the effects that they have on biobehavioral functioning, provide a context for understanding how and why stress has a number of consequences that affect health and well-being. This basic syndrome is present in many species. The elements of response fit together well, and they appear to have been selected because of their benefits for adaptation to the environment. In addition, such a process began before humans had appeared and unfolded through thousands of years of human development. Some have suggested that, because the world that was the basis for evolution of stress responses was the world of thousands of years ago, the nature of the selected responses may not be that useful or adaptive in our modern world. The stressors were different and "successful" responses different as well. At the time these integrated responses evolved, the earth was likely filled with immediate threats such as those posed by predators, geological or meteorological events, and famine. If the primary stressors in one's life include avoiding predators and providing food, the "fight or flight" responses described by Cannon (1939) would clearly confer an advantage and facilitate survival. In modern settings, though, where stressors may include sensory overload, alienation, crowding, and financial and occupational worries that ultimately may threaten one's ability to provide, the value of some of these energizing effects may be less. Even though these basic responses are still useful for some stressors (e.g., sudden life threat, accidents, challenges), they may not be effective in resolving others, and may produce unneeded and persistent and/or unusually intense responses, which may damage the body and cause distress, disease, and disability.

The activity of the stress "drivers" described above can be expected to have broad effects on the body, mood, and behavior. Basically, these may be considered to be stress responses or consequences. The distinction between them is generally derived from the relevance of the change for adaptation. Stress responses are changes, mostly mediated directly by SNS or HPA activation, that are either part of the emergency response or that are directly related to coping or adaptation to stressful circumstances. As was noted above, these changes are related to meeting the metabolic demands of strong and/or rapid responding, or to strengthening physical response, early identification of stressors, and coping. However, this arousal may also cause feelings of discomfort and may affect bodily systems that are not directly related to adaptation, or may cause "wear and tear" on systems used too often. These latter aspects of stress are more readily considered to be consequences, and form a basis for the pathophysiology of disease and mental health problems. Although the discomfort associated with stress arousal clearly motivates people to address the sources of stress, it does not directly increase one's ability to overcome them and may engender anxiety, depression, fear, anger, or irritability. In the workplace, this may contribute to absenteeism, poorer performance, conflict with co-workers, etc. Thus, stress responses, usually thought of as facilitating adaptation, may do so if the stressors in question are addressable with the kinds of physical responses selected. However, if the stressors are unusually strong or persistent, adaptation may not be achieved, and stress responses may actually increase in a maladaptive way. Under such conditions, unusually intense or prolonged SNS and HPA arousal, as well as arousal of the systems of the body affected by these neuroendocrine systems, may cause significant stress consequences. Excessive use of these systems, often at high levels of activity, can cause aging of the cells and systems of the body. In most cases, the major sources of stress are more readily avoided, accommodated, or eliminated, and responses may not engender severe consequences.

Behavioral Pathogens

Finally, another important area of concern for occupational health and illness are behavioral habits that have health-impairing consequences. These health-impairing habits have been called *behavioral pathogens* (Matarazzo, 1984). In fact, early reports focusing on the importance of behavioral factors in health had estimated that 50 % of the mortality from the 10 leading causes of death could be attributed to lifestyle habits (U.S. Department of Health, Education, and Welfare, 1979). For example, cigarette smoking had been linked with more than 350,000 deaths a year from heart disease, cancers, and chronic lung diseases (Grunberg, 1988). An analysis of international data by Peto, Boreham, Lopez, Thun, and Heath (1992) also projected that three million deaths worldwide each year can be attributed to smoking. About 200,000 deaths a year can be attributed to excessive consumption of alcohol, and fatal injuries (many alcohol-related were caused by driver error and preventative by the use of seatbelts) claimed more than 100,000 each year in the USA (U.S. Department of Health and Human Services, 1990). Other estimates suggest that seven of the ten leading causes of death in this country (heart disease, cancer, stroke, automobile accidents, diabetes, cirrhosis of the liver, and arteriosclerosis) could be reduced significantly if vulnerable individuals would change just five behaviors: smoking, alcohol abuse, nutrition, exercise, and compliance to medications to control hypertension (U.S. Department of Health and Human Services—*Healthy People 2000*).

Prevention Approaches

The significant relationships between the above mentioned major chronic diseases and modifiable behavioral pathogens that are under the individual's control have fostered prevention-oriented research and practice in clinical health psychology. It is now common to classify preventive efforts into three broad types. The first is *primary prevention* which refers to the modification of risk factors before the disease develops. In many respects, this is a highly cost-effective and beneficial strategy because, in the long term, the potential cost of life in dollars of treating disease are likely to outweigh the cost of preventing unhealthy habits. Examples of primary prevention efforts include educational campaigns to prevent adolescents from smoking or to encourage "safe sex" practices to prevent AIDS. Primary prevention is effective, but it is particularly challenging since it is often difficult to motivate otherwise healthy people to make changes in their behavior that may not have immediate benefits, despite the promise of long-term gains (Baum et al., 1997).

The terms *secondary prevention* and *tertiary prevention* refer, respectively, to interventions taken to arrest the progress of an illness already in the asymptomatic stages, and the rehabilitation and treatment interventions to stop the progression of disease that is symptomatic. Although less cost-effective and perhaps less beneficial in the long run, secondary and tertiary prevention activities may be easier to accomplish in the appropriate target groups (e.g., those that are ill) because they can be easily identified and are more motivated to change their behavior.

There are tremendous health-care cost savings, to both the government and industry in general, for initiating such primary, secondary, and tertiary intervention programs in the workplace. Indeed, the advent of the field of Occupational Health Psychology, which had with its initial roots highlighted in the document "Healthy People: The Surgeon General's Report on Health Promotion and Disease Prevention" (Surgeon General, 1979), first signaled the importance of taking human psychological well-being in occupational settings as an important goal for preventing disease states. As a result, the number of employers offering workplace wellness programs with financial incentives to employees has been steadily rising in the USA, despite the recent economic recession (National Business Group on Health, 2012).

The Transdisciplinary Model of Occupational Health and Wellness

Its Roots: The Biopsychosocial Perspective of Illness

During the Renaissance, the increased scientific knowledge in the areas of anatomy, biology, and physiology was accompanied by a *biomedical reductionism*, or a "dualistic" viewpoint, that mind and body function separately and independently. Unfortunately, this perspective dominated medicine until quite recently. However, a more comprehensive biopsychosocial approach to medicine was initially

Fig. 1.3 Engel's biopsychosocial model of illness

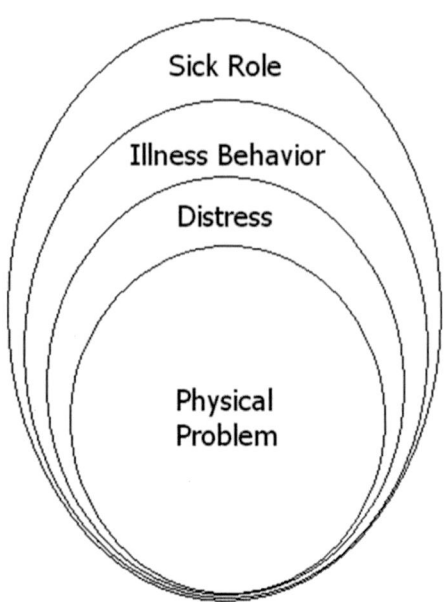

introduced by Engel (1977). This biopsychosocial model viewed physical disorders as the result of a dynamic interaction among physiologic, psychological, and social factors that perpetuates and may even worsen the clinical presentation. A range of psychological and socioeconomic factors can interact with physical pathology to modulate a patient's reports of symptoms and subsequent disability. This biopsychosocial model was subsequently more fully elaborated in the area of chronic pain management (Gatchel, 2005; Turk & Monarch, 2002). The biopsychosocial model focuses on both *disease* and *illness*, with illness being viewed as a complex interaction of biological, psychological, and social variables. According to Turk and Monarch, disease is defined as "an objective biological event" involving the destruction of specific body structures or organ systems by either anatomical, pathological, or physiological changes. Illness, in contrast, is generally defined as a "subjective experience or self attribution" that a disease is present. Thus, illness refers to how a sick individual and members of his or her family live with, and respond to, symptoms and disability. As originally proposed by Engel (1977), such a biopsychosocial model focuses primarily on illness. With this perspective, a diversity of illness expression (including its severity, duration, and psychosocial consequences) can be expected. The interrelationships among biological changes, psychosocial status, and the socioeconomic context all need to be considered if the patient's perception and response to illness are to be fully understood. Any model or treatment approach that focuses on only one of these core sets of factors would be incomplete. As can be seen in Fig. 1.3, Engel's conceptual model of illness includes factors that include not only the initial physical problem, but the subsequent psychosocial factors (such as emotional distress, illness behavior, and adopting the "sick role").

This biopsychosocial model has been demonstrated to be especially heuristic in the area of chronic pain and its management. Indeed, the most promising work on pain conducted thus far has embraced a biopsychosocial, interdisciplinary approach in which the psychosocial needs of patients require careful evaluation and treatment, along with the concurrent physical problems (Gatchel, 2004). This interdisciplinary approach requires the coordinated involvement of physicians, psychologists, physical therapists, vocational rehabilitation specialists, etc., in order to comprehensively deal with the full gamut of potential issues present in treating a chronic illness. Relatedly, many of these common chronic illnesses (such as diabetes mellitus, hypertension, cardiovascular disorders, asthma, gastrointestinal disorders, and chronic pain) cannot be "cured," but merely managed. Indeed, with the advent of the biopsychosocial model, there has been a move away from the traditional biomedical reductionist "curative" model to a more realistic and comprehensive biopsychosocial "management" model of care. Indeed, as noted by Dubos (1978):

> To heal does not necessarily imply to cure. It can simply mean helping to achieve a way of life compatible with their individual aspirations—to restore their freedom to make choices—even in the presence of continuing disease.

Ray (2004) has also provided an excellent overview of mind–body relationships and how social and behavioral factors can act on the brain to influence health, illness, and even death. In another earlier influential review, Cohen and Rodriguez (1995) pointed out important pathways linking mental and physical illness.

There have been a number of reviews that have documented the clinical effectiveness of such an interdisciplinary treatment approach, especially with chronic pain patients (Gatchel, 2005; Gatchel & Okifuji, 2006). These programs are needed for people with chronic pain who have complex needs and requirements. One variant of such program—functional restoration—has been comprehensively described in detail in a number of publications (Gatchel, 2005; Gatchel & Mayer, 1988; Mayer et al., 1987b). Clinical research has clearly demonstrated that the functional restoration program is associated with substantive improvements in various important socioeconomic outcomes (e.g., return-to-work and resolution of outstanding medical issues), as well as improvement in psychosocial functioning in patients who are chronically disabled with spinal disorders in 1-year follow up studies (Hazard et al., 1989; Mayer et al., 1985), as well as in a 2-year follow-up study (Mayer et al., 1987a). It should also be noted that this original functional restoration program has been independently replicated by others in this country, as well as by investigators in Denmark, France, Germany, Canada, and Japan (Gatchel & Okifuji, 2006). The fact that different clinical treatment teams, functioning in different States and countries, with markedly different economic/social conditions and workers' compensation systems, produced comparable outcome results speaks highly for the robustness of the clinical research finding and the utility, as well as the fidelity, of this functional restoration approach. Such interdisciplinary approaches involve a comprehensive team approach. Table 1.2 presents the different disciplines involved in such an approach, as well as how they function in an interdisciplinary program.

Beyond the Interdisciplinary Approach

There is now a growing appreciation that an interdisciplinary approach is essential for solving the complex problems of societal health care and wellness. It is worthwhile here to distinguish the differences among *multidisciplinary*, *interdisciplinary,* and *transdisciplinary* models. As noted by Dyer (2003) in the context of nursing care/education, a *multidisciplinary* model involves the use of different disciplines that individually conducts separate assessment, planning, treatment, etc., but with little coordination across the disciplines. In contrast, an *interdisciplinary* model expands the multidisciplinary approach through an ongoing shared collaborative process where all members of the different disciplines are "under one roof" at a facility, with careful daily collaborations and decision making as a team. The *transdisciplinary* model is the result of the further evolution of the interdisciplinary team approach, and values the knowledge and skill of all team members. Indeed, with the now recognized requirement of multiple health-care providers for dealing with the complex needs often associated with the comprehensive treatment health problems, especially when they become chronic in nature (such as chronic pain), it is viewed as extremely important to have a "teamwork" approach. This teamwork approach recognizes that no one particular health-care provider has all the requisite

Table 1.2 Interdisciplinary treatment team members

Physician	Serves as the medical director for all the patient's care
Nurse	Serves as a physician-extender, case manager, and provider of additional education
Psychologist	Completes psychosocial evaluations, and facilitates treatment planning and delivery
Physical therapist	Deals with physical conditioning/evaluation needs of patients
Occupational therapist	Deals with the occupational aspects of the patient's care, as well as help in returning to work and/or activities of daily living

skills and knowledge to deliver the best high-quality care. This type of teamwork was successfully incorporated in the interdisciplinary approach, as discussed above. The transdisciplinary model takes this approach one step farther in that each team member becomes so knowledgeable with the roles and responsibilities of the other team members that their tasks and functions become almost interchangeable (Cartmill, Soklaridis, & David Cassidy, 2011; Ellingson, 2002; Klein, 2008; Sinclair, Lingard, & Mohabeer, 2009). Thus, for example, a physical therapist becomes well versed in the approach of an occupational therapist, who then also both develop working knowledge of issues faced by case managers (such as insurance authorization and work-return plans). Likewise, physicians and psychologists on the team acquire the same knowledge base and can "fill in" for each other when needed. This results in coordinated staff team meetings where everyone is always "on the same page" and knowledgeable about barriers to recovery issues when they occur for any particular patient.

Throughout this Handbook, different areas of occupational health and wellness will be reviewed for which this transdisciplinary model is embraced. The relative degree of interactive and coordinated teamwork may vary, but its core ingredients will be seen as vital for success, both in the treatment and theory-building arenas.

Summary and Conclusions

As was reviewed in this chapter, there is now an ever growing body of clinical research evidence relating to the field of occupational health and wellness. This is partly due to the fact that we are in the midst of rapid global economic growth, with the associated complex international and financial systems that produce a wide range of potentially significant problems (e.g., environmental and occupational hazards/diseases; workers' safety and compensation issues; psychosocial stress). Moreover, we are now in the midst of an international recession that is causing a great deal of emotional distress and health problems triggered by high unemployment rates (which will be discussed in the last chapter of this Handbook). A brief historical overview of events that have led to the development of this field was provided, starting with the early European efforts to deal with occupational compensation issues that eventually spread to the USA during the last century. Moreover, with the rapid industrialization and scientific advances in the nineteenth century, many "unhealthy" work environments were unknowingly developed that had to subsequently be more closely monitored by the government through agencies such as the Environmental Protection Agency. With the backdrop of those potentially physical hazards in the occupational setting, it was not until relatively recently (during the last couple of decades) that the potentially significant problem of occupational psychosocial stress became an important area of concern and investigation. This was first recognized as a major health problem by research demonstrating that broad types of working conditions had been associated with coronary heart disease risk. Factors such as job demands, job autonomy, and job satisfaction were found to particularly heighten job-related stress and associated medical problems. The construct of stress, which underlies many of the topics included in the present Handbook, was then reviewed. Basic physiological processes involved in stress, such as two major neuroendocrine systems (the SNS and the HPA axis) were reviewed. How these stress-induced physiological underpinnings can be translated into health problems was then discussed. The topic of behavioral pathogens (e.g., health-impairing habits such as smoking, alcohol use, and diet) were also discussed as they relate to health-impairing consequences. Finally, the importance of prevention approaches was also touched upon.

We end this chapter with a discussion of the transdisciplinary model of occupational health and wellness. The roots of this model began with the biopsychosocial perspective of illness which was initially introduced by Engel (1977), and then subsequently elaborated in the area of chronic pain management by Gatchel (2005) and Turk and Moncarch (2002). This biopsychosocial perspective emphasizes the complex interaction of biological, psychological, and social variables, for better understanding the diversity of illness expression. This perspective led to the development of interdisciplinary treatment programs that required the coordinated involvement of physicians, psychologists, physical therapists, vocational rehabilitation specialists, etc., in order to comprehensively deal with the full gamut of potential problems present in treating a chronic illness. This approach also emphasized a "management" model of care rather than the outdated "curative" model of care. One example of such an interdisciplinary program is the functional restoration approach to chronic pain assessment and management, which has been demonstrated to be therapeutically effective. This interdisciplinary approach led directly into the now transdisciplinary model which has taken this approach one step farther in that each team member involved in the assessment-treatment process becomes so knowledgeable with the roles and responsibilities of the other team members that their tasks and functions become almost interchangeable. Throughout this Handbook, we will be discussing different areas of occupational health and wellness for which this transdisciplinary model is, or should be, embraced.

References

American Psychiatric Association. (2000). *Diagnostic and statistical manual of mental disorders* (4th ed.). Washington, DC: Author.
Anderson, G. B. J. (1991). Impairment evaluation issues and the disability system. In T. G. Mayer, V. Mooney, & R. J. Gatchel (Eds.), *Contemporary conservative care for painful spinal disorders*. Philadelphia: Lea & Febiger.
Baum, A., Gatchel, R. J., & Krantz, D. S. (Eds.). (1997). *An introduction to health psychology* (3rd ed.). New York: McGraw-Hill.
Bellamy, R. (1997). Compensation neurosis: Financial reward for illness as nocebo. *Clinical Orthopaedics and Related Research, 336*, 94–106.
Bryson, B. (2003). *A short history of nearly everything*. New York: Broadway Books.
Butcher, J. N., Dahlstrom, W. G., Graham, J. R., Tellegen, A. M., & Kaemmer, B. (1989). *MMPI-2: Manual for the administration and scoring*. Minneapolis, MN: University of Minnesota Press.
Cannon, W. B. (1939). *The wisdom of the body*. New York: Norton.
Cartmill, C., Soklaridis, S., & David Cassidy, J. (2011). Transdisciplinary teamwork: the experience of clinicians at a functional restoration program. *Journal of Occupational Rehabilitation, 21*(1), 1–8.
Cohen, S., & Rodriguez, M. S. (1995). Pathways linking affective disturbances and physical disorders. *Health Psychology, 14*, 371–373.
Conroy, M. A., & Kwartner, P. P. (2006). Malingering. *Applied Psychology in Criminal Justice, 2*(3), 29–51.
Dersh, J., Gatchel, R. J., & Kishino, N. (2005). The role of tertiary gain in pain disability. *Practical Pain Management, 5*, 13–28.
Dersh, J., Polatin, P., Leeman, G., & Gatchel, R. J. (2009). Secondary gains and losses in the medicolegal setting. In I. Z. Schultz & R. J. Gatchel (Eds.), *Handbook of complex occupational disability claims: early risk identification, intervention and prevention*. New York: Springer.

Dickerson, S. S., & Kemeny, M. E. (2004). Adult stressors and cortisol responses: A theoretical integration and synthesis of laboratory research. *Psychological Bulletin, 130*, 355–391.

Dubos, R. (1978). Health and creative adaptation. *Human Nature, 1*, 82.

Dyer, J. A. (2003). Multidisciplinary, interdisciplinary, and transdisciplinary educational models and nursing education. *Nursing Education Perspectives, 24*(4), 186–188.

Ellingson, L. (2002). Communication, collaboration, and team work among health care professionals. *Community Research Trends, 21*(3), 1–43.

Engel, G. L. (1977). The need for a new medical model: A challenge for biomedicine. *Science, 196*(4286), 129–136.

Engels, F. (1845). *The condition of the working class in England*. London: Penguin.

Finneson, B. (1976). Modulating effect of secondary gain on the low back syndrome. *Advances in Pain Research and Therapy, 1*, 949–952.

Fishbain, D. A. (1994). Secondary gain concept: Definition problems and its abuse in medical practice. *APS Journal, 3*(4), 264–273.

Fishbain, D. (1999). The association of chronic pain and suicide. *Seminars in Clinical Neuropsychiatry, 4*, 221–227.

Fishbain, D. A., Cutler, R. B., Rosomoff, H. L., & Rosomoff, R. S. (1999). Validity of self-reported drug use in chronic pain patients. Clinical Journal of Pain, 15(3), 184–191.

Fishbain, D. A., Rosomoff, H. L., Cutler, R. B., & Rosomoff, R. S. (1995). Secondary gain concept: A review of the scientific evidence. *Clinical Journal of Pain, 11*(1), 6–21.

Freud, S. (1917). *Introductory lectures on psychoanalysis*. London: Hogarth Press (1959).

Gatchel, R. J. (2004). Psychosocial factors that can influence the self-assessment of function. *Journal of Occupation Rehabilitation, 14*(3), 197–206.

Gatchel, R. J. (2005). *Clinical essentials of pain management*. Washington, DC: American Psychological Association.

Gatchel, R. J., & Baum, A. (2009). Biobehavioral mediators of stress and quality of life in occupational settings. In A. M. Rossi, J. C. Quick, & P. Perrewé (Eds.), *Stress and quality of working life: The positive and the negative*. Charlotte, NC: Information Age Publishing.

Gatchel, R. J., & Mayer, T. G. (1988). *Functional restoration for spinal disorders: The sports medicine approach*. Malvern, PA: Lea & Febiger.

Gatchel, R. J., & Okifuji, A. (2006). Evidence-based scientific data documenting the treatment- and cost-effectiveness of comprehensive pain programs for chronic nonmalignant pain. *Journal of Pain, 7*(11), 779–793.

Greene, R. L. (1997). Assessment of malingering and defensiveness by multiscale personality inventories. In R. Rogers (Ed.), *Clinical assessment of malingering and deception* (2nd ed.). New York: Guilford Press.

Grunberg, N. E. (1988). Behavioral factors in preventive medicine and health promotion. In W. Gordon, A. Herd, & A. Baum (Eds.), *Perspectives on behavioral medicine* (Vol. 3). New York: Academic.

Hadler, N. (1996). If you have to prove you are ill, you can't get well: The object lesson of fibromyalgia. *Spine, 20*, 2397–2400.

Harder, G., Veilleux, M., & Suissa, S. (1998). The effect of socio-demographic and crash-related factors on the prognosis of whiplash. *Journal of Clinical Epidemiology, 51*, 377–384.

Hazard, R. G., Fenwick, J. W., Kalisch, S. M., Redmond, J., Reeves, V., Reid, S., & Frymoyer, J. (1989). Functional restoration with behavioral support. A one-year prospective study of patients with chronic low-back pain. *Spine, 14*(2), 157–161.

Howard, K. J., Kishino, N. D., Johnston, V. J., Worzer, W. E., & Gatchel, R. J. (2010). Malingering and pain: is this a major problem in the medicolegal setting? *Psychological Injury and Law, 3*, 203–211.

Karasek, R. A., & Theorell, T. G. (1990). *Healthy work*. New York: Basic Books.

Karasek, R. A., Theorell, T. G., Schwartz, J., Schnall, P., Pieper, C. F., & Michela, J. L. (1988). Job characteristics in relation to the prevalence of myocardial infarction in the US Health Examination Survey (HES) and the Health and Nutrition Examination Survey (HANES). *American Journal of Public Health, 78*(8), 910–918.

Klein, J. T. (2008). Evaluation of interdisciplinary and transdisciplinary research: a literature review. *American Journal of Preventive Medicine, 35*(2, Supplement 1), S116–S123. doi:10.1016/j.amepre.2008.05.010.

Margoshes, B. G., & Webster, B. S. (2000). Why do occupational injuries have different health outcomes? In T. G. Mayer, R. J. Gatchel, & P. B. Polatin (Eds.), *Occupational musculoskeletal disorders*. Philadelphia: Lippincott, Williams & Wilkinson.

Marx, K. (1867). *Das Kapital*. Oxford: Oxford University Press.

Matarazzo, J. D. (1984). Behavioral immunogens and pathogens in health and illness. In B. L. Hammonds & C. J. Scheirer (Eds.), *Psychology and health: The master lecture series* (Vol. 3). Washington, DC: American Psychological Association.

Mayer, T. G., Gatchel, R. J., Kishino, N., Keeley, J., Capra, P., Mayer, H., Barnett, J., & Mooney, V. (1985). Objective assessment of spine function following industrial injury: a prospective study with comparison group and one-year follow-up. *Spine, 10*, 482–493.

Mayer, T. G., Gatchel, R. J., Mayer, H., Kishino, N., Keeley, J., & Mooney, V. (1987a). A prospective two-year study of functional restoration in industrial low back injury. *JAMA, 258*, 1181–1182.

Mayer, T. G., Gatchel, R. J., Mayer, H., Kishino, N. D., Keeley, J., & Mooney, V. A. (1987b). Prospective two year study of functional restoration in industrial low back injury. *JAMA, 258*(13), 1763–1767.

McIntosh, G., Melles, T., & Hall, H. (1995). Guidelines for the identification of barriers to rehabilitation of back injuries. *Journal of Occupational Rehabilitation, 5*(3), 195–201.

Mittenberg, W., Patton, C., Canyock, E. M., & Condit, D. C. (2002). Base rates of malingering and symptom exaggeration. *Journal of Clinical and Experimental Neuropsychology, 24*, 1094–1102.

National Business Group on Health. (2012). *Performance in an era of uncertainty: 17th Annual Towers Watson/National Business Group on Health Employer Survey on Purchasing Value in Health Care*. Washington, DC: Author.

Peto, R., Boreham, J., Lopez, A. D., Thun, M., & Heath, C. (1992). Mortality from tobacco in developed countries: indirect estimation from national vital statistics. *The Lancet, 339*(8804), 1268–1278. doi:10.1016/0140-6736(92)91600-D.

Rainville, J., Sobel, J., Hartigan, C., & Wright, A. (1997). The effect of compensation involvement of the reporting of pain and disability by patients referred for rehabilitation of chronic low back pain. *Spine, 22*(17), 2016–2024.

Ray, Q. (2004). How the mind hurts and heals the body. *American Psychologist, 59*, 29–40.

Robinson, J. P., Rondinelli, R. D., Scheer, S. J., & Weinstein, S. M. (1997). Industrial rehabilitation medicine. 1. Why is industrial rehabilitation medicine unique? *Archives of Physical medicine and Rehabilitation, 78*(suppl), S3–S9.

Rogers, R. (1997). *Clinical assessment of malingering and deception* (2nd ed.). New York: Guilford Press.

Rogers, R., Bagby, R. M., & Dickens, S. E. (1992). *Structured interview of reported symptoms: Professional manual*. Odessa, FL: Psychological Assessment Resources.

Rogers, R., Harrell, E., & Liff, C. (1993). Feigning neuropsychological impairment: A clinical review of methodological and clinical considerations. *Clinical Psychology Review, 13*, 255–274.

Schnall, P. L., Pleper, C., Schwartz, J. E., Karasek, R. A., Schlussel, Y., Devereux, R. B., Warren, K., & Pickering, T. G. (1990). The relationship between "job strain," workplace diastolic blood pressure, and left ventricular mass index. *JAMA, 263*(14), 1929–1935.

Schrader, H., Bovim, G., Sand, T., Obelieniene, D., Siurkiene, D., Mickevicience, D., & Miseviciene, I. (1996). Natural evolution of late whiplash syndrome outside the medicolegal context. *Lancet, 347*, 1207–1211.

Sinclair, L. B., Lingard, L. A., & Mohabeer, R. N. (2009). What's so great about rehabilitation teams? An ethnographic study of interprofessional collaboration in a rehabilitation unit. *Archives of Physical Medicine and Rehabilitation, 90*(7), 1196–1201. doi:10.1016/j.apmr.2009.01.021.

Sumanti, M., Brauer Boone, K., Savodnik, I., & Gorsuch, R. (2006). Noncredible psychiatric and cognitive symptoms in a workers' compensation "stress" claim sample. *The Clinical Neuropsychologist, 20*, 754–765.

Surgeon General. (1979). *Smoking and health (DHEW Publication No. [PHS] 79-50066)*. Washington, DC: GPO.

Terrill, A. L., Garofalo, J. P., Soliday, E., & Craft, R. (2012). Multiple roles and stress burden in women: a conceptual model of heart disease risk. *Journal of Applied Biobehavioral Research, 17*, 4–22.

Turk, D. C., & Monarch, E. S. (2002). Biopsychosocial perspective on chronic pain. In D. C. Turk & R. J. Gatchel (Eds.), *Psychological approaches to pain management: a practitioner's handbook* (2nd ed.). New York: Guilford.

U.S. Department of Health and Human Services. (1990). *Healthy people 2000: National health promotion and disease preventions objectives (DHHS Publication No. PHS 91-50212)*. Washington, DC: U.S. Government Printing Office.

U.S. Department of Health, Education, and Welfare. (1979). *Healthy people: Surgeon General's report on health promotion and disease prevention (DHEW Publication No. 79-55071)*. Washington, DC: US Government Printing Office.

Worzer, W. E., Kishino, N. D., & Gatchel, R. J. (2009). Primary, secondary and tertiary losses in chronic pain patients. *Psychological Injury and Law, 2*, 215–224.

Theories of Psychological Stress at Work

Philip J. Dewe, Michael P. O'Driscoll, and Cary L. Cooper

Introduction

This chapter is about theories of work-related stress. Of course, throughout this Handbook, stress-related topics are discussed. However, in order to understand different theories and to give them a sense of time, place, and meaning, we attempt to explore them against the changes in how stress has come to be defined. The importance of exploring stress theories in this way lies in the way it gives a sense of history: of why different theories prevailed (Cooper, Dewe, & O'Driscoll, 2001), whether they are "worthy of the intellectual resources focused on them" (Kaplan, 1996, p. 374), whether they adequately express the nature of the experience itself (Newton, 1995) and, despite the knowledge and understanding they have provided, whether they are still capable of expressing "the stress of the stress process" (Lazarus, 1990, p. 4). We also explore whether we can distil from them what should now become the organizing concept of the future around which such theories should focus. Liddle (1994) describes an organizing concept as one with "sufficient logic and emotional resonance to yield systematic theoretical and research enquiry that will make a lasting solution" (p. 167). Finally, we explore the different theories in terms of how they have influenced our measurement strategies, where our current methodologies are taking us, what this means for understanding the richness of the stress experience, and the type of evidence they provide in terms of work stress and well-being. However, this chapter does not review all the different theories of stress. In order to explore how they have evolved, we have selected a number that best express this evolutionary process, although all theories have an evolutionary element to them. A comprehensive review of stress theories can be found in

P.J. Dewe, Ph.D.
Department of Organizational Psychology, Birkbeck, University of London,
London, UK
e-mail: p.dewe@bbk.ac.uk

M.P. O'Driscoll, Ph.D. (✉)
Department of Psychology, University of Waikato,
Hamilton, New Zealand
e-mail: m.odriscoll@waikato.ac.nz

C.L. Cooper, CBE
Management School Office, Lancaster University Management School, Lancaster University,
Lancaster, UK
e-mail: c.cooper1@lancaster.ac.uk

Cooper (2000). This book is as "a compendium of theory rich in diversity and range" (p. 4) emphasising not just the need for theories to capture the essence of the work experience itself, but also help us as researchers fulfil our moral responsibility to those whose working lives we study. This chapter begins by first exploring the evolutionary milestones in the way stress has been defined. It then uses this as the context for exploring the development of selected stress theories. The chapter concludes by exploring what this means in terms of our understanding of work stress, those elements that should now be reflected in our theories of stress and the issues we now need to consider as researchers and practitioners.

Definitions of Stress and Their Evolutionary Role

Definitions of stress are, of course, products of their time. They produce a state of knowledge built around a research agenda that expressed the issues of the day. In this way, all definitions give us a sense of time and place, and it is through this sense that we get an understanding of why different definitions emerged, their influence on the development of theory, how we engaged in research and the way our results were interpreted. It is no wonder then that, as stress definitions first expressed the nature of stress in terms of its different components, these components provided the building blocks for our theories. What perhaps is critical to our understanding of how different theories emerged lies less in the different components that provided our theories with structure, although this makes them no less important, but in the way in which those components are arranged in terms of the relationship they expressed. Distinguishing between structure and relationship allows the emphasis to shift to "the sequencing of events that culminate in the experience of stress" (Kaplan, 1996, p. 387), and contributes to our understanding not just in terms of how definitions of stress have evolved but how the nature of that relationship has found expression in different theoretical models.

It is tempting when considering how stress has been defined to describe different definitions as reflecting different stages in our understanding of the term with each stage representing the research emphasis of the time. Describing stress definitions as progressing through a series of stages gives, perhaps, a more orderly feel to the way they evolved than actually occurred. Researchers, depending on their own agenda, followed different paths, influenced somewhat by the demands of their own discipline and nudged along by social, economic, and political issues, helping to explain why different approaches often were unacknowledged. Moreover, whenever the word stress was mentioned, or attempts made to define it, a fairly robust debate followed (Cooper et al., 2001; Dewe, 2001). Early definitions of stress defined it in terms of a stimulus, response, or the interaction between the two. Without doubt, these definitions have provided much needed information and a considerable body of knowledge now exists as to the nature and characteristics of these different components and their interaction (Dewe, O'Driscoll, & Cooper, 2010). This is not to say that such definitions should now be assigned to the annals of history, even though they do possess this quality of time and context. Such definitions also possess an evolutionary quality, allowing researchers to continue to explore their nature and evaluate their characteristics in terms of their relevance to contemporary work experiences, as well as continuing to explore whether the interaction between the two is best expressed as some sort of imbalance between the person and the environment (Cooper et al., 2001). The importance of these traditional definitions now lies less in the knowledge they provide and continue to provide, and more in whether they have the capacity to offer an understanding of the complexity and richness of the stress process itself (Dewe, 2001; Dewe et al., 2010).

In order to understand the full influence of definitions of stress on our stress-related theories, it is necessary to consider two further developments in the evolution of such definitions. These include the need to think of stress in transactional terms (Lazarus, 1990, 1999), as well as whether it is now time to shift our attention away from the somewhat contentious term "stress" to thinking more in terms of discrete emotions (Lazarus, 2001). This is because it is "discrete emotions experienced at work [that] constitute the coin of the realm" (Lazarus & Cohen-Charash, 2001, p. 45) when attempting to understand the dynamics of a stressful encounter. Turning first to the transactional nature of stress, such a definition takes the view that no one component can be said to define stress because each has to be viewed relationally as part of a more complex process where, ultimately, all become part of the context within which the stressful encounter takes place (Lazarus, 1999). Transaction implies that stress resides neither solely in the person nor solely in the environment, but in the transaction between the two (Lazarus 1991). The power of the transactional approach to defining stress lies in the fact that transaction implies process, and in order to understand the nature of that transaction commits researchers to exploring those cognitive processes that link the individual to the environment (Dewe et al., 2010). It is, as Lazarus (1999) suggests, the process of appraisal that provides that link and, in so doing, provides the "conduit" between the stressful encounter and the emotions that follow. The authority of appraisals lies in the fact that they act as a bridge to what one experiences and how one feels in a particular encounter (Lazarus, 2001). This also provides a conceptual pathway for more closely examining the role of discrete emotions.

If appraisals trigger the emotion response then, as Lazarus and Cohen-Charash (2001) suggest, stress always implies emotion so "stress and emotion should be treated as a single topic" as "emotion encompasses all the phenomena of stress" (p. 53). In this way, as Lazarus (1999, 2001) suggests, we can turn our attention away from the troublesome concept of stress and embrace discrete emotions as better expressing the nature of what it is individuals are experiencing. If, as researchers, we are interested in understanding whether our definitions (and therefore our theories of stress) represent the individual experience, then it is now time to develop definitions that more explicitly capture the reality of the emotional experience (Dewe et al., 2010). Thus, as definitions of stress have evolved, it is now time to think in terms of the different components to the stress transaction operating within a relational process (Lazarus, 1999, 2001). Our definition of stress should now lead us towards theories that point to the mechanisms that underlie and best express the nature of the stress process, and the manner in which those mechanisms provide a causal pathway that expresses the nature of the experience. In this way, when we think of the word "stress," we no longer think in terms of "detachable entities" (Coyne & Gottlieb, 1996, p. 966) like simply a stimulus and response, but more in terms of a process where the emphasis is on "tracing out" (Aldwin, 2000, p. 42) the transactional nature of that process. Such causal pathways will lead us in a more focused direction to the specific nature of what is being experienced, allowing us to abandon solely using the term "stress," and focus more on the emotional quality of the experience.

There are, of course, numerous definitions of stress, just as there are numerous theories of stress. A fine line exists between theory and definitions. Definitions are more likely to be products of our theories, and they express the evolving nature of our knowledge and the direction that research has led us. While each theory adopts its own particular focus, all are generally structured around a common set of components that are basically linked together in a relationship that is process-oriented. The idea of process is, more often than not, expressed through the ideas of "fit or balance" and is, now, more likely to be transactional rather than interactional in nature. Indeed, as Cooper (2000) suggests, the volume of empirical research using an interactional theoretical framework has "massively outstripped our ability to understand the implications of that research" (p. 2), and to place it within some theoretical framework seeking to develop theories that allow an understanding to emerge about those mechanisms that drive that process. Our aim, Cooper (1998, p. 4) concludes, must be to "understand those linkages" that not just give expression to the stress process, but also provide a context for exploring individual well-being. By presenting various theories that illustrate in their own way how such "linkages" have been conceptualized and researched, we wish simply to illustrate the creativity that exists in our field, the richness and complexity of the stress process, and the direction future research may wish to take. We begin with one of the earliest and most fundamental perspectives on psychological stress—Lazarus's transactional model.

Lazarus and the Transactional Model of Stress

The transactional model defines stress as arising from the appraisal that particular environmental demands are about to tax individual resources, thus threatening well-being (Holroyd & Lazarus, 1982). This definition of stress encompasses a number of themes that capture the transactional nature of stress and those processes that best express the nature of that transaction. These themes involve the following:

- Stress is a product of the transaction between the individual and the environment.
- The authority and power of the transaction lies in the process of appraisal that binds the person and the environment and, it is this "relational meaning" (Lazarus, 1999, 2001) that the person constructs from the transaction and that lies at the heart of the stress process.
- There are two types of appraisal—primary and secondary. It is through these appraisals that the focus is shifted to what people think and do in a stressful encounter, representing a process-oriented approach (Lazarus, 1999, 2001). This reflects the "the changing person–environment relationship" (Lazarus, 1990, p. 4), and provides an insight into the nature of the stress process itself.
- It is the appraisal process that offers a causal pathway—a bridge to those discrete emotions that best express the nature of the stress experience (Lazarus, 2001; Lazarus & Cohen-Charash, 2001).

As noted above, there are two types of appraisal (Lazarus, 1999). The first describes primary appraisal. This is where the person acknowledges that there is something at stake (Lazarus, 2001). The idea of whether "anything is at stake" is, as Lazarus (1999, p. 76) points out, fundamental and it is where the person asks, for example, "do I have a goal at stake, or are any on my core values engaged or threatened? "It is where the person considers the significance of the encounter and evaluates it in terms of its personal meaning. Lazarus identifies three types of primary appraisals (p. 76): *harm/loss*—something that has already occurred; *threat*—the possibility of some harm in the future; and *challenge*—where the person engages with the demand. Later, Lazarus (2001) added another appraisal that he described as *benefit*, where individuals search for the benefit in a demanding encounter. Negatively and positively toned appraisals (Lazarus) are associated with different types of emotions, and they provide the pathway through which as much emphasis can now be given to positive emotions as has been given to negative emotions (Dewe et al., 2010). It is these appraisals that operate as the "cognitive underpinnings" for coping as they are part of "an active search for information and meaning on which to predicate action" (Lazarus, 1999, p. 76).

It is secondary appraisal where the focus turns to "what can be done about it" (Lazarus, 1999). This is where the person evaluates the availability of coping resources (Lazarus, 2001). While much debate surrounds the definition of coping (Dewe et al., 2010), the definition put forward by Lazarus describes coping in terms of a process that embraces the "constantly changing cognitive and behavioural efforts a person makes to manage specific external or internal demands that are appraised as taxing or exceeding the resources of the person" (Lazarus, 1999, p.110). Lazarus and his colleague Folkman (1980) went on to identify two types of coping. These they described as problem-focused (where the focus is on managing the encounter), and emotion-focused (where the focus is on regulating the emotion) coping. Classifying coping strategies as either problem- or emotion-focused offered what Folkman and Moskowitz (2004, p. 751) described as a "broad brush approach." Since then, researchers have taken the opportunity to consider a range of ways of classifying coping strategies, expanding the original work to include, for example, strategies that include meaning-centred coping and relationship-social coping (Folkman, 2011). While no consensus has yet been reached as to the number of coping categories, researchers do agree that no category should be regarded as inherently better than another, because each needs to be considered within the context of a stressful encounter and how that encounter is appraised. Whether or not a consensus will ever be reached as to the way coping strategies should be classified is a moot point, as coping is always context specific.

Classifying coping strategies is one thing but, when considered in terms of the way they are being used in a particular encounter, illustrates the richness and complexity of the coping process and suggests that researchers may wish to explore the way in which different strategies are used before labelling them as simply falling into one category or another. Also, there is the vexed question of coping effectiveness. Two theoretical approaches offer an understanding as to how to best judge coping effectiveness. The first focuses on whether "personally significant" and appropriate outcomes have been successfully achieved (Folkman & Moskowitz, 2004, p. 754), whereas the second considers effectiveness in terms of the "fit" between the type of coping and the nature of the encounter. Folkman and Moskowitz suggest a number of refinements to these two approaches. The first is in terms of developing a better understanding of what we need to investigate when it comes to the nature of outcomes, such as their qualities and characteristics and, similarly, when it comes to "fit" developing a more refined analysis of those environmental characteristics that may influence the nature of coping. While as other authors (Dewe et al., 2010) point out, it may also be time to consider just exactly what we mean when we talk about coping effectiveness, starting perhaps from the proposition raised by Lazarus (1999): the issue of effectiveness for *whom* and at *what cost*; whatever position we take, "the issue of determining coping effectiveness remains one of the most perplexing in coping research" (Folkman & Moskowitz, 2004, p. 753).

The term "secondary" appraisal is not meant to suggest that it is of any less importance than "primary" appraisal. The difference between the two appraisals is, as Lazarus (1999, p. 78) points out, "not about timing but the contents of the appraisal." Lazarus goes on to add that it is the "distinctly different content of each type of appraisal" (p. 78) that requires each to be investigated separately. But, as he cautions, each is part of a "common process," where together they each help to shape a stressful encounter as the manner in which individuals give meaning to an encounter is further refined through the process of secondary appraisal. While coping research has captured the imagination of many researchers, there is still considerable debate as to just where current methodologies are taking us in terms of how coping is measured, and what it is that alternative measures may provide (Coyne, 1997; Dewe 2001; Folkman, 2011; Folkman & Moskowitz, 2004; Lazarus, 2000; Somerfield & McCrae, 2000). What is clear from this debate is that researchers are already looking towards how coping measures can move away from simply relying on checklists (Folkman & Moskowitz, 2004), to exploring process-driven longitudinal designs (Lazarus, 2000), and more ecologically driven methods that explore daily processing measures such as daily diaries and "intensive day-to-day monitoring of phenomena" (Tennen, Affleck, Armeli, & Carney, 2000, p. 627). What is encouraging, as Lazarus points out, is that there is "more reason to hope that the field of coping is maturing" with researchers using more creative approaches to measurement that "could add substantially to understanding and contribute to practical application" (Lazarus, 2000, p. 673).

While coping research has continued to grow, the role of primary appraisal and the meaning individuals give to demanding encounters has not, at least in work stress research, received the attention it deserves. Work stress research (Dewe, 1993; Dewe & Ng, 1999; Lowe & Bennett, 2003) has, when exploring work stressors, illustrated that individuals can distinguish between the objective nature of a stressor and its meaning, and explored whether underlying appraisals like challenge and hindrance help to better distinguish among common work stressors (Cavanaugh, Boswell, Roehling, & Boudreau, 2000). However, some researchers have questioned whether, by focusing on intra-individual process like appraisal, such individual-level analysis takes us away from what should be our primary goal of identifying work stressors that affect the working lives of most workers (Brief & George, 1991). Also, questions have been raised as to the utility of this approach in terms of how such information informs decisions about how to intervene (Schaubroeck, 1999). Nevertheless, far from questioning the theoretical rigor and empirical significance of Lazarus' transactional theory, with its emphasis on the appraisal process, most critics observe that there are, in the work stress agenda, opportunities for all aspects of the stress process to be studied (Frese & Zapf, 1999). Also, work stress research might profit from "reflecting more carefully on how such [appraisals] processes follow (Schaubroeck, 1999, p. 759), and that when investigating work stress it is, as Perrewe and Zellars (1999) suggest, not just important to explore individual appraisals but "it is *essential* in order to understand the stress process" (p. 749).

Person–Environment Fit

Another theoretical model which has been in existence for a considerable amount of time, and which to a large extent has underpinned other approaches to stress and well-being, is the *Person–Environment Fit* (P–E fit) perspective. This account of the stress process stems from the early work and theorizing of Lewin (1935) and Murray (1938). For example, reacting to prevailing mechanistic views of human behaviour which attributed the causes of behaviour solely to the environment, and psychodynamic approaches which tended to conceive behaviour as emerging from personality characteristics (traits), Lewin conceptualized the interaction between the person and environment (P×E) as the key to understanding people's cognitive, affective and behavioural reactions. His early thinking therefore provided the foundation for the modern perspective of P–E fit. In particular, he foreshadowed the notion that optimal fit between the person and his/her environment is needed for effective human functioning. Numerous descriptions of P–E fit are available in the literature, although perhaps the most comprehensive account is that offered by Edwards (1998), who also described earlier constructions of P–E fit, such as those initiated by French, Caplan, and Harrison (1982). Here we do not attempt to provide an exhaustive account of this theory and its applications; rather, we summarize the main elements of this perspective, and illustrate how it has been applied, along with its strengths and some limitations. It should also be noted that the tenets of P–E fit theory also underlie several other theoretical models of stressor–strain relationships, including the cybernetic theory (Cummings & Cooper, 1979; Edwards, 1998), which will not be discussed in this chapter. One specific advantage of the P–E fit conceptualization over some other (more specific) theories is that P–E fit is based essentially on the idea of employee adjustment in the work setting, which has been illustrated as being critical for overall well-being (Dawis & Lofquist, 1984).

We begin with the notion of "fit" itself. Synonyms for fit are "match," "congruence," and "correspondence." In the occupational stress and well-being literature, the fit concept has been characterized as having two components: (a) the degree of match, congruence, or correspondence between the demands people confront at work and their abilities to meet those demands, referred to as *demands–ability fit*; and (b) the match, congruence or correspondence between the person's needs (including physical and psycho-social needs) and the resources available to him/her. The latter is referred to as *needs–supplies fit*. Most research on the relationship between P–E fit and stress or well-being has focused on the second of these types of fit, as it is assumed that a lack of fit (that is, misfit) between needs and resources will have a pronounced impact on stress levels and overall well-being. However, demands–ability fit can also be important in terms of a person's well-being. For instance, if person's workload is high and they do not have the time or energy to perform what is expected from them, this can induce a high level of psychological strain. A (very simplified) depiction of the basic theory relating to P–E fit is provided in Fig. 2.1. The theory hinges on the amount of a "stimulus" (for example, workload, work complexity, level of authority,

		Preferred	
		High	Low
Received	High	Low strain	High strain?
	Low	High strain	Low strain

Fig. 2.1 Levels of psychological strain predicted by P–E fit theory

and social interaction with work colleagues) that an individual prefers to have, and the actual level of the various stimuli (referred to in this figure as "received"). There are two conditions in which the level of fit is high: when the preferred levels and the received levels are both high; or when they are both low. Consider, for instance, the level of social contact people have with their work colleagues. An individual may wish to have an extensive amount of contact with colleagues, and may actually experience this amount. This situation clearly is one where there is a strong match between what people want and what they receive; that is a strong fit, and they should (at least theoretically) experience low strain (and high psychosocial well-being). Alternatively, the individual may not actually want very much contact at all with work colleagues, and does not have substantial interpersonal contact. Again, this situation reflects a high degree of fit, and one might expect the levels of strain to be low. However, this situation is not as clear-cut as the high–high condition, because here social interaction may not be important for individuals and other factors may have more impact on their stress and well-being levels.

Conversely, P–E fit theory postulates that high strain will occur when there is a mismatch between the person's needs and what they receive or confront at work. The condition which (theoretically) should create highest levels of strain will be one where the person strongly desires a particular feature (such as interpersonal contact), but does not receive it (the high-low box in Fig. 2.1). Under these circumstances, strain will be at its highest level. On the other hand, when people do not have a strong preference for an attribute (in this case, interpersonal contact), but they do receive it, there is some ambiguity over whether this situation will be stressful for them. Strictly speaking, they should experience strain, as there is a mismatch between their preference and what they are supplied with. However, this is likely to depend on numerous other factors, including whether the attribute interferes with other activities or things the individual would prefer to be engaged in. For example, having frequent contact with work colleagues may distract the person from core job activities, leading to frustration and a sense of lack of achievement, in which case high strain might be anticipated. In contrast, even though they may not desire it, interpersonal contact may serve as a welcome distraction from a challenging task; hence, they may not feel stressed by it. In sum, although the P–E fit model predicts that misfit (of either kind) will increase levels of strain, in practice the amount of strain experienced in the high–low condition in Fig. 2.1 may be substantially greater than that felt in the low–high situation.

In summary, the basic notion underlying P–E fit theory is that there needs to be a match between what people want and what they receive, as well as a match between their abilities (knowledge, skills) and the demands placed upon them. Lack of match (misfit) creates strain and (ultimately) reduces their sense of psychosocial well-being. However, demands–ability and needs–supply match are considerably more relevant to people when the stimuli are important to them. Edwards (1995, 2000) has referred to this as dimension importance, and is related to Maslow's need-hierarchy principle. Using the example given above, if work performance is important to the person, then frequent interpersonal contact may be viewed as a substantial interference which reduces the ability of the person to achieve what he/she desires. On the other hand, if individuals are not concerned about how well they perform at work, frequent non-work related social interaction with work colleagues may not be considered a distraction and, hence, will not increase strain. As we have noted above, increased psychological strain and decreased psychosocial well-being are two major outcomes of misfit in the work context. Other potential outcomes have also been identified in the literature, including job dissatisfaction, reduced commitment to the organization, and greater turnover intentions. It is also evident that the notion of P–E fit is relevant across various domains, including life outside of work. For the purposes of this chapter, however, we concentrate on its relationship with work-related strain and well-being. Numerous studies have confirmed that misfit (mainly in respect of needs–supplies, but also in terms of demands–abilities) can have serious consequences for worker well-being. A good illustration of this relationship comes from a fairly recent study by Yang, Hongsheng, and Spector (2008). These researchers explored the actual and preferred conditions at work, with respect to two key issues—career advancement and relationships at work—in a sample of Chinese workers. Expectations concerning career development are clearly salient to many employees, and opportunities for advancement within their career are typically important. Yang and colleagues hypothesized that correspondence between the preferred level of career advancement and perceptions of opportunities available to employees would enhance job satisfaction, mental and physical well-being, whereas misfit between preferred levels and perceived opportunities would predict reductions in these criterion variables. A similar prediction was proffered by Yang and colleagues in relation to social relationships at work. They suggested that maintenance of harmonious social relationships is a critical need (perhaps even more so in a collectivist culture such as China), and that good social relationships will enable people to fulfil their need for affiliation and need for belonging. These researchers argued that a better fit between preferred levels of social relationship and actual levels would be related to greater job satisfaction and reduced turnover intentions.

An important consideration raised by this above study is how best to assess (measure) fit, in this case needs–supply fit. Early studies of fit tended to utilize the difference between actual and preferred levels of an attribute as the index of fit (or misfit). However, as pointed out by Edwards (1995), there are several difficulties with this computation, and techniques such as polynomial regression may be more appropriate for the assessment of levels of fit. This was the approach used by Yang and colleagues. Their findings confirmed the expected curvilinear relationships between actual and preferred levels of both career advancement and social relationships at work, although the "nature of fit-strain associations is contingent on the specific content dimension of fit and the specific indicator of stress outcome" (p. 581). For example, for career advancement, there was an increase in job satisfaction as the actual level of advancement approached the desired level, but when supply exceeded people's preferences, job satisfaction declined. The trend for turnover intention was in the opposite direction, as expected. A somewhat different pattern emerged with respect to relationships at work. In this case, job satisfaction and mental well-being were consistently higher when actual relationship quality was high, irrespective of preferred relationship quality. These findings illustrate that fit is a relative concept, and that the salience of fit per se may vary depending on the attribute (component) being investigated. In some circumstances, the extent of fit between needs and supplies may be critical, whereas in other situations the actual levels of a component may override the importance of perceived fit.

In summary, the concept of P–E fit has received widespread recognition in the occupational health and well-being literature, and numerous investigations have been designed (either explicitly or implicitly) around this concept. There is no doubt that this model occupies an important position in conceptualizations of both work stress (strain) and work-related well-being, and that the theory has several practical applications. This model has generated critical lessons for organizations in relation to stress-management interventions and occupational health and well-being promotions. As with all other perspectives, there are certainly limitations, including the relative salience of perceived fit versus actual levels of components, but these limitations are clearly outweighed by the significant contributions which the model has made to theorizing and practical application.

Conservation of Resources Theory

Another very popular theoretical model of the stress process is that developed by Stevan Hobfoll (1989), known as the *Conservation of Resources* (COR) theory. This perspective bears marked similarity with the P–E fit model, specifically in that both approaches examine the interaction of the person and the environment, and the degree of correspondence between demands in the environment and the individual's resources to deal with those demands. One key difference (outlined by Hobfoll, 2001) is that the P–E fit model focuses predominantly on people's perceptions of fit, whereas COR theory incorporates more objective indicators of actual fit. Nevertheless, there is considerable overlap between these approaches. The fundamental tenet of COR theory is that "individuals strive to obtain, retain, protect and foster those things that they value" (Hobfoll, p. 341). That is, people endeavour to both preserve resources and to accumulate resources in order to better navigate their way through life's demands and challenges. A "resource" is anything that is important to the person, contributes positively to their well-being and enables them to adjust. In his overview of COR theory and its applications, Hobfoll indicated that 74 different types of resources have been identified through research. Some of these are what he referred to as "personal" resources, whereas others are features of the environment (external resources). Personal resources include attributes such as personal values (e.g., the importance of achievement), personality traits (e.g., internal locus of control, hardiness, dispositional optimism, generalized self-esteem) and other characteristics, including positive affect (Nelson & Simmons, 2003). Environmental resources will vary depending on the kind of environment the person functions in. In a work context, for example, features such having autonomy in one's job, the amount (and type) of feedback received on one's job performance, and the level of rewards obtained for successful job performance, are all illustrations of environmental resources (Hakanen, Perhoniemi, & Toppinen-Tanner, 2008). Social support from work colleagues and organizational support for individuals (accommodating their needs) also represent major environmental resources, which can reduce stress and burnout (Halbesleben, 2006), as well as enhancing positive well-being (Luszczynska & Cieslak, 2005).

As just mentioned, a key feature of COR theory is its simultaneous consideration of both environmental elements and the individual's cognitions. In this theory, these dimensions are given relatively equal weight in determining whether or not the person will experience conservation of resources. Hobfoll suggests that Lazarus' transactional model gives too much emphasis to personal appraisals (of threat) and not enough consideration of why people appraise events in particular ways. His contention is that the transactional model over-emphasizes the role of cognitive processes, and gives insufficient attention to the environment itself. In contrast, COR theory delves into environmental characteristics that contribute to conservation of resources and, hence (according to Hobfoll), has more practical application. The basic idea underlying COR theory is that stressful circumstances lead to resource losses. For example, conflict with other people at work can drain the individual's energy, take time to deal with, and distract them from their basic job tasks, all of which will result in resource losses. In contrast, favourable conditions will lead to resource gains; for instance, when people receive positive feedback on their work from their supervisor, this will increase their positive affect and enhance their self-esteem, as well as confirming that their job performance is acceptable. However, although COR theory incorporates both resource losses (due to stressful environmental conditions) and resource gains (from favourable events occurring), the major emphasis is on losses. Hobfoll has also suggested that, because resource losses represent a major threat to survival, they have primacy over resource gains when the person is contending with unfavourable (stressful) circumstances. He also argued that individuals tend to focus more on resource losses than gains, again because losses can undermine the person's ability to survive and thrive in their world. Nevertheless, resource gains are important for the person to develop and to increase their overall level of psycho-social well-being.

Two other principles of COR theory are important to note: (a) resource spirals and (b) resource caravans. The concept of *spirals* is based on the notion that, when individuals lack resources to deal with stressful events, they are not only more vulnerable in that situation but also "loss begets further loss" of resources (Hobfoll, 2001, p. 354). Several studies have obtained support for this spiralling of resource losses. For instance, King, King, Foy, Keane, and Fairbank (1999) found that resource deficits experienced by combat personnel in Vietnam "spilled over" into a reduced ability to cope with post-combat trauma, reducing their opportunities for recovery. Similarly, resource gains can also spiral, such as when successful performance leads to further achievement, although Hobfoll has suggested that loss spirals typically have more impact on people's well-being than do gain spirals. In addition to gain/loss spirals, COR theory also includes the concept of resource *caravans*. This notion suggests that resources can aggregate and build upon each other. An example provided by Hobfoll is the caravanning of self-efficacy with optimism. For example, if the self-efficacy of individuals is enhanced by effective job performance, they will also become more optimistic concerning their ability to perform effectively in the future. Similarly, the availability of social support may bolster feelings of self-esteem of individuals, leading them to feel more comfortable about seeking further social support in the future. Extending the caravan metaphor, Hobfoll (2001) commented that "the retinue of resources tends to travel together over time unless some inner or outside forces are specifically directed to alter the constellation of resources" (p. 350).

As noted above, there is considerable empirical support for the COR principles and logic, and this theory has made a significant contribution to both the theoretical and applied literature. A recent study example (Xanthopoulou, Bakker, Demerouti, & Schaufeli, 2009) illustrates the applicability of COR theory. In a two-wave longitudinal investigation among employees in an electrical engineering and electronics firm in the Netherlands, Xanthopoulou and colleagues examined reciprocal relationships between job resources (namely autonomy, social support, supervisory coaching, performance feedback, and opportunities for professional development), personal resources (self-efficacy, organization-based self-esteem and optimism) and work engagement (based on Schaufeli, Bakker, & Salanova, 2006). They observed that when employees had high levels of resources, their work engagement increased and, conversely, high levels of engagement were also associated with greater resources at the second time period. Xanthopoulou and associates concluded that both role (job) resources and personal resources play an important role in facilitating work engagement. Their study also demonstrated the concept of gain spirals in respect of work engagement.

The Job Demands–Control–Support Model of Work Design

A somewhat different, but nonetheless complementary approach to those outlined above, is a theory of work design proposed initially by Karasek (1979) and later expanded by Karasek and Theorell (1990). It should be noted that Theorell has provided a more detailed description of this work in another chapter of the present Handbook. The initial proposition put forward by Karasek is referred to as the Job Demands–Control (JDC) Model, although the term "discretion" was also used by Karasek as a synonym for control. He proposed that, although excessive job demands or pressures (both physical and psychosocial) can have an impact on stress levels (especially psychological strain), by themselves these demands are not the most important contributors to strain experiences. Rather, the amount of strain people experience in their work will be determined by whether or not they have any control over the demands they have to deal with. That is to say, according to Karasek (1979), there will be interactive effects of Demands × Control (or discretion) on stress levels. Put another way, control will buffer (moderate) the impact of demands (pressures) on strain. This relationship is depicted in Fig. 2.2.

	Low Job Demands	High Job Demands
Low Control	Passive Job	High-strain Job
High Control	Low-strain Job	Active Job

Fig. 2.2 The job demands–job control model

Several issues remained unresolved with respect of this model. One is whether the effects of demands and control are additive or multiplicative (that is, there is an interactive effect between them). Researchers are divided on this question, and there is support for both points of view. A second issue which has not been fully resolved is whether *objective* control or *subjective* (perceived) control is the critical factor in determining stress reactions. In some studies, proxy variables have been used to determine some kind of "objective" measure of control, but most research on this model has focused on workers' perceptions of control, arguing that how much control the individual feels they have over their work environment is more critical than some kind of objective index of control. Although objective and subjective control are clearly correlated with each other, they do not necessarily coincide.

Empirical support for the JDC model has been produced, with several studies demonstrating a moderating influence of discretion or control on the relationship between job demands and psychological strain (Beehr, Glaser, Canali, & Wallwey, 2001). Nevertheless, there has been controversy about whether the approach is universally applicable. For example, a very recent study (Panatik, O'Driscoll, & Anderson, 2011) did not obtain moderator effects for perceived job control in a sample of Malaysian technical workers, but rather found that feelings of self-efficacy functioned as a moderator of demands–strain relations. It is possible that the Western emphasis on personal control (at work and in other aspects of life) does not generalize to non-Western cultures, which may value more group-oriented mechanisms.

The revised formulation of this perspective, proposed by Johnson and Hall (1988) and Karasek and Theorell (1990), added social support to the mix of factors which will influence a person's levels of psychological strain (and ultimately their psychosocial well-being) at work. The model then became known as the Job Demands–Control–Support (JDCS) model. Karasek and Theorell suggested that the beneficial effects of control (discretion) will be further enhanced when the individual receives social support (either practical or emotional) from his/her work colleagues and supervisor. The addition of social support to the model was based on extensive evidence that this variable can play a substantial role in alleviating stress in workers (Cooper et al., 2001), although there has been considerable debate over whether its impact is direct (that is, more support is directly associated with reduced strain) or indirect (that is, support will buffer the impact of stressors on strain). The latter view, known as the *buffering hypothesis*, intuitively makes a lot of sense, but has not always been confirmed empirically

(Cranford, 2004; Kickul & Posig, 2001). For instance, although some studies have obtained the predicted moderator (buffering) effects of social support, others have reported direct negative relationships between support and strain or, in some cases, a positive relationship between social support and strain, which is referred to as "reverse buffering" (Kickul & Posig).

Some research has also confirmed a three-way interaction among demands, control, and social support. Indeed, Daniels, Beesley, Cheyne, and Wimalasiri (2008) argued that the reason that control and support have a positive impact on reducing strain and enhancing well-being is that they enable the individual to cope more effectively with stressors (including work demands), and that these benefits accumulate over time. Daniels and his colleagues found that control and support facilitated both problem-focused and emotional-approach coping which, in turn, were related to factors such as fatigue, error rates and reduction of risky decisions. This study is especially important as it has further elucidated a mechanism by which control and support exert beneficial effects; that is, via their contribution to effective coping mechanisms. Other research, however, has reported very mixed support for the JDCS model, and there are unresolved issues. One particular problem which has been discussed for some time (see Wall, Jackson, Mullarkey, & Parker, 1996) concerns the methods of assessing perceived control. Some studies have measured very general control, which does not necessarily match up with the type of stressor (demands) being confronted by the person. For instance, if individuals are experiencing excessive time pressure to get work completed, having control over other aspects of their work domain, such as office layout, may be largely irrelevant, whereas control over the work itself will be critical. Similar arguments can be made with respect to social support. As noted above, social support from work colleagues and supervisors may be beneficial to a person, but is not always so and, in some cases, may actually be detrimental to their well-being (the reverse-buffering effect). In addition, the effects of different types of social support may vary depending on their appropriateness and whether the person wishes to receive any support (and, if so, what kind of support). However, despite the various controversies and unresolved questions in terms of the JDC and JDCS models, there is no doubt that they have had considerable "traction" in research on psychological strain and well-being. There has also been research on the interactive effects of job demands, control and support on physiological strains, such as cardiovascular disease and other physical strains (see, for instance, Shirom, Toker, Berliner, & Shapira, 2008). The theory has numerous practical applications, in that it suggests procedures for enhancing well-being at work and reducing the impact of stressors. Finally, it is linked with other theoretical accounts of the work stress process (which we do not cover in this chapter), such as the Effort–Reward Imbalance Model (Siegrist, 2009).

Different Perspectives, Different Theories

We have not attempted in this chapter to cover all of the (numerous) theories relating to work stress, but rather to discuss a few major ones that have highlighted, different, albeit complementary, different perspectives. Each of the theories discussed offers a different perspective for understanding the transaction between the individual and the environment. Other theories have taken up the issues of "process." For instance, the theory of stress outlined by Shupe and McGrath (2000) describes "a dynamic, adaptive process theory" (Cooper, 2000, p. 3) which, when focused at the individual level, suggests a complex cycle connected by four processes: the appraisal process (interpreting events); the choice process (the choice of a coping response); the performance process (the coping phase); and the outcome process (the consequences for the individual; Shupe & McGrath, 2000, pp. 86–88). Shupe and McGrath go on to outline the complexity of these interconnected process and the implications this complexity has for researchers in terms of measurement and interpretation. Similarly, Cummings and Cooper (2000) offer a "cybernetic theory" of work stress. The emphasis here is on time, information, and feedback.

These constructs are viewed as essential, and they are regarded as underlying the stress process as it moves from "the detection of strain, through the choice of adjustment processes to cope with the threat situation, and on to the subsequent feedback about coping effects" (p. 3). Cummings and Cooper also go on to outline the complexity of the process, such as the operational and measurement issues involved as the processes moves through its four (detection, choice, adjustment, and affects) phases. At the heart of this theory is the idea that "individuals are active purposive managers of stress and that knowledge can help them anticipate and manage stress" (Wethington, 2000, p. 642). The cybernetic approach is further developed by Edwards (2000) through the idea that the goal of "self regulating systems" is to regulate discrepancies between the individual and the environment. Discrepancies are expressed in terms of a negative feedback loop, and so stress, coping and well being are crucial elements in this self-regulating process.

The idea of process as expressed through some sort of transaction between the person and the environment lies at the heart of these different theoretical approaches. This is not to say that researchers, whilst still grappling with the issues of process and transaction, have not explored and developed other theoretical approaches. We briefly turn to two of these to illustrate the continuing creative way in which the stress process has been investigated. Warr (2007) explored the way in which work leaves us feeling happy or unhappy. While acknowledging the definitional difficulties surrounding terms like happiness and unhappiness, and the preference at times to use the term well-being, Warr (Warr & Clapperton, 2010) suggests that happiness should be considered not just in terms of its energising and tranquil forms, but also in terms of whether it is being used in a contextual (work) sense or even a facet (work component) sense. When exploring work and happiness, Warr (2007) draws attention to the transaction between the person and the environment. When considering the environment, Warr (Warr & Clapperton, 2010) identifies 12 sources of work happiness, but recognizes that there is no correct number of work sources, as these will differ across and within jobs, and will depend also on individual differences. Discussing these work sources, Warr (1997) suggests that the best way to think about these different sources is to liken them to vitamins where, in much the same way as vitamins, they are good for the person but only up to a certain level. Warr (2007) outlined how, like vitamins, moderate levels of these work sources produce happiness, but beyond a certain level there is a "tipping point" (Warr & Clapperton, 2010, p. 73) where the demands of some of these work sources reduce happiness and well-being and where, for other work sources, providing more does not produce more happiness as you have already reached as much as you want. The absence of these work sources does, of course, produce unhappiness.

The role of individual differences also plays a part in the work–happiness equation. While Warr (2007) and Warr and Clapperton (2010) point out the way different personality traits influence happiness, and how happiness also depends on the different sorts of comparisons individuals make about themselves in relation to others, they also raise the issue of whether individuals have a consistency in their levels of happiness—"a baseline" that they keep coming back to (Warr & Clapperton, p. 10). This brief overview cannot capture the level of analysis, the scope of the research or the complexity that resides within Warr's (2007) vitamin theory. The "overall message" that flows from this approach, however, is that happiness–unhappiness comes not just from the different work sources, but is also derived from within and that "possible improvements must be sought for both directions" (Warr & Clapperton, 2010, p. 177).

Another approach is offered by Nelson and Simmons (2003, 2004) and Simmons and Nelson (2007), who integrate into their holistic stress model the positive qualities of eustress and propose that the appraisal of any encounter can produce positive or negative meanings. This model "focuses on the positive responses and their effects on performance and health" (Simmons & Nelson, p. 40). Interestingly, these authors go on to point to their concept of "savouring the positive" (p. 40), and how this adds a new perspective on how people cope. Similarly, when individual differences are considered in terms of how they trigger positive beliefs, these authors point to how such beliefs aid individuals, create positive appraisals, develop resources for managing demanding encounters, and shift the focus towards those aspects of the work environment that help create the context for positive opportunities. While arguing that it is now time to include the positive as well as the negative into our theories of stress, these authors suggest that studying work stress should be "best thought of as a constellation of theories and models that each addresses a meaningful process or phenomenon" (Simmons & Nelson, p. 50).

Conclusions and Future Directions

If we have this constellation of theories, where do we go from here? The different theories reflect a number of perspectives, but all offer a lens through which the person–environment transaction can be explored. Each offers a dynamic view of the stress process, emphasising the importance of the context within which the transaction between the person and the environment takes place. Many of these theories draw attention not just to the "contribution of the person as opposed to the environment, in creating organizational stress" (Wethington, 2000, p. 641), but also to the way in which the demands of an encounter are appraised. If individuals are active participants in the stress process and if this "activity," as seems generally agreed, is initiated through the process of appraisal, then perhaps by focusing on these meanings that individuals give to demanding encounters will help us identify an "organizing concept" for the future. Capturing the meaning individuals give to stressful encounters cannot, of course, be separated from measurement. So, it is important for researchers to continually evaluate whether current measurement practices allow these meanings to emerge, expressed in a way that captures their explanatory richness. In the future, if our theories are to continue to develop our understanding of process, then our measurement practices will need to evolve to develop creative approaches that involve narratives, person-focused techniques and qualitative methods that allow such meanings to be captured. It is not that appraisals have been ignored, but it is more that they have yet to receive the attention they deserve. It is clear that appraisals provide the conduit through which coping and the emotional consequences emerge. It is the appraisal process that has the potential to provide a rich explanatory pathway, and one that enables us to begin the process of working towards the role of discrete emotions and away from the troublesome concept of stress fulfilling our moral responsibility to those who's working lives we explore.

References

Aldwin, C. M. (2000). *Stress, coping, and development: An integrative perspective*. New York: The Guilford Press.
Beehr, T. A., Glaser, K. M., Canali, K. G., & Wallwey, D. A. (2001). Back to basics: Re-examination of the demand-control theory of occupational stress. *Work and Stress, 15*(115–130).
Brief, A. P., & George, J. M. (1991). Psychological stress and the workplace: A brief comment on Lazarus' outlook. In P. L. Perrewé (Ed.). Handbook on job stress [Special Issue]. *Journal of Social Behaviour and Personality, 6*, 15–20.
Cavanaugh, M. A., Boswell, W. R., Roehling, M. V., & Boudreau, J. W. (2000). An empirical examination of self-reported work stress among U.S. managers. *Journal of Applied Psychology, 85*, 65–74.
Cooper, C. L. (Ed.). (2000). *Theories of stress*. Oxford: Oxford University Press.
Cooper, C. L., Dewe, P., & O'Driscoll, M. (2001). *Organizational Stress: A review and critique of theory, research, and applications*. Thousand Oaks: Sage.
Coyne, J. C. (1997). Improving coping research: Raze the slum before any more building! *Journal of Health Psychology, 2*, 153–155.
Coyne, J. C., & Gottlieb, B. H. (1996). The mismeasure of coping by checklist. *Journal of Personality, 64*, 959–991.
Cranford, J. A. (2004). Stress-buffering or stress-exacerbation? Social support and social undermining as moderators of the relationship between perceived stress and depressive symptoms among married people. *Personal Relationships, 11*(1), 23–40.

Cummings, T. G., & Cooper, C. L. (1979). *Cybernetic framework for studying occupational stress*. Minneapolis: Minnesota Press.

Cummings, T. G., & Cooper, C. L. (2000). A cybernetic theory of organizational stress. In C. L. Cooper (Ed.), *Theories of stress* (pp. 101–121). Oxford: Oxford University Press.

Daniels, K., Beesley, N., Cheyne, A., & Wimalasiri, V. (2008). Coping processes linking the demands-control-support model, affect and risky decisions at work. *Human Relations, 61*(6), 845–874.

Dawis, R. V., & Lofquist, L. H. (1984). *A psychological theory of work adjustment*. Minneapolis: University of Minnesota Press.

Dewe, P. (2001). Work stress, coping and well-being: implementing strategies to better understand the relationship. In P. Perrewe & D. Ganster (Eds.), *Research in occupational stress and well-being: Exploring theoretical mechanisms and perspectives 1* (pp. 63–96). Amsterdam: JAI Press.

Dewe, P., & Ng, A. (1999). Exploring the relationship between primary appraisal and coping using a work setting. *Journal of Social Behavior and Personality, 14*, 397–418.

Dewe, P., O'Driscoll, M., & Cooper, C. (2010). *Coping with work stress: A review and critique*. Chichester: Wiley-Blackwell.

Edwards, J. R. (1995). Alternatives to difference scores as dependent variables in the study of congruence in organizational research. *Organizational Behavior and Human Decision Processes, 64*, 307–324.

Edwards, J. R. (2000). Cybernetic theory of stress, coping and well-being. In C. L. Cooper (Ed.), *Theories of stress* (pp. 122–152). Oxford: Oxford University Press.

Folkman, S. (2011). Stress, health, and coping: Synthesis, commentary, and future directions. In S. Folkman (Ed.), *The Oxford handbook of stress, health, and coping* (pp. 453–462). Oxford: Oxford University Press.

Folkman, S., & Lazarus, R. S. (1980). An analysis of coping in a middle-aged community sample. *Journal of Health and Social Behaviour, 21*, 219–239.

Folkman, S., & Moskowitz, J. T. (2004). Coping: Pitfalls and promise. *Annual Review of Psychology, 55*, 745–774.

Frese, M., & Zapf, D. (1999). On the importance of the objective environment in stress and attribution theory. Counterpoint to Perrewe and Zellars. *Journal of Organizational Behavior, 20*, 761–765.

Hakanen, J. J., Perhoniemi, R., & Toppinen-Tanner, S. (2008). Positive gain spirals at work: From job resources to work engagement, personal initiative and work-unit innovativeness. *Journal of Vocational Behavior, 73*(1), 78–91.

Halbesleben, J. R. B. (2006). Sources of social support and burnout: A meta-analytic test of the conservation of resources model. *Journal of Applied Psychology, 91*(5), 1134–1145.

Hobfoll, S. E. (2001). The influence of culture, community and the nested-self in the stress process: Advancing conservation of resources theory. *Applied Psychology: An International Review, 50*, 337–421.

Holroyd, K., & Lazarus, R. (1982). Stress, coping and somatic adaptation. In L. Goldberger & S. Breznitz (Eds.), *Handbook of stress: Theoretical and clinical aspects* (pp. 21–35). New York: Free Press.

Johnson, J., & Hall, E. (1988). Job strain, work place social support and cardiovascular disease: A cross-sectional study of a random sample of the working population. *American Journal of Public Health, 78*, 1336–1342.

Kaplan, H. (1996). Themes, lacunae and directions in research on psychological stress. In H. Kaplan (Ed.), *Psychosocial stress: Perspectives on structure, theory, life courses and methods* (pp. 369–401). New York: Academic.

Karasek, R. A. (1979). Job demands, job decision latitude and mental strain: Implications for job redesign. *Administrative Science Quarterly, 24*, 285–308.

Karasek, R. A., & Theorell, T. (1990). *Healthy work: Stress, productivity and the reconstruction of working life*. New York: Basic Books.

Kickul, J., & Posig, M. (2001). Supervisory social support and burnout: An explanation of reverse buffering effects. *Journal of Managerial Issues, 13*, 328–344.

King, D. W., King, L. A., Foy, D. W., Keane, T. M., & Fairbank, J. A. (1999). Post-traumatic stress disorder in a national sample of male and female Vietnam veterans: Risk factors, war-zone stressors and resilience-recovery variables. *Journal of Abnormal Psychology, 108*, 164–170.

Lazarus, R. S. (1990). Theory based stress measurement. *Psychological Inquiry, 1*, 3–12.

Lazarus, R. S. (1999). *Stress and emotion: a new synthesis*. London: Free Association.

Lazarus, R. S. (2000). Toward better research on stress and coping. *American Psychologist, 55*, 665–673.

Lazarus, R. S. (2001). Relational meaning and discrete emotions. In K. Scherer, A. Schorr, & T. Johnstone (Eds.), *Appraisal processes in emotion: Theory, methods, research* (pp. 37–67). New York: Oxford University Press.

Lazarus, R. S., & Cohen-Charash, Y. (2001). Discrete emotions in organizational life. In R. Payne & C. Cooper (Eds.), *Emotions at work: theory, research and applications for management* (pp. 45–81). Chichester: John Wiley.

Liddle, H. A. (1994). Contextualizing resiliency. In M. C. Wong & E. W. Gordon (Eds.), *Educational resilience in inner-city America* (pp. 167–177). Hillsdale, N.Y.: Earlbaum.

Lowe, R., & Bennett, P. (2003). Exploring coping reactions to work stress: application of an appraisal theory. *Journal of Occupational and Organizational Psychology, 676*, 393–400.

Luszczynska, A., & Cieslak, R. (2005). Protective, promotive, and buffering effects of perceived social support in managerial stress: The moderating role of personality. *Anxiety, Stress and Coping, 18*(3), 227–244.

Murray, H. (1938). *Explorations in personality*. Boston, MA: Houghton Mifflin.

Nelson, D. L., & Simmons, B. L. (2003). Health psychology and work stress: A more positive approach. In J. C. Quick & L. E. Tetrick (Eds.), *Handbook of occupational psychology* (pp. 97–119). Washington, DC: American Psychological Society.

Nelson, D. L., & Simmons, B. L. (2004). Eustress: An elusive construct, an engaging pursuit. In P. L. Perrewe & D. C. Ganster (Eds.), *Research in occupational stress and well being* (Vol. 3, pp. 265–322). Amsterdam: Elsevier JAI.

Newton, T. (1995). *Managing' stress: Emotion and power at work*. London: Sage.

Panatik, S. A., O'Driscoll, M. P., & Anderson, M. H. (2011). Job demands and employee work-related psychological responses among Malaysian technical workers: The moderating effects of self-efficacy. *Work and Stress, 25*(4), 355–371.

Schaufeli, W. B., Bakker, A. B., & Salanova, M. (2006). The measurement of work engagement with a short questionnaire: A cross-national study. *Educational and Psychological Measurement, 66*(4), 701–716.

Shirom, A., Toker, S., Berliner, S., & Shapira, I. (2008). The job demand-control-support model and stress-related low-grade inflammatory responses among healthy employees: A longitudinal study. *Work and Stress, 22*(2), 138–152.

Shupe, E. I., & McGrath, J. E. (2000). Stress and the sojourner. In C. L. Cooper (Ed.), *Theories of stress* (pp. 86–100). Oxford: Oxford University Press.

Siegrist, J. (2009). Job control and reward: Effects on well-being. In S. Cartwright & C. L. Cooper (Eds.), *The Oxford handbook of organizational well-being* (pp. 109–132). Oxford: Oxford University Press.

Simmons, B. L., & Nelson, D. L. (2007). Eustress at work: Extending the holistic stress model. In D. L. Nelson & C. L. Cooper (Eds.), *Positive organizational behaviour* (pp. 40–53). London: Sage.

Somerfield, M., & McCrae, R. (2000). Stress and coping research: Methodological challenges, theoretical advances. *American Psychologist, 55*, 620–625.

Tennen, H., Affleck, G., Armeli, S., & Carney, M. (2000). A daily process approach to coping. *American Psychologist, 55*, 626–636.

Wall, T., Jackson, P., Mullarkey, S., & Parker, S. (1996). The demands-control model of job strain: A more specific test. *Journal of Occupational and Organizational Psychology, 69*, 153–166.

Warr, P. B. (2007). *Work, happiness and unhappiness*. Mahwah, NJ: Lawrence Erlbaum.

Warr, P. B., & Clapperton, G. (2010). *The joy of work: Jobs, happiness, and you*. London: Routledge.

Wethington, E. (2000). Theories of organizational stress: Book review. *Administrative Science Quarterly, 45*, 640–642.

Xanthopoulou, D., Bakker, A. B., Demerouti, E., & Schaufeli, W. B. (2009). Reciprocal relationships between job resources, personal resources, and work engagement. *Journal of Vocational Behavior, 74*(3), 235.

Yang, L.-Q., Hongsheng, C., & Spector, P. E. (2008). Job stress and well-being: An examination from the view of person-environment fit. *Journal of Occupational and Organizational Psychology, 81*(3), 567–587.

# The Growth of Occupational Health Psychology

Heather Graham, Krista J. Howard, and Angela Liegey Dougall

Introduction

With the above preamble in mind, it should be noted that the prevention of work-related illnesses is not just a matter of physical safety anymore. The health and well-being of modern day employees demands an interdisciplinary approach including psychology, medicine, business, and engineering (Maclean, Plotnikoff, & Moyer, 2000). The World Health Organization (WHO) has identified psychosocial factors as major occupational health concerns, in addition to problems associated with exposure to biochemical and physical hazards and unemployment (WHO, 2007). The field of occupational health psychology is growing in practice and acceptance to answer this need. Now, an institutionalized discipline, occupational health psychology has produced multiple handbooks and journals including *Stress* (Cox, 1978), *The Journal of Occupational Health Psychology* (American Psychological Association [APA], 1996), *The Handbook of Occupational Health Psychology* (Quick & Tetrick, 2003, 2010), and now the current *Handbook of Occupational Health and Wellness* (Gatchel & Schultz, 2012).

While the term organizational health used to refer to the resilience and strength of an organization, occupational health psychologists have expanded that definition to include, if not emphasize, the health of the employees within an organization (Tetrick & Quick, 2003). The prevention of illness or injury and the promotion of the physical, mental, and social well-being of employees is now the ultimate objective of occupational health researchers and practitioners alike. As such, the field has benefited from a positive health platform including healthy leadership practices, awareness of stress, strain and stressors, and a push toward proactive interventions (Tetrick & Quick, 2010).

The American Institute of Stress elevated work stress to an epidemic in the first part of this century based on self-reports, unscheduled absence data, violent incidents at work, and job loss statistics (Rosch, 2001). Sadly, the statistics are both supportive of this designation and startling. Now more

H. Graham, Ph.D. • A.L. Dougall, Ph.D. (✉)
Department of Psychology, The University of Texas at Arlington,
501 S. Nedderman Dr., LS313, Box 19528, Arlington, TX 76019, USA
e-mail: heather.graham@mavs.uta.edu; adougall@uta.edu

K.J. Howard, Ph.D.
Department of Psychology, Texas State University,
Psy 214C, 601 University Drive, San Marcos, TX 78666, USA
e-mail: krista.howard@txstate.edu

than ever, American workers have reported that they are more stressed over money and workplace concerns due to the tumultuous economy. According to a recent survey, the percentage of employees that reported stress due to job instability increased from 42 % in 2008 to 49 % in 2010 (APA, 2010). Furthermore, a startling 76 % of workers reported feeling stress and anxiety about money, while 70 % reported feeling stressed about work. The medical field points to stress for 60–90 % of all illnesses, as 75–80 % of Americans reported that their jobs are very or extremely stressful (American Institute of Stress, 2007; National Institute for Occupational Safety and Health [NIOSH], 2007). In this chapter, we briefly describe the emergence of occupational health psychology to date. Then, the changing nature of work due to the emergence of technology and globalization is discussed. Lastly, we will review common workplace stressors, the theoretical models of workplace stress, and how we can utilize our body of knowledge in a preventative framework. Many of these issues will be discussed in greater detail in other chapters of this handbook.

A Historical Perspective of Occupational Health Psychology

Healthy organizations, a term once used to describe companies that financially survive and cope with the turbulent ups and downs of the economy, have now taken a broader meaning that includes the health and wellness of the company's employees. While the origins of organizational health psychology date back to the early twentieth century, it was not until the American Psychological Association (APA) and the United States National Institute for Occupational Safety and Health (NIOSH) jointly identified job-related psychological disorders as one of the top ten employee health concerns, that the larger majority of organizations really began to understand the concern (Sauter, Murphy, & Hurrell, 1990). At present, most researchers ascribe to the World Health Organization's (1948) definition that health is not just an absence from disease. In fact, the discipline of organizational health psychology has expanded to include the social, physical, and psychological well-being of employees that results in optimal functioning (Hofmann & Tetrick, 2003; Macik-Frey, Quick, & Nelson, 2007; Schaufeli, 2004). However, throughout history, health has not always been a priority for organizational researchers.

The Principles of Scientific Management

The idea that work is a potential source of stress, illness, and physical strain began to appear in the literature detailing the dehumanizing mentality of factories in the late nineteenth century (Barling & Griffiths, 2010; Engels, 1845/1987; Marx, 1967/1845). One of the early organizational researchers that contributed to the mechanistic, dehumanizing perspective of factory workers was Fredrick Taylor, who authored the book, *The Principles of Scientific Management* (1911). In his book, Taylor suggested that factories could increase efficiency by taking control and discretion away from the employees. He was the first to compartmentalize workers into those that "think about work" and those that "do the work." Within the scientific management approach, one level of employees, the managers, would have control to plan what the other level of employees had to do, with no input from the employees themselves. In fact, many of the managers had been promoted from the ranks and had received little to no proper training as leaders. These newly appointed managers were given complete control over the workplace and were allowed to hire and fire employees at their own discretion, and were in charge of determining production and pay. The scientific management philosophy did not view the workers as humans but rather as machines. This type of work environment degraded the front-line employees and likely created a lot of stress, dissention, and illness.

Following the period of scientific management, a new approach was developed that focused more on the physical and psychological needs of the individual workers. Termed the human relations approach, this new leadership style allowed workers to be active participants in the decision-making processes of the organization (Schultz & Schultz, 2010). Research conducted following the period of scientific management has redirected the current focus in occupational health psychology on increasing worker control and taking into account employees' emotions.

The Hawthorne Effect

One of the first organizational psychology experiments to gain widespread attention was conducted by the Western Electric Company in Hawthorne, Illinois (Mayo, 1933, Roethlisberger & Dickson, 1939). Elton Mayo, an Industrial Research professor at Harvard University developed a series of experiments to evaluate how physical factors of the work environment affected work production. In efforts to maximize productivity, the working conditions were manipulated by altering the amount of light in the factory. The hope was to identify the optimal amount of light that factory workers needed to be most productive; however, the results of these studies were rather surprising. Researchers discovered that any change to the working conditions resulted in an increase in productivity. For example, when the researchers dimmed the lights by measurable increments, productivity increased. However, when the researchers then increased the light emitted within the factory, productivity continued to increase. Soon enough, it was apparent that the employees responded to the increased attention they felt from being the focus of an experiment, a phenomenon now appropriately referred to as the "Hawthorne Effect." Notably, this series of studies were critical to the human relations movement; managers and researchers began to understand the human side of employment. Counter to Taylor's scientific management model that essentially removed emotions and attitudes from the workplace, the focus began to shift to the promotion of happy, healthy workers.

Occupational Health Researchers

About 10 years after the ground-breaking Hawthorne studies, other areas of psychology were also highlighting the importance of motivation and mental health. For instance, Maslow published his theory of self-actualization that emphasized the importance of meeting the basic human needs before expecting employees to reach their full potential (Maslow, 1943). Similarly, Herzberg (1966) argued that increased productivity and satisfaction could be obtained by perfecting job design and providing realistic challenges and ongoing recognition. These ideas laid the groundwork for later models such as the Person-Environment Fit Model (Edwards & Cooper, 1990; French, Caplan, & Van Harrison, 1982; Kahn, Wolfe, Quinn, Snoek, & Rosenthal, 1964; Lofquist & Dawis, 1969), Demand–Control Model (Karasek, 1979; Karasek & Theorell, 1990), and Effort–Reward Model (Siegrist, 1996). These models will be further discussed later in the chapter.

Along with the increased interest in the ideal working conditions that support health and well-being, European researchers were also starting to investigate the impact of job design, job decision latitude (control), and job demands. In a series of studies, a psychologist by the name of Bertil Gardell posited that Taylor's scientific management approach created withdrawal and alienation within workforces (1971, 1977). Without a concern for the humanistic side of the employees, work became monotonous and fragmented and the workers felt isolated and underappreciated. Researchers then began to understand the influence of psychosocial work factors on health outcomes. For example, factors such as person–environment fit, role ambiguity, and role-conflict were empirically linked to the development of coronary heart disease (Katz & Kahn, 1966).

One of Gardell's students, Robert Karasek carried Gardell's research to new levels with his work on the cardiovascular health of a sample of Swedish men. In the book entitled *Healthy Work*, Karasek and Theorell (1990) suggested that the same psychosocial components of work that were important for satisfaction were also strongly associated with increased job performance. Furthermore, this work highlighted the importance of the ratio between job demands and job control when predicting work-related stress with workers who had low control and high demand experiencing the most stress and health problems (Barling & Griffiths, 2010; Theorell & Karasek, 1996). These findings were the impetus for a large body of research that has since demonstrated that factors which predict better physical and psychosocial health also promote increased productivity and better organizational outcomes. In another chapter in this handbook, Theorell provides a comprehensive review of that research.

Occupational Health Organizations

Standing on the shoulders of so many years of research, multiple national organizations have been organized and continue to play a significant role in the development of organizational health psychology. Since the 1990s, the United States National Institute for Occupational Safety and Health (NIOSH) has supported research to ensure that working conditions remain safe for USA employees. NIOSH has developed strategies to promote and protect the psychological well-being of employees based on the recommendations of researchers in the field. Further, NIOSH has partnered with another well-known organization, the American Psychological Association (APA), to fund organizational health graduate programs, as well as international conferences that have continued to promote work in this area. Another well-known organization in the field of occupational health is the Institute of Work, Health and Organisations (I-WHO). I-WHO has made significant contributions, particularly within the field of work stress (e.g., Cox, 1978). Utilizing the Cognitive Appraisal Model (Lazarus, 1966; Lazarus & Folkman, 1984; to be discussed in detail later in the chapter) as the basis of reasoning, the I-WHO concentrates on the processes through which people evaluate an event as being stressful or not. With this approach, Cox, the lead researcher, catalyzed a risk-management approach to understanding work stress.

Summary

Throughout the history of occupational health psychology there has been a flux of ideas. The field started with a focus on increased worker productivity that, in turn, decreased employee participation and ignored the psychological well-being of the employees. In stark contrast, today, the focus includes environmental and psychosocial factors that not only improve employee well-being and health but also ultimately increase productivity. These changes have been attributed to a number of prominent researchers throughout many disciplines and around the globe that have been supported by leading organizations devoted to enhancing occupational health. One influential factor in this climate change has been the changing nature of today's work environments.

The Changing Nature of Work

Throughout the growth of organizational health psychology as a discipline, researchers have had to shift gears as the nature of work continues to evolve. The revolutionizing world of technology is arguably the most influential factor in the changing nature of work. With every new technological advancement, job design, task duties, competition, and work conditions are affected in just about every industry all over the world. The competitive market is far more dynamic than it was at the birth of occupational health psychology.

Technology

Advancements in manufacturing technology have led to quicker and more efficient production, but have also placed higher demands on individual employees. One of the most noticeable shifts is the increase, over the past 50 years, in the number of service and professional jobs that are largely computer-driven (Tetrick & Quick, 2010). While there are still jobs that require rudimentary skill and physical endurance, there are now many more jobs that are cognitively demanding. Advances in technology have also been associated with organizational downsizing and restructuring, which have resulted in smaller work teams that are often required to deal with more ambiguity rather than doing the same task every day. Similarly, there are also more managerial jobs as teams have become more specialized. For instance, instead of one first-line supervisor for every 100 employees working on an assembly line, it is not uncommon for organizations to now operate with one manager for every ten departmental employees. This organizational structure translates to more managers with the added stress of managing and developing others (Sulsky & Smith, 2005). Likewise, the role of the leader has become much more personal and influential for the employees. Rather than perceive a supervisor and company as one unifying source of stress, the more personal social-exchange relationships that occur with smaller work teams allows employees to distinguish between the two potential sources of stress (Lavelle, Brockner, et al., 2009; Lavelle, McMahan, & Harris, 2009). Research has demonstrated that now the organization and the manager often serve as two individual sources of stress that interact with one another (Graham, Lopez, & Dougall, 2008; Greenberg, 2004). Furthermore, these studies indicated that the leader is often the most influential source of stress for employees over and above other organizational influences.

Globalization

The influx of technology has also vastly expanded the market-place to a globalized level. On one hand, globalization has the potential to widen the pool of buyers, increase time of productivity to a 24-h day, and reduce labor and over-head costs. On the other hand, globalization also increases the number of competitors, decreases job security, increases workforce diversity, and increases the amount of stress for individual employees. Increased levels of stress are often observed because of the circumstances surrounding globalization such as job-relocation, job-reassignment, unemployment, cultural clashes, and difficulties communicating (Brislin, 2008; Sharma & Sharma, 2010). In addition to globalization, the turbulent economy has forced many organizations to "do more with less."

Work Practices

Almost mimicking the 100-year old Principles of Scientific Management (Taylor, 1911), new organizational practices that seek to maximize productivity with minimal labor costs have recently emerged. These new-age practices, including Total Quality Management (Cua, McKone, & Schroeder, 2001), Lean Production, and Six Sigma, are often implemented to increase productivity and quality without regard for the employees' health and well-being (Shoaf, Genaidy, Karwowski, & Huang, 2004). In fact, these practices may add undue stress due to increased demands and unwanted stretch assignments (Seppälä & Klemola, 2004).

Summary

The shift to increased cognitively demanding jobs, globalization, and high-demand organizational processes brings about different types of health concerns for the field of occupational health psychology. For instance, rather than physical ailments and chemical exposures, most of the major threats to our modern workforce are chronic, degenerative diseases that are much more difficult to detect (Levi, 2011). Unfortunately, stress has been shown to be either the cause or an accelerator to both short- and long-term illnesses, even life-threatening diseases (Dougall & Baum, 2012; Levi, 2011). Furthermore, the relationship between work and stress, or rather the common outcomes of stress, such as illness, turnover and accidents, has been well established in the literature (Greenberg, 2010; Lax, Grant, Maanetti, & Klein, 1998). In essence, work-related stress is just as concerning, if not more so, as the first health and safety concerns that triggered the occupational health movement.

Job-Related Stressors

A prominent focus of occupational health research is to identify the factors that contribute to job-related stress and to understand how those factors affect the employees' health and occupational outcomes. The factors often considered by occupational health psychologists can be viewed from a job-specific approach, such that the job itself is hazardous and stressful, or from a psychosocial approach, such that leadership, organizational support, and perceived equity can have a negative effect on health and occupational outcomes. The following section will provide an overview of the various occupational factors that have been found to not only contribute to poor health and illness but also to be linked with poor occupational outcomes, such as low job satisfaction, productivity and organizational commitment, higher rates of absenteeism, and turnover.

Workplace Characteristics

The physical work environment is a major factor that affects not only the health and safety of the organization's employees, but it also can influence general job satisfaction and productivity. Various elements within the work environment have been researched and found to contribute to employee stress. Environmental factors, such as lighting, noise, and temperature, have been identified to have significant effects on productivity and job satisfaction. Also, employee work schedules have been studied to determine what types of schedules are beneficial or detrimental to productivity and health. Likewise, efforts have been made to reduce the likelihood of illnesses and injuries on the job that can often be prevented. Organizational health researchers have examined such stressors to identify what types of professions and individuals are at higher risks of adverse outcomes. Through this process, occupational health researchers can then create prevention and intervention strategies to reduce and eliminate harmful effects from poorly designed workplace environments.

Physical Working Conditions

Environmental work factors have been systematically studied within various industries to determine the effects on employees' health, stress levels, and productivity. The physical working conditions commonly studied in occupational health psychology can include general workplace conditions, such as noise, lighting and temperature, but have also focused on the physical demands for the job. These physical demands include exposure to noxious materials and dangerous work environments, which have been correlated with long-term illnesses, disabilities, and fatalities. Again, the National Institute for Occupational Safety and Health (NIOSH), a federally funded agency that conducts research and develops recommendations and guidelines for prevention of workplace injuries and illnesses, has sponsored numerous studies on workplace factors such as noise, lighting, and temperature. One factor that has been investigated extensively in the work-place settings is noise. Not only has noise been shown to affect productivity at work by causing distractions and increasing errors (Evans & Johnson, 2000), but exposure to noise, both high levels and prolonged duration, has been linked with permanent hearing loss and chronic stress (Morata, Byrne, & Rabinowitz, 2011; Szalma & Hancock, 2011). Another element of the workplace that has been studied considerably in the field of industrial and occupational health is lighting. In fact, high intensity, poor distribution, glare, and artificial sources of light have been correlated with decreased employee job satisfaction, lower productivity, poor vision and increased workplace injuries (Anshel, 2006; Juslen, Wouters, & Tenner, 2007; Schultz & Schultz, 2010). Temperature is another work-place factor that has been broadly studied by occupational health researchers. In a poll asking office employees about their physical work conditions, the top two complaints were that it was either too cold or too hot (Schultz & Schultz, 2010). While some studies have evaluated the effects of moderate changes within the workplace on job satisfaction and morale (Lan, Lian, & Pan, 2010), others have focused on the negative health effects associated with prolonged exposure to extreme temperature conditions (Bortkiewicz et al., 2006; Kovats & Hajat, 2008).

Exposure to hazardous substances is another factor within the workplace that is considered to be stressful to employees. For example, individuals who work in mining, textiles, industrial chemicals, and oil refinery are often exposed to chemicals linked with various lung cancers and other terminal diseases. Medical technicians and power plant workers who are exposed to radiation are at increased risks of various cancers, including thyroid, lung and bone cancer (Schultz & Schultz, 2010). First responders are oftentimes exposed to harmful environmental conditions during rescue and recovery efforts and can experience injuries, respiratory illness, skin irritations, and the like (Centers for Disease Control and Prevention, 2002, 2006). The Occupational Safety and Health Act (OSHA) was passed in 1970 to enforce federal standards ensuring that preventative safety measures are in place to reduce and eliminate the likelihood of diseases and accidents in the workplace. Mandatory provision of personal protective equipment to employees has greatly reduced the incidence of hazardous exposure (Howie, 2008), but other factors also play a role in worker safety.

Scheduling Factors

A substantial amount of research has been conducted on productivity, safety, and satisfaction of employees whose work schedules fall out of the typical 9-to-5 days. Occupational health researchers have evaluated the extent to which changes in traditional work schedules not only affects stress and health outcomes for the employee but also relates to changes in productivity and injuries on the job. The Fair Labor Standards Act was passed in 1938 (US Department of Labor) which established the 5-day, 40 h-per-week work schedule for all employees. However, alternative schedules have become more prominent in recent years. Part-time work, for example, has been correlated with reduced stress and burnout in higher-stress professions. Other variations to traditional scheduling, such as a 4-day workweek, telecommuting and flexible work schedules, have also been linked with improved productivity and job satisfaction (Schultz & Schultz, 2010).

On the other hand, research on shift work has been shown to have negative effects on health and productivity (this topic will be discussed in greater detail in another chapter of the handbook). The disruption of the circadian rhythm for shift workers is directly linked to changes in physiological functions, such as body temperature, heart rate, and blood pressure (Sulsky & Smith, 2005). In fact, gastrointestinal disorders, specifically gastric ulcers, are more prevalent in night-time and rotating shift workers as compared to those with traditional daytime schedules (Costa, 1996). Shift workers are also more likely to gain weight and be obese, putting them at risk for cardiovascular disease and diabetes (Antunes, Levandovski, Dantas, Caumo, & Hidalgo, 2010). Furthermore, shift work can have detrimental consequences, for both the worker and the organization. Shift workers report greater levels of stress, including less autonomy and more work conflicts as compared to employees with traditional work schedules (Parkes, 2003). Likewise, employees with night work schedules commonly report conflict in their personal lives, such that the decreased interactions with spouses and children cause excess stress for family members (Jackson, Zedeck, & Summers, 1985). In fact, Tepas, Armstron, Carlson, and Duchon (1985) reported that shift workers are 50 % more likely to divorce than workers with traditional schedules.

Research on performance for employees who work nights or rotating shifts has also shown that there is an increase in errors and accidents, particularly during late night and early morning hours (Folkard, 1990). Factors that contribute to these errors and accidents include not only general sleep deprivation, but also arise from the type of work being done. For example, employees who monitor equipment, such as air traffic controllers and power plant personnel, are more likely to fall asleep on the job as compared to employees whose tasks are more active (Folkard, 1990). It is through the work of occupational health researchers that these work-place factors are identified and the appropriate interventions are developed, such as alternative schedules and rotating shifts. Effective interventions can reduce the likelihood of injuries and lost productivity for the organization while promoting better health outcomes for the employees.

Ergonomics and Occupational Injuries

Research on ergonomic design within the workplace has identified factors related to physical strain and stress on the employee for which better workplace designs and equipment have been developed. A subset of Occupational Health Psychology, known as Engineering Psychology, focuses on ergonomics and how physical stressors can lead to reduced productivity and the development of serious health conditions. For hundreds of years, ergonomics were never a consideration, as long as workers performing manual labor were easily replaced if injured. Not until the early 1900s was there an interest in the biomechanics in the occupational setting; yet, during this time, productivity, as opposed to human safety, was the main interest. Frederick Winslow Taylor, a mechanical engineer in the late 1800s, helped to transform this point of view from employing "disposable" workers to recognizing how improving working conditions could actually improve productivity (Kanigel, 1997). Taylor's initiative, termed *industrial efficiency*, put forth recommendations specifically for managers to supervise and organize production processes, to train workers to execute functions more systematically, to allow for routine breaks to avoid excessive fatigue and reduced productivity, and to supply the appropriate equipment necessary for optimal performance. This was the first of its kind to address concerns of biomechanics within the industry setting. This positive contribution was from the same person (Taylor) referenced earlier in the chapter, who also had a negative impact on the field by advocating industrial efficiency at the expense of workers. Thus, his contributions were both positive and negative, with the negative greatly outweighing the positive.

One of the most noted contributors to biomechanics and ergonomics was Lillian Gilbreth, who further developed a classification system of motions in skilled labor settings. Like F.W. Taylor, Gilbreth studied motions and timing of movements associated with skilled labor. The focus was on improving performance time by changing aspects of certain jobs to limit musculoskeletal stress. Since the 1970s, the view of occupational injuries has changed. In response to the high prevalence rates and escalating costs associated with occupational injuries, workplace interventions geared at ergonomics and employee safety have taken precedence. In many larger corporations, teams of engineers, health and safety experts, and experienced workers are created to develop comprehensive evaluations of workplace ergonomics (Chaffin, 2009).

According to the Bureau of Labor Statistics, there were approximately 4,500 workplace fatalities and approximately 3.3 million nonfatal workplace injuries reported in 2009 (Bureau of Labor and Statistics, 2010). Occupational health psychologists have conducted extensive research on risk factors for workplace injuries and have designed preventative measures to reduce the likelihood of accidents occurring. Occupational injuries are thought to be caused by several factors, such as physical biomechanics, ergonomics, and psychosocial and cognitive constituents (Boocock et al., 2007; Schachter, Busch, & Peloso, 2003; Waling, Javholm, & Sundelin, 2002). Developing preventions for occupational musculoskeletal injuries can be a difficult task considering individual differences and the influence of psychosocial factors. Many of the factors considered as risk factors for occupational injuries include the type of industry, hours of work, lighting, temperature, equipment design, safety devices, and work pressure. Furthermore, personal factors such as cognitive ability, physiological and psychological fatigue, general health, work experience, job involvement, and job insecurity have been evaluated as contributors to the incidence of accidents in the workplace. Furthermore, occupational health psychologists have also evaluated the extent to which the individuals' personality characteristics can contribute to workplace injuries (Salminen, 2010; Schultz & Schultz, 2010; Vanroelen, Levecque, Moors, Gadeyne, & Louckx, 2009; Villanueva & Garcia, 2011; Wallace & Chen, 2005).

Psychology Factors

Occupational health researchers have also identified numerous psychosocial factors that are related to increased stress, which correlate with reduced productivity, increased absenteeism, and greater likelihood of turnover. Many of these factors are related to the job itself, including such issues as role conflict, role ambiguity, supervisor and social support, and perceived equity among colleagues. Other factors are of a personal nature, such as work-life balance and family issues. The following section provides an overview of a few of the commonly assessed psychosocial factors, both work-related and personal, that occupational health researchers have identified as potential stressors for employees.

Job-Related Psychosocial Stressors

Research has shown that a major contributor to low job satisfaction is job-related stress, and low job satisfaction is directly correlated with poor occupational outcomes, such as increased absenteeism, low organizational commitment, and turnover (Petterson & Arnetz, 1997). Therefore, by identifying the psychosocial job-related factors that are deemed highly stressful, occupational health psychologists can put forth intervention strategies aimed at training management to recognize and actively work to eliminate common work-place psychosocial stressors.

Work-role demands describe both the formal responsibilities of the job along with the informal responsibilities. Oftentimes, stress occurs when the employee encounters discord within the work-role demands. Role conflict, a leading work-place stressor, describes situations for which the employee is faced with contradicting demands. For example, an employee may be asked to increase productivity while simultaneously cutting resources, or an employee may be given conflicting directives by two different supervisors. Another example of role conflict is when an employee's job requirements violate his or her own personal ethics. In such situations, employees have a greater likelihood of experiencing stress (Sulsky & Smith, 2005). Ambiguity is another work-role demand issue that can cause stress. Workers without clear descriptions of their roles often experience role ambiguity. Task ambiguity occurs when an employee is not given the appropriate training or tools to fulfill his or her responsibilities (Sulsky & Smith, 2005). Furthermore, both work overload, which is described as having too many job demands, and work underload, for which the employee has too few responsibilities, have been linked to occupational stress and poor health outcomes (Dewa, Thompson, & Jacobs, 2011; Lindfors, Berntsson, & Lundberg, 2006; Shultz, Wang, & Olson, 2010). More recently, research has shown how employees who manage others experience high levels of stress. Being responsible for other individuals can create a great amount of stress and anxiety for not only managers but also for teachers, health care workers, law enforcement, etc. (Sulsky & Smith, 2005).

Another workplace factor that has been linked to stress relates to organizational change, which can lead to downsizing and job loss. Research has shown that job insecurity is a major stressor for employees. More recent studies have focused on how organizational survivors, that is, those who did not lose their jobs during a time of organizational change, still exhibit high levels of stress and anxiety. One study showed that employees who had higher levels of control over their work before the layoffs found the reorganization to be more fair as compared to survivors who did not perceive high control (Davy, Kinicki, & Scheck, 1991). Other researchers have found that employee's levels of job commitment and job involvement were likely to decrease for survivors of downsizing (Allen, Freeman, Russell, Reizenstein, & Rentz, 2001).

External Stress-Related Factors

Occupational health researchers do not only limit their studies to the workplace itself but also investigate external factors that increase the likelihood of poor occupational outcomes. For example, many studies have shown that females are more likely to report higher levels of stress as compared to males (Schultz & Schultz, 2010). However, in a more thorough investigation, Galanakis, Stalikas, Kallia, Karagianni, and Karela (2009) found that when controlling for age, education level and marital status, males and females did not differ on levels of stress. The authors of this study suggest that one reason females tend to report higher levels of stress is because of other mediating factors related to holding multiple roles. Indeed, work-life balance is a factor that has been studied more recently and findings have shown that having poor work–family balance is linked not only to increased stress and poor health but also with reduced work productivity increased absenteeism and general job dissatisfaction (Schultz & Schultz, 2010). In a recent longitudinal study, Kinnunen, Feldt, Mauno, and Rantanen (2010) examined the effects of how work influences family conflict and how family influences work conflict. In this study, high family interference in work conflict was shown to have long-term effects, such that there was both a decrease in job satisfaction and an increase in work influence in family conflict. Additionally, crossover effects were also identified, such that when one partner experienced a stress or psychological strain, it was shown to have an effect on the other partner. Another study demonstrated that there is a bidirectional, or reciprocal, effect such that work–family conflict can increase burnout and that burnout can increase work–family conflict (Innstrand, Langballe, Espnes, Falkum, & Aasland, 2008).

Occupational health researchers have focused on factors that lead to burnout. Several factors that have been identified include emotional exhaustion, depersonalization and inefficacy (Maslach, Schaufeli, & Leiter, 2008), high levels of time pressure, role conflict, role ambiguity and reduced social support (Schultz & Schultz, 2010), and high work–family conflict and low job satisfaction (Thompson, Brough, & Schmidt, 2006). Burnout affects individuals both physically and psychologically, and has important reciprocal relationships with family roles affecting home and family life (Innstrand et al., 2008). It is important to recognize the symptoms of burnout so that both the organization and the individual can take proactive steps to reduce the stressors.

Summary

It is widely recognized that workplace stress not only affects occupational outcomes, such as reduction in productivity, lower job satisfaction, and increased absenteeism and turnover, but workplace stress is also linked to poor health outcomes. Occupational health researchers are interested in not only identifying these stressors and determining the various individual risk factors for experiencing poor consequences because of these stressors, but are also interested in developing prevention and intervention strategies for reducing the occurrence of these stressors. Some of these stressors are specific to the workplace environment. Such examples include the physical characteristics of the workplace, such as noise, lighting, temperature, and even dangerous job demands. Other stressors include factors inherent to the work itself, such as scheduling, leadership, and work-role factors. External stressors, such as work–family balance, can also contribute to poor health and work productivity.

Many organizations offer some type of stress-management program to help employees experiencing stressors that affect both their job and their health. From an organizational perspective, providing opportunities for control, reducing role conflict, ambiguity and overload, along with providing social support are ways that the employer can help their employees reduce the likelihood of being stressed and experiencing the negative physical and psychological effects of stress.

Theoretical Models of Work Stress

In addition to understanding the nature of work and work-related stressors, occupational health psychologists work to understand the theoretical underpinnings of perceived stress. From a theoretical perspective, it is imperative to understand why certain situations are perceived as stressors, what types of stressors cause stress (or strain) and, with this knowledge, what recommendations can be made that will help organizations reduce the amounts of perceived stress within their workforce? For example, some of psychosocial stressors mentioned in the previous section of this chapter, such as work-role demands, demand–control conflict, and reduced social support were more thoroughly understood through theoretical models such as *Person-Organization Fit* (Edwards & Cooper, 1990; Kahn et al., 1964; Lofquist & Dawis, 1969), *Stress-at-Work* (Cooper & Marshall, 1976; Marshall & Cooper, 1979), *Demand–Control* (Karasek, 1997), Effort–Reward (Siegrist, 1996), and *Organizational Justice* (Greenberg, 2004). Notably, most occupational health-related theories are grounded in one of the most accepted and widely utilized stress models, the *Cognitive Appraisal Model* developed by Lazarus and Folkman (1984). After a review of the Cognitive Appraisal Model, the following sections will highlight each of these theoretical models with regard to work stress (see Table 3.1).

Cognitive Appraisal Model

The Cognitive Appraisal Model suggests that demands are processed through two separate, but equally important, appraisals. The primary appraisal distinguishes a stimulus as being irrelevant, benign-positive, or stressful. Intuitively, an irrelevant stimulus is determined to be outside of the realm of importance for the appraiser, whereas a benign-positive demand is assumed to benefit the well-being of the individual. Stress appraisals are slightly more complicated as they include appraisals of potential losses, harmful events, threats, or challenges.

In the primary stress appraisal, a demand is considered to be a threat if it is indicative of imminent harm or loss (Lazarus & Folkman, 1984). Furthermore, an appraisal of a threat also indicates there is

Table 3.1 Summary of the major theoretical models of work stress

Theory	Brief description
Cognitive appraisal model (Lazarus & Folkman, 1984)	Stress is the result of the interaction between the person and his/her environment. Events that are appraised as a threat, harm/loss, or challenge during primary appraisal are deemed stressors. Secondary appraisal then involves the assessment of one's coping resources. Reappraisal occurs constantly as people choose coping strategies to eliminate or adapt to the event. Stress responses involve emotional, cognitive, behavioral, and physiological reactions
Person–environment fit (Van Harrison, 1978)	Discrepancies between a worker's capacities and the demands of the work environment produce stress. Dimensions of person–environment fit include person–occupation fit, person–group fit, person–job fit, and person–organization fit
Demand–control (Theorell & Karasek, 1996)	Job stress is the product of the quality and quantity of the job demands and the worker's ability to control the work environment and amount of decision latitude
Effort–reward (Siegrist, 1996)	Builds on the Demand–Control Model by adding the concept of status control. Concerns about status control may be more stressful than low task-related control especially if demands are high
Organizational justice (Greenberg, 2004)	Based on the cognitive appraisal model, stress is the product of perceived injustice in the workplace that consists of four dimensions: distributive justice, procedural justice, interpersonal justice, and informational justice

some room for adaptation or preemptive coping to take place in preparation of the looming harm or loss. A challenge appraisal is similar in anticipatory nature; however, a challenge appraisal is more optimistic with regard to implications. Challenges are typically characterized by positive expectations and excitement about the demand outcomes. It is important to note that both challenges and threat appraisals can happen simultaneously and they are not considered to be polar opposites. Once a demand is appraised to be a challenge or threat, the secondary appraisal of an individual's resources and coping capabilities becomes salient (Lazarus & Folkman, 1984). A thorough evaluation of coping capabilities at this stage includes both the expectation that one encompasses the required coping option (i.e., efficacy expectation), and the expectation that it will work to diminish the threat (i.e., outcome expectation, Bandura, 1977, 1982). After people are given the opportunity to assess the potential impact an event may have, given the extent of the demand and their abilities to overcome it, they respond in a manner indicative of their evaluation (Greenberg, 2004). Stress responses are comprised of emotional, biochemical, physiological, cognitive, and behavioral changes aimed at reducing or adapting to a stressful event and its effects (Baum, 1990). Many researchers have relied upon Lazarus and Folkman's cognitive appraisal model to explain sources of work-related stress.

Person–Environment Fit

Perhaps one of the most salient characteristics of stress involves individuals' evaluation of their own capabilities (Lazarus & Launier, 1978; Vermunt & Steensma, 2005). Often described in terms of person–environment fit, the interaction between an individual's capabilities with the demands of a situation can lead to perceived stress (Kahn, 1970; Lewin, 1938). The misfit between the demands of the environment and the resources of the individual is typically determined by the individual's appraisal of his/her own internal and external resources (Lazarus & Launier, 1978). To the extent there is a discrepancy between a person's capacities and the demands or challenges of the environment, the situation is deemed a stressor (Kahn, 1970; Lazarus & Launier, 1978; Lewin, 1938). Researchers and practitioners are more readily evaluating person–environment fit with a contextual framework by considering components such as organizational conditions (e.g., culture, technology, industry), as well as environmental conditions (e.g., legal requirements, labor markets, economy; Russell, 2001; Van Harrison, 1978). In fact, person–environment fit has been broken down into four distinct fit indices including: person–occupation fit (evaluates industry and vocation; Holland, 1959), person–group fit (evaluates coworkers and peer groups; Higgins & Sekiguchi, 2006; Kristof, 1996), person–job fit (evaluates job demands; Dawis, 1992; Edwards, 1991), and person–organization fit (evaluates company climate and values; Kristof, 1996). Further, some researchers go as far as to use two frameworks to evaluate person–environment fit: the demand-abilities fit and the needs-supply fit (Cable & Judge, 1994; Kristof, 1996; Sekiguchi, 2004a, 2004b). Recent research has demonstrated that these multiple dimensions of fit can have independent effects on job satisfaction, commitment, and intention to leave (Edwards & Billsberry, 2010). Therefore, the multidimensional nature of person–environmental fit should be routinely taken into consideration when examining work-related stress.

Demand–Control

The Demand–Control Model, another framework used to describe job stress, points to the amount of decision latitude an employee has, relative to the demands being placed on them in their job role (Karasek & Theorell, 1990). In this model, the term job demands refers to the mental workload, including interpersonal interactions, qualitative demands, and quantitative demands, rather than any physical demands included in the role. Control refers to the ability to influence others in order to reduce threats, which is particularly useful as a coping mechanism in reference to the Cognitive Appraisal Model (Ganster, 1989; Lazarus & Launier, 1978). Autonomy, a sub-factor of control, refers to the amount of decision latitude that includes the authority to make decisions about work schedules and methods, and also having the possibility to utilize skills and develop other skills as needed (Connell, Lee, & Spector, 2004). The additional component of decision latitude to job demands allowed this model to be one of the first to view the risk of psychosocial stressors on nonexecutive populations, particularly the working class (Theorell & Karasek, 1996). Using the Demand–Control Model as a framework, these authors demonstrated that the combination of a highly psychologically demanding job, with low control or decision latitude, is a health risk factor that has been linked to cardiovascular disease (Theorell & Karasek, 1996). Additionally, further research has demonstrated that limited decision latitude (low control) can also be a risk factor for distress in and of itself (Hemingway & Marmot, 1999).

Effort–Reward

The Effort–Reward Model, proposed by Siegrist (1996), was developed to reflect the stress that is perceived due to an imbalance of high efforts and low rewards. Built upon the premise of equity and reciprocity, societal norms regarding social exchange suggest that efforts should be matched with a fair reward of some type (e.g., money, esteem, status control, etc.). Often referred to as costs (effort) and gains (reward), the Effort–Reward Model posits that an imbalance between these two constructs indicates a lack of reciprocity, which triggers the response of emotional distress.

The Effort–Reward Model was not suggested to replace the Demand–Control Model (Karasek, 1979; Karasek & Theorell, 1990), but it was proposed to explain observed differences that the Demand–Control Model could not. For instance, the Effort–Reward Model introduces the term *status control* to operationalize the need for self-regulation in terms of self-esteem, efficacy, and sense of mastery or accomplishment (Siegrist, 1996). As Siegrist explains, occupational position serves as a social role for most people; therefore, a threat to that role would likely produce emotional distress. In that sense, any indication of job insecurity would indicate low status control.

The Effort–Reward Model differs from the Demand–Control Model in that the costs of adapting to a lack of control that is task-related is less than the costs of adapting to a lack of status control (Siegrist, 1996). As such, Siegrist argues that, particularly due to the changing nature of work through globalization and technology, concerns about status control (i.e., threats of job termination or lack of promotional opportunities) may override low task-related control, particularly if high efforts are exerted.

Organizational Justice

Organizational justice, one of the most widely studied areas with regard to job-related stress, is still relatively new. Despite its novelty in the field, there is sufficient evidence that is indicative of the consistent and compelling dynamic between injustice and stress (Greenberg, 2010). Justice was first conceived by Adams (1965) who investigated negative responses (i.e., psychological distress) to inequitable rewards (i.e., perceived unfair decisions). In his study, Adams measured the psychological distress in terms of behavioral reactions, such as a reduction in effort, rationalizing that the participant reduced the inputs to balance out the effort to output ratio. Outcome fairness, appropriately labeled distributive justice, was expanded to include allocation rules such as equity and need (Leventhal, 1976). In 1980, Leventhal introduced the importance of procedural justice, described as the fairness of the procedures that determine outcomes (Leventhal, Karuza, & Fry, 1980). Almost a decade later, a third justice variable was introduced by Bies and Moag (1986). They coined the term *interactional justice* and defined it as the interpersonal treatment people receive in organizations, qualified by the distributive and procedural justice within the organization. Recently, interactional justice has separated into two further dimensions labeled *interpersonal justice* and *informational justice*. Interpersonal justice refers to the interactional factors related to distributive justice, whereas informational justice encompasses the interactional factors related to procedural justice (Colquitt, Conlon, Wesson, Porter, & Ng, 2001; Greenberg, 1993).

Firmly grounded within the Cognitive Appraisal Model, Greenberg (2004) proposed a theory entitled the *Justice Salience Hierarchy* (JSH), in which the organizational justice variables act as the events for which the cognitive appraisals of harm/loss, threat, or challenge occur. Greenberg suggested that people evaluate their outcomes (i.e., distributive justice) through their fairness appraisals of the processes that designate those outcomes (i.e., procedural justice). Studies depicting this interaction reported lower levels of stress, exhaustion, anxiety, and depression in those that experienced negative outcomes followed by fair procedures than those that the negative outcomes were followed by unfair procedures (e.g., Janssen, 2004; Tepper, 2000, 2001).

The secondary appraisal within the JSH then points to the moderating effects of interactional justice (Greenberg, 2004). In his theoretical paper, Greenberg suggested that the interpersonal nature of this third justice variable could either increase or diminish the perceived stress, thus resulting in an interaction. In totality, the JSH proposes that an outcome (i.e., distributive justice) is first evaluated as a threat to the extent that the procedures determining the outcome (i.e., procedural justice) are unfair and secondly assessed to the extent that the interpersonal treatment surrounding the event (i.e., interactional justice) is unjust (Greenberg, 2004). To our knowledge, the only study to directly test both the primary and secondary appraisal levels of the JSH was conducted on a cross-sectional sample of working college students (Graham, Lopez, & Dougall, 2008). In their study, informational justice, a component of interactional justice moderated the negative relationships of both the distributive and procedural justice and stress. The negative associations increased when informational injustice was present; however, it was less intense when participants perceived informational justice from their supervisors.

Summary

A number of theories have been developed to conceptualize the experience of work-related stress. Most of these theories have evolved from Lazarus and Folkman's (1984) theory of stress, appraisal, and coping and include important modifiers of stress, such as person–environment fit, work demand, perceived control, balance of effort and reward, and employees' appraisals of justice in the work place. Theories on work stress will continue to develop as researchers work to identify important risk and resiliency factors in occupational stress and health. These theories are also the guiding principles for preventative stress management interventions designed to decrease worker stress and promote well-being.

Preventative Stress Management

Adverse psychosocial stressors can be as serious as other health risks; however, they are also the least understood, likely due to their hidden and indirect nature (Everson-Rose & Lewis, 2004). In that regard, it is important that both organizations and researchers investigate the depth of this relationship for both humanitarian and economic reasons. In other words, organizations should strive to reduce the levels of perceived stress among their workforce simply because they care about their employees, but also to realize the economic returns of stress reduction through fewer counter-productive behaviors, lower rates of absenteeism, and increased commitment and productivity. In fact, studies have reported that workers with high stress levels were over two times more likely to be absent 5 or more days a year (Jacobson, Aldana, Goetzel, & Vardell, 1996). Job stress is responsible for an estimated cost of $10,000 per worker, which translates to $300 billion for the US economy. For our nation's top executives, outcomes linked directly to stress such as absence, illness, and early death, account for an estimated $10–20 billion annually (AIS, 2007).

Preventative stress management, one of the leading models of stress management within the business world, may be helpful if applied through an organizational justice framework. Preventative stress management purports that, if job stress is truly an epidemic, then prevention is the best policy for addressing the issue at hand (Elkin & Rosch, 1990; Quick, Quick, Nelson, & Hurrell, 1997). The guiding principle behind preventative stress management involves interpreting the public health notions of prevention through an organizational framework (Quick, Quick, & Nelson, 1998). Within the preventative stress management framework, there are three key points of intervention, intuitively labeled the primary, secondary, and tertiary levels, respectively (see Fig. 3.1; Quick, Cooper, Nelson, Quick, & Gavin, 2003).

Primary prevention targets the front-line demands of the work environment to ensure that work demands are manageable for the employee. At this level, the goal is to address the cause of the problem before it becomes an issue. At this level of intervention, public health training, promotions, and campaigns are deployed in organizations for the entire population, regardless of those at risk or not (Tetrick & Quick, 2003).

The secondary level of prevention targets those that are suspected of being at risk of heightened stress. This level of intervention focuses more on managing the individual's responses to the demands placed on them (Quick & Quick, 1997; Quick, Simmons, & Nelson, 2000). At this level, the demands are held constant, but the intervention comes about in helping individuals' cope with and manages the stress they may feel. Typically, this level includes stress reduction techniques that help employees

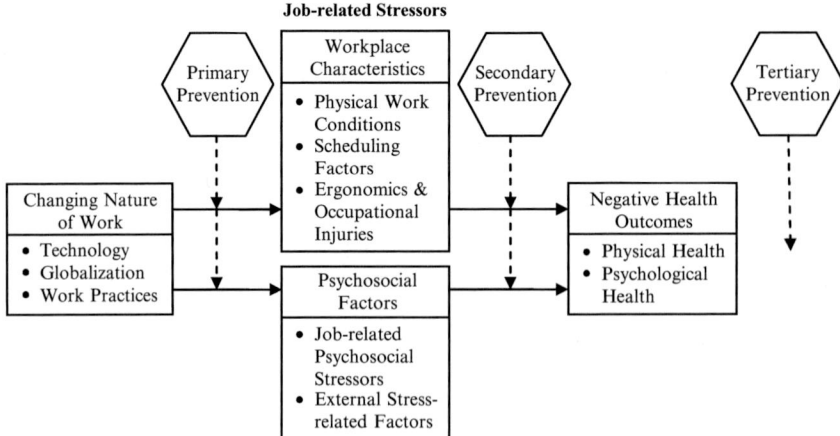

Fig. 3.1 Conceptual model of the application of primary, secondary, and tertiary prevention interventions to prevent or alleviate work-related stress and its negative health outcomes

manage their potentially adverse reactions prior to the escalation of the stress response. Likewise, this level of prevention can also be conducted with either groups or individuals.

The final, tertiary level of prevention targets individuals who have shown signs of degenerative health due to stress (Quick et al., 2003). This level of intervention is primarily therapeutic through either a psychosocial or medicinal approach. Notably, the primary and secondary levels of prevention fit well within occupational health psychology as they are best approached from a multidisciplinary framework; however, the tertiary level of prevention is often delegated to clinical, counseling, or rehabilitative psychology (Tetrick & Quick, 2003).

Conclusions

Occupational health psychology has made great strides in the past 100 years. Employees are no longer perceived as emotionless, mechanistic workers whose sole purpose is to increase organizational productivity. The field now acknowledges that productivity is most effectively maximized by enabling happy and healthy workers. The focus is now on increasing both worker and organizational health in today's changing work environments. Many researchers and organizational health psychology organizations across the World have identified important risk and resilience factors for predicting employees' physical, mental, and social well-being. Most of these factors can be linked to the experience of stress in the work place. Theories of work-related stress have emerged that help to conceptualize the process and suggest targets for interventions aimed at reducing stress and its adverse health effects. The field of occupational health psychology has made amazing contributions to occupational health, but it is still growing. It will be exciting to see what new developments occur in the next 100 years as the nature of work continues to change with continued advancements in technology and globalization.

Future Directions

Research in occupational health psychology has led to improvements in most employees' work conditions. However, there is limited dissemination of many effective occupational health interventions, including stress management. Some countries like Sweden and those in the European Union have or are developing legislation to promote employee participation in decisions related to their jobs and performance. In the USA, NIOSH makes similar recommendations, but there are no laws in place. Public health policy changes aimed at creating legislation can be further supported with continued research by occupational health psychologists. Additionally, even when employees have access to interventions, they may not follow the appropriate procedures, thereby decreasing the effectiveness of the interventions or eschewing the intervention efforts altogether. For example, many employees in the USA work in environments with hazardous noise exposure, yet some employees do not wear the personal protective equipment that is provided to prevent hearing loss (Tak, Davis, & Calvert, 2009). Clearly, research efforts need to focus on teaching organizations about the effectiveness of existing occupational health programs and creating feasible interventions that can be easily disseminated, possibly through the creation of wellness centers and programs. After organizations adopt appropriate interventions, organizational health psychologists need to devise ways to educate employees and increase their use of such interventions.

Additionally, new priority areas in occupational health are regularly identified by national organizations. In the USA, the National Occupational Research Agenda was developed in 1996 to identify high priority research needs and to help provide a research framework for occupational health (Rosenstock, Olenec, & Wagner, 1998). These research priorities vary by the type of workforce sector, acknowledging the complexity and uniqueness of each type of job and the person–environment fit. Organizational health psychology teams are perfect for addressing these high priority needs. They bring interdisciplinary perspectives from a rich history of research that inspires innovative research designs to develop creative solutions.

Given the nature of the ever-changing work environment, new concerns and needs will continue to arise in occupational health, as well as those current needs that researchers are only beginning to understand. Some of these emerging needs are discussed in later chapters of this handbook and include work-place bullying (Chap. 11), presenteeism (Chap. 8), workforce diversity (Chap. 24), the reciprocal nature of work and family conflicts (Chap. 15), among others. Of prime importance, researchers need to more fully explore the bidirectional relationships between organizational health and employee health, promoting well-being in both dimensions simultaneously.

References

Adams, J. S. (1965). Inequity in social exchange. In L. Berkowitz (Ed.), *Advances in experimental social psychology* (Vol. 2, pp. 267–299). New York, NY: Academic.
Allen, T. D., Freeman, D. M., Russell, J. E. A., Reizenstein, R. C., & Rentz, J. O. (2001). Survivor reactions to organizational downsizing: Does time ease the pain? *Journal of Occupational and Organizational Psychology, 74*, 145–164.
American Institute of Stress. (n.d.). *Job stress*. Retrieved October 10, 2007 from http://www.stress.org/job.htm
American Psychological Association (1996). *Journal of Occupational Health Psychology*. Washington DC: APA.
American Psychological Association. (2010). *Stress in America findings*. Retrieved from the American Psychological Association website. http://www.apa.org/news/press/releases/stress/national-report.pdf
Anshel, J. (2006). Visual ergonomics in the workplace: Improving eyecare and vision can enhance productivity. *Professional Safety, 51*(8), 20–25.
Antunes, L. C., Levandovski, R., Dantas, G., Caumo, W., & Hidalgo, M. P. (2010). Obesity and shift work: Chronobiological aspects. *Nutrition Research Reviews, 23*, 155–168.
Bandura, A. (1977). Self-efficacy: Toward a unifying theory of behavioral change. *Psychological Review, 84*, 191–215.
Bandura, A. (1982). The self mechanisms of agency. In J. Suls (Ed.), *Social psychological perspectives on the self* (pp. 3–39). Hillsdale, NJ: Lawrence Erlbaum.
Barling, J., & Griffiths, A. (2010). A history of occupational health psychology. In J. C. Quick & L. E. Tetrick (Eds.), *Handbook of occupational health psychology* (2nd ed., pp. 21–34). Washington, DC: APA Books.
Baum, A. (1990). Stress, intrusive imagery, and chronic distress. *Health Psychology, 9*(6), 653–675.
Bies, R. J., & Moag, J. F. (1986). Interactional justice: Communication criteria of fairness. In R. J. Lewicki, B. H. Sheppard, & M. H. Bazerman (Eds.), *Research on negotiations in organizations* (Vol. 1, pp. 43–55). Greenwich, CT: JAI Press.

Boocock, M. G., McNair, P. J., Larmer, P. J., Armstrong, B., Collier, J., Simmonds, M., et al. (2007). Interventions for the prevention and management of neck/upper extremity musculoskeletal conditions: A systematic review. *Occupational Environmental Medicine, 64*, 291–303.

Bortkiewicz, A., Gadzicka, E., Szymczak, W., Szyjkowska, A., Koszada-Wlodarczyk, W., & Makowiec-Dabrowska, T. (2006). Physiological reaction to work in cold microclimate. *International Journal of Occupational Medicine and Environmental Health, 19*(2), 123–131.

Brislin, R. W. (2008). *Working with cultural differences: Dealing effectively with diversity in the workplace*. Westport, CT: Praeger Publishers.

Bureau of Labor and Statistics. (2010). *Workplace injuries and illnesses report*. Publication no. http://www.bls.gov/iif/

Cable, D., & Judge, T. (1994). Pay preferences and job search decisions: A person–organization fit perspective. *Personnel Psychology, 47*, 317–348.

Centers for Disease Control and Prevention (CDC). (2002). Injuries and illnesses among New York City Fire Department rescue workers after responding to the World Trade Center attacks. *Morbidity and Mortality Weekly Report, 51*, 1–5.

Centers for Disease Control and Prevention (CDC). (2006). Health hazard evaluation of police officers and firefighters after Hurricane Katrina—New Orleans, Louisiana, October 27–28 and November 30–December 5, 2005. *Morbidity and Mortality Weekly Report, 55*, 456–458.

Chaffin, D. B. (2009). The evolving role of biomechanics in prevention of overexertion injuries. *Ergonomics, 52*(1), 3–14.

Colquitt, J. A., Conlon, D. E., Wesson, M. J., Porter, C. O., & Ng, K. Y. (2001). Justice at the millennium: A meta-analytic review of 25 years of organizational research. *Journal of Applied Psychology, 86*(3), 425–445.

Connell, P., Lee, V. B., & Spector, P. E. (2004). Job stress assessment methods. In J. C. Thomas (Vol. Ed.) and M. Hersen (Ed.), *Comprehensive handbook of psychological assessment: Industrial and organizational assessment* (Vol. 4, pp. 455–469). Hoboken, NJ: Wiley.

Cooper, C. L., & Marshall, J. (1976). Occupational sources of stress: A review of the literature relating to coronary heart disease and mental ill health. *Journal of Occupational Psychology, 49*(1), 11–28.

Costa, G. (1996). The impact of shift and night work on health. *Applied Ergonomics, 27*(1), 9–16.

Cox, T. (1978). *Stress*. London: Macmillan.

Cua, K. O., McKone, K. E., & Schroeder, R. G. (2001). Relationships between implementation of TQM, JIT, and TPM and manufacturing performance. *Journal of Operations Management, 19*(6), 675–694.

Davy, J. A., Kinicki, A. J., & Scheck, C. L. (1991). Developing and testing a model of survivor responses to layoffs. *Journal of Vocational Behavior, 38*, 302–317.

Dawis, R. (1992). Person–environment fit and job satisfaction. In C. Cranny, P. Smith, & E. Stone (Eds.), *Job satisfaction: How people feel about their jobs and how it affects their performance* (pp. 69–88). New York, NY: Lexington Books.

Dewa, C. S., Thompson, A. H., & Jacobs, P. (2011). Relationships between job stress and worker perceived responsibilities and job characteristics. *International Journal of Occupational Medicine and Environmental Medicine, 2*(1), 37–46.

Dougall, A. L., & Baum, A. (2012). Stress, health, and illness. In A. Baum, T. A. Revenson, & J. E. Singer (Eds.), *Handbook of health psychology* (2nd ed.). New York, NY: Taylor & Francis. (pp. 53–78)

Edwards, J. (1991). Person–job fit: A conceptual integration, literature review, and methodological critique. In N. C. Cooper & I. Robertson (Eds.), *International review of industrial/organizational psychology* (Vol. 6, pp. 282–327). London: Wiley.

Edwards, J., & Billsberry, J. (2010). Testing a multidimensional theory of person–environment fit. *Journal of Managerial Issues, 22*(4), 476–493.

Edwards, J. R., & Cooper, C. L. (1990). The person–environment fit approach to stress: Recurring problems and some suggested solutions. *Journal of Organizational Behavior, 11*(4), 293–307.

Elkin, A. J., & Rosch, P. J. (1990). Promoting mental health at the workplace: The prevention side of stress management. *Occupational Medicine, 5*(4), 739–754.

Engels, F. (1845/1987). *The condition of the working class in England*. London: Penguin Books.

Evans, G. W., & Johnson, D. (2000). Stress and open-office noise. *Journal of Applied Psychology, 85*, 779–783.

Everson-Rose, S. A., & Lewis, T. T. (2004). Psychosocial factors and cardiovascular diseases. *Annual Review of Public Health, 26*, 469–500.

Folkard, S. (1990). Circadian performance rhythms: Some practical and theoretical implications. *Philosophical Transactions of the Royal Society of London: Biological Sciences, 327*, 543–553.

French, J. R. P., Caplan, R. D., & Van Harrison, R. (1982). *The mechanisms of job stress and strain*. New York, NY: Wiley.

Gatchel, R. J., & Schultz, I. Z. (2012). *Handbook of occupational health and wellness*. New York: Springer Science.

Galanakis, M., Stalikas, A., Kallia, H., Karagianni, C., & Karela, C. (2009). Gender differences in experiencing occupational stress: The role of age, education and marital status. *Stress and Health, 25*, 397–404.

Ganster, D. C. (1989). Worker control and well-being: A review of research in the workplace. In S. L. Sauter, J. J. Hurrell, & C. L. Cooper (Eds.), *Job control and worker health* (pp. 3–24). New York, NY: Wiley.

Gardell, B. (1971). Alienation and mental health in the modern industrial environment. In L. Levi (Ed.), *Society, stress and disease* (Vol. 1, pp. 148–180). Oxford: Oxford University Press.

Gardell, B. (1977). Autonomy and participation at work. *Human Relations, 30*, 515–533.

Graham, H.E., Lopez, N., & Dougall, A. (2008). Organizational justice and stress: An investigation of the justice salience hierarchy using the four-factor model. Unpublished master's thesis, University of Texas at Arlington, Arlington, Texas.

Greenberg, J. (1993). The social side of fairness: Interpersonal and informational classes of organizational justice. In R. Cropanzano (Ed.), *Justice in the workplace: Approaching fairness in human resource management* (pp. 79–103). Hillsdale, NJ: Erlbaum.

Greenberg, J. (2004). Stress fairness to fare no stress: Managing workplace stress by promoting organizational justice. *Organizational Dynamics, 33*, 352–365.

Greenberg, J. (2010). Organizational injustice as a health risk. *Academy of Management, 4*, 205–243.

Hemingway, H., & Marmot, M. (1999). Psychosocial factors in the etiology and prognosis of coronary heart disease: Systematic review of prospective cohort studies. *British Medical Journal, 318*, 1460–1467.

Herzberg, F. (1966). Work and the nature of man. Cleveland: World Publishing Co.

Higgins, C., & Sekiguchi, T. (2006). To influence or adjust: A dynamic model of person–group fit. In C. Schriesheim & L. Neider (Eds.), *Power and influence in organizations: New empirical and theoretical perspectives* (pp. 129–154). Charlotte, NC: Information Age Publishing.

Hofmann, D. A., & Tetrick, L. E. (2003). *Health and safety in organizations: A multilevel perspective*. San Francisco, CA: Jossey-Bass.

Holland, J. L. (1959). A theory of vocational choice. *Journal of Counseling Psychology, 6*(1), 35–45.

Howie, R. M. (2008). Personal protective equipment. In K. Gardiner & J. M. Harrington (Eds.), *Occupational hygiene* (3rd ed.). Oxford: Blackwell Publishing Ltd.. doi:10.1002/9780470755075.ch31.

Innstrand, S. T., Langballe, E. M., Espnes, G. A., Falkum, E., & Aasland, O. G. (2008). Positive and negative work–family interaction and burnout: A longitudinal study of reciprocal relations. *Work & Stress, 22*(1), 1–15.

Jackson, S. E., Zedeck, S., & Summers, E. (1985). Family life disruptions: Effects of job-induced structural and emotional interference. *Academy of Management Journal, 28*, 574–586.

Jacobson, B. H., Aldana, S. G., Goetzel, R. Z., & Vardell, K. D. (1996). The relationship of perceived stress and self-reported illness-related absenteeism. *American Journal of Health Promotion, 11*, 54–61.

Janssen, O. (2004). How fairness perceptions make innovative behavior more or less stressful. *Journal of Organizational Behavior, 25*(2), 201–215.

Juslen, H. T., Wouters, M. C., & Tenner, A. D. (2007). Lighting level and productivity: A field study in the electronics industry. *Ergonomics, 50*(4), 615–624.

Kahn, R. L. (1970). Some propositions toward a reachable conceptualization of stress. In J. E. McGrath (Ed.), *Social and psychological factors in stress* (pp. 97–103). New York, NY: Holt, Rinehart, and Wilson.

Kahn, R. L., Wolfe, D. M., Quinn, R. P., Snoek, J. D., & Rosenthal, R. A. (1964). *Organizational stress: Studies in role conflict and ambiguity*. New York, NY: Wiley.

Kanigel, R. (1997). *The one best way—Frederick Winslow Taylor and the enigma of efficiency*. New York, NY: Viking.

Karasek, R. A., Jr. (1979). Job demands, job decision latitude, and mental strain: Implications for job redesign. *Administrative Science Quarterly, 24*(2), 285–308.

Karasek, R. (1997). Labor participation and work quality policy: Requirements for an alternative economic future. *Scandinavian Journal of Work, Environment & Health, 23*(Suppl. 4), 55–65.

Karasek, R., & Theorell, T. (1990). *Healthy work: Stress, productivity, and the reconstruction of working life*. New York, NY: Basic Books.

Katz, D., & Kahn, R. (1966). *Social psychology of organizations*. New York, NY: Wiley.

Kinnunen, U., Feldt, T., Mauno, S., & Rantanen, J. (2010). Interface between work and family: A longitudinal individual and crossover perspective. *Journal of Occupational and Organizational Psychology, 83*, 119–137.

Kovats, R. S., & Hajat, S. (2008). Heat stress and public health: A critical review. *Annual Review of Public Health, 29*(1), 41–55.

Kristof, A. (1996). Person–organization fit: An integrative review of its conceptualization, measurement, and implications. *Personnel Psychology, 49*, 1–49

Lan, L., Lian, Z., & Pan, L. (2010). The effects of air temperature on office workers' well-being, workload and productivity—Evaluated with subjective ratings. *Applied Ergonomics, 42*(1), 29–36.

Lavelle, J. J., Brockner, J., Konovsky, M. A., Price, K. H., Henley, A. B., Taneja, A., & Vishnu, V. (2009). Commitment, procedural fairness, and organizational citizenship behavior: A multifoci analysis. *Journal of Organizational Behavior, 30*, 337–357.

Lavelle, J. J., McMahan, G. C., & Harris, C. M. (2009). Fairness in human resource management, social exchange relationships, and citizenship behavior: Testing linkages of the target similarity model using nurses in the United States. *The International Journal of Human Resource Management, 20*, 2419–2434.

Lax, M. B., Grant, W. D., Manetti, F. A., & Klein, R. (1998). Recognizing occupational disease: Taking an effective occupational history. *American Family Physician, 58*, 935–944.

Lazarus, R. S. (1966). *Psychological stress and the coping process*. New York, NY: McGraw-Hill.

Lazarus, R. S., & Folkman, S. (1984). *Stress, appraisal, and coping*. New York, NY: Springer.

Lazarus, R., & Launier, R. (1978). Stress-related transactions between person and environment. In L. Pervin & M. Lewis (Eds.), *Perspectives in interactional psychology* (pp. 287–327). New York, NY: Plenum.

Leventhal, G. S. (1976). The distribution of rewards and resources in groups and organizations. In L. Berkowitz & W. Walster (Eds.), *Advances in experimental social psychology* (Vol. 9, pp. 91–131). New York, NY: Academic.

Leventhal, G. S., Karuza, J., & Fry, W. R. (1980). Beyond fairness: A theory of allocation preferences. In G. Mikula (Ed.), *Justice and social interaction* (pp. 167–218). New York, NY: Springer.

Levi, L. (2011). Towards a Europe of health: Perspectives for future health policies [Editorial]. *The European Journal of Psychiatry, 25*(1), 5–7.

Lewin, K. (1938). *The conceptual representation and measurement of psychological forces*. Durham, NC: Duke University Press.

Lindfors, P., Berntsson, L., & Lundberg, U. (2006). Total workload as related to psychological well-being and symptoms in full-time employed female and male white-collar workers. *International Journal of Behavioral Medicine, 13*(2), 131–137.

Lofquist, L. H., & Dawis, R. V. (1969). *Adjustment to work: A psychological view of man's problems in a work-oriented society*. New York, NY: Appleton-Century-Crofts.

Macik-Frey, M., Quick, J. C., & Nelson, D. L. (2007). Advances in occupational health: From a stressful beginning to a positive future. *Journal of Management, 33*(6), 809–840.

Maclean, L. M., Plotnikoff, R. C., & Moyer, A. (2000). Transdisciplinary work with psychology from a population health perspective: An illustration. *Journal of Health Psychology, 5*(2), 173–181.

Marshall, J., & Cooper, C. L. (1979). *Executives under pressure: A psychological study*. London: MacMillan.

Marx, K. (1967/1845). The German ideology. In L. D. Easton, & K. H. L. Guddat (Eds. and Trans.), *Writings of the young Marx on philosophy and society*. Garden City, NY: Doubleday.

Maslach, C., Schaufeli, W., & Leiter, M. (2008). Job burnout. *Annual Review of Psychology, 52*, 397–422.

Maslow, A. H. (1943). A theory of human motivation. *Psychological Review, 50*, 370–396.

Mayo, E. (1933). *The human problems of an industrial civilization*. New York, NY: MacMillan.

Morata, T. C., Byrne, D. C., & Rabinowitz, P. M. (2011). *Noise exposure and hearing disorders* (6th ed.). New York, NY: Oxford University Press.

National Institute for Occupational Safety and Health. (n.d.). *Stress...at work*. Retrieved October 10, 2007 from http://www.cdc.gov/niosh/docs/99-101/

Parkes, K. (2003). Shiftwork and environment as interactive predictors of work perceptions. *Journal of Occupational Health Psychology, 8*(4), 266–281.

Petterson, I., & Arnetz, B. (1997). Measuring psychosocial work quality and health: Development of health care measures of measurement. Journal of Occupational Health Psychology, 2, 229–241.

Quick, J. C., Cooper, C. L., Nelson, D. L., Quick, J. D., & Gavin, J. H. (2003). Stress, health, and well-being at work. In J. Greenberg (Ed.), *Organizational behavior: The state of the science* (2nd ed.). Mahwah, NJ: Lawrence Erlbaum Associates Publishers.

Quick, J. C., & Quick, J. D. (1997). Stress management programs. In L. H. Peters, S. A. Youngblood, & C. R. Greer (Eds.), *The Blackwell encyclopedia of human resource management* (pp. 338–339). Oxford: Basil Blackwell Ltd.

Quick, J. D., Quick, J. C., & Nelson, D. L. (1998). The theory of preventive stress management in organizations. In C. L. Cooper (Ed.), *Theories of organizational stress* (pp. 246–268). Cambridge: Oxford University Press.

Quick, J. C., Quick, J. D., Nelson, D. L., & Hurrell, J. J., Jr. (1997). *Preventative stress management in organizations*. Washington, DC: American Psychological Association.

Quick, J. C., Simmons, B., & Nelson, D. L. (2000). Work conditions. In A. Kazdin (Ed.), *Encyclopedia of psychology* (Vol. 8, pp. 269–274). Washington, DC: American Psychological Association and Oxford University Press.

Quick, J. C., & Tetrick, L. E. (2003). *Handbook of occupational health psychology*. Washington, DC: American Psychological Association.

Quick, J. C., & Tetrick, L. E. (2010). *Handbook of occupational health psychology* (2nd ed.). Washington, DC: American Psychological Association.

Roethlisberger, F., & Dickson, W. J. (1939). *Management and the worker*. Cambridge, MA: Harvard University Press.

Rosch, P. J. (2001). The quandary of job stress compensation. *Health and Stress, 3*, 1–4.

Rosenstock, L., Olenec, C., & Wagner, G. R. (1998). The National Occupational Research Agenda: A model of broad stakeholder input into priority setting. *American Journal of Public Health, 88*, 353–356.

Russell, C. J. (2001). A longitudinal study of top-level executive performance. *Journal of Applied Psychology, 86*(4), 560–573.

Salminen, S. (2010). Shift work and extended working hours as risk factors for occupational injury. *Ergonomics Open Journal, 3*, 14–18.

Sauter, S. L., Murphy, L. R., & Hurrell, J. (1990). Prevention of work-related psychological disorders: A national strategy proposed by the National Institute for Occupational Safety and Health (NIOSH). *American Psychologist, 45*(10), 1146–1158.

Schachter, C. L., Busch, A. J., & Peloso, P. M. (2003). Effects of short versus long bouts of aerobic exercise in sedentary women with fibromyalgia: A randomized controlled trial. *Physical Therapy, 83*, 340–358.

Schaufeli, W. B. (2004). The future of occupational health psychology. *Applied Psychology, 53*(4), 502–517.

Schultz, D., & Schultz, S. E. (2010). *Psychology and work today* (10th ed.). Englewood Cliffs, NJ: Prentice Hall.

Sekiguchi, T. (2004a). Person–organization fit and person–job fit in employee selection: A review of the literature. *Osaka Keidai Ronshu, 54*, 179–196.

Sekiguchi, T. (2004b). Toward a dynamic perspective of person–environment fit. *Osaka Keidai Ronshu, 55*, 177–190.

Seppälä, P., & Klemola, S. (2004). How do employees perceive their organization and job when companies adopt principles of lean production? *Human Factors and Ergonomics in Manufacturing, 14*(2), 157–180.

Sharma, S., & Sharma, M. (2010). Globalization, threatened identities, coping and well-being. *Psychological Studies, 55*(4), 313–322.
Shoaf, C., Genaidy, A., Karwowski, W., & Huang, S. H. (2004). Improving performance and quality of working life: A model for organizational health assessment in emerging enterprises. *Human Factors and Ergonomics in Manufacturing, 14*(1), 81–95.
Shultz, K., Wang, M., & Olson, D. A. (2010). Role overload and underload in relation to occupational stress and health. *Stress and Health, 26*, 99–1111.
Siegrist, J. (1996). Adverse health effects of high-effort/low-reward conditions. *Journal of Occupational Health Psychology, 1*(1), 27–41.
Sulsky, L., & Smith, C. (2005). *Work stress*. Belmont, CA: Wadsworth.
Szalma, J. L., & Hancock, P. A. (2011). Noise effects on human performance: A meta-analytic synthesis. *Psychological Bulletin, 137*(4), 682–707.
Tak, S., Davis, R. R., & Calvert, G. M. (2009). Exposure to hazardous workplace noise and use of hearing protection devices among US workers—NHANES, 1999–2004. *American Journal of Industrial Medicine, 52*(5), 358–371.
Taylor, F. W. (1911). *The principles of scientific management*. New York, NY: Harper.
Tepas, D. I., Armstrong, D. R., Carlson, M. L., & Duchon, J. C. (1985). Changing industry to continuous operations: Different strokes for different plants. *Behavior Research Methods, Instruments and Computers, 17*(6), 670–676.
Tepper, B. J. (2000). Consequences of abusive supervision. *The Academy of Management Journal, 43*(2), 178–190.
Tepper, B. J. (2001). Health consequences of organizational injustice: Tests of main and interactive effects. *Organizational Behavior and Human Decision Processes, 86*(2), 197–215.
Tetrick, L. E., & Quick, J. C. (2003). Prevention at work: Public health in occupational settings. In J. C. Quick & L. Tetrick (Eds.), *Handbook of occupational health psychology* (pp. 3–17). Washington, DC: American Psychological Association.
Tetrick, L. E., & Quick, J. C. (2010). Overview of occupational health psychology: Public health in occupational settings. In J. C. Quick & L. Tetrick (Eds.), *Handbook of occupational health psychology* (2nd ed., pp. 3–20). Washington, DC: American Psychological Association.
Theorell, T., & Karasek, R. A. (1996). Current issues relating to psychosocial job strain and cardiovascular disease research. *Journal of Occupational Health Psychology, 1*(1), 9–26.
Thompson, B., Brough, P., & Schmidt, H. (2006). Supervisor and subordinate work–family values. *International Journal of Stress Management, 13*, 45–62.
US Department of Labor. *The Fair Labor Standards Act* of 1938, as amended 29 U.S.C. § 201, et seq.
Van Harrison, R. (1978). Person–environment fit and job stress. In C. L. Cooper & R. Payne (Eds.), *Stress at work*. Chichester: Wiley.
Vanroelen, C., Levecque, K., Moors, G., Gadeyne, S., & Louckx, F. (2009). The structuring of occupational stressors in a Post-Fordist work environment. Moving beyond traditional accounts of demand, control and support. *Social Science and Medicine, 68*(6), 1082–1090.
Vermunt, R., & Steensma, H. (2005). How can justice be used to manage stress in organizations? In J. Greenberg & J. A. Colquit (Eds.), *Handbook of organizational justice* (pp. 383–410). Mahwah, NJ: Lawrence Erlbaum Associates Publishers.
Villanueva, V., & Garcia, A. M. (2011). Individual and occupational factors related to fatal occupational injuries: A case–control study. *Accident Analysis and Prevention, 43*(1), 123–127.
Waling, K., Javholm, B., & Sundelin, G. (2002). Effects of training on female trapezius myalgia: An intervention study with a 3-year follow-up period. *Spine, 27*, 789–796.
Wallace, J.C., & Chen, G. (2005). Development and validation of a work-specific measure of cognitive failure: Implications for occupational safety. *Journal of Occupational and Organizational Psychology, 78*: 615–632.
World Health Organization. (1948). *Preamble to the Constitution of the World Health Organization as adopted by the International Health Conference*, New York, 19 June–22 July 1946; signed on 22 July 1946 by the representatives of 61 States (Official Records of the World Health Organization, no. 2, p. 100) and entered into force on 7 April 1948.
World Health Organization. (2007). *Workers' health: Global plan of action*. Sixtieth World Health Assembly. Retrieved from the World Health Organization website: http://www.who.int/occupational_health/WHO_health_assembly_en_web.pdf

Part II

Major Symptoms and Disorders in the Workplace

Work-Related Musculoskeletal Disorders and Pain

Ann Marie Hernandez and Alan L. Peterson

Abbreviations

BLS	Bureau of Labor Statistics
CT	Computerized tomography
CTS	Carpal tunnel syndrome
MRI	Magnetic resonance imaging
NIH	National Institutes of Health
NIOSH	National Institute of Occupational Safety and Health
NRC	National Research Council
NSAID	Nonsteroidal inflammatory medication
TENS	Transcutaneous electrical nerve stimulation
WRMDs	Work-related musculoskeletal disorders

Introduction

Work-related musculoskeletal disorders (WRMDs) have intrigued and challenged clinicians and researchers since the beginning of the eighteenth century. These disorders are generally characterized as injuries or dysfunctions that primarily involve the major supporting structures of the body, including the nerves, muscles, bones, joints, and cartilage (National Institute of Occupational Safety and Health [NIOSH], 1997). These disorders have been attributed to the cumulative impact of repetitive movements and/or prolonged awkward postures that often occur in the work environment and ultimately result in overuse, sprains, strains, tears, hernias, and/or other connective tissue injuries (NIOSH, 2001). It is

---

A.M. Hernandez, Ph.D. (✉) • A.L. Peterson, Ph.D., A.B.P.P.
Department of Psychiatry, University of Texas Health Sciences Center at San Antonio,
7550 IH 10 West, Suite 1325, San Antonio, TX 78229, USA

Department of Psychiatry—Mail Code 7792, University of Texas Health Sciences Center at San Antonio,
7703 Floyd Curl Drive, San Antonio, TX 78229-3900, USA
e-mail: hernandezam@uthscsa.edu; petersona3@uthscsa.edu

important to distinguish WRMDs from general pain disorders that are attributed to off-duty injuries (e.g., falls, motor-vehicle accidents, etc.), autoimmune disease, and/or other etiological factors unrelated to occupational duties.

Clinicians and researchers refer to these painful and oftentimes disabling afflictions using a variety of terms including repetitive motion injuries, repetitive strain injuries, cumulative trauma disorders, overuse syndrome, regional musculoskeletal disorders, soft tissue disorders, ergonomic disorders, etc. (Gatchel, Peng, Peters, Fuchs, & Turk, 2007; Huang, Feuerstein, & Sauter, 2002). Examples of more commonly recognized WRMDs include low back pain, neck pain, tennis elbow, and carpel tunnel syndrome. The inconsistent nomenclature can be attributed to the fact that these disorders largely defy traditional disease classification systems (NIOSH, 2001). Furthermore, there is significant disagreement regarding the causal mechanisms underlying the development and/or maintenance of musculoskeletal disorders in the workplace. The current literature largely emphasizes the impact of occupational duties on the development and maintenance of musculoskeletal disorders. For instance, the impact of computerized work environments, subsequent repetitive upper limb movement, and a prolonged sedentary posture on musculoskeletal disorders of the upper limbs has garnered significant empirical support (Griffiths, Mackey, & Adamson, 2007). In fact, the NIOSH (1997) stated that multiple studies have demonstrated evidence of a causal relationship between physical activity at work and WRMDs, based on a review of the most rigorous epidemiological research available. Still, the relationship between musculoskeletal disorders and work-related factors remains the subject of substantial debate due to the multiple factors (e.g., physical, occupational, organizational, psychosocial, individual, and sociocultural) that contribute to the development and maintenance of such disorders (World Health Organization, 1985). The current chapter provides an overview of the most commonly studied WRMDs, including those injuries and diseases that are the result of events and exposures in the work environment that cause or contribute to the condition.

Epidemiology

The incidence and prevalence rates of WRMDs vary greatly across epidemiological studies due to differences in study populations and diagnostic criteria. The US Department of Labor's Bureau of Labor Statistics (BLS) provides what may be the most representative and comprehensive data currently available on the prevalence of WRMDs in the USA. Estimates are calculated from the BLS Annual Survey of Occupational Injuries and Illnesses, which surveys over 230,000 private industry establishments across 44 US states and territories. *The epidemiological evidence suggests that musculoskeletal disorders represent the single largest category of illnesses recorded as occupational diseases in the USA* (Bureau of Labor Statistics [BLS], 2010; National Research Council [NRC], 1999). A recordable case includes work-related injuries, disorders, or illnesses that result in medical treatment, restricted activity or job transfer, loss of consciousness, days away from work, and a diagnosis by a physician or other licensed health professional. More specifically, WRMDs accounted for 28 % of the 3.3 million reported cases of nonfatal occupational injuries and illnesses reported in 2009 (BLS, 2010). Of the 3.3 million nonfatal occupational injury and illnesses reported, over 1.2 million workers required time away from work to recover (BLS; see Fig. 4.1).

Of these occupations, the specific occupations that reported the highest incidence of WRMDs were among psychiatric aides (256.0 per 10,000 full-time workers), emergency medical technicians and paramedics (233.5 per 10,000 full-time workers), and nursing aides and orderlies (232.5 per 10,000 full-time workers). As indicated in Fig. 4.2, the vast majority of WRMD cases occur to the back, followed by injuries to the upper extremities.

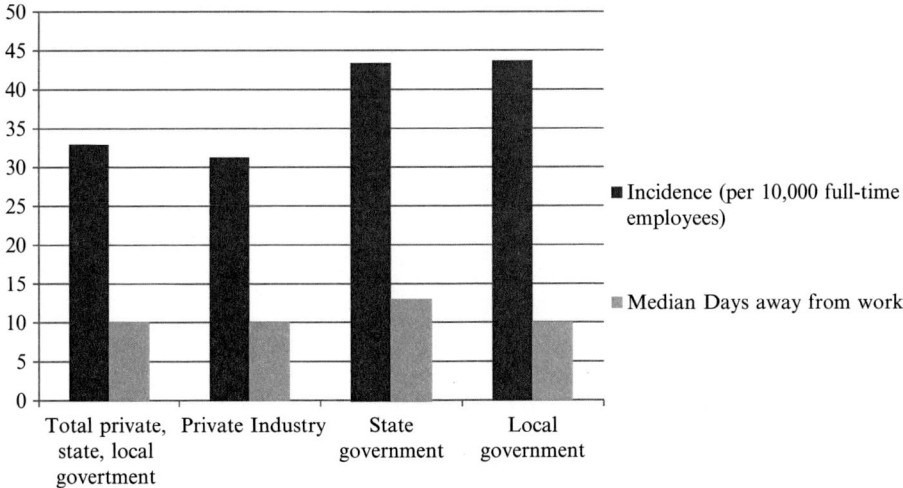

Fig. 4.1 Incidence and median days of work missed across private industry, local government, and state government, 2009. *Source*: Bureau of Labor Statistics, 2010

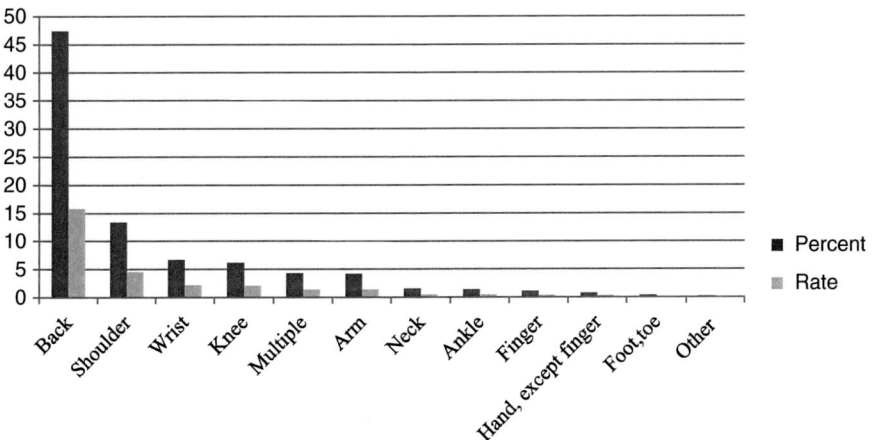

Fig. 4.2 Percent and incidence rate (per 10,000) of part of body affected, 2008. *Source*: Bureau of Labor Statistics, 2010

Sprains, strains, and tears of various connective tissues account for three quarters of the 236,260 musculoskeletal disorders cases reported in the private industry, with similar patterns exhibited among government employees (Fig. 4.3).

Economic Burden of Work-Related Musculoskeletal Disorders

WRMDs account for more disability and costs to the US health care system and commercial industries than any other condition (NIOSH, 2001). Within the Department of Defense, WRMDs result in more missed duty day, medical profiles, and medical discharges from active duty than any other medical condition (Amoroso & Canham, 1999; Feuerstein, Berkowitz, & Peck, 1997; Jones, Amoroso, Canham, Schmitt, & Weyandt, 1999). Given the aging population, the economic burden of WRMDs is likely to increase. WRMDs affect the economy by contributing to increased absenteeism, health

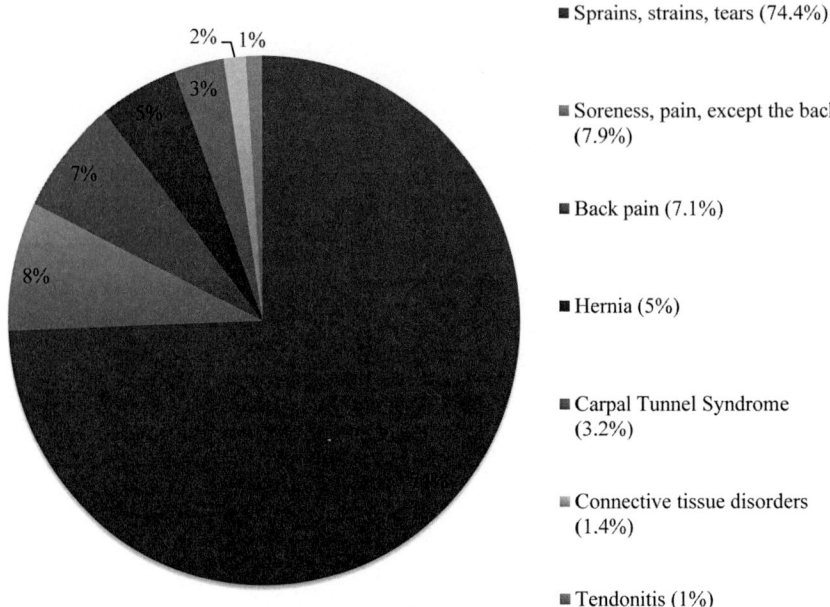

Fig. 4.3 Distribution of musculoskeletal disorders in the private industry by nature of injury or illness, 2008. *Source*: Bureau of Labor Statistics, 2010

care costs, and worker compensation expenditures. For example, nearly one million people each year report taking time away from work for treatment to recover from WRMDs, with most individuals returning to work within 31 days (BLS, 2010). In 2008, WRMDs required a median of 10 days away from work, with significant variability across disorders. For instance, carpal tunnel syndrome (CTS) accounted for a substantial percentage of absenteeism where an average of 28 days of leave were taken per incident, whereas more commonly reported disorders, such as low back pain, accounted for 7 days of leave per incident (BLS, 2010). Health care and compensation expenditures related to WRMDs continue to increase and place a significant burden on private and public industries. WRMDs account for nearly 70 million physician office visits in the USA annually, and an estimated 130 million total health care encounters including outpatient, hospital, and emergency room visits. In 2007, the National Academy of Social Insurance reported that cash benefits to injured workers and medical payments for their health care exceeded $55 billion, with total costs to employers reaching approximately $85 million (Sengupta, Reno, & Burton, 2009). These figures are conservative and represent only reported cases, as many disorders that can be attributed to work go unreported and therefore are not counted in any of the existing databases. Regardless of the estimates used, the problem is large both in terms of health and economic impact.

Conceptual Model for the Development of Work-Related Musculoskeletal Disorders

Several conceptual models have been created to delineate the potential relationships between external and internal factors that impact the development of WRMDs. The majority of models for the development of WRMDs take into account individual, social, organizational, and occupational factors. One of the most oft-cited models was provided by the National Institute for Occupational Safety and Health (NIOSH, 2001). The NIOSH synthesized numerous reviews of the literature on WRMDs, and

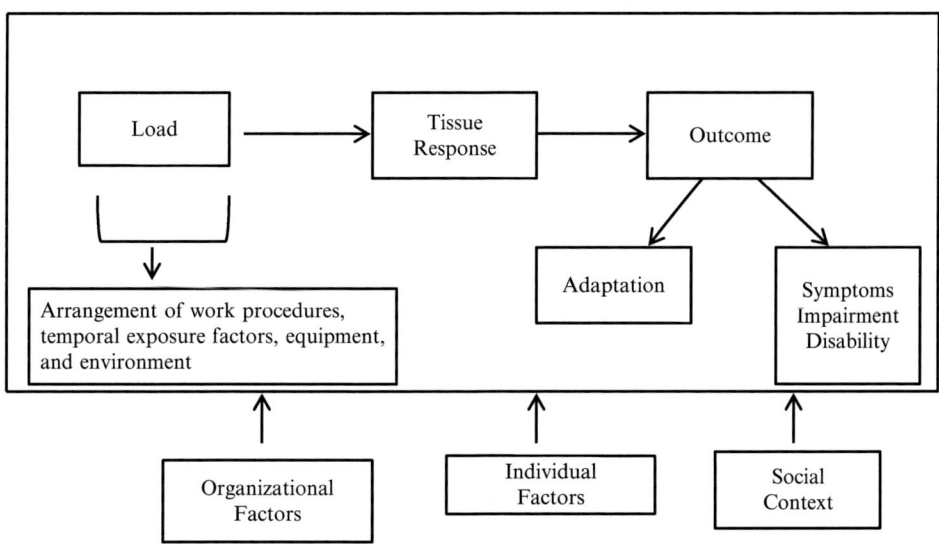

Fig. 4.4 Conceptual model for work-related musculoskeletal disorders development. *Source*: National Institute of Occupational Safety and Health, 2001

proposed that the physical activities that place an individual at increased risk for the development of musculoskeletal disorders are impacted by individual, social, and organizational factors (Buckle & Devereux, 1999; Frank, Pulcins, Kerr, Shannon, & Stansfeld, 1995; Frank et al., 1996; Katz et al., 1998; Krause, Dasinger, & Neuhauser, 1998; Moore, 1992; Szabo, 1998; see Fig. 4.4).

In this model, the initial load (e.g., static or dynamic muscle load) to which an individual is exposed to is dependent upon work requirements, duration of exposure, and the environment in which the individual is interacting. This initial load is applied to the musculoskeletal system either by external or by internal forces, which lead to internal tissue responses in the muscles, ligaments, and at the joint surfaces. Depending upon the magnitude of the load and other individual, organizational, or social factors, one or more outcomes may result. These may include adaptation effects (such as increases in strength, fitness, or conditioning) or potentially harmful outcomes (such as pain or other symptoms, and structural damage to tendons, nerves, muscles, joints, or supporting tissues) that may result in symptoms, impairment, or disability. Whether the exposure leads to a WRMD depends upon the physical demands of the job, the adaptation response of the worker, and other individual physical and psychological factors. These factors, in turn, may regulate the effects of the external load.

Recent findings largely support the assertions made by this model, in which physical occupational requirements, organizational influences, individual characteristics, and psychosocial factors contribute to increased risk of WRMDs (Bigos et al., 1992; Hoogendoorn, van Poppel, Bongers, Koes, & Bouter, 2000). For instance, several studies have demonstrated the negative impact that excessive physical load has on the musculoskeletal system using three-dimensional modeling of physical load on various joints and measures of tissue disintegration and inflammatory processes (Marras, Cutlip, Burt, & Waters, 2009). More recently, research has also demonstrated the association of individual (e.g., personality traits), organizational (e.g., job satisfaction and safety climate), and psychosocial factors (e.g., social support and work stress) with both lower extremity and upper extremity musculoskeletal disorders (Andersen et al., 2003; Bigos et al., 1992; Hoogendoorn et al., 2000, Marras, Davis, Ferguson, Lucas, & Gupta, 2001; NRC, 1999). Psychosocial factors include nonphysical influences that concern the mental stress response of the worker in the workplace. Reviews of epidemiological studies indicate that between 11 and 80 % of low-back injuries and 11–95 % of extremity injuries are attributable to workplace physical factors, whereas between 14 and 63 % of injuries to the low back and between 28 and 84 % of injuries of the upper extremity are attributable to psychosocial factors (NRC, 1999). It is understood that the contribution of each factor to the risk of a WRMD varies with the nature of the disorder and the anatomical area involved.

Types of Work-Related Musculoskeletal Disorders

Much confusion surrounds the accurate classification and diagnosis of these conditions. As a result, a variety of classification schemes have been proposed, but none has been universally adopted (Buckle & Devereux, 2002). This significantly hinders clinicians' and researchers' ability to communicate in a consistent, accurate, and meaningful manner about these disorders, thereby preventing progression towards the identification of the most effective strategies for their prevention and treatment. For the purposes of this chapter, the most commonly reported WRMDs will be described and organized by affected anatomical area, as this is the manner in which they are classified in the literature. It is understood that individual, biomechanical, and psychosocial risk factors vary with the nature of the disorder and the anatomical area involved. It is important to note that the current state of the science is such that the temporal relationship between risk factor and disorder cannot be clearly established. As such, the risk factors associated with each category of musculoskeletal disorders will be addressed separately within each category.

Work-Related Musculoskeletal Disorders of the Upper Body

Neck and/or Shoulder

Musculoskeletal complaints in the neck and/or shoulder (part of the cervicobrachial area) are common among adults in developed nations and are showing increasing trends. Common symptoms associated with WRMDs of the neck and/or shoulder include pain, tenderness, and stiffness at the base of neck and upper back; signs of hardened muscle bands or nodularity; headaches due to tension in neck muscles; intermittent muscle spasms in neck muscles; and/or dull pain referred to the upper limbs. These contribute to the demand for medical services and the economic burden of absence from work due to sickness. Population-based studies suggest a lifetime prevalence of over 70 %, and point-prevalence rates ranging from 12 to 34 % (NIOSH, 1997; van Rijn, Huisstede, Koes, & Burdorf, 2010). More than 40 epidemiological studies have been published that focus on the relationship between neck and shoulder pain and occupation. The studies are heterogeneous in design, classification of disorder (e.g., neck pain, tension neck syndrome, rotator cuff syndrome, cervical strain, tension myalgia, etc.), population (e.g., dental professionals, automobile assembly workers, computer workers, factory workers, secretaries, poultry workers, scissor makers, sewing machine operators, healthcare employees, grocery checkers, etc.), symptom assessment (e.g., self-report, physician examination, etc.), outcome measurement (neck pain, neck, and/or shoulder pain, physical examination), and analysis.

Biomechanical Risk Factors
The majority of these studies investigated the impact of repetitive work movements and/or improper static postures on neck and/or shoulder disorders. Repetitive work activities are defined as continuous head, neck, arm, and/or hand movements that affect the muscles of the neck and shoulder areas. Multiple studies have shown that employees who are exposed to prolonged and improper postures involving the neck and/or shoulder muscles and to forceful and/or repetitive tasks, are at significantly

greater risk for neck and/or shoulder WRMDs. For example, Morse et al. (2007) noted that dental hygienists frequently work with their neck flexed over 30 °, while leaning sideways or rotating their shoulders. These prolonged static postures create high static loads and fatigue within the trapezius muscles (Finsen, Christensen, & Bakke, 1998). These repeated exposures have been tied to self-reported pain symptoms and to abnormal physician exam findings, suggesting that these demands place employees at greater risk of developing neck and/or shoulder WRMDs. Similar findings have been demonstrated among individuals across a variety of occupations, including computer workers, factory employees, and other employees who are exposed to similar biomechanical risk factors in their respective work setting.

Psychosocial Risk Factors

Greater emphasis has been placed on psychosocial risk factors that may contribute to the development of WRMDs. Research suggests that several psychosocial factors place workers at risk for neck pain, including poor workplace support from supervisors/colleagues, high occupational demands, and poor control over working patterns (Cagnie, Danneels, Van Tiggelen, De Loose, & Cambier, 2007; Griffiths et al., 2007). For instance, Cagnie et al. (2007) found that individuals who perceived a shortage of personnel and an inability to meet company demands were at increased risk of reporting neck pain. This may be an indirect reflection of work overload which, in turn contributed to increased opportunity for the development of WRMDs. Furthermore, a review conducted by Griffiths et al. (2007) suggests that multiple risk factors place workers at increased risk for pain, including excessive workload, time/deadline pressures, and reduced opportunities for social interactions. These issues are particularly salient among nonprofessional office workers due to low levels of job control, social support, and task clarity (Griffiths et al.). These factors are assumed to interact with other individual and biomechanical factors to increase a person's individual risk factors. For example, the cumulative stress placed on the neck and shoulder area, as a result of longer hours at a computer terminal due to personnel shortage or increase work demands, is one example of combinations of factors that contribute to the development of WRMDs. Taken together, therefore, the evidence suggests that neck pain and neck disorders are associated with mechanical and psychosocial workplace factors.

Individual Risk Factors

Cross-sectional and prospective studies have provided inconsistent evidence for associations between individual factors among workers (e.g., gender, age, physical activity, and personality factors) and neck and/or shoulder pain symptoms (Viikari-Juntura et al., 2001). Individual factors are largely conceptualized as confounding factors that influence the relation between environmental demands of the job and the occurrence of neck pain in the employee. Studies suggest that women are at greater risk of reported neck and/or shoulder pain compared to men; however, the mechanisms underlying this relationship are not fully understood (Cagnie et al., 2007; Korhonen et al., 2003; Leclerc et al., 1999). More specifically, prevalence rates suggest that neck pain is twice as common among female full-time employees compared to their male counterparts (Cagnie et al., 2007; Korhonen et al., 2003; Leclerc et al., 1999; Marcus et al., 2002). However, these higher rates are not exclusive to neck and shoulder pain, as this pattern is found across most forms of body pain. Research suggests that smaller stature and lower muscular strength in the neck and shoulder areas explain the gender differences (Korhonen et al., 2003). Several other physical, cultural, and sociological factors have been proposed as explanations, although none have been supported in the empirical literature (Guez, Hildingsson, Nilsson, & Toolanen, 2002). In addition, an inverse U-shaped relationship has been demonstrated between age and prevalence of neck pain, where the risk of neck pain increases until approximately 50 years of age, and decreases slightly thereafter (Bot et al., 2005; Leclerc et al., 1999; Viikari-Juntura et al., 2001). Research suggests that increased pain is associated with increased degeneration of the cervical spine. However, the decrease in neck and/or shoulder complaints may be attributed to other, more debilitating disorders taking precedence later in life (Bot et al., 2005).

A relationship between physical activity and neck and/or shoulder pain has been identified in observational studies. For example, Korhonen et al. (2003) found in their cohort study that employees who exercised less frequently demonstrated a higher risk of neck pain. However, it is unclear if individuals do not engage in physical activity as a result of the pain or are at greater risk for the development of WRMDs due to poor muscle strength and sedentary lifestyle. This may have some clinical implications, as an increase in physical activity may be one way to of reduce musculoskeletal morbidity in sedentary workers (Hildebrandt, Bongers, Dul, van Dijk, & Kemper, 2000). Finally, the study of personality traits and neck and/or shoulder pain among workers has yielded inconsistent results. Some studies found an association between neck and shoulder pain symptoms and Type A behavior (Malchaire, Cock, & Vergracht, 2001), while others did not (Andersen et al., 2003). Also, introversion (Malchaire et al., 2001) and neurotic perfectionist traits (van Eijsden-Besseling, Peeters, Reijnen, & de Bie, 2004) were reported to be associated with WRMDs of the neck and upper limbs. It is hypothesized that these individual factors interact with biomechanical and psychosocial mechanisms in the development and maintenance of WRMDs. However, additional research is warranted given the sparse and inconsistent literature investigating the impact of personality factors on WRMDs.

Assessment and Diagnosis

WRMDs of the neck and/or shoulder are assessed using a variety of methods across research and clinical settings, suggesting a lack of agreement regarding the appropriate way to assess for the presence of these particular disorders. Epidemiological studies utilize data gathered from interviews or questionnaires to assess the intensity, frequency, and duration of pain, tingling, and/or numbing in the neck and shoulder region. The criterion used to diagnose the presence of a neck and/or shoulder WRMD varies across studies, accounting for the wide-ranging prevalence rates. General recommendations regarding the clinical assessment of musculoskeletal disorders include inspection of the affected area; testing for range of motion, pain, and muscle strength; palpitation of muscle tendons; and specific tests including computerized tomography (CT). CT scans are usually reserved for individuals who experienced a blunt trauma or are at high risk for more serious pathology. Despite the availability of assessment techniques, the majority of clinicians utilize a clinical physical examination in determining the presence of a disorder in the neck and/or shoulder region (Nordin et al., 2009).

Treatment Approaches

Researchers, clinicians, and occupational health professionals have prescribed numerous interventions in an attempt to limit the disabling and costly effects of neck and shoulder pain on employees (Gatchel et al., 2007; Schultz, Stowell, Feuerstein, & Gatchel, 2007). The vast majority of WRMDs interventions focus on modifying the ergonomics, or design, of the workplace or equipment in an attempt to minimize the load placed on the neck and/or shoulder muscles (Hurwitz et al., 2008; Leyshon et al., 2010). Ergonomic interventions aim to decrease the strain on the neck and/or shoulder muscles by altering the workstation and the environment. For instance, employers have utilized improved lighting, lumbar support, alternative keyboards, and pointing devices among computer users. Unfortunately, evidence supporting the effectiveness of these conservative approaches is largely inconsistent. While some reviews lend support to the use of ergonomic interventions (Boocock et al., 2007), other reviews failed to find associations (Kennedy et al., 2010). Other conservative approaches include the use of chiropractic manipulation, massage, frequent rest breaks, exercise, and biofeedback. However, these interventions lack long-term effects, as indicated by the high rate of recurring neck and/or shoulder pain symptoms after treatment (Hurwitz et al., 2008). More recent research has investigated the potential benefit of incorporating a cognitive-behavioral approach to the management of WRMDs (Leon et al., 2009). Preliminary research suggests that a cognitive-behavioral intervention, which included psychoeducation, cognitive restructuring, and breathing retraining in conjunction with standard rheumatic care, can significantly decrease pain ratings and prevent relapse (Leon et al.). More recently, *Transcutaneous Electrical Nerve Stimulation (TENS)* units have also been used to treat neck and/or shoulder WRMDs. A TENS unit is a device that provides light electrical current via electrodes attached to the skin surrounding the painful area. It is hypothesized that the electrical stimulation interrupts and modulates the pain signals sent from the affected area to the brain; however, there is no consensus regarding the pain relief mechanism(s). One study suggests that relief from neck pain symptoms can be reached with a single TENS session (Maayah & Al-Jarrah, 2010). As with the other interventions mentioned above, the long-term efficacy of the TENS unit is undetermined. Furthermore, neck and/or shoulder WRMD intervention studies are plagued by small sample sizes, non-random assignment, lack of comparison groups, and inconsistent classification and diagnosis of disorders. These limitations—combined with the prevalence and physical, emotional, and economic costs of neck and/or shoulder WRMDs—highlight the need for further high-quality intervention research.

Elbow

Epicondylitis is one of the most common disorders of the elbow, and it is associated with significant pain, functional impairment, and a reduction in productivity (da Costa & Vieira, 2010; NIOSH, 2001). Epicondylitis can be further classified as medial or lateral epicondylitis, conditions commonly referred to as "golfer's or tennis elbow," respectively. Epicondylitis is attributed to the overuse of the extensor and flexor muscles in the elbow, which often leads to inflammation of the tendon (Park, Lee, & Lee, 2008). However, specifics regarding the pathogenesis of medial and lateral epicondylitis are not well understood. Epicondylitis is also one of the most costly WRMDs and contributes to lost workdays, decreased productivity, and worker's compensation claims (Kurppa, Viikari-Juntura, & Kuosma, 1991; Verhaar, 1994). For example, work-related epicondylitis had an annual workers' compensation incidence rate of 4.7 per 10,000 full-time employees in the state of Washington alone. This translated to an average of 136 lost workdays per claim, and more than $12 million in direct costs (Foley, Silverstein, & Polissar, 2007; Foley, Silverstein, Polissar, & Neradilek, 2009; Silverstein & Adams, 2007). Employees in certain industries are said to be at greater risk for developing medial and/or lateral epicondylitis including, but not limited to, assembly line workers, cashiers, cooks, and packaging workers. Research suggests that biomechanical, psychosocial, and individual factors interact with the physical and environmental demands of these occupations and contribute to the development of WRMDs of the elbow.

Biomechanical Risk Factors

Research largely emphasizes the role of biomechanical risk factors in the work place in relation to WRMDs of the elbow. Numerous biomechanical risk factors have been identified, including forceful and repetitive physical work, extreme nonneutral position of the hands and arms, high grip forces, and vibrating hand tools (da Costa & Vieira, 2010; Shiri, Viikari-Juntura, Varonen, & Heliövaara, 2006). Many manufacturing and service industries require that employees engage in activities that require prolonged engagement in these types of movements. For example, assembly workers are often required to the use force, tight grips, and vibrating hand tools for several hours a day when assembling products. Research suggests that the risk of developing medial or lateral epicondylitis increases as the frequency and duration of such physical exertion increases (Shiri et al., 2006; van Rijn et al., 2010). While multiple systematic reviews support these findings, researchers are cautious in establishing a causal link between these biomechanical factors and medial and lateral epicondylitis, as the vast majority of these studies are cross-sectional (da Costa & Vieira, 2010; Shiri et al., 2006).

Psychosocial Risk Factors

Less is known about the potential role that psychosocial risk factors play in the development of epicondylitis. There are some cross-sectional data to suggest that factors such as poor job control, negative affectivity, dissatisfaction with work, and high psychosocial demands place employees at greater risk for developing WRMDs of the elbow (Macfarlane et al., 2009; NIOSH, 1997; Shiri et al., 2006). These factors are not unique to epicondylitis and are apparent risk factors for the development of several other WRMDs. Interestingly, there are preliminary data to suggest that psychosocial factors may influence lateral and medial epicondylitis differently. For instance, a review by van Rijn et al. (2010) found that psychosocial factors, such as low job control and low social support, were related to lateral but not medial epicondylitis. This suggests that, while the majority of studies focus on lateral or both lateral and medial disorders together, future research may benefit from investigating potential unique risk factors.

Individual Risk Factors

Studies have identified several individual factors that may place an individual at greater risk for the development of lateral and/or medial epicondylitis. For instance, research suggests that risk factors include older age, female gender, smoking, obesity, and diabetes (Shiri et al., 2006; da Costa & Vieira, 2010). However, the manner in which these factors place a worker at greater risk is unclear. The association between age and WRMDs of the elbow is believed to be due to the fact that this is a more common disorder among individuals who are of working age, as opposed to younger individuals (e.g., 30–64). Female gender has also been found to be associated with WRMDs of the elbow, but potential mediators have not been identified (Macfarlane et al., 2009; NIOSH, 1997 Shiri et al., 2006). In addition, interestingly, research suggests that smoking serves as a risk factor for epicondylitis. Smoking may interference with the circulation of tendons, which not only places the tissue at risk for injury but also slows or prevents their healing during recovery period. This pattern is also found in previous tobacco users, suggesting that tobacco may have a persistent effect on the vascular system (Shiri et al.). Other factors, such as obesity and diabetes, have been associated with the development of epicondylitis among workers; however, it is unclear as to the manner in which these variables are related. Researchers propose that obesity contributes to insulin resistance, a component of a metabolic syndrome, which may lead to Type II diabetes and increase the risk of developing WRMDs in general (Shiri et al., 2006; van Rijn et al., 2010). Further research is needed to clarify the potential relationship between smoking, obesity, and epicondylitis.

Assessment and Diagnosis

Assessment of lateral and medial epicondylitis disorders requires a thorough patient history, physical examination, and radiographic and imaging studies. However, radiographic and imaging studies are primarily utilized to rule out more serious pathology. Diagnostic criteria differ slightly across clinical settings and research studies, but generally require the presence of local pain at the elbow, tenderness at the epicondyle on palpitation, and pain at the epicondyle on resisted isometric extension or flexion of the wrist. More specifically, a lateral epicondylitis diagnosis requires the presence of pain in the lateral epicondyle that is exacerbated by resisted forearm pronation and wrist and digital flexion. Medial epicondylitis is characterized by pain along the medial elbow, which is also worsened by resistance to forearm pronation and wrist and digital flexion (Shiri et al., 2006). The duration in which symptoms must be present range from 1 week to 6 months, depending on the clinical or research guideline being used.

Treatment Approaches

While a wide range of treatments for lateral and medial epicondylitis are available, there is no consensus among clinicians and researchers regarding the most efficacious treatments. This is largely due to the fact that large-scale randomized clinical trials have not been conducted. As such, clinicians are unable to confidently prescribe one treatment over another, as there are no data to support the relative effectiveness of a particular treatment. First-line treatments for lateral and medial epicondylitis are largely conservative in nature and are used in combination with one another. The most important components of these conservative approaches include rest from the aggravating activity, activity modification, watchful waiting, and the use of nonsteroidal inflammatory medications (NSAIDs). Various orthotic devises, such as elastic bands placed on the forearm, have also been utilized, but numerous reviews have been unable to find support for their effectiveness. While some researchers suggest that bracing alleviates pain and improves grip strength, there is no evidence to suggest that it is better than sham bracing and other conservative therapies, and it may in fact be inferior to topical NSAIDs and corticosteroid injections (Bisset, Paungmali, Vicenzino, & Beller, 2005; Struijs et al., 2001). Individuals with chronic, reoccurring elbow pain that is unresponsive to more conservative approaches also have the option to use more aggressive procedures, including physical therapy, corticosteroid injections, *extracorporeal shock therapy*, and acupuncture. Corticosteroid injections have been shown to alleviate painful symptoms and improve grip strength for approximately 2–6 weeks. While corticosteroids are effective in the short term, their long-term effectiveness and advantages over more conservative approaches are uncertain. Technological advances have led clinicians to experiment with extracorporeal shock therapy, which delivers low- or high-frequency electrical current to the affected area. It is believed that these electrical currents trigger a healing response in the damaged tendon. However, research to date does not support the efficacy of this form of treatment for epicondylitis (Bisset et al., 2005; Trudel et al., 2004). Exercise is commonly prescribed as a way to manage and treat elbow pain. Physical therapy regimens used to treat WRMDs of the elbow typically involve strength training and stretching. While these exercises have been effective in reducing pain, there is less evidence to suggest that it results in improved grip strength (Bisset et al.; Trudel et al.). Acupuncture has garnered some attention as a potential treatment for epicondylitis. Interestingly, the National Institutes of Health (NIH, 1998) released a consensus statement supporting the use of acupuncture in the treatment of epicondylitis despite conflicting evidence of its efficacy.

Given the often self-limiting nature of the disorder, and the effectiveness of some conservative approaches, most individuals do not need to undergo surgery. However, epicondylitis can be a chronic and debilitating disorder for a small minority of sufferers. Surgery is usually reserved for those cases where conservative approaches have not provided any relief over the previous 6 months to a year. While various surgical procedures are utilized in the treatment of epicondylitis, the main objective is to remove abnormal tissue within the tendon or release the tendon altogether. While there is some evidence that such invasive procedures provide relief, more stringent research testing the relative effectiveness of surgery to more conservative approaches is lacking. Interestingly, one of the few randomized controlled trials conducted in this area suggest that more conservative approaches, such as watchful waiting and rest combined with NSAIDs, were more effective, relative to aggressive approaches such as corticosteroid injections (Smidt et al., 2002). While many interventions for lateral and medial epicondylitis exist and are commonly put into practice, little is known about best practices for managing this disorder. This is unfortunate given the high prevalence and economic impact of epicondylitis. For chronic elbow pain, a comprehensive interdisciplinary treatment approach will provide the best chance of decreasing pain, increasing function, and returning to work (Gatchel & Okifuji, 2006; Gatchel et al., 2007; Schultz et al., 2007).

Hand and Wrist

There are few occupations that do not require use of the hands as a major part of daily work requirements. As a result, WRMDs of the hand and wrist have a greater impact on work attendance, productivity, and wages than WRMDs affecting any other region of the body (BLS, 2010). One of the most costly and prevalent WRMDs of the hand and wrist is CTS. CTS is caused by a combination of biomechanical and biobehavioral work-related factors involving excessive and repetitive forceful use of the hand, such as higher levels of computer keyforce during typing (Feuerstein, Armstrong, Hickey, & Lincoln, 1997; Harrington & Feuerstein, 2010; Nicholas, Feuerstein, & Suchday, 2005; Palmer, 2011). This excessive force results in compression of the median nerve in the wrist that supplies feelings and movement to the hand, which in turn leads to sensorimotor dysfunction in parts of the hand (Patijn et al., 2011). Individuals with CTS endorse symptoms such as numbness, tingling, weakness, or pain in the hand and fingers. Prevalence estimates indicate that about 14 % of the general US population reports symptoms of recurring pain, numbness, and/or tingling in the median nerve distribution in the hands (Atroshi et al., 1999). Upon clinical and electrophysiological examination, about 4 % of the population meets diagnostic criteria for CTS. While CTS can be caused by a variety of chronic illnesses, such as rheumatoid arthritis, gout, and diabetes, this disorder has been primarily linked to workplace factors. In fact, it is estimated that half of all medically diagnosed cases of CTS are work-related (Lawrence et al., 2008). Estimates suggest that employers expend approximately $45,000–$89,000 per CTS claimant when losses of earning, productivity, and workers compensation claims are taken into account (Foley et al., 2007). Employee health stakeholders are highly motivated to identify and potentially modify those variables that contribute to the development of WRMDs of the hand and wrist such as CTS.

Biomechanical Risk Factors

As is the case of other WRMDs, the majority of the literature surrounding WRMDs of the hand and wrist focuses on mechanical forces that act on the body as a result of occupational duties (Palmer, 2011; Patijn et al., 2011; Viikari-Juntura & Silverstein, 1999). For example, a significant amount of force is placed upon, and exerted from, the tendons of the hand and wrist by factory workers, who oftentimes are required to manually assemble products using repetitive forceful movements of the hand and wrist. The research has identified several biomechanical risk factors across various occupations that increase the likelihood of the development of hand and wrist WRMDs, including awkward static and dynamic forearm, wrist, and finger postures; repetitive work; hand and/or wrist vibration; and prolonged computer work (NIOSH, 1997). Researchers hypothesize that hand and wrist WRMDs occur in the tendons as a result of movements that stimulate an acute inflammatory response. This response may resolve with tissue repair or tissue degeneration depending on the use of appropriate interventions. Barr, Barbe, and Clark (2004) suggest that CTS is due to central nervous system reorganization, which occurs after the performance of repetitive hand and wrist movements. This repeated activation or overstimulation of nociceptive afferents causes a greater release of excitatory neuropeptides and amino acids. These nociceptors become hypersensitive and increase the excitability of secondary neurons in the spinal cord, thereby contributing to the hyperalgesia associated with chronic pain and inflammation (Dubner & Ruda, 1992; McCarson, 1999). The underlying mechanisms that account for the associations between biomechanical force and WRMDS of the hand and wrist continue to be debated. As such, there is no consensus regarding the independent influence of biomechanical factors on the hand and wrist.

Psychosocial Risk Factors

Studies indicate that psychosocial factors in the workplace, such as intense deadlines, a poor social work environment, and low levels of job satisfaction, are major contributors to CTS pain. Research suggests that psychosocial conditions are more likely to be important factors in contributing to CTS in office workers, although they also complicate the condition in employees whose work is primarily physical (Nordstrom, Vierkant, DeStefano, & Layde, 1997). For example, people reporting the least influence at work had 2.86 times the risk (95 % CI, 1.10–7.14) as those with the most influence at work (Nordstrom et al., 1997). Therefore, the risk of developing CTS appears to be more prevalent in occupations where employees lack control or influence over their work environment and responsibilities. Such psychosocial issues have been repeatedly noted in many other chapters of this Handbook.

Individual Risk Factors

The most significant individual risk factor for CTS is the use of excessive force in the performance of work-related duties involving the hands (Feuerstein et al., 1997; Harrington & Feuerstein, 2010; Nicholas et al., 2005). For example, the generation of excessive force while working on a computer keyboard has been shown to directly contribute to the severity of CTS symptoms (Feuerstein et al., 1997). Similar findings have been reported in professional sign language interpreters with CTS (Feuerstein & Fitzgerald, 1992). By comparison with the control group, those working with CTS pain exhibited fewer rest breaks, more frequent hand/wrist deviations from a neutral position, more frequent lateral excursions from an optimal work envelope, and more rapid finger/hand movements while interpreting. Many of the additional individual risk factors for CTS have also been identified for other WRMDs. For instance, individual risk factors, such as older age, female gender, smoking, overweight, and diabetes, have been shown to place a worker at increased risk for CTS. As with other pain disorders, studies indicate that women have a significantly higher risk for CTS than men. While an explanation for this greater risk has not been determined, it is hypothesized to be related to smaller wrist size. However, there are some individual risk factors that are unique to WRMDS of the hand and wrist, including pregnancy (Burt et al., 2011). Hormonal changes also appear to play a major role in the development of CTS in women who are pregnant. CTS that begins during pregnancy is not usually severe and persistent enough to require treatment, as most cases go away on their own after delivery. Being overweight has been highlighted frequently as a risk factor for CTS and may play a direct causal role on CTS. Greater body mass appears to reduce nerve flow speed into the hand. Obesity is also related to poor physical fitness, which may also increase risk. A 2005 analysis indicated that weight is strongly linked to the onset of CTS in patients under the age of 63, but it may be a less important factor as patients increase in age (Bland, 2005).

Assessment and Diagnosis

Assessment of WRMDs of the hand and wrist can take various forms. For example, CTS is diagnosed using a combination of techniques, including self-report, physical examination, and imaging studies. A physical examination typically entails inspection of the wrist for tenderness, swelling, warmth, and discoloration. Specific tests, such as the *Tinel* and *Phalen tests*, are also used to reproduce the symptoms of CTS (Dale, Descatha, Coomes, Franzblau, & Evanoff, 2010). The Tinel test requires that the health professional tap or place moderate pressure on the median nerve in the patient's wrist. The test is positive for CTS when symptoms such as pain and/or tingling occurs in the hand and fingers. The Phalen, or wrist-flexion, test involves having the patient hold his or her forearms upright by pointing the fingers down and pressing the backs of the hands together. The presence of CTS is suggested if one or more symptoms, such as tingling or increasing numbness, are felt in the fingers within 1 min. Often, it is necessary to confirm the diagnosis by use of electrodiagnostic tests that include nerve conduction tests, ultrasounds, and magnetic resonance imaging (MRI). In a nerve conduction study, electrodes are placed on the hand and wrist. Small electric shocks are applied and the speed with which nerves transmit impulses is measured and used to determine the presence of CTS. Ultrasound imaging can show impaired movement of the median nerve, while MRI can show the anatomy of the wrist and help identify any abnormalities.

Some disease-specific self-report questionnaires have been developed for use in research and clinical settings. Levine et al. (1993) introduced the first disease-specific questionnaire—called the *Boston*

Carpal Tunnel Questionnaire—to assess the outcome after carpal tunnel release. Since then, various other upper-limb outcome measures have been used in the assessment of carpal tunnel patients. Some of the commonly used outcomes measures include the *Disability of Arm, Shoulder and Hand* (Greenslade, Mehta, Belward, & Warwick, 2004); *Patient Evaluation Measure* (Dias, Bhowal, Wildin, & Thompson, 2001); *Michigan Hand Outcome Questionnaire* (Chung, Pillsbury, Walters, & Hayward, 1998); and *Upper Extremity Functional Scale* (Pransky, Feuerstein, Himmelstein, Katz, & Vickers-Lahti, 1997). These self-administered questionnaires assess severity of symptoms and functional status. Despite the numerous assessment strategies, there is no consensus regarding a formal assessment of CTS.

Treatment Approaches

Treatment of hand and wrist WRMDs can be broadly divided in nonsurgical and surgical approaches. Initial treatment generally involves resting the affected hand and wrist for at least 2 weeks, avoiding activities that may worsen symptoms, and immobilizing the wrist with a splint in order to avoid further damage from twisting or bending. Nonsteroidal anti-inflammatory drugs, such as aspirin, ibuprofen, and other nonprescription pain relievers may ease symptoms that have been present for a short time or have been caused by strenuous activity. Corticosteroids, such as prednisone, can be injected directly into the wrist or taken by mouth to relieve pressure on the median nerve and provide immediate, temporary relief to persons with mild or intermittent symptoms. In addition, stretching and strengthening exercises can be helpful in people whose symptoms have abated. Behavioral interventions can also be used for individuals using excessive force in the performance of their work-related duties involving the hands (Feuerstein et al., 2004; Nicholas et al., 2005; Sullivan, Feuerstein, Gatchel, Linton, & Pransky, 2005). For example, feedback and training to use appropriate amounts of force and to promote self-management of rest breaks has been found to decrease CTS symptoms. In addition, the use of frequent *micro-breaks* during computer use can allow for sufficient muscle recovery while typing, and to allow for sustained performance without muscle fatigue and over-use symptoms (Henning et al., 1996; Henning, Jacques, Kissel, Sullivan, & Alteras-Webb, 1997). As with other treatments for WRMDS, little is known regarding the long-term effectiveness of these interventions. For chronic CTS, the best chance of decreasing pain, increasing function, and returning to work is likely to come from a multicomponent, interdisciplinary treatment approach (Gatchel & Okifuji, 2006; Gatchel et al., 2007; Schultz et al., 2007).

Surgical options for WRMDs of the hand and wrist vary widely and are one of the most commonly conducted surgical procedures in the USA (Huisstede et al., 2010). Generally, surgery is recommended if symptoms persist for 6 months after all conservative treatments have failed. Surgery involves severing the band of tissue around the wrist to reduce pressure on the median nerve. Although symptoms may be relieved immediately after surgery, full recovery from carpal tunnel surgery can take months as the wrist may lose strength because the carpal ligament was cut. Patients oftentimes undergo physical therapy after surgery to restore wrist strength. Recurrence of CTS following treatment is rare, as the majority of patients recover completely. This suggests that surgery may be a viable option for individuals suffering from chronic CTS symptoms.

Work-Related Musculoskeletal Disorders of the Lower Body

Lower Back

WRMDs of the lower back, as is the case with all other WRMDS, originate in the context of work and/or are exacerbated by occupational duties. Lifetime prevalence rates of low back pain are as high as 84 % in the general adult population (Cassidy, Carroll, & Côté, 1998). It is estimated that up to 95 %

of low back pain cases in the working population are the result of muscle, tendon, and ligament strain or sprain (Agency for Health Care Policy and Research, 1994). Health-care costs associated with low back pain were estimated at $85.9 billion in the USA in 2005 (Martin et al., 2008). However, the majority of cases are classified as "nonspecific" low back pain, as our current knowledge does not allow health care providers to determine, by clinical, laboratory, and/or imaging tests, the exact cause of pain in most cases. Multiple risk factors have been identified and are presented below.

Biomechanical Risk Factors

Most of the published literature examining biomechanical risk factors for work-related low back pain is based on cross-sectional data, thereby limiting our understanding of the potential causal relationships between work-related physical activity and low back pain. While some studies suggest an association between workplace biomechanical exposures such as heavy lifting, motor vehicle driving, and whole-body vibration, nonneutral postures and low back pain, methodological flaws prevent any inferences regarding causality (Marras et al., 2001; Punnett, Fine, Keyserling, Herrin, & Chaffin, 1991). A case–control study by Punnett et al. (1991) used detailed assessments of the postures of individual automobile assembly line workers and demonstrated a fivefold increase in low back pain risk from prolonged bending and twisting on the job. Similar work by Marras et al. (2001) also has demonstrated an increased risk among people working in jobs with higher biomechanical demands (a combination of lifting frequency, load moment, and trunk motion). In general, these studies have found that biomechanical factors produced large risk estimates, underscoring the risk associated with the physical demands of work in the context of low back pain.

Psychosocial Risk Factors

There is limited but growing empirical evidence linking psychosocial risk factors to the occurrence of low back pain (Hoogendoorn et al., 2000). However, the complex relationship between work-related psychosocial factors (such as job dissatisfaction) and the physical demands of work (such as spinal loading) make it difficult to reach definitive conclusions about their relative risk of developing low back disorders. Still, research suggests that high perceived workload and time pressure are related to low back pain. One of the most often cited studies conducted by Bigos et al. (1992) found that worker dissatisfaction was the only work-related risk factor associated with subsequent reporting of low back pain, while none of the variables assessing the physical demands of work significantly predicted back pain. Still, it may be premature to conclude that psychosocial factors are a more important predictor of low back pain than the physical demands of work given the paucity of corroborative research.

Individual Risk Factors

Observational studies have identified potential individual risk factors for low back pain, including younger age, female gender, smoking, and obesity (Garg & Moore, 1992; NIOSH, 1997). However, these risk factors are not unique to low back pain, as they also place workers at risk for other WRMDs. Additionally, the underlying mechanisms that account for the associations between low back pain and age, gender, smoking, and obesity are unknown. Further research is needed to clarify the relationship between individual risk factors and the various WRMDs described above before any conclusions regarding causality can be made.

Assessment and Diagnosis

The Clinical Efficacy Assessment Subcommittee of the American College of Physicians and the American Pain Society has established a clinical practice guideline for the assessment and diagnosis of low back pain through their *Low Back Pain Guidelines Panel* (Chou et al., 2007). These guidelines recommend that clinicians conduct a focused history and physical examination to help place patients with low back pain into one of three broad categories: (1) nonspecific low back pain, (2) back pain potentially associated with radiculopathy or spinal stenosis, or (3) back pain potentially associated with another specific spinal cause. The clinical assessment should include a review of psychosocial risk factors, which have been found to predict risk for chronic disabling back pain (Gatchel, Polatin, & Mayer, 1995). It is also recommended that clinicians *not* routinely obtain imaging or other diagnostic tests in patients with nonspecific low back pain. Imaging and other testing for patients with low back pain should only be conducted when severe or progressive neurologic deficits are present, or in cases when serious underlying conditions are suspected on the basis of history and physical examination.

Treatment Approaches

The *Low Back Pain Guidelines Panel* (Chou et al., 2007) also provides specific treatment recommendations for low back pain. The Panel recommends that clinicians consider the use of medications with proven benefits, in conjunction with back care information and self-care. The first-line medication options for most patients are acetaminophen or nonsteroidal anti-inflammatory drugs. The Panel also recommends that clinicians assess the severity of baseline pain and functional deficits, as well as the potential risks and benefits before initiating therapy. For patients who do not improve with self-care, the Panel recommends that clinicians consider the addition of non-pharmacologic therapy, such as intensive interdisciplinary rehabilitation, exercise therapy, cognitive-behavioral therapy, or progressive relaxation (Gatchel & Okifuji, 2006; Gatchel et al., 2003).

Knee, Foot, and Ankle

The majority of the WRMD research literature focuses on the upper limbs or lower back. By comparison, there has been limited research on disorders of the knee, ankle, and foot. The most likely explanation for this is the significantly higher prevalence of upper-extremity and lower-back WRMDs. A review of the available occupational literature suggests that certain disorders of the knee (e.g., bursitis, meniscal lesions or tears, and osteoarthritis), ankle (e.g., osteoarthritis), and foot (e.g., plantar fasciitis, heal pain, osteoarthritis) are more common among people in occupations with high physical demands, such as carpet and floor layers, painters, and construction workers (Kivimäki, Riihimäki, & Hanninen, 1994; Reid, 2010). Heel pain is the most common complaint presented to foot and ankle specialists and may be seen in upwards of 11–15 % of adults (Thomas et al., 2010). Heel pain most often has a mechanical pathology, but it can also include arthritic, neurologic, traumatic, or other systemic conditions.

Biomechanical Risk Factors

Biomechanical risk factors identified for the development of WMSD of the lower body include prolonged kneeling or squatting, climbing, and lifting heavy loads.

Psychosocial Risk Factors

There is limited research on psychosocial and occupational factors related to musculoskeletal knee, ankle, and foot disorders.

Individual Risk Factors

Individual risk factors, similar to those found among WRMDS of the upper body, have been identified in disorders of the lower body, including smoking and obesity (D'Souza, Franzblau, & Werner, 2005; Merlino, Rosecrance, Anton, & Cook, 2003). However, these associations are based on a very limited cross-sectional research base. As such, conclusions surrounding potential aggravating factors are hindered until further research is conducted.

Assessment and Diagnosis

Assessment and diagnosis of disorders of the knee, ankle, and foot are generally accomplished by orthopedic, foot, and ankle specialists according to a variety of clinical practice guidelines. A complete review of assessment and diagnosis approaches for all of the different WRMDs for the knee, ankle, and foot are beyond the scope of this Chapter.

Treatment Approaches

Treatments for such disorders of the knee, ankle, and foot parallel those of the upper limb in that the majority consist of rest, avoidance of aggravating activities, and analgesic use. More aggressive treatments are administered when conservative approaches fail and may include cortisone shots, physical therapy, and surgery. The American Academy of Orthopedic Surgeons (Richmond et al., 2009) has published a clinical practice guideline for the nonsurgical treatment of osteoarthritis of the knee. The guidelines recommend that patients with symptomatic osteoarthritis of the knee participate in self-management educational programs and engage in self-care. Self-care consists primarily of weight loss, engaging in regular physical exercise, and quadriceps strengthening. The guideline also recommends taping of the knee for short-term pain relief, as well as the use of analgesics and intra-articular corticosteroids. The guidelines do not recommend the use of glucosamine or chondroitin.

Heel pain is one of the most common forms of foot pain. The American College of Foot and Ankle Surgeons Heel Pain Committee has published clinical practice guidelines for the diagnosis and treatment of heel pain (Thomas et al., 2010). The Clinical Practice Guideline outlines three tiers of treatment for heel pain. The first tier includes conservative treatments, such as stretching, home-based physical therapy, over-the counter orthotics, and oral anti-inflammatory medication. Second tier treatments include corticosteroid injections, prescriptive physical therapy, and custom orthotics. Surgery for heel pain is included in the third tier, and is only recommended for chronic symptoms and after more conservative treatments have been used for at least 6 months. However, the long-term effectiveness of most of these interventions for pain resulting from WRMDs of the lower limbs has yet to be determined. Clearly, further high-quality research to include prospective studies and intervention trials is needed in this area.

Summary

WRMDs are painful afflictions that result from injury to or dysfunction of nerves, tendons, and muscles largely due to repetitive movements and/or prolonged nonneutral postures required by the work environment. Epidemiological data suggest that WRMDs, such as muscle strains, low back pain, and CTS, account for the vast majority occupational diseases in the USA. In fact, these disorders account for more human suffering, loss of productivity, and economic burden than any other condition. The establishment of a causal relationship between musculoskeletal disorders and occupational duties remains a source of significant controversy. Research suggests that multiple factors (e.g., physical, occupational, organizational, psychosocial, individual, and sociocultural) contribute to the development and maintenance of such disorders. Researchers and clinicians have tested and utilized a wide variety of interventions to include conservative approaches, such as ergonomic modifications, and more invasive procedures, such as surgery. The short- and long-term effectiveness of such interventions varies greatly across conditions. Furthermore research investigating causal mechanisms and potential sources of intervention is necessary in order to limit the disabling and costly effects of these conditions.

Recommendations for Future Research

As people live longer and the average age of the US work force increases, the impact of aging on work-related loading, tolerance, psychosocial stress, and their interactions must be better investigated. Traditionally, high-force, highly repetitive loading of the musculoskeletal system has been the hallmark of work. However, the workplace and the nature of the work are changing rapidly and, as a result, so are the type and frequency of WRMDs. For instance, the number of employees working on a traditional assembly line is decreasing. However, those who remain employed in these environments are increasingly exposed to more frequent but less forceful motions (Punnett et al., 1991). Collectively, these trends indicate that the nature of physical exposure is rapidly evolving to a low force, highly repetitive environment (Westgaard & Winkel, 1997). Improved quantification of physical risk factors, rather than reliance on self-reported measures, would strengthen our knowledge of the relationship between various types of exposure and development of WRMDs (Waters, Dick, Davis-Barkley, & Krieg, 2007). Furthermore, studies evaluating the quantitative link among epidemiological, biomechanical, individual, and psychosocial factors should be pursued to establish a better understanding of the pathways of injury and resultant preventive strategies. Moreover, problems such as different diagnostic criteria (due to lack of a gold standard for the clinical diagnosis of most WRMD), different outcome assessments, and different methods for measuring exposure make the establishment of risk factors a very difficult task to accomplish (Punnett & Wegman, 2004). It is recommended that multidisciplinary investigators collaborate in order to standardize the conduct, assessment, and reporting of WMSD research trials. Finally, a continuing need exists for high-quality randomized clinical trials (Frank et al., 1996). In summary, understanding the current body of WRMDs research, and the identification of research gaps, is necessary for the development of more robust and clinically relevant models for assessment and treatment. This will aid in better workplace design, exposure assessments, diagnosis and, ultimately, lower risk, reduced medical costs, and healthier workers.

Acknowledgment We would like to thank Julie Collins for her editorial support in preparation of this book chapter.

References

Agency for Health Care Policy and Research. (1994). *Clinical Practice Guideline Number 14: Acute low back problems in adults*. Rockville, MD: U.S. Department of Health and Human Services.

Amoroso, P. J., & Canham, M. L. (1999). Chapter 4: Disabilities related to the musculoskeletal system: Physical Evaluation Board data. In P. J. Jones, P. J. Amoroso, M. L. Canham, M. B. Weyandt, & J. B. Schmitt (Eds.), *Atlas of injuries in the U.S. Armed Forces. Military medicine, 164*(8 suppl), 4-1 to 4-73. Retrieved from http://www.dtic.mil/cgi-bin/GetTRDoc?AD=ADA367256&Location=U2&doc=GetTRDoc.pdf

Andersen, J. H., Thomsen, J. F., Overgaard, E., Lassen, C. F., Brandt, L. P., Vilstrup, I., et al. (2003). Computer use and carpal tunnel syndrome: A 1-year follow-up study. *Journal of the American Medical Association, 289*, 2963–2969. doi:10.1001/jama.289.22.2963.

Atroshi, I., Gummesson, C., Johnsson, R., Ornstein, E., Ranstam, J., & Rosén, I. (1999). Prevalence of carpal tunnel syndrome in a general population. *Journal of the American Medical Association, 282*, 153–158. doi:10.1001/jama.282.2.153.

Barr, A. E., Barbe, M. F., & Clark, B. D. (2004). Work-related musculoskeletal disorders of the hand and wrist: Epidemiology, pathophysiology, and sensorimotor changes. *Journal of Orthopedic and Sports Physical Therapy, 34*, 610–627. Retrieved from http://www.jospt.org/.

Bigos, S. J., Battié, M. C., Spengler, D. M., Fisher, L. D., Fordyce, W. E., Hannson, T., et al. (1992). A longitudinal, prospective study of industrial back injury reporting. *Clinical Orthopaedics and Related Research, 279*, 21–34. Retrieved from http://www.springer.com/medicine/orthopedics/journal/11999.

Bisset, L., Paungmali, A., Vicenzino, B., & Beller, E. (2005). A systematic review and meta-analysis of clinical trials on physical interventions for lateral epicondylalgia. *British Journal of Sports Medicine, 39*, 411–422. doi:10.1136/bjsm.2004.016170.

Bland, J. D. P. (2005). The relationship of obesity, age, and carpal tunnel syndrome: More complex than was thought? *Muscle and Nerve, 32*, 527–532. doi:10.1002/mus.20408.

Boocock, M. G., Mcnair, P. J., Larmer, P. J., Armostrong, B., Collier, J., Simmonds, M., & Garrett, N. (2007). Interventions for the prevention and management of the neck/upper extremity musculoskeletal conditions: a systemic review. *Occupational and Environmental Medicine, 64*, 291–303. doi:10.1136/oem.2005.025593.

Bot, S. D. M., van der Waal, J. M., Terwee, C. B., van der Windt, D. A., Schellevis, F. G., Bouter, L. M., & Dekker, J. (2005). Incidence and prevalence of complaints of the neck and upper extremity in general practice. *Annals of the Rheumatic Diseases, 64*, 118–123. doi:10.1136/ard.2003.019349.

Buckle, P., & Devereux, J. (1999). *Work-related neck and upper limb musculoskeletal disorders*. Luxembourg: European Agency for Safety and Health at Work.

Buckle, P. W., & Devereux, J. J. (2002). The nature of work-related and upper limb musculoskeletal disorders. *Applied Ergonomics, 33*, 202–217. Retrieved from.

Bureau of Labor Statistics. (2010). *Workplace injuries and illnesses—2010: Annual report*. Washington, DC: United States Department of Labor.

Burt, S., Crombie, K., Jin, Y., Wurzelbacher, S., Ramsey, J., & Deddens, J. (2011). Workplace and individual risk factors for carpal tunnel syndrome. *Occupational and Environmental Medicine, 61*, 928–933. doi:10.1136/oem.2010.063677.

Cagnie, B., Danneels, L., Van Tiggelen, D., De Loose, V., & Cambier, D. (2007). Individual and work related risk factors for neck pain among office workers: a cross sectional study. *European Spine Journal, 16*(5), 679–686. doi:10.1007/s00586-006-0269-7.

Cassidy, J. D., Carroll, L. J., & Côté, P. (1998). The Saskatchewan health and back pain survey: The prevalence of low back pain and related disability in Saskatchewan adults. *Spine, 23*, 1860–1866. doi:10.1097/00007632-199809010-00012.

Chou, R., Qaseem, A., Snow, V., Casey, D., Cross, T., Jr., Shekelle, P., et al. (2007). Diagnosis and treatment of low back pain: A joint clinical practice guideline from the American College of Physicians and the American Pain Society. *Annals of Internal Medicine, 147*, 478–491. Retrieved from http://www.annals.org/.

Chung, K. C., Pillsbury, M. S., Walters, M. R., & Hayward, R. A. (1998). Reliability and validity testing of the Michigan Hand Outcomes Questionnaire. *The Journal of Hand Surgery, 23*, 575–587. doi:10.1016/s0363-5023(98)80042-7.

da Costa, B. R., & Vieira, E. R. (2010). Risk factors for work-related musculoskeletal disorders: A systematic review of recent longitudinal studies. *American Journal of Industrial Medicine, 53*, 285–323. doi:10.1992/ajim.20750.

Dale, A. M., Descatha, A., Coomes, J., Franzblau, A., & Evanoff, B. (2010). Physical examination has a low yield in screening for carpal tunnel syndrome. *American Journal of Industrial Medicine*. doi:10.1002/ajim.20915.

Dias, J. J., Bhowal, B., Wildin, C. J., & Thompson, J. R. (2001). Assessing the outcome of disorders of the hand. Is the patient evaluation measure reliable, valid, responsive and without bias? *Journal of Bone and Joint Surgery, 83*, 235. doi:10.1302/0301-620X.83B2.10838.

D'Souza, J. C., Franzblau, A., & Werner, R. A. (2005). Review of epidemiologic studies on occupational factors and lower extremity musculoskeletal and vascular disorders and symptoms. *Journal of Occupational Rehabilitation, 15*, 129–165. doi:10.1007/s10926-005-1215-y.

Dubner, R., & Ruda, M. A. (1992). Activity-dependent neuronal plasticity following tissue injury and inflammation. *Trends in Neurosciences, 15*, 96–103. doi:10.1016/0166-2236(92)90019-5.

Feuerstein, M., & Fitzgerald, T. E. (1992). Biomechanical factors affecting upper extremity cumulative trauma disorders in sign language interpreters. *Journal of Occupational and Environmental Medicine, 34*, 257–264. doi:10.1097/00043764-199203000-00009.

Feuerstein, M., Armstrong, T., Hickey, P., & Lincoln, A. (1997). Computer keyboard force and upper extremity symptoms. *Journal of Occupational and Environmental Medicine, 39*, 1144–1153. doi:10.1097/00043764-199712000-00008.

Feuerstein, M., Berkowitz, S. M., & Peck, C. A., Jr. (1997). Musculoskeletal-related disability in US Army personnel: Prevalence, gender, and military occupational specialties. *Journal of Occupational and Environmental Medicine, 39*, 68–78. doi:10.1097/00043764-199701000-00013.

Feuerstein, M., Nicholas, R. A., Huang, G. D., Dimberg, L., Ali, D., & Rogers, H. (2004). Job stress management and ergonomic intervention for work-related upper extremity symptoms. *Applied Ergonomics, 35*, 565–574. doi:10.1016/j.apergo.2004.05.003.

Finsen, L., Christensen, H., & Bakke, M. (1998). Musculoskeletal disorders among dentists and variation in dental work. *Applied Ergonomics, 29*, 119–125. Retrieved from http://www.journals.elsevier.com/applied-ergonomics/.

Foley, M., Silverstein, B., & Polissar, N. (2007). The economic burden of carpal tunnel syndrome: long-term earnings of CTS claimants in Washington state. *American Journal of Industrial Medicine, 50*, 155–172. doi:10.1002/ajim.20430.

Foley, M., Silverstein, B., Polissar, N., & Neradilek, B. (2009). Impact of implementing the Washington state ergonomics rule on employer reported risk factors and hazard reduction activity. *American Journal of Industrial Medicine, 52*(1), 1–16.

Frank, J. W., Pulcins, J. R., Kerr, M. S., Shannon, H. S., & Stansfeld, S. A. (1995). Occupational back pain: An unhelpful polemic. *Scandinavian Journal of Work, Environment and Health, 21*, 3–14. doi:10.5271/sjweh.2.

Frank, J. W., Kerr, M. S., Brooker, A.-S., DeMaio, S. E., Maetzel, A., Shannon, H. S., et al. (1996). Disability resulting from occupational low back pain: Part I: What do we know about primary prevention? A review of the scientific evidence on prevention before disability begins. *Spine, 21*, 2908–2917. doi:10.1097/00007632-199612150-00024.

Garg, A., & Moore, J. S. (1992). Epidemiology of low-back pain in industry. *Occupational Medicine, 7*, 593–608.

Gatchel, R. J., & Okifuji, A. (2006). Evidence-based scientific data documenting the treatment and cost-effectiveness of comprehensive pain programs for chronic nonmalignant pain. *The Journal of Pain, 7*, 779–793.

Gatchel, R. J., Polatin, P. B., & Mayer, T. G. (1995). The dominant role of psychosocial risk factors in the development of chronic low back pain disability. *Spine, 20*, 2702–2709.

Gatchel, R. J., Polatin, P. B., Noe, C., Gardea, M., Pulliam, C., & Thompson, J. (2003). Treatment- and cost-effectiveness of early intervention for acute low-back pain patients: A one-year prospective study. *Journal of Occupational Rehabilitation, 13*, 1–9.

Gatchel, R. J., Peng, Y. B., Peters, M. L., Fuchs, P. N., & Turk, D. C. (2007). The biopsychosocial approach to chronic pain: scientific advances and future directions. *Psychological Bulletin, 133*, 581–624.

Greenslade, J. R., Mehta, R. L., Belward, P., & Warwick, D. J. (2004). DASH and Boston questionnaire assessment of carpal tunnel syndrome outcome: What is the responsiveness of an outcome questionnaire? *The Journal of Hand Surgery: British and European Volume, 29*, 159–164. doi:10.1016/j.jhsb.2003.10.010.

Griffiths, K. L., Mackey, M. G., & Adamson, B. J. (2007). The impact of a computerized work environment on professional occupational groups and behavioural and physiological risk factors for musculoskeletal symptoms: A literature review. *Journal of Occupational Rehabilitation, 17*, 743–765.

Guez, M., Hildingsson, C., Nilsson, M., & Toolanen, G. (2002). The prevalence of neck pain. *Acta Orthopaedica, 73*, 455–459. doi:10.1080/00016470216329.

Harrington, C. B., & Feuerstein, M. (2010). Workstyle in office workers: Ergonomic and psychological reactivity to work demands. *Journal of Occupational and Environmental Medicine, 52*, 375–382. doi:10.1097/JOM.0b013e3181d5e51d.

Henning, R. A., Callaghan, E. A., Ortega, A. M., Kissel, G. V., Guttman, J. I., & Braun, H. A. (1996). Continuous feedback to promote self-management of rest breaks during computer use. *International Journal of Industrial Ergonomics, 18*, 71–82. doi:10.1016/0169-8141(95)00032-1.

Henning, R. A., Jacques, P., Kissel, G. V., Sullivan, A. B., & Alteras-Webb, S. (1997). Frequent short rest breaks from computer work: Effects on productivity and well-being at two field sites. *Ergonomics, 40*, 78–91. doi:10.1080/001401397188396.

Hildebrandt, V. H., Bongers, P. M., Dul, J., van Dijk, F. J., & Kemper, H. C. (2000). The relationship between leisure time, physical activities and musculoskeletal symptoms and disability in worker populations. *International Archives of Occupational and Environmental Health, 73*, 507–518. doi:10.1007/s004200000167.

Hoogendoorn, W. E., van Poppel, M. N. M., Bongers, P. M., Koes, B. W., & Bouter, L. M. (2000). Systematic review of psychosocial factors at work and private life as risk factors for back pain. *Spine, 25*, 2114–2125. doi:10.1097/00007632-200008150-00017.

Huang, G. D., Feuerstein, M., & Sauter, S. L. (2002). Occupational stress and work-related upper extremity disorders: Concepts and models. *American Journal of Industrial Medicine, 41*, 298–314. doi:10.1002/ajim.10045.

Huisstede, B. M., Randsdorp, M. S., Coert, J. H., Glerum, S., van Middelkoop, M., & Koes, B. W. (2010). Carpal tunnel syndrome. Part II: Effectiveness of surgical treatments: A systematic review. *Archives of Physical Medicine and Rehabilitation, 91*, 1005–1024. doi:10.1016/j.apmr.2010.03.023.

Hurwitz, E. L., Carragee, E. J., van der Velde, G., Carroll, L. J., Nordin, M., Guzman, J., et al. (2008). Treatment of neck pain: Noninvasive interventions: Results of the bone and joint decade 2000–2010 task force on neck pain and its associated disorders. *Spine, 33*(4S), S123–S152. doi:10.1097/BRS.0b013e3181644b1d.

Jones, B. H., Amoroso, P. J., Canham, M. L., Schmitt, J. B., & Weyandt, M. B. (1999). Chapter 9: Conclusions and recommendations of the DoD Injury Surveillance and Prevention Work Group. In P. J. Jones, P. J. Amoroso, M. L. Canham, M. B. Weyandt, & J. B. Schmitt (Eds.), *Atlas of injuries in the U.S. Armed Forces. Military medicine, 164* (8 suppl), 9-1 to 9-26. Retrieved from http://www.dtic.mil/cgi-bin/GetTRDoc?AD=ADA367256&Location=U2&doc=GetTRDoc.pdf

Katz, J. N., Lew, R. A., Bessette, L., Punnett, L., Fossel, A. H., Mooney, N., & Keller, R. B. (1998). Prevalence and predictors of long-term work disability due to carpal tunnel syndrome. *American Journal of Industrial Medicine, 33*, 543–550. doi:10.1002/(sici)1097-0274(199806)33:6<543::aid-ajim4>3.0.co;2-r.

Kennedy, C. A., Amick, B. C., III, Dennerlein, J. T., Brewer, S., Catli, S., Williams, R., et al. (2010). Systematic review of the role of occupational health and safety interventions in the prevention of upper extremity musculoskeletal symptoms, signs, disorders, injuries, claims and lost time. *Journal of Occupational Rehabilitation, 20*, 127–162. doi:10.1007/s10926-009-9211-2.

Kivimäki, J., Riihimäki, H., & Hanninen, K. (1994). Knee disorders in carpet and floor layers and painters: Part II: Knee symptoms and patellofemoral indices. *Scandinavian Journal of Rehabilitation Medicine, 26*, 97–101.

Korhonen, T., Ketola, R., Toivonen, R., Luukkonen, R., Häkkänen, M., & Viikari-Juntura, E. (2003). Work related and individual predictors for incident neck pain among office employees working with video display units. *Occupational and Environmental Medicine, 60*, 475–482. doi:10.1136/oem.60.7.475.

Krause, N., Dasinger, L. K., & Neuhauser, F. (1998). Modified work and return to work: A review of the literature. *Journal of Occupational Rehabilitation, 8*, 113–139. doi:10.1023/a:1023015622987.

Kurppa, K., Viikari-Juntura, E., & Kuosma, E. (1991). Incidence of tenosynovitis or peritendinitis and epicondylitis in a meat-processing factory. *Scandinavian Journal of Work, Environment and Health, 17*, 32–37. doi:10.5271/sjweh.1737.

Lawrence, R. C., Felson, D. T., Helmick, C. G., Arnold, L. M., Choi, H., Deyo, R. A., et al. (2008). Estimates of the prevalence of arthritis and other rheumatic conditions in the United States: Part II. *Arthritis and Rheumatism, 58*, 26–35. doi:10.1002/art.23176.

Leclerc, A., Niedhammer, I., Landre, M. F., Ozguler, A., Etore, P., & Pietri-Taleb, F. (1999). One-year predictive factors for various aspects of neck disorders. *Spine, 24*, 1455–1462. doi:10.1097/00007632-199907150-00011.

Leon, L., Jover, J. A., Candelas, G., Lajas, C., Vadillo, C., Blanco, M., et al. (2009). Effectiveness of an early cognitive-behavioral treatment in patients with work disability due to musculoskeletal disorders. *Arthritis Care and Research, 61*, 996–1003. doi:10.1002/art.24609.

Levine, D. W., Simmons, B. P., Koris, M. J., Daltroy, L. H., Hohl, G. G., & Fossel, A. H. (1993). A self-administered questionnaire for the assessment of severity of symptoms and functional status in carpal tunnel syndrome. *Journal of Bone and Joint Surgery, 75*, 1585–1592. Retrieved from http://www.jbjs.org.

Leyshon, R., Chalova, K., Gerson, L., Savtchenko, A., Zakrzewski, R., Howie, A., & Shaw, L. (2010). Ergonomic interventions for office workers with musculoskeletal disorders: A systematic review. *Work, 35*, 335–338. doi:10.3233/WOR-2010-0994.

Maayah, M., & Al-Jarrah, M. (2010). Evaluation of transcutaneous electrical nerve stimulation as a treatment of neck pain due to musculoskeletal disorders. *Journal of Clinical Medicine Research, 2*, 127–136. doi:10.4021/jocmr2010.06.370e.

Macfarlane, G. J., Pallewatte, N., Paudyal, P., Blyth, F. M., Coggon, D., Crombez, G., et al. (2009). Evaluation of work-related psychosocial factors and regional musculoskeletal pain: Results from a EULAR Task Force. *Annals of the Rheumatic Diseases, 68*, 885–891. doi:10.1136/ard.2008.090829.

Malchaire, J., Cock, N., & Vergracht, S. (2001). Review of the factors associated with musculoskeletal problems in epidemiological studies. *International Archives of Occupational and Environmental Health, 74*, 79–90. doi:10.1007/s004200000212.

Malchaire, J. M., Roquelaure, Y. R., Cock, N. C., Piette, A. P., Vergracht, S. V., & Chiron, H. C. (2001). Musculoskeletal complaints, functional capacity, personality and psychosocial factors. *International Archives of Occupational and Environmental Health, 74*, 549–557. doi:10.1007/s004200100264.

Marcus, M., Gerr, F., Monteilh, C., Ortiz, D. J., Gentry, E., Cohen, S., et al. (2002). A prospective study of computer users: II. Postural risk factors for musculoskeletal symptoms and disorders. *American Journal of Industrial Medicine, 41*, 236–249. doi:10.1002/ajim.10067.

Marras, W. S., Davis, K. G., Ferguson, S. A., Lucas, B. R., & Gupta, P. (2001). Spine loading characteristics of patients with low back pain compared with asymptomatic individuals. *Spine, 26*, 2566–2574. doi:10.1097/00007632-200112010-00009.

Marras, W. S., Cutlip, R. G., Burt, S. E., & Waters, T. R. (2009). National Occupational Research Agenda (NORA) future directions in occupational musculoskeletal disorder health research. *Applied Ergonomics, 40*, 15–22. doi:10.1016/j.apergo.2008.01.018.

Martin, B. I., Deyo, R. A., Mirza, S. K., Turner, J. A., Comstock, B. A., Hollingworth, W., & Sullivan, S. D. (2008). Expenditures and health status among adults with back and neck problems. *Journal of the American Medical Association, 299*, 656–664. doi:10.1001/jama.299.6.656.

McCarson, K. E. (1999). Central and peripheral expression of neurokinin-1 and neurokinin-3 receptor and substance P-encoding messenger RNAs: Peripheral regulation during formalin-induced inflammation and lack of neurokinin receptor expression in primary afferent sensory neurons. *Neuroscience, 93*, 361–370. doi:10.1016/S0306-4522(99)00102-5.

Merlino, L. A., Rosecrance, J. C., Anton, D., & Cook, T. M. (2003). Symptoms of musculoskeletal disorders among apprentice construction workers. *Applied Occupational and Environmental Hygiene, 18*, 57–64. doi:10.1080/10473220301391.

Moore, J. S. (1992). Carpal tunnel syndrome. *Occupational Medicine, 7*, 741–763.

Morse, T., Bruneau, H., Michalak-Turcotte, C., Sanders, M., Warren, N., Dussetschleger, J., et al. (2007). Musculoskeletal disorders of the neck and shoulder in dental hygienists and dental hygiene students. *Journal of Dental Hygiene, 81*(1), 10. Retrieved from http://adha.publisher.ingentaconnect.com/content/adha/jdh.

National Institutes of Health (NIH) Consensus Development Panel on Acupuncture. (1998). Acupuncture. *Journal of the American Medical Association, 280*, 1518–1524. doi:10.1001/jama.280.17.1518.

National Institute of Occupational Safety and Health (NIOSH), Centers for Disease Control and Prevention, Public Health Service, U.S. Department of Health and Human Services. (1997). *Musculoskeletal disorders and workplace factors. A critical review of epidemiologic evidence for work-related musculoskeletal disorders of the neck, upper extremity, and low back* (DHHS [NIOSH] Publication No. 97–41). Retrieved from http://www.cdc.gov/niosh/docs/97-141/.

National Institute of Occupational Safety and Health (NIOSH), Centers for Disease Control and Prevention, Public Health Service, U.S. Department of Health and Human Services. (2001). *National occupational research agenda: Research topics for the next decade* (DHHS [NIOSH] Publication No. 2001–117). Retrieved from http://www.cdc.gov/niosh/docs/2001-117/.

National Research Council (NRC). (1999). *Work related musculoskeletal disorders: Report, workshop summary, and workshop papers*. Washington, DC: National Academy Press. Retrieved from http://www.nap.edu/openbook.php?record_id=6431&page=R1.

Nicholas, R. A., Feuerstein, M., & Suchday, S. (2005). Workstyle and upper-extremity symptoms: A biobehavioral perspective. *Journal of Occupational and Environmental Medicine, 47*, 352–361. doi:10.1097/01.jom.0000158705.50563.4c.

Nordin, M., Carragee, E. J., Hogg-Johnson, S., Weiner, S. S., Hurwitz, E. L., Peloso, P. M., et al. (2009). Assessment of neck pain and its associated disorders: Results of the bone and joint decade 2000–2010 task force on neck pain and its associated disorders. *Journal of Manipulative and Physiological Therapeutics, 32*(2 Suppl), S117–S140. doi:10.1016/j.jmpt.2008.11.016.

Nordstrom, D. L., Vierkant, R. A., DeStefano, F., & Layde, P. M. (1997). Risk factors for carpal tunnel syndrome in a general population. *Occupational and Environmental Medicine, 54*, 734–740. doi:10.1136/oem.54.10.734.

Palmer, K. T. (2011). Carpal tunnel syndrome: The role of occupational factors. *Best Practice and Research. Clinical Rheumatology, 25*, 15–29. doi:10.1016/j.berh.2011.01.014.

Park, G. Y., Lee, S. M., & Lee, M. Y. (2008). Diagnostic value of ultrasonography for clinical medial epicondylitis. *Archives of Physical Medicine and Rehabilitation, 89*, 738–742. doi:10.1016/j.apmr.2007.09.048.

Patijn, J., Vallejo, R., Janssen, M., Huygen, F., Lataster, A., van Kleef, M., & Mekhail, N. (2011). Carpal tunnel syndrome. *Pain Practice, 11*, 297–301. doi:10.1111/j.1533-2500.2011.00457.x.

Pransky, G., Feuerstein, M., Himmelstein, J., Katz, J. N., & Vickers-Lahti, M. (1997). Measuring functional outcomes in work-related upper extremity disorders: Development and validation of the upper extremity function scale. *Journal of Occupational and Environmental Medicine, 39*, 1195–1202. doi:10.1097/00043764-199712000-00014.

Punnett, L., Fine, L. J., Keyserling, W. M., Herrin, G. D., & Chaffin, D. B. (1991). Back disorders and nonneutral trunk postures of automobile assembly worker. *Scandinavian Journal of Work, Environment and Health, 17*, 337–346. doi:10.5271/sjweh.1700.

Punnett, L., & Wegman, D. H. (2004). Work-related musculoskeletal disorders: The epidemiologic evidence and the debate. *Journal of Electromyography and Kinesiology, 14*(1), 13–23.

Reid, C. R. (2010). A review of occupational knee disorders. *Journal of Occupational Rehabilitation, 20*, 489–501. doi:10.1007/s10926-010-9242-8.

Richmond, J., Hunter, D., Irrgang, J., Jones, M. H., Levy, B., Marx, R., et al. (2009). Treatment of osteoarthritis of the knee (nonarthroplasty). *Journal of the American Academy of Orthopaedic Surgeons, 17*, 591–600. Retrieved from http://www.jaaos.org/.

Schultz, I. Z., Stowell, A. W., Feuerstein, M., & Gatchel, R. J. (2007). Models of return to work for musculoskeletal disorders. *Journal of Occupational Rehabilitation, 17*, 327–352. doi:10.1007/s10926-007-9071-6.

Sengupta, I., Reno, V., & Burton, J. F. (2009). *Workers' compensation: Benefits, coverage, and cost*. Washington, DC: National Academy of Social Insurance. Retrieved from www.nasi.org/research/workers-compensation.

Shiri, R., Viikari-Juntura, E., Varonen, H., & Heliövaara, M. (2006). Prevalence and determinants of lateral and medial epicondylitis: A population study. *American Journal of Epidemiology, 164*, 1065–1074. doi:10.1093/aje/kwj325.

Silverstein, B., & Adams, D. (2007). *Work-related musculoskeletal disorders of the neck, back, and upper extremity in Washington State, 1997–2005 Technical Report Number 40-11-2007*. Washington, DC: Washington State Department of Labor & Industries.

Smidt, N., van der Windt, D. A., Assendelft, W. J., Devillé, W. L., Korthals-de Bos, I. B., & Bouter, L. M. (2002). Corticosteroid injections, physiotherapy, or a wait-and-see policy for lateral epicondylitis: A randomised controlled trial. *The Lancet, 359*(9307), 657–662. doi:10.1016/S0140-6736(02)07811-X.

Struijs, P. A., Smidt, N., Arola, H., van Dijk, C. N., Buchbinder, R., & Assendelft, W. J. (2001). Orthotic devices for tennis elbow: A systematic review. *British Journal of General Practice, 51*, 924–992. Retrieved from http://www.rcgp.org.uk/brjgenpract.aspx.

Sullivan, M. J., Feuerstein, M., Gatchel, R., Linton, S. J., & Pransky, G. (2005). Integrating psychosocial and behavioral interventions to achieve optimal rehabilitation outcomes. *Journal of Occupational Rehabilitation, 15*, 475–489. doi:10.1007/s10926-005-8029-9.

Szabo, R. M. (1998). Carpal tunnel syndrome as a repetitive motion disorder. *Clinical Orthopaedics and Related Research, 351*, 78–89. doi:10.1097/00003086-199806000-00011.

Thomas, J. L., Christensen, J. C., Kravitz, S. R., Mendicino, R. W., Schuberth, J. M., Vanore, J. V., et al. (2010). The diagnosis and treatment of heel pain: A clinical practice guideline-revision 2010. *The Journal of Foot and Ankle Surgery, 49*(3 Suppl), S1–S19. doi:10.1053/j.jfas.2010.01.001.

Trudel, D., Duley, J., Zastrow, I., Kerr, E. W., Davidson, R., & MacDermid, J. C. (2004). Rehabilitation for patients with lateral epicondylitis: A systematic review. *Journal of Hand Therapy, 17*, 243–266. doi:10.1197/j.jht.2004.02.011.

van Eijsden-Besseling, M. D. F., Peeters, F. P. M. L., Reijnen, J. A. W., & de Bie, R. A. (2004). Perfectionism and coping strategies as risk factors for the development of non-specific work-related upper limb disorders (WRULD). *Occupational Medicine, 54*, 122–127. doi:10.1093/occmed/kqh003.

van Rijn, R. M., Huisstede, B. M. A., Koes, B. W., & Burdorf, A. (2010). Associations between work-related factors and specific disorders of the shoulder—a systematic review of the literature. *Scandinavian Journal of Work, Environment and Health, 36*, 189–201. doi:10.5271/sjweh.2895.

Verhaar, J. A. N. (1994). Tennis elbow: Anatomical, epidemiological and therapeutic aspects. *International Orthopaedics, 18*, 263–267. doi:10.1007/BF00180221.

Viikari-Juntura, E., & Silverstein, B. (1999). Role of physical load factors in carpal tunnel syndrome. *Scandinavian Journal of Work, Environment and Health, 25*(3), 163–185. doi:10.5271/sjweh.423.

Viikari-Juntura, E., Martikainen, R., Luukkonen, R., Mutanen, P., Takala, E. P., & Riihimäki, H. (2001). Longitudinal study on work related and individual risk factors affecting radiating neck pain. *Occupational and Environmental Medicine, 58*, 345–352. doi:10.1136/oem.58.5.345.

Waters, T. R., Dick, R. B., Davis-Barkley, J., & Krieg, E. F. (2007). A cross-sectional study of risk factors for musculoskeletal symptoms in the workplace using data from the General Social Survey (GSS). *Journal of Occupational and Environmental Medicine, 49*, 172–184. doi:10.1097/JOM.0b013e3180322559.

Westgaard, R. H., & Winkel, J. (1997). Ergonomic intervention research for improved musculoskeletal health: A critical review. *International Journal of Industrial Ergonomics, 20*, 463–500. doi:10.1016/S0169-8141(96)00076-5.

World Health Organization (WHO) Expert Committee on Identification and Control of Work-Related Diseases. (1985). *Identification and control of work-related diseases: Report of a WHO expert committee*. Geneva: World Health Organization.

Cardiovascular Disease and the Workplace

5

Alexandra L. Terrill and John P. Garofalo

Overview

Cardiovascular disease (CVD) is the leading cause of morbidity and mortality worldwide, representing 30 % of all global deaths. According to the American Heart Association (AHA), roughly one out of three Americans has some form of CVD, including high blood pressure and coronary heart disease (CHD). The total direct and indirect cost of CVD is an estimated $300 billion in the USA in 2007 alone (Roger et al., 2011). These numbers are expected to rise in the next decade, thereby underscoring the need to identify contributing mechanisms to the pathogenesis of all forms of CVD. Several models proposed to date have framed their findings examining the interaction between physiological mechanisms and psychosocial factors, replacing the outdated view that biological mechanisms alone account for this national epidemic.

CVD affect heart and blood vessels and usually have similar risk factors and mechanisms, with *atherosclerosis* as a common underlying cause. *Atherosclerosis* is a chronic inflammatory response that involves thickening and hardening of arterial walls due to plaque formation (Ross, 1999). Characteristic of CHD, the most common form of CVD, as the plaque enlarges, blood flow to the heart is reduced, which may cause insufficient blood flow to the heart tissue (i.e., *ischemia*) leading to chest discomfort and myocardial infarction (MI: heart attack). In addition, the plaque may rupture, creating a thrombus or a particle that may become lodged downstream creating an acute ischemic event distal to the blockage.

In addition to traditional risk factors, including but not limited to hypertension, hypercholesterolemia, and smoking, compelling evidence supports psychosocial risk factors as significant determinants of CVD development, progression, and morbidity and mortality (Chida & Hamer, 2008; Everson-Rose & Lewis, 2005; Smith & Ruiz, 2002). The psychosocial factor consistently linked with CVD and other health outcomes is stress (e.g., Chida & Hamer; Segerstrom & Miller, 2004).

A.L. Terrill, Ph.D. • J.P. Garofalo, Ph.D. (✉)
Department of Psychology, Washington State University Vancouver,
14204 NE Salmon Creek Avenue, Vancouver, WA 98686-9600, USA
e-mail: jgarofalo@vancouver.wsu.edu

Work-related stress is the most often studied source of chronic stress (Rozanski, Blumenthal, & Kaplan, 1999), and research findings indicate a strong association between this type of chronic stress and CVD, including atherosclerosis (Bosma, Peter, Siegrist, & Marmot, 1998; Lynch, Krause, Kaplan, Salonen, & Salonen, 1997) and the prediction of cardiac events (Aboa-Eboule et al., 2007; Karasek et al., 1988; Theorell et al., 1998). According to a recent comprehensive meta-analysis of prospective cohort studies, work stress is associated with ~50 % excess risk of CHD (Kivimäki et al., 2006). The central goal of this chapter is to review the role of work-related stress in CVD.

Models of Work Stress and Cardiovascular Disease

Two theoretical models—the "job strain" model and the "effort–reward imbalance (ERI)" model—have received the most attention in research on chronic psychosocial stress in the work environment and CVD. Literature reviews indicate that, in most cases, either the full models or their components are associated with increased CVD risk (Eller et al., 2009; Kivimäki et al., 2006; Siegrist, 2005).

Job Strain Model

The job strain, or demand-control, model posited by Karasek, Baker, Marxer, Ahlbom, and Theorell (1981) is the most widely used conceptual framework used to evaluate the effect of psychosocial factors in the work environment on cardiovascular health. It should be noted that another chapter in this Handbook, by Theorell, has summarized a great deal of this work. Karasek developed this model for work environment stressors that do not present initially as life-threatening but, instead, represent a chronic source of stress as a product of the ongoing sophisticated human organizational decision-making process (1979). The model comprises two components: psychological demands and decision latitude (or control). The concept of psychological demands refers to the quantity of work, mental requirements, and time constraints, and may be defined by questions such as "working very fast," "working very hard," and not "enough time to get the job done." Job decision latitude is defined as both the ability to use skills on the job and the decision-making authority available to the worker. Being able to determine one's pace, timed breaks, and scheduled hours, as well as being creative and developing skills, increases people's decision latitude or control. Job strain occurs when people contend with high levels of psychological demands while simultaneously being deprived of control over the work environment. A burgeoning literature reveals that high-strain or high demand–low control work environments pose the most significant health risk. Occupations typically higher in job strain are machine-paced (including assemblers and freight handlers) and service-based (such as waiters and cooks). Conversely, low-strain work environments have fewer psychological demands and high levels of control, and are predicted to have lower psychological strain and adverse health effects. Examples of low-strain jobs are self-paced occupations such as repairmen. "Active work" environments are associated with high psychological demands but also high decision latitude. As a result of this high level of job control, people in an active work environment are able to problem-solve and mobilize to meet demands; psychological growth and learning often result. Typical active work jobs may include lawyers, nurses, and managers. Low demand–low control, or "passive work," environments, on the other hand, tend to lack a strong motivational component and may promote disengagement. Examples of passive work jobs include clerical workers and service personnel.

In addition to the original two components, a third component, social support, was later added to the job strain model (Johnson & Hall, 1988). Notably, receiving instrumental and/or emotional support from supervisors and coworkers can potentially buffer the effect of high demands and low control job environments. According to this modified version of the job strain model, the highest level of strain is expected in "iso-strain" work environments characterized by high demand, low control, and low social support (or social isolation).

Measurement

In this context of health research, job strain is often assessed using self-report measures, such as the *job content questionnaire* (JCQ) and the psychological job strain questionnaire (PSJSQ) (Karasek, 1985; Karasek et al., 1998), or external assessment of job characteristics via an expert observer. The demand and control components of the model are typically both considered, and are either used to create the four categories, or quadrants, of work environment (*high strain, low strain, active*, and *passive*) or dichotomized into high versus low job strain.

Evidence for Job Strain Model

Over the past 20 years, a considerable body of research has investigated the effect of job strain on CVD risk, including MI, CHD, and CVD-related mortality. From the first application of the job strain model to CVD in the 1970s (Karasek, 1979), literature findings on the relationship between these high demand/low control work environments and increased risk for cardiovascular morbidity and mortality have yielded largely mixed results (Haynes, Feinleib, & Kannel, 1980; Karasek et al., 1988; Kuper & Marmot, 2003; Lynch, Krause, Kaplan, Salonen, et al., 1997, Lynch, Krause, Kaplan, Tuomilehto, & Salonen, 1997; Marmot, Bosma, Hemingway, Brunner, & Standfeld, 1997; Steenland et al., 2000; Theorell et al., 1998). Several studies observed a direct association between job strain and CHD (Aboa-Eboule et al., 2007; Bosma et al., 1998; Haynes et al., 1980; Hintsanen et al., 2005; Karasek et al., 1988; Kivimäki et al., 2002; Kuper & Marmot, 2003; Netterstrøm, Kristensen, & Sjol, 2006; Steenland et al., 2000; Theorell et al., 1998). For example, in the *Whitehall Study II*, which collected data on 10,000 British civil servants, job strain was associated with the risk of CHD events, even after adjusting for other risk factors, and was stronger among younger participants (Kuper & Marmot, 2003). Of the two components, high demands were predictive of all CHD events, especially fatal CHD and non-fatal MI for both men and women. Conversely, low control was associated with CHD events in men only. In a prospective cohort study of men and women who had sustained their first MI and returned to work, chronic job strain was found to be an independent predictor of recurrent CHD after 2.2 years or more of follow-up (Aboa-Eboule et al., 2007). Other studies, primarily from the USA, showed no direct association between job strain and CHD (Amick et al., 2002; Greenlund et al., 1995; Hlatky et al., 1995; Lee, Colditz, Berkman, & Kawachi, 2002; Netterstrøm, Kristensen, Jensen, & Schnor, 2010).

Other findings have been more mixed, supporting an interaction between gender and the effect of job strain on CHD (Eaker, Sullivan, Kelly-Hayes, D'Agostino, & Benjamin, 2004; Rosvall et al., 2002). For example, recent research results from the Framingham Offspring Study (Eaker et al., 2004) reveal no association between job strain and CHD incidence or mortality in men or women; instead, that particular study linked high demand/high control work environments to increased CHD risk in women. The investigators speculated that their findings may serve as a reflection of historical shifts in social status and roles for women in this cohort (mid-1980s), where breaking into traditional "men's roles" of authority and control has encountered opposition and social pressures that could have negatively impacted their cardiovascular health.

Iso-Strain Model

Studies testing the *iso-strain* variant of the job strain model have also yielded mixed results (e.g., Aboa-Eboule et al., 2007; Hammar, Alfredsson, & Johnson, 1998; Kuper & Marmot, 2003). A study testing the *iso-strain* model in a sample of Swedish employees found no support for the *iso-strain* model. However, low social support and a low demand/low control work environment predicted MI and stroke in women but not in men (André-Petersson, Engström, Hedblad, Janzon, & Rosvall, 2007).

Subclinical Indicators of Cardiovascular Disease

Studies examining the relationship between job strain and subclinical CVD indicators have yielded mixed results (Hintsanen et al., 2005; Nordstrom, Dwyer, Merz, Shircore, & Dwyer, 2001; Rosvall et al., 2002;). In the *Cardiovascular Risk in Young Finns Study*, which comprised Finnish schoolchildren followed over a 20-year period, the investigators observed an association between adult job strain and *intima-media thickness* (an indicator of atherosclerosis) independent of adult risk factors and occupational status (Hintsanen et al.). However, this association was limited to men. Furthermore, a follow-up study found that preemployment influences, adolescent risk factors including biological, familial, and socioeconomic factors, did not confound the association between job strain and atherosclerosis (Kivimaki et al., 2007). Similarly, Nordstrom et al. found an association between early atherosclerosis in men only, whereas Rosvall et al. found job strain to be associated with increased carotid IMT and plaque in women but not in men. The aforementioned studies, some of which are prospective, struggle in capturing the cumulative effects of the biological factors, as well as the variability of self-reports of physical and leisure activity, thereby limiting investigators in articulating potential causal associations.

Hypertension

Perhaps the strongest empirical evidence linking job strain to cardiovascular risk factors is found for hypertension, and both cross-sectional and longitudinal studies have demonstrated that exposure to job strain is associated with significantly higher blood pressure. For example, in a study that followed 3,200 initially normotensive, employed young adults (20–32 years old), job strain was significantly associated with the incident hypertension over 8 years (Markovitz, Matthews, Whooley, Lewis, & Greenlund, 2004). Similarly, in another study examining the cumulative exposure to job strain over 3 years, both men and women were found to have significantly higher systolic and diastolic blood pressures as opposed to workers who were not exposed to job strain (Schnall, Schwartz, Landsbergis, Warren, & Pickering, 1998).

Similar to other findings in the job strain-CVD risk literature, findings for job strain and hypertension are also more mixed in women. In a prospective study of over 8,000 white-collar workers, the job strain model was tested to evaluate the effects of cumulative job strain on blood pressure over 7 years (Guimont et al., 2006). Findings indicated that cumulative exposure was significantly associated with higher systolic blood pressure in men only, and this effect was similar in magnitude to effects of age and sedentary lifestyle, two well-known traditional risk factors for high blood pressure. In addition, having low social support at work increased the risk for high blood pressure in both men and women. A study examining the effects of job strain over 6.5 years in Swedish workers only found a significant positive relationship between job strain and blood pressure for men (Ohlin, Berglund, Rosvall, &

Nilsson, 2007). Also, men who were employed for more than 25 years and were exposed to job strain for half of their working life tended to have higher blood pressure compared to women in similar work conditions (Landsbergis, Schnall, Pickering, Warren, & Schwartz, 2003). Some research also suggests that job strain, specifically high demand/high control, is associated with masked hypertension in men but not in women (Trudel, Brisson, & Milot, 2010).

Effort–Reward Imbalance Model

The ERI model (Siegrist, 1996) assesses the balance between rewards and effort in the work environment. An individual's occupation is often a source of social status and identity in adulthood, and one's work role potentially confers important benefits, including being rewarded. The ERI model is based on the application of social reciprocity in the context of a work contract (Siegrist, 2010); specifically, in exchange for defined obligations and tasks, rewards such as money (salary), esteem, and opportunities (e.g., promotion, job security) are expected. Work stress is a result of an imbalance, or failed reciprocity, between high effort and low control over long-term rewards (Siegrist, 2005). Effort can stem from factors that are extrinsic or intrinsic. Extrinsic factors are conceptually similar to Karasek's psychological demands, and involve specific demands and obligations of the job, such as time pressure, increased workload, and mandatory overtime (Siegrist et al., 2004). Intrinsic sources of effort include factors such as overcommitment and need for control. Overcommitment is the inability to withdraw from work obligations, and is assumed to enhance the deleterious effect of ERI on health (Siegrist et al., 2004). According to this model, having a demanding but unstable job, or achieving at a high level without prospects of promotion, leads to distress that could be potentially harmful to one's physical health.

Measurement

ERI is measured with a self-report questionnaire that contains the scales effort, reward, and overcommitment (Siegrist et al., 2004). Similar to the job strain model, observations from an outside observer may also be used. Most often, the scales of effort and reward are considered independently. However, in a recent study, Aboa-Eboule et al. (2011) calculated an effort–reward ratio.

Evidence for Effort–Reward Imbalance Model

As compared to the job strain model, studies testing the ERI model have been less numerous. Studies primarily conducted in Europe have shown that ERI at work predicts CHD (Kivimäki et al., 2002). For example, in the British Whitehall study, men exposed to high effort–low reward work environments doubled their risk of CHD over 5 years (Bosma et al., 1998). High ERI continued to predict increased CHD risk, as well as general poor physical and mental health, at the 11-year follow-up (Kuper, Singh-Manoux, Siegrist, & Marmot, 2002). Similarly, in a prospective study of Finnish men, having high work demands, low work resources, and low salary more than doubled the risk of MI or CHD-related death after 8 years (Kivimäki et al., 2002). In a case–control study conducted in China, working men and women in high effort, low reward, and high overcommitment were five times as likely to belong in the MI group (Xu, Zhao, Guo, Guo, & Gao, 2009). Aboa-Eboule et al. (2011) demonstrated that ERI at work was significantly associated with recurrent CHD in a 4-year prospective study of post-MI patients. In the *Finnish Kuopio Ischaemic Heart Disease Risk Study*, the combination of high demand and low income was significantly associated with atherosclerosis progression over 4 years (Lynch, Krause, Kaplan, Salonen et al., 1997, Lynch, Krause, Kaplan, Tuomilehto, et al., 1997), as well as MI risk (Lynch, Krause, Kaplan, Tuomilehto, et al.).

ERI has also been found to be significantly associated with hypertension in women and men (Gilbert-Ouimet, Brisson, Vézina, Milot, & Blanchette, 2012; Peter et al., 1998; Peter, Alfredsson, Knutsson, Siegrist, & Westerholm, 1999). Two studies also linked high ERI with increased ambulatory blood pressure (Steptoe, Siegrist, Kirschbaum, & Marmot, 2004; Vrijkotte, van Doornen, & de Geus, 2000).

Comparing and Combining Job Strain and Effort–Reward Imbalance Models

While the two models have conceptual and operational differences, there is also considerable overlap, and the models complement each other (Siegrist, 2010). In the context of a high effort work environment, low control and low reward are stressful experiences that elicit negative emotions and enhanced physiological stress responses that may result in long-term health consequences including CVD. Preliminary evidence suggests that the effects of job control and ERI are statistically independent in predicting CHD (Bosma et al., 1998). A study that tested both the job strain and ERI models on 812 Finnish employees over 25 years found that those who were exposed to environments high in job strain and high in ERI increased their cardiovascular mortality risk 2.2- and 2.4-fold, respectively (Kivimäki et al., 2002). Combining the two models captures a broader range of stressors at work, and appears to improve CVD risk estimates (Peter et al., 2002). Moreover, combined effects of job strain and ERI on CVD are considerably stronger than effects of each alone (Xu et al., 2011). Some studies have sought to combine elements of the job strain and ERI models. An interesting finding in a study examining the effect of work stress in women indicated that the combination of exposure to job strain plus overcommitment was associated with significantly higher risk of MI than either job strain or overcommitment alone (Peter et al., 2002).

Explaining Inconsistent Findings on Job Stress and CVD

Although a bulk of the empirical evidence supports a relationship between job strain and CVD, many results are mixed. These inconsistent findings in study results could reflect differences in how the variables of job stress and CVD were assessed. For instance, one potential explanation for these differences is in the definition and measurement of the "job stress" construct; more specifically, the construct may be measured subjectively (using a self-report measure) or objectively (e.g., hours worked, salary, or by job description) or both, and may thus yield different results. Another important difference may be to consider longitudinal versus cross-sectional study designs. In theory, chronic exposure to job strain over many years would lead to more "wear and tear" of the body; cross-sectional studies are only able to indicate job stress at one period of time. A certain time lag may be needed for job strain to have an observable effect on cardiovascular health, a finding noted for other outcomes as well (de Lange, Taris, Kompier, Houtman, & Bongers, 2003). A review examining cross-sectional and longitudinal empirical studies (Belkic, Landsbergis, Schnall, & Baker, 2004) showed that of 17 longitudinal studies, 8 had a significant positive association, and 3 showed positive trends between job strain and CHD risk. Half of eight cross-sectional studies had significant positive results. However, other reviews of longitudinal studies indicated only moderate support for the job strain—CHD risk model (de Lange et al., 2003; Kivimäki et al., 2006). In spite of these mixed findings, the weight of the data leans in the direction that job strain poses as a risk factor that can influence cardiovascular functioning.

Other Models: Shift Work and Overtime Work and CVD

Epidemiological studies suggest a modest association between shift work and heart disease. In a Finnish study on cardiovascular risk in young adults, shift work was associated with increased subclinical atherosclerosis in men under age 40, but not in women (Puttonen et al., 2009). Shift workers may be at increased risk of CVD for a number of reasons: disrupting circadian rhythms and being associated with poorer lifestyle factors, including reduced physical activity and poorer diet, and greater job strain. Another chapter in this Handbook reviews this shift work phenomenon in greater detail.

Working overtime is commonly thought to be stressful and may impact sleep, thus involving similar mechanisms proposed for higher risk in shift work. Generally, being at work increases blood pressure and, therefore, more time at work implies elevated blood pressure over longer periods of time which, in turn, contributes to heart disease risk (Pieper, Warren, & Pickering, 1993). In Japan, "Karoshi," or death from overwork, is a publicly recognized phenomenon. Several studies, all from Japan, have attempted to examine the effect of long work hours on CVD, and report an association between longer hours worked and increased CVD risk, including higher blood pressure and MI (Hayashi, Kobayashi, Yamaoka, & Yano, 1996; Iwasaki, Takahashi, & Nakata, 2006; Sokejima & Kagamimori, 1998).

Work Stress and Gender

Much of the literature to date has focused on the effects of work stress on men's cardiovascular health (Schnall & Landsbergis, 1994). Although there are several studies that have tested the job strain model that have included women, female samples are lacking for ERI models (e.g., Kivimäki et al., 2006). It should be noted that most women and men are employed in jobs where their own gender is in the majority. The types of jobs primarily held by women may be characteristically different from men's, particularly with regard to job strain. Studies in Europe, the USA, and Canada have demonstrated that job strain is more prevalent in women than men (Bosma et al., 1998). Women typically contend with lower levels of control in their jobs, and some studies observed higher psychosocial demands (Bosma et al., 1997; Greenlund et al., 1995). In addition, some research suggests that the association between psychosocial risk and incident CHD is stronger in women than men, with the implication that women may be relatively more sensitive to psychosocial stressors than men (Hallman, Burell, Setterlind, Od'en, & Lisspers, 2001; Thurston & Kubzansky, 2007).

Although women appear to contend with higher levels of job strain, work stress is only moderately predictive of incidence and prognosis of CHD in women (Eaker, 1998; Eaker, Pinsky, & Castelli, 1992; Marmot et al., 1997; Orth-Gomer et al., 2000; Wamala, Mittleman, Horsten, Schenck-Gustafsson, & Orth-Gomér, 2000). Whereas occupational stress has been relatively consistently linked with CHD risk in men, other types of stress tend to be associated with heart disease risk in women (Everson-Rose & Lewis, 2005; Rosengren et al., 2004). Research examining physiological markers of stress supports the notion that men and women may respond differently to work stress: Separate studies of employed men and women found a significant positive relationship between perceived stress and physiological responses at work in men, but not in women (Frankenhaeuser et al., 1989; Orth-Gomér, Wenger, & Chesney, 1998). This suggests that limiting stress measures to the effects of paid employment alone may not accurately capture women's experience of stress or the physiological consequences of women's stress burden.

To date, 68 million women are active members of the US labor force, comprising nearly half of the total US labor force (Solis & Hall, 2009). However, equal involvement in paid employment does not necessarily translate into equality in domestic gender roles. Women from dual-career households continue to do a larger share of housework and childcare, and carry primary responsibility for these tasks (for a review, see Coltrane, 2000). The literature shows that, for women, being involved in paid work is associated with positive health outcomes (Artazcoz, Borrell, Benach, Cortès, & Rohlfs, 2004; Khlat, Sermet, & Le Pape, 2000; Kostiainen, Martelin, Kestilä, Martikainen, & Koskinen, 2009; Lahelma, Arber, Kivelä, & Roos, 2002; Lundberg & Frankenhaeuser, 1999; Martikainen, 1995), and may protect women from CHD (Brezinka & Kittel, 1995; Carson et al., 2009; Hazuda et al., 1986; Kritz-Silverstein, Wingard, & Barrett-Connor, 1992; Rose et al., 2004). However, the combination of employment and family appears to be associated with worse health outcomes, including increased risk of psychosomatic strain and physical illness (e.g., Arber, 1991; Arber & Lahelma, 1993; Lahelma et al.; McMunn, Bartley, & Kuh, 2006), and may also enhance CHD risk (Brezinka & Kittel, 1995; Haynes & Feinleib, 1980; Theorell, 1991). Findings from the *Framingham Heart Study* indicated that the incidence of CHD over 8 years was nearly twice as high in employed women with three or more children, relative to employed women without children (Haynes et al., 1980). A more recent study looking at 24-h ambulatory blood pressure, Brisson et al. (1999) found that a combination of larger amounts of family responsibilities and job strain among white-collar women had a greater effect on blood pressure levels than only one of these factors.

Inequalities in workload that are linked with traditional gender roles may also be tied to problems in recovery after MI. Research suggests that female patients tend to ignore symptoms of overexertion and resume contraindicated physically demanding household chores, such as vacuuming and doing the laundry within a shorter time period after hospital discharge than male patients (Hamilton & Seidman, 1993; Kristofferzon, Loefmark, & Carlsson, 2003; Lemos, Suls, Jenson, Lounsbury, & Gordon, 2003; Rose, Suls, Green, & Gordon, 1996). Women are also less likely to enter, and more likely to withdraw from, cardiac rehabilitation due to family obligations than other nonmedical reasons than men (Halm, Penque, Doll, & Beahrs, 1999; Jackson, Leclerc, Erskine, & Linden, 2005; Marzolini, Brooks, & Oh, 2008). This may increase women's risk of morbidity and mortality following an MI. In addition to stress associated with demands from household chores and childcare, marital strain has also been implicated in CVD in women. For instance, in female coronary patients, work stress did not predict coronary events. However, in women who experienced high marital stress, long-term survival was poorer (Orth-Gomer et al., 2000) and the combined effects of stress from both work and marriage was associated with the worst health outcome (Orth-Gomér & Leineweber, 2005). Similarly, prolonged exposure to combined marital and work stress has been linked with progression in atherosclerotic narrowing in female coronary patients (Blom, Janszky, Balog, Orth-Gomer, & Wamala, 2003; Wang et al., 2007).

Potential Mechanisms

Two pathways are generally considered as potential mediators of the relationship between work stress and CVD: health behaviors and psychobiological mechanisms. A recent study by Chandola et al. (2008), that sought to determine biological and behavioral factors linking work stress with CHD among male and female civil servants of the Whitehall II study, estimated that 32 % of the effect of work stress on CHD can be explained via the effects of work stress on health behaviors (particularly low physical activity and poor diet), and a clustering of biological risk factors collectively termed the *metabolic syndrome*. Furthermore, this association was stronger among participants under the age of 50.

Health behaviors. Work stress may indirectly influence CVD risk through increased health-risk behaviors, such as smoking, decreased physical activity, and poor diet and sleep (Choi et al., 2010; de Lange et al., 2009; Hellerstedt & Jeffery, 1997; Kouvonen et al., 2007; Kouvonen, Kivimäki, Cox, Cox, & Vahtera, 2005).

Psychobiological mechanism. A potential mechanism in the relationship between work stress and heart disease may be through chronic overactivation and dysregulation of the autonomic nervous system and the hypothalamus–pituitary–adrenal cortex (HPA) axis. Physiologically, stress evokes a set of "fight-or-flight" responses that include rapid heart rate, increased respiration, and vasoconstriction/vasodilation (Cannon, 1932). When faced with a threat, these responses are instrumental in ensuring an organism's survival. However, severe, prolonged stress eventually leads to tissue damage and disease (Selye, 1956). One possible pathway linking chronic stress to disease is physiological reactivity. The "reactivity hypothesis" suggests that larger, more frequent, and longer lasting physiological changes, such as increased blood pressure and heart rate, may contribute to the development and progression of stress-mediated disease (Kamarck & Lovallo, 2003; Krantz & Manuck, 1984; Manuck, 1994). Support for this hypothesis had been found in research on nonhuman primates (Manuck, Kaplan, Adams, & Clarkson, 1988), where monkeys that exhibited higher reactivity to stress had more extensive atherosclerosis. Subsequent research demonstrated a similar relationship between exaggerated cardiovascular reactivity response and development of atherosclerosis in humans (Barnett, Spence, Manuck, & Jennings, 1997; Jennings et al., 2004; Matthews, Zhu, Tucker, & Whooley, 2006). In fact, mounting evidence suggests that cardiovascular reactivity can contribute to some preclinical (e.g., increased blood pressure and left ventricular mass) states, as well as the onset and progression of coronary artery disease and the manifestations of CHD (Smith & Ruiz, 2002; Treiber et al., 2003).

The body's inherent ability to adapt to stressors and maintain homeostasis via fluctuating or heightened physiological responses, termed *allostasis*, is crucial to an organism's survival. The cumulative burden of stressors that increase physiological arousal over time results in "wear and tear" on the body, and can accelerate disease by contributing to *allostatic load* (McEwen, 1998). In addition, a genetic loading, combined with health behaviors, calibrates one's physiological response to adapt to daily living. A greater *allostatic load* will result in a disproportionately more reactive and/or a prolonged response, thereby increasing the susceptibility to disease. A comprehensive quantitative review of the literature has linked chronic exposure to psychosocial stress to poorer cardiovascular recovery (Chida & Hamer, 2008). Being chronically exposed to a stressful work environment may, therefore, contribute to the development of CVD via greater *allostatic load* and increased and prolonged reactivity to new stressors.

Empirical support. A recent review of psychophysiological biomarkers of work stress (Chandola, Heraclides, & Kumari, 2010) largely supports the notion that exposure to stressful work environments is associated with reduced heart rate variability (a biomarker for autonomic influences on the heart), as well as altered levels of catecholamine and cortisol secretion (biomarkers for the HPA axis). Similarly, a study that sought to identify an etiologic mechanism in the relationship between job strain and CVD examined heart rate variability as an autonomic index, and found that job strain was associated with a disturbed cardiovascular regulatory pattern, specifically a persistent reduction in cardiac vagal tone and elevations in sympathetic control during working hours (Collins, Karasek, & Costas, 2005). Other studies indicate reduced immune function, enhanced endogenous inflammation, and heightened acute inflammatory responsivity as potentially linking work stress and CVD (Bellingrath, Rohleder, & Kudielka, 2010; Hamer et al., 2006).

Emotion. Several findings in the literature also support an association between job stress and negative emotion, particularly depression (e.g., De Lange, Taris, & Kompier, 2004; Godin, Kittel, Coppieters, & Siegrist, 2005). A considerable body of literature documents the associations between negative emotions, such as depression, and CHD development, progression, and mortality (Everson-Rose & Lewis, 2005; Kubzansky & Kawachi, 2000). Negative emotions may play a role in mediating the relationship between job stress and CHD, perhaps through disturbance in cardiovascular reactivity and recovery (Chida & Hamer, 2008), or via inflammatory processes (Miller & Blackwell, 2006; Vaccarino et al., 2007) as outlined in the previous section.

Clinical Implications and Workplace Interventions

The proportion of CVD possibly due to job strain varies greatly between studies. However, Karasek and Theorell estimated that approximately one-quarter of heart disease could potentially be prevented, if job strain in occupations with the highest strain levels were reduced to the average of other occupations.

Health Promotion Programs

These interventions typically target healthy workers, and workers at risk for CVD, by obtaining self-reports of risky behaviors, including smoking, and biometric measures such as blood pressure and cholesterol. The objective of these programs is to target one particular CVD risk factor and assist employees in making lifestyle changes to reduce risk.

Stress-Management

Stress-management at the worksite may consist of environmental (e.g., chemical stressors), physical (e.g., noise, rotating shift work), and psychosocial interventions. Psychosocial interventions may include individual strategies to alleviate stress, such as progressive muscle relaxation, visualization, exercise, as well as interpersonal coping skills, including assertiveness training, conflict management, and communication skills. Another type of stress reduction intervention is through increasing intrapersonal awareness of cognitive and affective responses to work stress, including stress inoculation training and cognitive-behavioral skills training (cite71). Such programs have been shown to be effective in reducing cholesterol levels and high blood pressure, as well as favorably influence catecholamine ("stress hormones") levels and cardiac function.

Organizational Prevention Strategies

Rather than reducing traditional CVD risk factors (as in health promotion programs) and modifying an individual's perception and ability to cope with stress (stress-management), organizational prevention strategies focus on reducing or eliminating the source of the problem in the work environment (41). Potential strategies include job redesign, job enrichment, and participative management. Such reliance on the infrastructure of the work environment overcomes the traditional barriers of time and inconvenience for participating in any health promotion approach, the onsite. From an economic standpoint, industry would greatly benefit from assuming an active role in participating in healthcare promotion programs, as 25–30 % of companies' medical costs are directed towards patients with risk factors for CVD and other chronic physical morbidities (Anderson et al., 2000).

Health promotion interventions need to be delivered appropriately to those at increased risk. The translation of these interventions in the work environment, though, poses a formidable challenge. The AHA has defined a multidimensional approach in the work environment that would include a number of components to reduce the risk for heart disease (Carnethon et al., 2009). It is advocated that the following elements of wellness be included: tobacco cessation; enhancing physical activity; equipping workers with evidenced-based stress-management strategies; early detection/screening; nutrition education and promotion; weight management; disease management; and overall CVD education. The role of the employer can be viewed as a facilitator that offers health appraisals/checklists and reminders for employees.

Another recommendation for such health programs is for environmental modifications that actually facilitate the recommended health behaviors to occur. The modifications not only foster the opportunity to engage in health-enhancing behaviors but also eliminate the exposure to health-impairing behaviors (i.e., removal of vending machines with nutritionally lacking products). In addition, the AHA recommends that regulations and policy are designed to take into consideration the importance of health promotion in the work environment. For example, if financial incentives are available for participation in such a program, they are given directly to the employee, increasing the likelihood of successful participation. Finally, the AHA recommends that health promotion programs for CVD are made available to all employees. This effort would bypass the risk that a corporate hierarchy would prevent such programs from reaching the more vulnerable populations.

Effectiveness of Worksite Intervention Programs

To date, there have been a number of empirical efforts devoted towards examining the effectiveness of worksite interventions to reduce the likelihood of CVD. However, the findings have been variable and, overall, there tends to be little tailoring of these programs to maximize the breadth of their benefits. Racette et al. (2009) evaluated the effectiveness of a multifaceted worksite health promotion program targeting CVD risk factors over a 1-year period. Of note, the investigators observed improvements in terms of fitness, blood pressure, and total-, HDL-, and LDL-cholesterol. BMI and fat mass were different between worksites. They noted that many of these improvements were attained with worksite health assessments and personalized health reports rather than intervention itself.

In another study, the effectiveness of a lifestyle intervention program was evaluated in its ability to reduce risk factors for CVD and Type II Diabetes (Di Battista et al., 2011). Specifically, employees of a hospital and a steel mill met with a dietitian and an exercise specialist for eight sessions, focusing on bolstering motivation and providing education. The results suggest that the program facilitated behavioral change, and may be a viable, effective workplace-based strategy. Similarly, another study evaluated the effectiveness of a lifestyle intervention for male workers in the construction industry at risk of CVD. Specifically, standard care was compared to 6 months of individual counseling, aimed at enhancing health behaviors. The components in the aforementioned studies would ideally be used in concert towards a comprehensive intervention strategy aimed at reducing the risk factors for CVD. The results revealed that those receiving individual-based counseling experienced significant positive effects on body weight at 6- and 12-month assessments. In spite of these successes, however, more work is needed to determine the optimal strategies and the delivery mechanisms to prevent CVD for individuals regardless of their risk.

Conclusions and Future Directions

In a brief overview, we have underscored a number of pathways in which work-related stress can influence the risk of cardiovascular disease. In today's economic climate, the importance in developing prophylactic interventions to thwart disease matters greatly. Currently, the evidence supports taking into account both histological and psychosocial variables to prevent cardiovascular disease. Future research should address the issue of whether interventions centered on reducing work stress can contribute to positive psychological and physical outcomes. Moreover, the extent to which gender interacts with risk factors remains to be evaluated. Such interventions could ultimately become an integral part of comprehensive care for cardiovascular disease. Long-term investigations will determine the costs and benefits of such interventional efforts.

References

Aboa-Eboule, C., Brisson, C., Maunsell, E., Bourbonnais, R., Vezina, M., Milot, A., et al. (2011). Effort-reward imbalance at work and recurrent coronary heart disease events: A 4-year prospective study of post-myocardial infarction patients. *Psychosomatic Medicine, 73*, 436–447.

Aboa-Eboule, C., Brisson, C., Maunsell, E., Masse, B., Bourbonnais, R., Vezina, M., et al. (2007). Job strain and risk of acute recurrent coronary heart disease events. *Journal of the American Medical Association, 298*(14), 1652–1660.

Amick, B. C. I., McDonough, P., Chang, H., Rogers, W. H., Pieper, C. F., & Duncan, G. (2002). Relationship between all-cause mortality and cumulative working life course psychosocial and physical exposures in the United States labor market from 1968 to 1992. *Psychosomatic Medicine, 64*(3), 370–381.

André-Petersson, L., Engström, G., Hedblad, B., Janzon, L., & Rosvall, M. (2007). Social support at work and the risk of myocardial infarction and stroke in women and men. *Social Science & Medicine, 64*(4), 830–841.

Anderson, D. R., Whitmer, R. W., Goetzel, R. Z., Ozminkowski, R. J., Dunn, R. L., Wasserman, J., et al. (2000). The relationship between modifiable health risks and group-level health care expenditures. Health Enhancement Research Organization (HERO) Research Committee. American Journal of Health Promotion, 15, 45–52.

Arber, S. (1991). Class, paid employment and family roles: Making sense of structural disadvantage, gender and health status. *Social Science & Medicine, 32*(4), 425–436.

Arber, S., & Lahelma, E. (1993). Inequalities in women's and men's ill-health: Britain and Finland compared. *Social Science & Medicine, 37*, 1055–1068.

Artazcoz, L., Borrell, C., Benach, J., Cortès, I., & Rohlfs, I. (2004). Women, family demands and health: The importance of employment status and socio-economic position. *Social Science & Medicine, 59*(2), 263–274.

Barnett, P. A., Spence, D., Manuck, S. B., & Jennings, J. R. (1997). Psychological stress and the progression of carotid artery disease. *Journal of Hypertension, 15*, 49–55.

Belkic, K., Landsbergis, P. A., Schnall, P. L., & Baker, D. (2004). Is job strain a major source of cardiovascular disease risk? *Scandinavian Journal of Work, Environment and Health, 30*(2), 85–128.

Bellingrath, S., Rohleder, N., & Kudielka, B. M. (2010). Healthy working school teachers with high effort-reward-imbalance and overcommitment show increased pro-inflammatory immune activity and a dampened innate immune defence. *Brain, Behavior, and Immunity, 24*, 1332–1339.

Blom, M., Janszky, I., Balog, P., Orth-Gomer, K., & Wamala, S. P. (2003). Social relations in women with coronary heart disease: The effects of work and marital stress. *Journal of Cardiovascular Risk, 10*, 201–206.

Bosma, H., Marmot, M. G., Hemingway, H., Nicholson, A. C., Brunner, E., & Stansfeld, S. A. (1997). Low job control and risk of coronary heart disease in Whitehall II (prospective cohort) study. *BMJ, 314*(7080), 558–565.

Bosma, H., Peter, R., Siegrist, J., & Marmot, M. (1998). Two alternative job stress models and the risk of coronary heart disease. *American Journal of Public Health, 88*(1), 68–74.

Brezinka, V., & Kittel, F. (1995). Psychosocial factors of coronary heart disease in women: A review. *Social Science & Medicine, 42*(10), 1351–1365.

Brisson, C., Laflamme, N., Moisan, J., Milot, A., Masse, B., & Vezina, M. (1999). Effect of family responsibilities and job strain on ambulatory blood pressure among white-collar women. *Psychosomatic Medicine, 61*, 205–213.

Cannon, W. B. (1932). *The wisdom of the body*. New York: Norton.

Carson, A. P., Rose, K. M., Catellier, D. J., Diez-Roux, A. V., Muntaner, C., & Wyatt, S. B. (2009). Employment status, coronary heart disease, and stroke among women. *Annals of Epidemiology, 19*, 630–636.

Carnethon, M., Whitsel, L. P., Franklin, B. A., Kris-Etherton, P., Milani, R., Pratt, C. A., et al. (2009). Worksite wellness programs for cardiovascular disease prevention: a policy statement from the American Heart Association. Circulation, 120, 1725–1741.

Chandola, T., Britton, A., Brunner, E., Hemingway, H., Malik, M., Kumari, M., et al. (2008). Work stress and coronary heart disease: What are the mechanisms? *European Heart Journal, 29*, 640–648.

Chandola, T., Heraclides, A., & Kumari, M. (2010). Psychophysiological biomarkers of workplace stressors. *Neuroscience and Biobehavioral Reviews, 35*, 51–57.

Chida, Y., & Hamer, M. (2008). Chronic psychosocial factors and acute physiological responses to laboratory-induced stress in healthy populations: A quantitative review of 30 years of investigations. *Psychological Bulletin, 134*(6), 829–885.

Choi, B., Schnall, P. L., Yang, H., Dobson, M., Landsbergis, P., Israel, L., et al. (2010). Psychosocial working conditions and active leisure-time physical activity in middle-aged US workers. *International Journal of Occupational Medicine and Environmental Health, 23*(3), 239–253.

Collins, S. M., Karasek, R. A., & Costas, K. (2005). Job strain and autonomic indices of cardiovascular disease risk. *American Journal of Industrial Medicine, 48*(3), 182–193.

Coltrane, S. (2000). Research on household labor: Modeling and measuring the social embeddedness of routine family work. *Journal of Marriage and the Family, 62*, 1208–1233.

de Lange, A. H., Kompier, M. A., Taris, T. W., Geurts, S. A., Beckers, D. G., Houtman, I. L., et al. (2009). A hard day's night: A longitudinal study on the relationships among job demands and job control, sleep quality and fatigue. *Journal of Sleep Research, 18*(3), 374–383.

De Lange, A. H., Taris, T. W., & Kompier, M. A. (2004). The relationships between work characteristics and mental health. *Work and Stress, 18*(2), 149–166.

de Lange, A. H., Taris, T. W., Kompier, M. A., Houtman, I. L., & Bongers, P. M. (2003). "The very best of the millennium": Longitudinal research and the demand-control-(support) model. *Journal of Occupational Health Psychology, 8*(4), 282–305.

Di Battista, E. M., Williams, M., Rice, S., Bracken, R. M., & Mellalieu, S. D. (2011). An evaluation of the effect of a worksite delivered lifestyle intervention programme on anthropometric risk factors for type 2 diabetes and cardiovascular disease. Journal of Human Nutrition and Dietetics, 24, 385.

Eaker, E. D. (1998). Psychosocial risk factors for coronary heart disease in women. *Clinical Cardiology, 16*(1), 103–111.

Eaker, E. D., Pinsky, J., & Castelli, W. P. (1992). Myocardial infarction and coronary death among women: Psychosocial predictors from a 20-year follow-up of women in the Framingham Study. *American Journal of Epidemiology, 135*(8), 854–864.

Eaker, E. D., Sullivan, L. M., Kelly-Hayes, M., D'Agostino, R. B., Sr., & Benjamin, E. J. (2004). Does job strain increase the risk for coronary heart disease or death in men and women? The Framingham Offspring Study. *American Journal of Epidemiology, 159*, 950–958.

Eller, N. H., Netterstrøm, B., Gyntelberg, F., Kristensen, T. S., Nielsen, F., Steptoe, A., et al. (2009). Work-related psychosocial factors and the development of ischemic heart disease: A systematic review. *Cardiology in Review, 17*(2), 83–97.

Everson-Rose, S. A., & Lewis, T. T. (2005). Psychosocial factors and cardiovascular diseases. *Annual Review of Public Health, 26*, 469–500.

Frankenhaeuser, M., Lundberg, U., Fredrikson, M., Melin, B., Tuomisto, M., Myrsten, A. L., et al. (1989). Stress on and off the job as related to sex and occupational status in white-collar workers. *Journal of Organizational Behavior, 10*, 321–346.

Gilbert-Ouimet, M., Brisson, C., Vézina, M., Milot, A., & Blanchette, C. (2012). Repeated exposure to effort-reward imbalance, increased blood pressure, and hypertension incidence among white-collar workers Effort-reward imbalance and blood pressure. *Journal of Psychosomatic Research, 72*(1), 26–32.

Godin, I., Kittel, F., Coppieters, Y., & Siegrist, J. (2005). A prospective study of cumulative job stress in relation to mental health. *BMC Public Health, 5*, 67.

Greenlund, K. J., Liu, K., Knox, S., McCreath, H., Dyer, A. R., & Gardin, J. (1995). Psychosocial work characteristics and cardiovascular disease risk factors in young adults: The CARDIA study. Coronary artery risk disease in young adults. *Social Science & Medicine, 41*(5), 717–723.

Guimont, C., Brisson, C., Dagenais, G. R., Milot, A., Vézina, M., Mâsse, B., et al. (2006). Effects of job strain on blood pressure: A prospective study of male and female white-collar workers. *American Journal of Public Health, 96*, 1436–1443.

Hallman, T., Burell, G., Setterlind, S., Od'en, A., & Lisspers, J. (2001). Psychosocial risk factors for coronary heart disease, their importance compared with other risk factors and gender differences in sensitivity. *Journal of Cardiovascular Risk, 8*, 39–49.

Halm, M., Penque, S., Doll, N., & Beahrs, M. (1999). Women and cardiac rehabilitation: Referral and compliance patterns. *The Journal of Cardiovascular Nursing, 13*(3), 83–92.

Hamer, M., Williams, E., Vuonovirta, R., Giacobazzi, P., Gibson, E. L., & Steptoe, A. (2006). The effects of effort-reward imbalance on inflammatory and cardiovascular responses to mental stress. *Psychosomatic Medicine, 68*, 408–413.

Hamilton, G. A., & Seidman, R. N. (1993). A comparison of the recovery period for women and men after an acute myocardial infarction. *Heart & Lung, 22*, 308–315.

Hammar, N., Alfredsson, L., & Johnson, J. V. (1998). Job strain, social support at work, and incidence of myocardial infarction. *Occupational and Environmental Medicine, 55*(8), 548–553.

Hayashi, T., Kobayashi, Y., Yamaoka, K., & Yano, E. (1996). Effect of overtime work on 24-h ambulatory blood pressure. *Journal of Occupational and Environmental Medicine, 38*(10), 1007–1011.

Haynes, S. G., & Feinleib, M. (1980). Women, work and coronary heart disease: Prospective findings from the Framingham Heart Study. *American Journal of Public Health, 70*, 133–141.

Haynes, S. G., Feinleib, M., & Kannel, W. B. (1980). The relationship of psychosocial factors to coronary heart disease in the Framingham Study. III. 8-year incidence of coronary heart disease. *American Journal of Epidemiology, 111*(1), 37–58.

Hazuda, H. P., Haffner, S. M., Stern, M. P., Knapp, J. A., Eifler, C. W., & Rosenthal, M. (1986). Employment status and women's protection against coronary heart disease. Findings from the San Antonio Heart Study. *American Journal of Epidemiology, 123*(4), 623–640.

Hellerstedt, W. L., & Jeffery, R. W. (1997). The association of job strain and health behaviours in men and women. *International Journal of Epidemiology, 26*(3), 575–583.

Hintsanen, M., Kivimäki, M., Elovainio, M., Pulkki-Råback, L., Keskivaara, P., Juonala, M., et al. (2005). Job strain and early atherosclerosis: The Cardiovascular Risk in Young Finns Study. *Psychosomatic Medicine, 67*(5), 740–747.

Hlatky, M. A., Lam, L. C., Lee, K. L., Clapp-Channing, N. E., Williams, R. B., Pryor, D. B., et al. (1995). Job strain and the prevalence and outcome of coronary artery disease. *Circulation, 92*(3), 327–333.

Iwasaki, K., Takahashi, M., & Nakata, A. (2006). Health problems due to long working hours in Japan: Working hours, workers' compensation (Karoshi), and preventive measures. *Industrial Health, 44*(4), 537–540.

Jackson, L., Leclerc, J., Erskine, Y., & Linden, W. (2005). Getting the most out of cardiac rehabilitation: A review of referral and adherence predictors. *Heart, 91*(1), 10–14.

Jennings, J. R., Kamarck, T. W., Everson-Rose, S. A., Kaplan, G. A., Manuck, S. B., & Salonen, J. T. (2004). Exaggerated blood pressure responses during mental stress are prospectively related to enhanced carotid atherosclerosis in middle-aged Finnish men. *Circulation, 110*, 2198–2203.

Johnson, J. V., & Hall, E. M. (1988). Job strain, workplace social support and cardiovascular disease: A cross-sectional study of a random sample of the Swedish working population. *American Journal of Public Health, 78*, 1336–1342.

Kamarck, T. W., & Lovallo, W. R. (2003). Cardiovascular reactivity to psychological challenge: Conceptual and measurement considerations. *Psychosomatic Medicine, 65*, 9–21.

Karasek, R. (1979). Job demands, job decision latitude and mental strain: Implications for job redesign. *Administrative Science Quarterly, 24*, 285–307.

Karasek, R. (1985). *Job content questionnaire and user's guide: Department of Industrial and Systems Engineering.* Los Angeles, CA: University of Southern California.

Karasek, R. A., Baker, D., Marxer, F., Ahlbom, A., & Theorell, T. (1981). Job decision latitude, job demands, and cardiovascular disease: A prospective study of Swedish men. *American Journal of Public Health, 71*(7), 694–705.

Karasek, R., Brisson, C., Kawakami, N., Houtman, I., Bongers, P., & Amick, B. (1998). The job content questionnaire (JCQ): An instrument for internationally comparative assessments of psychosocial job characteristics. *Journal of Occupational Health Psychology, 3*, 322–355.

Karasek, R. A., Theorell, T., Schwartz, J. E., Schnall, P. L., Pieper, C. F., & Michela, J. L. (1988). Job characteristics in relation to the prevalence of myocardial infarction in the US Health Examination Survey (HES) and the Health and Nutrition Examination Survey (HANES). *American Journal of Public Health, 78*(8), 910–918.

Karasek Theorell 1990 Healthy Work. New York: Basic Books (5, p. 167)

Khlat, M., Sermet, C., & Le Pape, A. (2000). Women's health in relation with their family and work roles: France in the early 1990s. *Social Science & Medicine, 50*(12), 1807–1825.

Kivimäki, M., Leino-Arjas, P., Luukkonen, R., Riihimäki, H., Vahtera, J., & Kirjonen, J. (2002). Work stress and risk of cardiovascular mortality: Prospective cohort study of industrial employees. *BMJ, 325*(7369), 857.

Kivimäki, M., Virtanen, M., Elovainio, M., Kouvonen, A., Väänänen, A., & Vahtera, J. (2006). Work stress in the etiology of coronary heart disease—a meta-analysis. *Scandinavian Journal of Work, Environment and Health, 32*(6), 431–442.

Kivimaki, M., Hintsanen, M., Keltikangas-Jarvinen, L., Elovainio, M., Pulkki-Raback, L., Vahtera, J., et al. (2007). Early risk factors, job strain, and atherosclerosis among men in their 30s: the Cardiovascular Risk in Young Finns Study. Am J Public Health, 97(3), 450–452.

Kostiainen, E., Martelin, T., Kestilä, L., Martikainen, P., & Koskinen, S. (2009). Employee, partner, and mother: Women's three roles and their implications for health. *Journal of Family Issues, 30*(8), 1122–1150.

Kouvonen, A., Kivimäki, M., Cox, S. J., Cox, T., & Vahtera, J. (2005). Relationship between work stress and body mass index among 45,810 female and male employees. *Psychosomatic Medicine, 67*(4), 577–583.

Kouvonen, A., Kivimäki, M., Väänänen, A., Heponiemi, T., Elovainio, M., Ala-Mursula, L., et al. (2007). Job strain and adverse health behaviors: The Finnish Public Sector Study. *Journal of Occupational and Environmental Medicine, 49*(1), 68–74.

Krantz, D. S., & Manuck, S. B. (1984). Acute psychophysiologic reactivity and risk of cardiovascular disease: A review and methodologic critique. *Psychological Bulletin, 96*(3), 435–464.

Kristofferzon, M.-L., Loefmark, R., & Carlsson, M. (2003). Myocardial infarction: Gender differences in coping and social support. *Journal of Advanced Nursing, 44*(4), 360–374.

Kritz-Silverstein, D., Wingard, D. L., & Barrett-Connor, E. (1992). Employment status and heart disease risk factors in middle-aged women: The Rancho Bernardo Study. *American Journal of Public Health, 82*(2), 215–219.

Kubzansky, L. D., & Kawachi, I. (2000). Going to the heart of the matter: Do negative emotions cause coronary heart disease? *Journal of Psychosomatic Research, 48*, 323–337.

Kuper, H., & Marmot, M. (2003). Job strain, job demands, decision latitude, and risk of coronary heart disease within the Whitehall II study. *Journal of Epidemiology and Community Health, 57*(2), 147–153.

Kuper, H., Singh-Manoux, A., Siegrist, J., & Marmot, M. (2002). When reciprocity fails: Effort-reward imbalance in relation to coronary heart disease and health functioning within the Whitehall II study. *Occupational and Environmental Medicine, 59*(11), 777–784.

Lahelma, E., Arber, S., Kivelä, K., & Roos, E. (2002). Multiple roles and health among British and Finnish women: The influence of socioeconomic circumstances. *Social Science & Medicine, 54*, 727–740.

Landsbergis, P. A., Schnall, P. L., Pickering, T. G., Warren, K., & Schwartz, J. E. (2003). Life-course exposure to job strain and ambulatory blood pressure in men. *American Journal of Epidemiology, 157*, 998–1006.

Lee, S., Colditz, G., Berkman, L. F., & Kawachi, I. (2002). A prospective study of job strain and coronary heart disease in US women. *International Journal of Epidemiology, 31*(6), 1147–1153.

Lemos, K., Suls, J., Jenson, M., Lounsbury, P., & Gordon, E. E. I. (2003). How do female and male cardiac patients and their spouses share responsibilities after discharge from the hospital? *Annals of Behavioral Medicine, 25*(1), 8–15.

Lundberg, U., & Frankenhaeuser, M. (1999). Stress and workload of men and women in high-ranking positions. *Journal of Occupational Health Psychology, 4*(2), 142–151.

Lynch, J. W., Krause, N., Kaplan, G. A., Salonen, R., & Salonen, J. T. (1997). Workplace demands, economic reward, and progression of carotid atherosclerosis. *Circulation, 96*(1), 302–307.

Lynch, J. W., Krause, N., Kaplan, G. A., Tuomilehto, J., & Salonen, J. T. (1997). Workplace conditions, socioeconomic status, and the risk of mortality and acute myocardial infarction: The Kuopio Ischemic Heart Disease Risk Factor Study. *American Journal of Public Health, 87*(4), 617–622.

Manuck, S. B. (1994). Cardiovascular reactivity in cardiovascular disease: "Once more unto the breach". *International Journal of Behavioral Medicine, 1*(1), 4–31.

Manuck, S. B., Kaplan, J. R., Adams, M. R., & Clarkson, T. B. (1988). Studies of psychosocial influences on coronary artery atherosclerosis in cynomolgus monkeys. *Health Psychology, 7*, 113–124.

Markovitz, J. H., Matthews, K. A., Whooley, M., Lewis, C. E., & Greenlund, K. J. (2004). Increases in job strain are associated with incident hypertension in the CARDIA study. *Annals of Behavioral Medicine, 28*(1), 4–9.

Marmot, M. G., Bosma, H., Hemingway, H., Brunner, E., & Standfeld, S. (1997). Contribution of job control and other risk factors to social variations in coronary heart disease incidence. *350*(9073), 235–239.

Martikainen, P. (1995). Women's employment, marriage, motherhood and mortality: A test of the multiple role and role accumulation hypotheses. *Social Science & Medicine, 40*(2), 199–212.

Marzolini, S., Brooks, D., & Oh, P. I. (2008). Sex differences in completion of a 12-month cardiac rehabilitation programme: An analysis of 5922 women and men. *European Journal of Cardiovascular Prevention and Rehabilitation, 15*, 698–703.

Matthews, K. A., Zhu, S., Tucker, D. C., & Whooley, M. A. (2006). Blood pressure reactivity to psychological stress and coronary calcification in the Coronary Artery Risk Development in Young Adults Study. *Hypertension, 47*, 391–395.

McEwen, B. S. (1998). Stress, adaptation, and disease: Allostasis and allostatic load. *Annals of the New York Academy of Science, 840*, 33–44.

McMunn, A., Bartley, M., & Kuh, D. (2006). Women's health in mid-life: Life course social roles and agency as quality. *Social Science & Medicine, 63*, 1561–1572.

Miller, G. E., & Blackwell, E. (2006). Turning up the heat: Inflammation as a mechanism linking chronic stress, depression, and heart disease. *Current Directions in Psychological Science, 15*, 269–272.

Netterstrøm, B., Kristensen, T. S., Jensen, G., & Schnor, P. (2010). Is the demand-control model still a useful tool to assess work-related psychosocial risk for ischemic heart disease? Results from 14 year follow up in the Copenhagen City Heart Study. *International Journal of Occupational Medicine and Environmental Health, 23*(3), 217–224.

Netterstrøm, B., Kristensen, T. S., & Sjol, A. (2006). Psychological job demands increase the risk of ischaemic heart disease: A 14-year cohort study of employed Danish men. *European Journal of Cardiovascular Prevention and Rehabilitation, 13*, 414–420.

Nordstrom, C. K., Dwyer, K. M., Merz, C. N. B., Shircore, A., & Dwyer, J. H. (2001). Work related stress and early atherosclerosis. *Epidemiology, 12*(2), 180–185.

Ohlin, B., Berglund, G., Rosvall, M., & Nilsson, P. M. (2007). Job strain in men, but not in women, predicts a significant rise in blood pressure after 6.5 years of follow-up. *Journal of Hypertension, 25*(3), 525–531.

Orth-Gomér, K., & Leineweber, C. (2005). Multiple stressors and coronary disease in women. The Stockholm Female Coronary Risk Study. *Biological Psychology, 69*(1), 57–66.

Orth-Gomer, K., Wamala, S. P., Horsten, M., Schenck-Gustafsson, K., Schneiderman, N., & Mittleman, M. A. (2000). Marital stress worsens prognosis in women with coronary heart disease. The Stockholm Female Coronary Risk Study. *Journal of the American Medical Association, 284*, 3008–3014.

Orth-Gomér, K., Wenger, N. K., & Chesney, M. (1998). *Women, stress, and heart disease*. Mahwah, NJ: Erlbaum.

Peter, R., Alfredsson, L., Hammar, N., Siegrist, J., Theorell, T., & Westerholm, P. (1998). High effort, low reward, and cardiovascular risk factors in employed Swedish men and women: Baseline results from the WOLF study. *Journal of Epidemiology and Community Health, 52*(9), 540–547.

Peter, R., Alfredsson, L., Knutsson, A., Siegrist, J., & Westerholm, P. (1999). Does a stressful psychosocial work environment mediate the effects of shift work on cardiovascular risk factors? *Scandinavian Journal of Work, Environment and Health, 25*(4), 376–381.

Peter, R., Siegrist, J., Hallqvist, J., Reuterwall, C., Theorell, T., & Group, t. S. S. (2002). Psychosocial work environment and myocardial infarction: Improving risk estimation by combining two complementary job stress models in the SHEEP study. *Journal of Epidemiology and Community Health, 56*, 294–300.

Pieper, C. F., Warren, K., & Pickering, T. G. (1993). A comparison of ambulatory blood pressure and heart rate at home and work on work and non-work days. *Journal of Hypertension, 11*(2), 177–183.

Puttonen, S., Kivimäki, M., Elovainio, M., Pulkki-Råback, L., Hintsanen, M., Vahtera, J., et al. (2009). Shift work in young adults and carotid artery intima-media thickness: The Cardiovascular Risk in Young Finns study. *Atherosclerosis, 205*(2), 608–613.

Racette, S. B., Deusinger, S. S., Inman, C. L., Burlis, T. L., Highstein, G. R., Buskirk, T. D., et al. (2009). Worksite opportunities for wellness (WOW): Effects on cardiovascular disease risk factors after 1 year. Preventive Medicine, 49, 108–114.

Roger, V. L., Go, A. S., Lloyd-Jones, D. M., Adams, R. J., Berry, J. D., Brown, T. M., et al. (2011). Heart disease and stroke statistics—2011 update: A report from the American Heart Association. *Circulation, 123*, e18–e209.

Rose, K. M., Carson, A. P., Catellier, D., Diez Roux, A. V., Muntaner, C., Tyroler, H. A., et al. (2004). Women's employment status and mortality: The Atherosclerosis Risk in Communities Study. *Journal of Women's Health, 13*(10), 1108–1118.

Rose, G. L., Suls, J., Green, P. J., & Gordon, E. E. I. (1996). Comparison of adjustment, activity, and tangible social support in men and women patients and their spouses during the 6 months post-myocardial infarction. *Annals of Behavioral Medicine, 18*(4), 264–272.

Rosengren, A., Hawken, S., Ounpuu, S., Sliwa, K., Zubaid, M., Almahmeed, W. A., et al. (2004). Association of psychosocial risk factors with risk of acute myocardial infarction in 11 119 cases and 13 648 controls from 52 countries (the INTERHEART study): Case–control study. *364*, 953–962.

Ross, R. (1999). Mechanisms of disease: Atherosclerosis—an inflammatory disease. *The New England Journal of Medicine, 340*, 115–126.

Rosvall, M., Ostergren, P. O., Hedblad, B., Isacsson, S. O., Janzon, L., & Berglund, G. (2002). Work-related psychosocial factors and carotid atherosclerosis. *International Journal of Epidemiology, 31*(6), 1169–1178.

Rozanski, A., Blumenthal, J. A., & Kaplan, J. (1999). Impact of psychological factors on the pathogenesis of cardiovascular disease and implications for therapy. *Circulation, 99*, 2192–2217.

Schnall, P. L., & Landsbergis, P. A. (1994). Job strain and cardiovascular disease. *Annual Review of Public Health, 15*, 381–411.

Schnall, P. L., Schwartz, J. E., Landsbergis, P. A., Warren, K., & Pickering, T. G. (1998). A longitudinal study of job strain and ambulatory blood pressure: Results from a 3-year follow-up. *Psychosomatic Medicine, 60*, 697–706.

Segerstrom, S. C., & Miller, G. E. (2004). Psychological stress and the human immune system: A meta-analytic study of 30 years of inquiry. *Psychological Bulletin, 130*(4), 601–630.

Selye, H. (1956). *The stress of life*. New York: McGraw-Hill.

Siegrist, J. (1996). Adverse effects of high-effort/low reward conditions. *Journal of Occupational Health Psychology, 1*, 27–41.

Siegrist, J. (2005). Social reciprocity and health: New scientific evidence and policy implications. *Psychoneuroendocrinology, 30*(10), 1033–1038.

Siegrist, J. (2010). Effort-reward imbalance at work and cardiovascular disease. *International Journal of Occupational Medicine and Environmental Health, 23*(3), 279–285.

Siegrist, J., Starke, D., Chandola, T., Godin, I., Marmot, M., & Niedhammer, I. (2004). The measurement of effort–reward imbalance at work: European comparisons. *Social Science & Medicine, 58*, 1483–1499.

Smith, T. W., & Ruiz, J. M. (2002). Psychosocial influences on the development and course of coronary heart disease: Current status and implications for research and practice. *Journal of Consulting and Clinical Psychology, 70*, 548–568.

Sokejima, S., & Kagamimori, S. (1998). Working hours as a risk factor for acute myocardial infarction in Japan: Case–control study. *BMJ, 19*, 775–780.

Solis, H. L., & Hall, K. (2009). *Women in the labor force: A databook* (Rep. No. 1018). Washington, DC: US Department of Labor and US Bureau of Labor Statistics.

Steenland, K., Fine, L., Belki , K., Landsbergis, P., Schnall, P., Baker, D., et al. (2000). Research findings linking workplace factors to CVD outcomes. *Occupational Medicine, 15*(1), 7–68.

Steptoe, A., Siegrist, J., Kirschbaum, C., & Marmot, M. (2004). Effort–reward imbalance, overcommitment, and measures of cortisol and blood pressure over the working day. *Psychosomatic Medicine, 66*, 323–329.

Theorell, T. (1991). Psychosocial cardiovascular risks–on the double loads in women. *Psychotherapy and Psychosomatics, 55*, 81–89.

Theorell, T., Tsutsumi, A., Hallquist, J., Reuterwall, C., Hogstedt, C., Fredlund, P., et al. (1998). Decision latitude, job strain, and myocardial infarction: A study of working men in Stockholm. The SHEEP Study Group. Stockholm heart epidemiology program. *American Journal of Public Health, 88*(3), 382–388.

Thurston, R. C., & Kubzansky, L. D. (2007). Multiple sources of psychosocial disadvantage and risk of coronary heart disease. *Psychosomatic Medicine, 69*, 748–755.

Treiber, F. A., Kamarck, T. W., Schneiderman, N., Sheffield, D., Kapuku, G., & Taylor, T. (2003). Cardiovascular reactivity and developement of preclinical and clinical disease states. *Psychosomatic Medicine, 65*, 46–62.

Trudel, X., Brisson, C., & Milot, A. (2010). Job strain and masked hypertension. *Psychosomatic Medicine, 72*(8), 786–793.

Vaccarino, V., Johnson, B. D., Sheps, D. S., Reis, S. E., Kelsey, S. F., Bittner, V., et al. (2007). Depression, inflammation, and incident cardiovascular disease in women with suspected coronary ischemia: The National Heart, Lung, and Blood Institute-sponsored WISE study. *Journal of the American College of Cardiology, 50*(21), 2044–2050.

Vrijkotte, D. G. M., van Doornen, L. J. P., & de Geus, E. J. C. (2000). Effect of work stress on ambulatory blood pressure, heart rate, and heart rate variability. *Hypertension, 35*, 880–886.

Wamala, S. P., Mittleman, M. A., Horsten, M., Schenck-Gustafsson, K., & Orth-Gomér, K. (2000). Job stress and the occupational gradient in coronary heart disease risk in women. The Stockholm Female Coronary Risk Study. *Social Science & Medicine, 51*(4), 481–489.

Wang, H.-X., Leineweber, C., Kirkeeide, R., Svane, B., Schenck-Gustafsson, K., Theorell, T., et al. (2007). Psychosocial stress and atherosclerosis: Family and work stress accelerate progression of coronary disease in women. The Stockholm Female Coronary Angiography Study. *Journal of Internal Medicine, 261*, 245–254.

Xu, W., Yu, H., Gao, W., Guo, L., Zeng, L., & Zhao, Y. (2011). When job stress threatens Chinese workers: Combination of job stress models can improve the risk estimation for coronary heart disease–the BADCAR study. *Journal of Occupational and Environmental Medicine, 53*(7), 771–775.

Xu, W., Zhao, Y., Guo, L., Guo, Y., & Gao, W. (2009). Job stress and coronary heart disease: A case–control study using a Chinese population. *Journal of Occupational Health, 51*, 107–113.

Challenges Related to Mental Health in the Workplace

6

Carolyn S. Dewa, Marc Corbière, Marie-José Durand, and Jennifer Hensel

Introduction

Over the past decade, growing attention has been paid to the mental health of workers and its effects on the workplace. For example, the European Ministers of Health have advocated that employers include mental health programs as part of occupational health and safety (World Health Organization, 2005). The Australian Human Rights Commission (2010) acknowledged the need for workplaces to support workers with mental illnesses. Similar interests have taken root in the USA and Canada. In the USA, the President's New Freedom Commission on Mental Health (2003) suggested that employment for people with mental illnesses should be a national goal. The Canadian Standing Senate Committee on Social Affairs, Science and Technology (2006) raised prevention, promotion and treatment of mental illness as critical national issues. They identified the workplace as the intersection where "the human and economic dimensions of mental health and mental illness come together most evidently."

C.S. Dewa (✉)
Centre for Research on Employment and Workplace Health, Centre
for Addiction and Mental Health, 455 Spadina, Suite 300, M5S 2G8 Toronto, ON, Canada

Department of Psychiatry, University of Toronto,
Toronto, ON, Canada M5S 2G8
e-mail: carolyn.dewa@camh.ca

M. Corbière
Department Centre for Action in Work Disability Prevention and Rehabilitation, Université de Sherbrooke - Campus de Longueuil, 1111, rue St Charles Ouest, Longueuil, QC, Canada J4K 5G4
e-mail: marc.corbiere@usherbrooke.ca

M.-J. Durand
Department Faculty of Medicine and Health Sciences, University of Sherbrooke,
Longueuil, Université de Sherbrooke - Campus de Longueuil,
150 Place Charles-Le Moyne, bureau 200, Longueuil, QC, Canada, J4K 0A8
e-mail: marie-jose.durand@usherbrooke.ca

J. Hensel
Department of Psychiatry, University of Toronto,
Toronto, ON, Canada,
e-mail: jennifer.hensel@camh.ca

What is the basis for the concern about mental health and the workplace? There are at least three main arguments on which it could be founded. The first stems from an interest in protecting basic human rights. Governments around the World have recognized work and employment as a fundamental right of all people who want to work. In 1948, the United Nations (UN) General Assembly adopted the *Universal Declaration of Human Rights* (United Nations, 1948) in which it proclaimed, "Everyone has the right to work, to free choice of employment, to just and favourable conditions of work and to protection against unemployment. (Article 23.1)" Second, health has also been recognized as a basic human right. In 1966, the UN ratified the *International Covenant on Economic, Social and Cultural Rights* (ICESCR) (United Nations, 1966) in which it describes government responsibilities with, "The States Parties to the present Covenant recognize the right of everyone to the enjoyment of the highest attainable standard of physical and mental health. (Article 12.1)" Article 12 goes on to describe that this responsibility involves, "The improvement of all aspects of environmental and industrial hygiene; (Article 12.2.b)" The ICESCR suggests that the workplace plays a role in the attainment of both physical and mental health.

Although many industrialized countries adopted the ICESCR in the 1970s, there seems to have been a lag in addressing mental illness in the working population. For example, this is evidenced by the need for the USA's 1996 and 2008 Mental Health Parity Acts that require equal insurance benefits (often paid for by employers) for both physical and mental disorders. The fact that almost two decades after the adoption of the ICESCR, the European Ministers of Health considered it necessary to reiterate the obligation employers have to ensure mental health (World Health Organization, 2005) also suggests that mental disorders remain at the frontiers of health. Some have gone so far as describing it as the "orphan child of healthcare" (Romanow, 2002). Part of the controversy surrounding the workplace's role arises because it is more difficult to pinpoint the cause of a mental illness than it typically is for a physical disorder (Goldberg & Steury, 2001). For example, in the case of an injury, one could presumably identify the crash or fall that caused it. In contrast, the case for a mental disorder could be less clear-cut. For instance, there are a number of biological risk factors for adult depression, including genetics, neurobiology and health status, as well as exposure to environmental risk factors encountered during childhood development, at home, as well as at work (Kendler, Gardner, & Prescott, 2002). It is not yet clear how each risk factor contributes and interacts such that an adult develops depression. As a result, there are questions about how employers should define their roles in promoting mental health.

In the face of the reticence to invest in mental health, there has also been growing awareness about the potential costs of continuing on this course. This brings us to the third argument for the focus on mental health of workers and its effects on the workplace. That is, it is costly not to address it. In North America, the estimated annual societal cost of mental illness range from $51 billion (CAD) (Lim, Jacobs, Ohinmaa, Schopflocher, & Dewa, 2008) to $83.1 billion (USD) (Greenberg et al., 2003). Between 30 % and 60 % of the societal cost of depression is related to losses associated with decreased work productivity (Greenberg et al., 2003; Stephens & Joubert, 2001). The third argument focuses on the costs of the disability associated with mental disorders. In this chapter, we consider the case for this third argument that focuses on the impact of disability related to mental disorders and their impact on the workplace. We begin by examining the components of the case: (1) the incidence and prevalence of mental disorders in the working-aged population; (2) the effects of work disability related to mental disorders; and (3) the current state of knowledge with regards to workplace interventions aimed at preventing mental disorders and decreasing disability.

A Case for the Concern About The Impact of Mental Illnesses for the Workplace

There are a number of ways to make a case for the magnitude of the impact of mental disorders on the workplace. One way would be to show that the incidence and prevalence of mental disorders in the working-aged population far exceeds that of other types of disorders for which the working population is at risk. Thus, the rationale would be that, because there are large numbers of workers affected by mental disorders, the impacts associated with mental disorders are as great as those for all other types of disorders. In turn, if workplaces invest in safety programs to prevent other types of disability such as those arising from injuries, it would also make sense for workplaces to invest in programs to prevent mental disorders. In the event that the incidence and prevalence of mental disorders does not surpass those of other types of disorders, it still may be beneficial to focus on mental illnesses if, although fewer workers are affected, the disability and the effects of the disability experienced by workers with mental illnesses are greater than those for other types of disorders.

A Review of the Incidence and Prevalence of Mental Illnesses

We begin our discussion by reviewing the evidence regarding the incidence and prevalence of mental disorders in the working population. Overall, during a 12-month period, about 10 % of the Canadian working population have at least one mental disorder (Dewa, Lin, Kooehoorn, & Goldner, 2007). This estimate includes the mood and anxiety disorders: depression, mania, agoraphobia, generalized anxiety disorder (GAD), and panic disorder. Also included are indicators for eating problems and problems with illicit drugs, alcohol, and gambling. In their review of the literature, Sanderson and Andrews (2006) identified depression and simple phobia as the most prevalent mental disorders experienced by the working population. Estimates from the USA, the Netherlands, Australia, and Canada indicate that between 2 and 7 % of the workforce experience depression (Birnbaum et al., 2010; Kessler & Frank, 1997; Laitinen-Krispijn & Bijl, 2000; Lim, Sanderson, & Andrews, 2000; Wang, Adair, & Patten, 2006). In addition, from 5 to 6 % of workers have simple phobia (Kessler & Frank, 1997; Laitinen-Krispijn & Bijl, 2000; Wang et al., 2006). Finally, between 1996 and 2001, Cherry, Chen, and McDonald (2006) observed that among workers, the largest number of cases of mental disorders that both occupational health physicians and psychiatrists treated were related to anxiety and/or depression (511/million and 95/million, respectively). Post-Traumatic Stress Disorder (PTSD) cases were about 42/million and 13/million, respectively. There were about three psychotic episode cases/million seen by psychiatrists and none by occupational health physicians.

Comorbidity of Mental Disorders

One of the challenges of understanding the prevalence of individual mental disorders is related to their comorbidity. For example, Wang et al. (2006) observed that among workers, 18 % had 1 diagnosis of a mental disorder, while 7 % had 2 diagnoses and 8 % had 3 or more diagnoses. Indeed, Dewa and Lin (2000) reported that mood disorders were more likely to have a comorbid mental disorder. The prevalence rates for mental disorders indicate that there is a significant proportion of workers who experience more than one mental disorder at a time.

Comparisons with Physical Disorders

But, the question remains, "How does this compare with other types of disorders?" Reports indicate that mental disorders are among the top five disorders for which workers are treated (Cherry & McDonald, 2002). Among UK workers treated by occupational health physicians, Cherry and McDonald (2002) observed the highest incidence rates for musculoskeletal disorders (men: 144/million and women: 127/million). The second highest was for mental disorders (men: 67/million and women: 71/million). Among Dutch workers, Buist-Bouwman, de Graaf, Vollebergh, and Ormel (2005) found the highest prevalence rates were for anxiety disorders (12.9 %), sinus infection (9.7 %), chronic back trouble (8.9 %), rheumatism (8.3 %), and mood disorders (8.1 %).

Dewa, Lin, Corbiere, and Shain (2010) reported that approximately 40 % of the Canadian working population had at least one type of chronic physical condition including: asthma, fibromyalgia, arthritis, high blood pressure, chronic bronchitis, emphysema/chronic obstructive pulmonary disease, epilepsy, heart disease, diabetes, cancer, stomach/intestinal ulcers, stroke, bowel disorder, chronic fatigue syndrome, or migraines. In comparison, 4 % had a mental disorder. At the same time, another 6 % had both a chronic physical and a mental disorder.

Comorbidity of Physical and Mental Disorders

It is also becoming clearer that the picture is further complicated by the fact that there appears to be an association between physical and mental disorders. For example, Alonso et al. (2004) observed, in a six European country population-based study, that lower physical health status was associated with major depression among workers. Similarly, Buist-Bouwman et al. (2005) found that workers with chronic physical disorders such as chronic back trouble, rheumatism, asthma, migraine headaches, and hypertension were significantly more likely to have a mood or anxiety disorder. Following a group of Canadian workers who had a work-related musculoskeletal disorder, Franche et al. (2009) reported that about 43 % of these workers had high levels of depressive symptoms which persisted among 27 % of the workers 6 months later.

Summary of the Incidence and Prevalence

These reports suggest that, while mental disorders are not necessarily the leading disorders experienced by workers, they appear to be among the top 10. In addition, they are often simultaneously present with physical disorders. This suggests that although the primary reason for treatment may be a physical disorder, there may also be a mental disorder that may or may not be recognized and vice versa (Dersh, Gatchel, Polatin & Mayer, 2002; Franche et al., 2009). The effects of comorbidities both with physical and other mental disorders will be discussed further in the following sections that explore the effects of mental disorders on disability.

Effects of Work Disability Related to Mental Disorders

The effects of mental disorders on the workplace primarily take the form of disability. But, disability can take a number of forms. To get a complete picture of the burden, we must consider each piece of the puzzle (Fig. 6.1). Disability can result in unemployment, decreased productivity at work, as well as short- and long-term work absences. In this section, we focus on these four types of work-related outcomes and their relationship to mental disorders.

Unemployment Related to Disability

Mental disorders often are barriers to employment for working age adults. This means that people with mental disorders are more likely to either be unemployed or to have left the labor force (Bowden, 2005; Ettner, Frank, & Kessler, 1997; Marwaha & Johnson, 2004; Mechanic, Bilder, & McAlpine, 2002; Patel, Knapp, Henderson, & Baldwin, 2002; Waghorn, & Lloyd, 2005). This may be the result of either an inability to obtain or retain employment (Lerner et al., 2004), or a reluctance by employers to hire people with mental disorders (Nicholas, 1998; Scheid, 1999).

In their review of the literature, Marwaha and Johnson (2004) found that UK studies report 70–80 % unemployment rates among people with schizophrenia, while other European studies suggest the range is from 80 to 90 %. In their review of the literature, McAlpine and Warner (2001) found four USA population-based studies reported that between 60 and 78 % of people with schizophrenia are unemployed. Employment rates of people with severe and persistent mental disorders (e.g., schizophrenia) in most countries are lower than those of people with severe physical disabilities (Kilian & Becker, 2007). These estimates indicate that the majority of people with severe and persistent mental

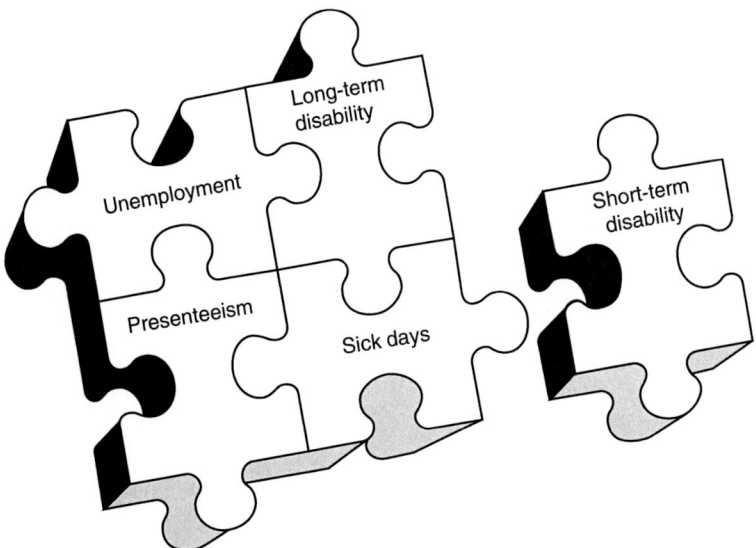

Fig. 6.1 Putting the pieces together—types of work disabilities

disorders are not working. In comparison, people with mood and anxiety disorders are more likely to be working than those with schizophrenia. However, when compared to people without either mood or anxiety disorders, they are less likely to be working (Alonso et al., 2004; Ettner & Grzywacz, 2001; Lerner & Henke, 2008; Marcotte, Wilcox-Gok, & Redmon, 2000; Marcotte, Wilcox-Gok, & Redmon, 1999). Comino et al. (2003) found that people who are unemployed are more likely to have anxiety, mood, and substance abuse disorders. Cohidon, Imbernon, and Gorldberg (2009) reported similar patterns in a French sample in which the prevalence of mood disorders was 10 % among the males who were working, and 22 % among males who were unemployed. In contrast, based on their literature review, McAlpine and Warner (2001) found that four USA population-based studies reported between 29 and 56 % of adults with depression are unemployed. From the USA National Comorbidity Survey Replicate, Birnbaum et al. (2010) estimated that about 26 % of people with Major Depressive Disorder were not working. Using a German population-based survey, Baune, Adrian, and Jacobi (2007) found that, compared to people without a major depressive disorder, those who had one were less likely to be working (32 % vs. 45 %). In addition, Simon, Ludman, Unutzer, Operskalski, and Bauer (2008) observed that about 34 % of people with bipolar disorder did not have paid employment. Using a USA population-based household survey, Bystritsky et al. (2010) noted that people who had a panic disorder during the past 12-months were half as likely to be employed than those who did not. In addition, the presence of mental disorders with physical disorders may also increase the risk of unemployment. For example, it has been estimated that between 15 % and 41 % of people with physical conditions are not working (McAlpine & Warner, 2001). When a physical condition occurs with a mental disorder, the unemployment increases to between 33 and 63 % (McAlpine & Warner, 2001). At the same time, there is literature suggesting that unemployment may contribute to the development of mental disorders. Maier et al. (2006) observed that workers who were unemployed for a year experienced a significant decrease in working capacity and increase in emotional disturbance during that first year of unemployment.

Decreased Productivity Among Workers

One of the primary work-related effects of mental disorders on workers is decreased productivity at work (Dewa & Lin, 2000; Kessler, Ormel, Demler, & Stang, 2003; Lim et al., 2000; Sanderson & Andrews,

2006). That is, workers come to work but are working with impairment. In the literature, this phenomenon has been referred to as *presenteeism* (there is a separate chapter in this Handbook on *presenteeism/absenteeism*). For a 2-week period, USA workers lose an estimated average of 4 h/week or 10 % of a 40-h work week due to depression-related presenteeism; this translated into $36 billion (USD) (Stewart, Ricci, Chee, Hahn, & Morganstein, 2003). Another study reported that major depression was associated with a 11 % decrease in productivity (Lerner et al., 2004). Greenberg et al. (2003) and Greenberg, Stiglin, Finkelstein, and Berndt (1993) estimated that, during a depressive episode, 20 % of lost work time takes the form of presenteeism. Kessler et al. (2006) observed that the USA annually loses the equivalent of 151 million days due to presenteeism related to major depressive disorder, which costs the country about $24.5 billion. In comparison, they found that annual presenteeism losses related to bipolar disorder total to about 52 million days or cost $7.6 billion.

In their review of the literature, Hoffman, Dukes, and Wittchen (2008) found that, compared to people with no disorders, those with obsessive compulsive disorders, GAD, panic disorders, and comorbid anxiety and depression, experienced significantly more work impairment. It also has been observed that depression comorbid with chronic physical disorders increases functional disability (Schmitz, Wang, Malla, & Lesage, 2007). The greatest interference with functioning was for depression occurring with heart diseases, ulcers, arthritis, and diabetes. Comorbid mental disorders also increase the likelihood of functional impairment such that, the more diagnoses a person had, the greater the interference they experience (Wang et al., 2006).

There are a number of ways in which mental disorders decrease productivity at work. They can interfere with a worker's social participation, understanding and communicating and day-to-day functioning (Wang et al., 2006). Workers with depressive symptoms are more likely to experience decreased effectiveness at work (Druss, Schlesinger, & Allen, 2001). This could be attributed to the fact that, on average, depression is found to limit performance of physical jobs 20 % of the time, and mental interpersonal demands 35 % of the time (Lerner & Henke, 2008). Workers with severe depression have more job performance deficits than those with moderate or mild depression, and individuals with dysthymia had fewer job performance deficits than patients with major depression (Lerner & Henke, 2008). In addition, Lerner et al. (2004) observed that workers with depression experience more impairment with time management. A 15-year longitudinal study found that work disability was one of the main persistent impairments that people with mood disorders experienced (Judd et al., 2008). Finally, Adler et al. (2008) found that workers with Attention Deficit Hyperactivity Disorder (ADHD) were more likely to have problems with concentration, organization, decreased efficiency, and increased boredom.

Work Loss Days

Among those who are employed, workplace productivity losses due to work absences among workers who have mental disorder are substantial. There are two basic types of absences from work. One type of absence is sporadic, such as sick days taken for a cold. The other is prolonged but taken with an intention to return to the position in the company from which the worker is absent; these types of absences are often referred to as disability absences. This section discusses recent findings regarding the former types of absences which we will refer to as work loss days.

Population-based surveys of workers estimate the annual average depression-related absenteeism productivity loss is about 1 h/week/worker; this is equivalent to $8 billion (USD) (Stewart et al., 2003). Kessler et al. (2006) observed lower numbers of lost work days. Their estimates indicate workers with major depressive disorders experience average annual work absences of 9 days; this totals about $24 billion (USD) or a total of 151 million days lost. In addition, $6 billion (USD) or a total of 41 million days are lost each year due to work days absences related to bipolar disorder (Kessler et al., 2006). The number of absences related to depression is also greater than those for many chronic medical conditions

(Buist-Bouwman et al., 2005; Druss, Rosenheck, & Sledge, 2000; Grzywacz & Ettner, 2000). Compared to people with physical conditions, those with mental disorders have, on average, more days during which they are not able to carry out their usual activities (Alonso et al. 2011). Data from one USA firm indicate that workers experience an annual average of almost 10 work loss days for depression, compared to 7 days for diabetes, heart problems, and back problems, and 3 days for all other problems (Druss et al., 2000). Using population-based data from the Netherlands, Buist-Bouwman et al. (2005) found that chronic back problems are associated with 25 additional work loss days, compared to 29 additional work loss days associated with mood disorder, and 18 days with anxiety disorders.

There is also increasing evidence that, when they occur together, mental and chronic physical disorders increase the risk of work loss. The odds of a mood or anxiety disorder are significantly greater when someone has a chronic physical disorder (Buist-Bouwman et al., 2005). Those with comorbid mental and chronic physical disorders experience more sick days (Braden, Zhang, Zimmerman, & Sullivan, 2008; Buist-Bouwman et al., 2005; Dewa et al., 2007; Druss et al., 2000). Workers with both mental and chronic physical disorders are at four times the odds of an absence day compared to a worker who has neither (Dewa et al., 2007). Buist-Bouwman et al. (2005) reported there were significant increases in work loss days for workers who have comorbid anxiety and mood disorders with chronic back problems or hypertension, relative to either type of condition alone. Workers with chronic pain disorders (e.g., migraine/chronic headache, arthritis, back problems) and a mental disorder are more likely to miss at least one work day in the past month (Braden et al., 2008). Holden et al. (2011) observed increased absenteeism among workers with comorbid psychological distress and either an injury, cancer, or arthritis.

Disability Absences

In contrast to work loss days, disability absences are absences from work that extend beyond what would be covered by "sick leave." Generally, it is an absence for which a worker must file an insurance claim for income replacement or disability benefits (i.e., short-term or long-term disability) while s/he is off from work. These benefits may be either publicly or privately sponsored. It should also be noted that the qualifications for disability benefits differ by disability insurance plans. As a result, it is difficult to estimate the precise costs associated with these types of disability benefits. That being said, it is possible to examine the trends in disability benefit claims. Disability claims for mental and nervous disorder have increased over time. Between 1989 and 1994, the Health Insurance Association of America (HIAA, 1995) found that disability claims doubled. HIAA (1995) also found respondent companies spend between $360 and $540 million on disability claims related to this group of disorders. Over half of short-term mental or nervous disorder disability claims are attributed to depression [Conti & Burton, 1994; Dewa, Goering, Lin, & Paterson, 2002; Health Insurance Association of America (HIAA), 1995].

In Canada, mental illness-related short- and long-term disability account for up to a third of claims and account for about 70 % of the total costs, translating into $15–$33 billion annually (Sroujian, 2003). For some companies, claims related to mental and nervous disorders account for 30–40 % of all short-term disability claims (Sairanen, Matzanki, & Smeall, 2011). In addition, it has been observed that at the end of a short-term disability episode, about 76 % of workers return to their jobs, while approximately 8 % go on to receive long-term disability benefits (Dewa et al., 2002). Although a small proportion of workers receive long-term disability benefits, a long-term disability episode could cost almost four times that of a short-term disability episode (Sairanen et al., 2011). There are suggestions that long-term disability episodes have increased by 0.5–1.0 % and account for as much as 30 % of total claims (Sairanen et al., 2011).

The total cost of disability claims depends on three factors: (1) the per diem disability absence cost; (2) the length of the absence; and (3) the number of disability absences. The cost of a single disability absence is a function of the first two factors. If the disability benefit serves as a salary replacement, the per diem cost will reflect the worker's salary. That is, the higher the salary, the more each day of the disability absence costs. Furthermore, each disability day is multiplied by per diem disability absence cost. Thus, the more disability absence days, the greater the total cost of the disability absence. Compared with other types of disability absences, those related to depression are relatively longer than those for other types of disorders such as rheumatoid arthritis, heart disease, and diabetes (Adler et al., 2006; Burton & Conti, 1998; Conti & Burton, 1994; Druss et al., 2000). Factors contributing to more disability absence days are a diagnosis of depression or anxiety, being over 50 years old and worker expectations (Nieuwenhuijsen, Verbeek, de Boer, Blonk, & van Dijk, 2006). In addition, females were also more likely to have a longer disability absence (Rytsala et al., 2007). It has been observed that, compared with the costs of the average disability episode related to physical disorders, those for mental/behavioral disorders can be double the cost per episode (Dewa et al., 2010). Higher rates of comorbid mental and physical disorders contribute to duration of disability leave. For example, Hensel, Bender, Bacchiochi, Pelletier, and Dewa (2010) observed that workers who experienced psychological trauma, and who had a permanent physical impairment also with multiple mental disorders, were significantly more likely to receive disability benefits than those with less complex cases.

The third factor contributing to the total costs of disability absences is the number of disability absences. This is related to the recurrence of a disorder. Workers who have previously been on a disability leave are more likely to have a future leave (Dewa, Chau, & Dermer, 2009; Lotters, Hogg-Johnson, & Burdorf, 2005; Rytsala et al., 2005). In comparison to workers who did not have a past disability, those who had one related to a mental disorder are seven times more likely to have another leave, and those with leaves for other types of disorders were twice as likely (Dewa, Chau, & Dermer, 2009). Relative to other disorders such as diabetes, hypertension, and asthma, workers who had a leave for depression are more likely to have another leave (Burton & Conti, 1998). Andrews (2008) identified one of the main factors that contribute to the enormity of the burden of depression is the high relapse rates.

Summary of the Effects of Work Disability Related to Mental Disorders

Work disability related to mental disorders take a number of forms, including unemployment, presenteeism, and work absences. We discussed the various work outcomes of disability, highlighting the fact that the greatest impacts are with people with mental disorders. The main points are summarized below.

- Mental disorders often create barriers to working. As a result, working age people with mental disorders are less likely to be working. Estimates suggest that the majority of people with schizophrenia and other severe and persistent mental disorders are not working. People with depression and anxiety disorders are at higher risks of unemployment than those who do not have them.
- One of the primary work-related disability outcomes of mental disorders is presenteeism. The decreased productivity experienced by workers is related to the symptoms of the mental disorders. While they do necessarily inhibit the ability to attend work, symptoms related to mental disorders can interfere with the performance of work tasks requiring concentration, communication, and social interaction.
- Although workers often experience relatively fewer work loss and disability days than presenteeism days, these work absences nevertheless represent significant productivity losses. Compared to workers with chronic physical disorders, workers with mental disorders can experience as many or more work loss days.
- Over time, there has been an increase in the short- and long-term disability claims related to mental disorders. Furthermore, the length of a disability absence appears to be longer for mental disorder

claims when compared to those for physical disorders. In addition, the length of the absence can be exacerbated with a comorbid physical disorder. Furthermore, workers who have had one disability absence related to a mental disorder are more at risk of another absence than those with absences for other types of disorders.

Work-Related Risk Factors for Mental Disorders and Disability

The previous section highlighted the burden of mental disorders in the workplace. A correlated question would be whether the work contributes to the burden of mental disorders. In this section, we will discuss the evidence regarding work-related risk factors for mental disorders and disability-related to mental disorders. Over the past 20 years, the literature about the negative relationship between work stress and mental health (Bourbonnais, Comeau, Vezina, & Dion, 1998; Clumeck et al., 2009; Ibrahim, Scott, Cole, Shannon, & Eyles, 2001) has been growing (indeed, many other chapters in this Hnadbook have documented this fact). For example, longitudinal studies have found that exposure to high job strain (Karasek & Theorell, 1990) leads to increased risk of depression and anxiety (Clays et al., 2007; Shields, 2006; Wang, Schmitz, Dewa, & Stansfeld, 2009). In addition, there are numerous cross-sectional studies reporting that high job strain is related to a higher risk of self-reported mental health problems (e.g., Amick et al., 1998; Parent-Thirion, Fernández Macías, Hurley, & Vermeylen, 2007). There is a twofold increase in the risk of any psychiatric condition among those experiencing work-related stress (Bourbonnais & Mondor, 2001). In addition the probability of disability among workers who have a mental disorder increases in the presence of chronic work stress (Dewa et al., 2007). These results suggest that addressing chronic work stress may be one of the key ways to decrease either the prevalence of mental disorders or disability among workers with mental disorders. An understanding of the work-related risk factors helps to better target interventions (Fig. 6.2). The following offers a short description about a selection of these factors.

Job Characteristics

A number of risk factors for chronic work stress and job strain have been identified. For instance, chronic work stress can be associated with a number of job characteristics, including high effort and low reward, as well as high job demands (Stansfeld, Fuhrer, Shipley, & Marmot, 1999). High job strain has been associated with a threefold risk of depression or anxiety disorders independent of other nonwork-related factors (Clark et al., 2012). A recent review of prospective studies found that exposure to a combination of high effort and low reward is associated with a 1.8 increased risk of depression (Siegrist, 2008). In addition, workers who viewed their work as a career, felt greater responsibility for their companies, having to work variable or extra hours, and were more likely to report that their jobs were highly stressful (Dewa, Thompson, & Jacobs, 2011a, 2011b). This suggests that meaningful work recognition may have a positive influence on mental health status (Dewa, Dermer et al. 2009).

One way to counter the potential negative impacts of stressful job characteristics could be to promote worker satisfaction. Workers with high work satisfaction are less likely to report high work stress (Dewa, Thompson, & Jacobs, 2011a, 2011b; Siegrist, 2008). There is also a significant body of work examining the relationship between work satisfaction and mental health status. A meta-analysis, based on 500 reported studies, found a strong correlation between job satisfaction and mental health status (Faragher, Cass, & Cooper, 2005). There also has been increasing awareness about the impacts of conflict at work and aggression, such as bullying in the workplace (which will be discussed in another chapter of this Handbook). Prospective studies have noted an association between experiences

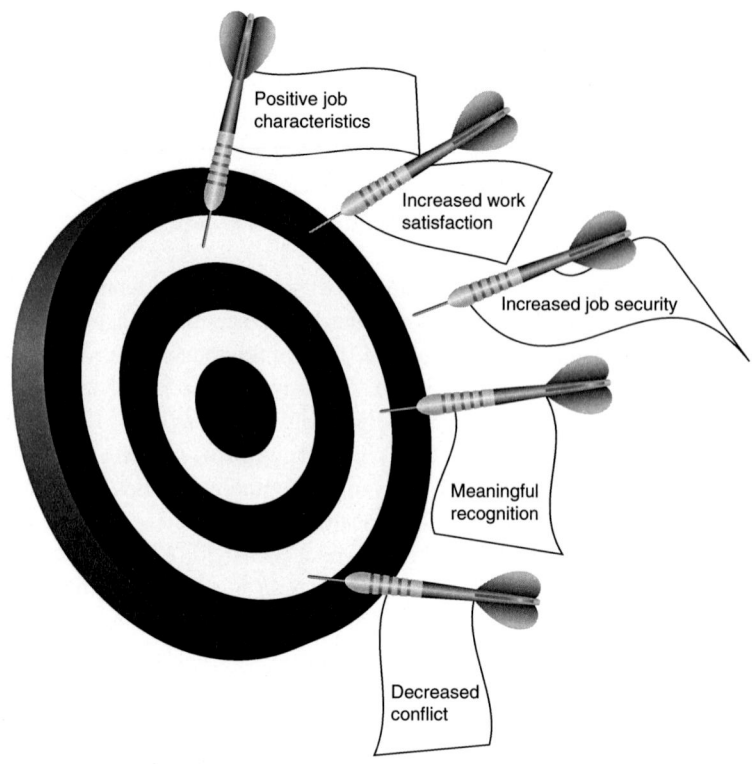

Fig. 6.2 Targeting factors contributing to chronic work stress

of bullying and depression (Kivimaki et al., 2003). A large longitudinal study of Finnish employees reported that employees who experienced recent interpersonal conflict at work, defined as "difficulties" with any coworker, supervisors, or supervisees in the past 6 months, had an elevated risk of mental health problems regardless of gender (Romanov, Appelberg, Honkasalo, & Koskenvuo, 1996), and that females had a higher association with work disability (early retirement on medical grounds; Romanov, Appleberg et al., 1996). Similarly, a study of young workers between 16 and 19 years old found a positive association between interpersonal conflict with coworkers and depression (Frone, 2000).

There also are differences in the chronic work stress experienced by occupation. There is accumulating evidence that within many contexts, professionals, and managers are at relatively greater risks of experiencing chronic work stress as are workers in clerical and secretarial positions (Cherry et al., 2006; Dewa et al., 2010). Thus, it may be important to ensure that "at risk" occupations can access programs and supports to help workers address work stress. Certain occupations are also at higher risk of being exposed to conditions that may precipitate negative psychosocial reactions. This is especially relevant for occupations at high risk of traumatic events, including emergency service workers (fire fighters, police, paramedics), military personnel, acute medical services staff, retail clerks potentially exposed to armed robbery, as well as transportation workers (i.e., train and subway drivers; McFarlane & Bryant, 2007). It should also be noted that job characteristics appear to have different impacts on men and women. For example, there is a high proportion of men with depression who have high job strain, whereas there is a high proportion of women with depression who have low social support in the workplace (Godin et al., 2009). Long working hours were associated with depression in women (Shields, 1999). These results suggest the need for workplaces to encourage activities that include team building.

Job Security

There is also a significant relationship between job insecurity and lower mental health status (Korten & Henderson, 2000). Job insecurity is associated with increasing the odds of depression by four times and the odds of anxiety by three times (D'Souza, Strazdins, Lim, Broom, & Rodgers, 2003). The relationship between job insecurity and depressive symptoms has been found to be especially significant for men (Rugulies, Bultmann, Aust, & Burr, 2006; Stansfeld & Candy, 2006). There also appears to be an interaction between job insecurity and job status. Workers who are in high or mid-status positions, and who have low job security, are at greater risk of poor mental health (D'Souza et al., 2003). Thus, in poor economic times as organizations seek ways to reduce staff, they may be inadvertently increasing the risk of mental health problems and disability among remaining staff. This suggests a need to balance austerity motivated measures with interventions to support the staff and decrease the risk of inadvertent negative impacts of those measures.

Summary of Work-Related Risk Factors for Mental Disorders and Disability

The current evidence suggests that work stress is one of the critical ways in which the workplace affects mental health and disability. A variety of job characteristics and job security significantly contribute to either increasing or decreasing work stress. The relationships among the factors suggest that there may be ways in which aspects of work could be modified to lower the risk of mental disorder and disability. Examples would be to ensure there is meaningful work recognition or promotion of activities that increase worker satisfaction. More work is needed to identify the most effective ways of addressing these factors and whether there are differences by occupations and industries. What is meaningful in different settings? The fact that workplaces play significant roles in worker health also calls to attention the complexity of the relationship between worker mental health and the workplace.

Interventions to Decrease Disability

Much of the work about mental disorders and the workplace focus on understanding the impact of mental disorders on the workplace, and the complex relationship between the worker and his/her work. There is less information about how evidence-based interventions can address work disability related to mental disorders. In this section, we highlight selected evidence-based interventions aimed at decreasing disability related to mental disorders.

Interventions for People Who Are Not Employed

We begin this section by discussing an evidence-based employment model for people with severe and persistent mental disorders who are unemployed. Although people who are not working or who are unemployed do not directly impact the workplace, their absence nevertheless has meaning. Admittedly, it may be difficult to imagine the counterfactual. However, there are at least two main reasons for considering workplace interventions for this group. First, unemployment may reinforce an infinite loop. As discussed above, unemployment may serve as a risk factor for mental disorders (Baumeister & Harter, 2007; Lindstrom, 2005; Maier et al., 2006). If unemployment can also contribute to the development of mental disorders, it could also prevent recovery. Second, there are evidence-based interventions designed for people with severe mental disorders who want to work. Supported employment (SE) programs are an example. SE programs are among the most widely studied and recognized evidence-based practices for supporting people with severe mental disorders to integrate or reintegrate into competitive employment (Burns et al., 2007; Cook et al., 2005; Corrigan, Mueser, Bond, Drake, & Solomon, 2008; Crowther, Marshall, Bond, & Huxley, 2001; Latimer et al., 2006; Wong et al., 2008). The SE model uses employment specialists who are available to accompany clients to job interviews and who provide continuous and time-unlimited support once clients are employed.

In a recent review of 11 randomized trials assessing the effectiveness of SE programs, Bond, Drake, and Becker (2008) found that, on average, work integration success rates for people with severe mental disorders were about 60 %, as compared to 25 % for other types of work reintegration programs. In their review, Bond et al. (2008) reported significant variations in reported success that ranged from 27 to 78 %. The variation in findings have been attributed to difficulties in the SE implementation process (Becker et al., 2007; Marshall, Rapp, Becker, & Bond, 2008; Rapp et al., 2010; Rinaldi, Miller, & Perkins, 2010; Sherring, Robson, Morris, Frost, & Tirupati, 2010; Swain, Whitley, McHugo, & Drake, 2010). Rinaldi et al. (2010) propose three main phases needed for implementation: (1) adoption in principle, (2) early implementation, and (3) persistence and perseverance in maintaining program fidelity. Numerous authors have identified strategies that should be considered during these phases. The strategies include (1) ensuring there is leadership for the SE program implementation, (2) a clear understanding about the SE program model, (3) training and supervision for SE program employment specialists, (4) SE program implementation staff have a recovery philosophy, and (5) use of fidelity scales to ensure implementation is consistent with the standardized model (Corbiere et al., 2010; Marshall et al., 2008; Rapp et al., 2010; Swain et al., 2010). These implementation strategies will be discussed below in the order of Rinaldi et al. (2010) proposed phases.

Phase 1: Adoption in Principle
Persuasive and assertive leadership is essential to demystifying mental illness and to convincing SE stakeholders that individuals with severe mental disorders can successfully be employed. Swain et al. (2010) refers to effective leaders as "champions." These champions are often supervisors or directors who are motivated by the belief that any person with a severe mental disorder can be integrated into the competitive work setting if appropriate measures are put in place. Rapp et al. (2010) point out that supervisors who adopt a "laissez faire" attitude with no particular expectations of the employment specialists will be counterproductive. In addition to having clinical skills, champions also should ideally have sales or marketing skills and should play a liaison role, developing collaborative relationships with influential community leaders (Marshall et al., 2008). They should also be able to offer sceptics concrete examples of successes in local workplaces with which all stakeholders are familiar.

Phase 2: Early Implementation
Implementation preparation seems to be an essential strategy for success. This training is essential given that it is difficult to find in-depth academic and clinical training on how to be an employment specialist (Loisel & Corbiere, 2011). Other authors recommend ensuring client follow-up during this phase so that the employment specialists can help their clients successfully obtain and maintain competitive work. Rigorous follow-up can be carried out by such means as systematic client evaluation, even after clients have obtained employment (Torrey, Bond, McHugo, & Swain, 2011).

Phase 3: Persistence and Perseverance in Maintaining Program Fidelity
Regular assessment of program fidelity to the standardized model helps to ensure the service quality. Drake and Bond (2008) assert that a high level of program fidelity can be attained within 6 months to a year if program activities are monitored. Several authors suggest that fidelity scales be used to

properly assess program fidelity (Campbell et al., 2007; Mowbray, Holter, Teague, & Bybee, 2003). One specific type of standardized SE (i.e., has well-defined criteria with which fidelity to the established model can be evaluated) is the Individual Placement and Support (IPS) program. Becker and Drake (1994) enumerate the principles of the IPS model as (1) enrolment based on client choice (zero exclusion); (2) competitive employment as the goal; (3) immediate job search upon enrolment in the program with the search lasting from 1 to 3 months; (4) employment specialists work in close collaboration with the client's mental health treatment team; (5) clients select workplace based on their vocational interests/preferences; (6) employment specialists are available for support and time unlimited follow-up; and (7) benefits counseling is offered to inform clients of potential financial consequences of earnings.

Interventions for Workers Experiencing Disability Related to Mental Disorders

Use of mental health services has been identified as an effective way of decreasing the impact of mental disorders among workers experiencing disability related to mental disorders (Dewa et al. in press). However, a recent population-based study observed that about 57 % of workers with a moderate depressive episode, and 40 % of workers with a severe depressive episode, did not use treatment (Dewa et al. in press). Yet, there is evidence that those with moderate and severe depressive episodes who receive treatment (as compared to those who do not) have a significantly greater likelihood of being highly productive at work (Dewa et al. in press). There is also evidence that early treatment can shorten the length of disability leave. For example, workers who received antidepressant treatment within the first 30 days of their disability leaves had significantly shorter disability episodes than those who did not (Dewa, Hoch, Lin, Paterson, & Goering, 2003). One of the impediments to receipt of care is out-of-pocket costs (Dewa, Hoch, & Goering, 2008). That is, in environments in which health care is not publically funded, workers must rely on the insurance benefits offered by their employers. Often, these benefits have cost-sharing arrangements such that workers must pay for part of the treatments they use. If this is the case, these costs can serve as deterrents to accessing services.

Another barrier to accessing early intervention can be related to difficulty in finding specialty care. This necessitates a reliance on primary care providers to handle cases of mental disorders regardless of the case's complexity. Collaborative care models have been suggested as an intervention to address this type of situation. In these models, specialists act as consultants to the primary care physicians. There is evidence that these models are cost-effective in workplace settings (Dewa, Hoch, Carmen, Guscott, & Anderson, 2009).

Interventions for Workers Returning to Work After a Disability Leave

In this section, we describe interventions that have been effective for people who are returning to work following a disability leave. The return-to-work process is complex, and only can be effectively achieved through a coordination and collaboration of a variety of actors and the development and use of an accommodation plan (Durand & Loisel, 2001; Loisel et al., 2001). Much of the current thinking about return-to-work is based on successes from the management of musculoskeletal disorders (Noordik, van Dijk, Nieuwenhuijsen, & van der Klink, 2009; van der Klink & van Dijk, 2003; van Oostrom, van Mechelen, Terluin, de Vet, & Anema, 2009). The hallmarks studies in this area have been conducted by Mayer et al. (1987). They developed the first comprehensive interdisciplinary pain management found to be therapeutically effective for chronic musculoskeletal disorders, such as low back pain (Mayer & Gatchel, 1988). Labeled as *functional restoration*, it became the "gold standard" of care for such musculoskeletal pain and disability disorders. The treatment- and cost-effectiveness of such programs have been well documented in the scientific literature (e.g., Gatchel & Okifuji, 2006; Turk & Swanson, 2007). Such programs requires an interdisciplinary team of clinicians (physician, psychologist/psychiatrist, physical therapist, occupational therapist) who work closely together, and set goals of restoring physical functional capacity and psychosocial performance in patients. A systematic review by Guzman et al. (2001) revealed that intensive interdisciplinary rehabilitation with functional restoration achieved its goal of pain reduction and functional restoration, relative to usual care. Support for the robustness of the findings on functional restoration programs include the fact that studies across economic and social conditions have produced positive and comparable outcomes not only in the USA but also in other countries such as Denmark (Bendix et al., 1996; Bendix & Bendix, 1994), Germany (Hildebrandt, Pfingsten, Saur, & Jansen, 1997), Canada (Corey, Koepfler, Etlin, & Day, 1996), France (Jousset et al., 2004), and even Japan (Shirado et al., 2005). Thus, Gatchel and Okifuji (2006) had concluded "The fact that different clinical treatment teams, functioning in different States and different countries, with markedly different economic and social conditions and workers' compensation systems produced comparable positive results speaks highly for the robustness of the research findings and the utility, as well as the fidelity, of this approach to pain management…" (p. 782). Moreover, the success of the functional restoration approach has been thoroughly documented, with over 40 studies now available through MEDLINE supporting the approach with dissemination Worldwide, including into the USA military.

The Sherbrooke Model is another later example of an effective approach (using functional restoration methods) for work disability related to musculoskeletal disorders that was tested using a randomized controlled trial. Its effective components include early intervention that has participative ergonomics (Loisel et al., 1997; Loisel et al., 2002), as well as systematic follow-up for all workers on disability leave and early detection of cases at risk of prolonged absence. Participative ergonomics involves collaboration among the worker on leave, the ergonomist, the immediate supervisors, and coworkers. Together, they identify work site risk factors and associated solutions. One of the strengths of the model seems to be the problem-solving aspect focused on the workplace.

Interventions for workers returning to work from a work disability leave related to a mental disorder have drawn from the examples such as the Sherbrooke Model. For example, van Oostrom et al. (2007) used the principles of the Sherbrooke Model to develop a program for workers with mental disorders that incorporated participative ergonomics, such as described above, along with a significant investment by the workers and their immediate supervisors in the problem-solving process. The program was effective for workers who had been absent from work for high psychosocial stress for 2 to 8 weeks (van Oostrom et al., 2010; van Oostrom et al., 2010). Two studies have looked at work-focused problem-solving interventions for people with adjustment disorders in which workers are prepared for stressors that they may encounter when they return. Both studies incorporated cognitive behavioral interventions focusing on stress management. Using a randomized trial design, van der Klink, Blonk, Schene, and van Dijk (2003) found that, compared with medical treatment alone and intervention that included gradual return to work, stress management activities (Meichenbaum, 1993), and a cognitive behavioral intervention that focused on developing worker skills to resolve work-related problems (Saunders, Driskell, Johnston, & Salas, 1996), resulted in increased rates of return-to-work and reduced the lengths of disability leaves. They also included a follow-up with workers in which a workplace physician helped to address factors to prevent relapse. Indeed, it has been reported that compared to those with no history of disability leaves, workers who have had a previous disability leave are significantly more at risk of a future episode (Dewa, Chau, & Dermer, 2009).

In their study, Blonk, Brenninkmeijer, Lagerveld, and Houtman (2006) observed a reduction of 200 days of absence for workers who had both a cognitive behavioral intervention and sessions focused on stress management, and preparing for obstacles and conditions that workers might encounter as they returned to work. In the Sherbrooke Model, if the absence continued after the participative ergonomics, the workers on disability leave for musculoskeletal disorders were encouraged to take part in an education and exercise program. If the leave continued, workers were referred to an interdisciplinary return-to-work program. This more intensive approach has also been adapted for workers on disability leave for mental disorders. An example is the Therapeutic Return-to-Work (TRW) program developed by Durand and Briand (2011). It has been feasibility tested in two Quebec contexts (Durand, Coutu, St-Arnaud, & Corbiere, 2009). Using an evidence-based approach (Durand, Loisel, & Charpentier, 2004; Durand et al., 2004; Durand, Vachon, Loisel, & Berthelette, 2003), the TRW program seeks to address the multiple factors contributing to a disability leave (Loisel et al., 2001), while taking a client-centered approach (Falardeau & Durand, 2002). It is based on the four critical steps in the return-to-work process identified by Briand, Durand, St-Arnaud, and Corbiere (2007) and used by other rehabilitation models (Anthony, Cohen, Farkas, & Gagne, 2002; de las Heras, Llerena, & Kielhofner, 2003; Farkas, Sullivan-Soydan, & Gagne, 2001; Fougeyrollas et al., 1998; Kielhofner, 2002). The four steps are (1) evaluate the work disability context, (2) increase the readiness to commit to return-to-work, (3) support active involvement (mobilization) in the return to work, and lastly, (4) decrease risk of relapse. These steps are briefly described below.

Evaluating the Work Disability Context
To clearly understand the worker's context, the program's clinical team is careful to identify, throughout the rehabilitation process, all the "levers and obstacles" to the worker's return-to-work. The worker's core clinical team consists of an occupational therapist with ergonomics training, and a psychologist trained in cognitive behavioral therapy. The core is supplemented with other clinicians, including the worker's physician, who performs the regular follow-up, and a psychiatrist who, as required, evaluates the worker and makes recommendations regarding diagnosis and treatment. Several tools may be used for this purpose, including the *Work Disability Diagnostic Interview for Common Mental Disorders* (WoDDI-CMD) (Durand et al., 2011). The WoDDI brings together information about the worker (medical, historical, psychological and related to lifestyle habits), his/her work environment, and his/her family and social situation. It is useful in helping to identify the combination and interaction of factors that may inhibit a worker's return to work. Because the worker's context may be changing throughout the disability leave and return, it is important to constantly note and adjust for these changes.

Increasing Readiness to Commit to Return-to-Work (Concept of Rehabilitation Readiness; Farkas et al., 2001)
Following a prolonged disability leave, the worker is often caught in a vicious circle of demotivation and deconditioning. In cases of a disability leave related to mental disorders, absence from work can be for several weeks to allow for stabilization of prescription drugs. At the same time, St-Arnaud, Saint-Jean, and Rhéaume (2003) suggested that absence from work can increase anxiety. As a result, the worker may then enter a spiral of avoidance that reinforces his/her fears about returning to work. Muschalla and Linden (2009) report that, in extreme situations, the events can lead to the development of ergophobia, a phobic anxiety reaction toward the work environment. Thus, part of the return-to-work process must target the worker's motivation and self-esteem. Therapeutic activities include interventions focused on increasing self-awareness, as well as cognitive behavioral approaches centered on adjusting perceptions and developing stress management strategies, but also interventions geared toward reintroducing the worker to the work context through a visit to the workplace and simulation of work tasks. Establishing a coherent discourse among the various stakeholders, including the worker, his/her supervisors, the clinicians involved (occupational therapist, psychologist, and physician) and the insurance company is also important.

Support Active Involvement (Mobilization) in the Return-to-Work

This step builds on the preceding one by actively supporting the collaboration of the employer, immediate supervisor, the clinicians involved (occupational therapist, psychologist, and physician), and the insurance company in the return-to-work process. A return-to-work coordinator can be effective in ensuring collaboration and communication among the stakeholders (Pomaki et al., 2010). A successful collaboration may require extensive negotiation (or mediation), as well as an investment in effective communication among all parties. This may mean helping employers and immediate supervisors to modify their expectations for the worker when s/he returns to work. There is a danger that when an employee returns to his/her regular work schedule after a long absence, there may be the expectation that s/he should have a level of productivity equal to that of the persons in good health occupying the same position. In order to address expectations, the TRW reframes the return-to-work as a therapeutic return to work rather than a gradual return to work. Whereas a gradual return-to-work is often the recommendation of general practitioners and focuses on the number of hours of work, the therapeutic return-to-work sees initial return as a way to condition the worker for an eventual resumption of his/her full tasks. Thus, in the TRW process, the supervisor is prepared for the fact that the worker will not immediately return to full productivity.

It should be noted that the quality of the relationship between the worker and his/her supervisor and coworkers could affect the success of the return-to-work attempt. The support of coworkers and supervisors is an important factor in decreasing job stress and increasing mental health status (D'Souza et al., 2005; Dewa, Dermer et al., 2009). Yet, prior to a disability leave, the relationship between the worker and his/her coworkers and supervisor could deteriorate because of the symptoms of the mental disorders. For example, Smith et al. (2002) observed that workers with depression experienced workplace conflict. Other studies have shown that workers suffering from depression are more likely to have difficulty focusing on tasks and meeting their quotas (Lerner et al., 2003; Wang et al., 2004). The impairment in functioning can also affect coworkers who may need to undertake the additional workload to meet a deadline or quota. In the process, resentment could develop because of the extra workload.

Ideally, the TRW program would intervene to reframe the negative perceptions and attempt to create a positive or at least neutral job atmosphere for the worker. But, workers do not always work in ideal contexts. In fact, the TRW program is sometimes confronted with the refusal by the worker to disclose his/her mental health problems to his/her coworkers and supervisor; this could complicate the clinician's intervention. This refusal is not unwarranted given evidence that people with mental disorders often face stigma and prejudice in the workplace (Marwaha & Johnson, 2004). One German study reported there were strong negative responses to people with schizophrenia returning to their jobs (Schulze & Angermeyer, 2003). In addition, employers have indicated a reluctance to either hire or to promote individuals with histories of mental illness (Nicholas, 1998; Scheid, 1999). It will be important for future research to either identify effective interventions that work around the problem of stigma or eliminate stigma all together. Once the collaboration has been established, progressive conditioning in the work environment can begin. Progressive conditioning involves gradually exposing the worker to the anxiety-provoking situation and putting him into action (as long as the work environment acts as a lever to his return-to-work rather than as an obstacle; Durand & Loisel, 2001). The worker can thus regain confidence in his/her work related skills, reclaim his/her place again at work, and reconstruct his/her socio-professional identity as a worker. The essential ingredient is the establishment of a favorable and flexible work environment. Supervision by a clinician, usually the occupational therapist, during the gradual return ensures a healthy balance between the worker's abilities (which will evolve during the process) and the work demands. To help the worker evolve toward a return to his/her full duties, a gradual increase in the work demands is essential, otherwise the risk of relapse is significant.

Decrease Risk of Relapse

Continuing the conditioning directly in the work environment is favored, as are meetings with core clinical team and the employer (and the insurance company, if necessary) to generate recommendations for work accommodations (modifying the work routine or work space, etc.). Thus, after the worker reassumes his/her full work schedule and related work demands, telephone conversations between the clinician and the worker could continue to take place for several weeks. These conversations provide a way of tracking the evolution and maintenance of the worker's condition. These supports are not only necessary in the first months of return-to-work, but could be useful on a continuous basis. Anecdotal evidence indicates that these activities help to defuse various work situations and avoid relapses. There is evidence that, although workers who have had a previous disability absence are more at risk of another one, most do not have a recurrent disability absence within the first year of their return to work (Dewa, Chen, Chau, & Dermer, 2011). This raises the question of whether the availability of ongoing support could decrease the risk of recidivism.

Summary of Interventions to Decrease Disability

While there are not copious evidence-based interventions from which to choose, the literature is growing and there seems to be common ingredients emerging from the evidence that we have. First, collaboration among stakeholders appears to be a critical component. At a minimum, it means that the worker, the worker's clinician, and the supervisor should be conferring about how to ensure successful employment. The involvement of the supervisor begins to raise a number of questions including, "What do managers need to know?" This is a question that middle managers often pose (Dewa, Burke, Hardaker, Caveen, & Baynton, 2006). Thus, thought must be put into developing a curriculum and training to prepare for this responsibility. Ongoing support and resources are useful for managers to consult about questions that arise (Dewa et al., 2006). The validation and offer of resources from an organization's leadership is also important to reinforcing that this is an important activity for managers to undertake (Caveen, Dewa, & Goering, 2006). More research is required to identify effective ways of enabling managers to support their employees both who are returning to work as well as their coworkers. In addition, the worker needs accessibility to services and supports. These services and supports include someone to consult if work becomes stressful or work-related problems are encountered. The support could come from a clinician in terms of medical treatment or ongoing counseling. Or, it could also be the worker if s/he is given the adequate tools to cope and problem solve. Future inquiry could focus on understanding the most effective designs for worker benefit plans that allow for access to continuous supports.

Conclusions: Deciding on a Course of Action

In this chapter, we looked at the case for the importance of mental health and the workplace. We discussed the incidence and prevalence of mental disorders in the working-aged population. Studies seem to indicate consistently that mental health disorders are not the leading disorders experienced by workers. However, as with musculoskeletal disorders, they appear to be among the top 10 disorders. In addition, they often accompany physical disorders. We also discussed the effects of work disability related to mental health disorders. The evidence indicates that mental disorders are associated with significant losses in the forms of unemployment, presenteeism, and work absences. The fact that mental disorders are not the only conditions that affect workplaces suggests that there are a number of concerns that might draw employers' attentions. This creates a dilemma about where to invest scarce workplace resources. One way of informing the decision is to begin by considering what it would cost to continue business as usual. For example, based on estimates from Dewa, Chau, and Dermer (2010), suppose the overall short-term disability absence rate for a company is 145 episodes/1,000 employees. The top two primary categories of disability absences were for musculoskeletal disorder (19/1,000 employees) and mental/behavioral disorders (21/1,000 employees). The average cost of a short-term disability absence for a musculoskeletal disorder is about $9,000 and $18,000 for a mental/behavioral absence. If the company of 1,000 employees did nothing, it would spend up to $171,000 a year for musculoskeletal disorders and $378,000 for mental/behavioral disorders. What can a company do? Hoch and Dewa (2008) summarize the considerations for making such decisions. In their chapter, they describe two main steps. First, a company might look for evidence-based interventions for both disorders. Once it finds interventions that could work in its context, it will be faced with at least two questions. The first is, "How much more/less could an intervention cost on average than current state and how much more/less on average could the company benefit?" The answer to this question allows the decision maker to be a wise shopper. It helps to clarify what it is getting, and at what it costs, versus the current practice. As an example, suppose Company A has 1,000 employees and disability claims that look like those we described above. The company spends up to $18,000 for a disability claim related to a mental/behavioral disorder. How much could it spend to prevent one disability absence related to a mental/behavioral disorder? If Company A wanted to break even, it would spend up to $18,000, to save $18,000.

If an intervention is a good deal, there is a second step that a company still must face. It is to answer the question of, "Is there a budget for the intervention?" Although the intervention appears to be a "good deal", it is not always possible to shift funds from one department to another or from one budget item such as disability insurance to occupational health. This example is not to suggest that the responsibility of the mental health of workers rests entirely with employers. Dewa, McDaid, and Ettner (2007) argue that it is a societal responsibility, with roles for workers, providers, employers, and government because each sector bears part of the burden. Consequently, it is in the best interest of each sector to contribute to its solution. But, because resources are scarce, choices must be made and there are multiple ways to address the challenge. To help each player make better informed decisions, future directions for the research community should include evaluations of interventions that include measures that are relevant to decision makers, including how interventions impact disability. There is increasing evidence about the "critical ingredients" of effective interventions. But, more work needs to be done understanding how those ingredients fit together, the most effective ways of combining them and the most effective adaptations for the multitude of work environments, occupations, and business sectors.

Acknowledgments The authors would like to acknowledge the excellent research assistance provided by Desmond Loong and Caitlin Finney. We would also like to thank Anja Kessler for her superb illustrations. Dr. Dewa gratefully acknowledges the support provided by her Canadian Institutes of Health Research/Public Health Agency of Canada Applied Public Health Chair. The Centre for Addiction and Mental Health receives funding from the Ontario Ministry of Health and Long-Term Care to support research infrastructure and do not reflect their views. Any remaining errors are the sole responsibility of the authors.

References

Adler, D. A., McLaughlin, T. J., Rogers, W. H., Chang, H., Lapitsky, L., & Lerner, D. (2006). Job performance deficits due to depression. *The American Journal of Psychiatry, 163*(9), 1569–1576.
Adler, L. A., Spencer, T. J., Levine, L. R., Ramsey, J. L., Tamura, R., Kelsey, D., et al. (2008). Functional outcomes in the treatment of adults with ADHD. *Journal of Attention Disorders, 11*(6), 720–727.
Alonso, J., Angermeyer, M. C., Bernert, S., Bruffaerts, R., Brugha, T. S., Bryson, H., et al. (2004). Prevalence of mental disorders in Europe: Results from the European Study of the Epidemiology of Mental Disorders (ESEMeD) project. *Acta Psychiatrica Scandinavica Supplementum, (420)*, 21–27.

Alonso, J., Petukhova, M., Vilagut, G., Chatterji, S., Heeringa, S., Ustun, T. B., et al. (2011). Days out of role due to common physical and mental conditions: Results from the WHO World Mental Health surveys. *Molecular Psychiatry, 16*(12), 1234–1246.

Amick, B. C., 3rd, Kawachi, I., Coakley, E. H., Lerner, D., Levine, S., & Colditz, G. A. (1998). Relationship of job strain and iso-strain to health status in a cohort of women in the United States. *Scandinavian Journal of Work, Environment and Health, 24*(1), 54–61.

Andrews, G. (2008). Reducing the burden of depression. *Canadian Journal of Psychiatry, 53*(7), 420–427.

Anthony, W. A., Cohen, M. R., Farkas, M. D., & Gagne, C. (2002). *Psychiatric rehabilitation* (2nd ed.). Boston: Massachusetts Boston University, Center for Psychiatric Rehabilitation.

Appelberg, K., Romanov, K., Heikkila, K., Honkasalo, M. L., & Koskenvuo, M. (1996). Interpersonal conflict as a predictor of work disability: A follow-up study of 15,348 Finnish employees. *Journal of Psychosomatic Research, 40*(2), 157–167.

Baumeister, H., & Harter, M. (2007). Prevalence of mental disorders based on general population surveys. *Social Psychiatry and Psychiatric Epidemiology, 42*(7), 537–546.

Baune, B. T., Adrian, I., & Jacobi, F. (2007). Medical disorders affect health outcome and general functioning depending on comorbid major depression in the general population. *Journal of Psychosomatic Research, 62*(2), 109–118.

Becker, D. R., Baker, S. R., Carlson, L., Flint, L., Howell, R., Lindsay, S., et al. (2007). Critical strategies for implementing supported employment. *Journal of Vocational Rehabilitation, 27*(1), 13–20.

Becker, D. R., & Drake, R. E. (1994). Individual placement and support: A community mental health center approach to vocational rehabilitation. *Community Mental Health Journal, 30*(2), 193–206.

Bendix, T., & Bendix, A. (1994). *Different training programs for chronic low back pain–A randomized, blinded one-year follow-up study*. Paper presented at the International Society for the Study of the Lumbar Spine, Seattle.

Bendix, A. E., Bendix, T., Vaegter, K., Lund, C., Frolund, L., & Holm, L. (1996). Multidisciplinary intensive treatment for chronic low back pain: A randomized, prospective study. *Cleveland Clinic Journal of Medicine, 63*(1), 62–69.

Birnbaum, H. G., Kessler, R. C., Kelley, D., Ben-Hamadi, R., Joish, V. N., & Greenberg, P. E. (2010). Employer burden of mild, moderate, and severe major depressive disorder: Mental health services utilization and costs, and work performance. *Depression and Anxiety, 27*(1), 78–89.

Blonk, R. W., Brenninkmeijer, V., Lagerveld, S. E., & Houtman, I. (2006). Return to work: A comparison of two cognitive behavioural interventions in cases of work-related psychological complaints among the self-employed. *Work and Stress, 20*(2), 129–144.

Bond, G. R., Drake, R. E., & Becker, D. R. (2008). An update on randomized controlled trials of evidence-based supported employment. *Psychiatric Rehabilitation Journal, 31*(4), 280–290.

Bourbonnais, R., Comeau, M., Vezina, M., & Dion, G. (1998). Job strain, psychological distress, and burnout in nurses. *American Journal of Industrial Medicine, 34*(1), 20–28.

Bourbonnais, R., & Mondor, M. (2001). Job strain and sickness absence among nurses in the province of Quebec. *American Journal of Industrial Medicine, 39*(2), 194–202.

Bowden, C. L. (2005). Bipolar disorder and work loss. *The American Journal of Managed Care, 11*(3 Suppl), S91–S94.

Braden, J. B., Zhang, L., Zimmerman, F. J., & Sullivan, M. D. (2008). Employment outcomes of persons with a mental disorder and comorbid chronic pain. *Psychiatric Services, 59*(8), 878–885.

Briand, C., Durand, M. J., St-Arnaud, L., & Corbiere, M. (2007). Work and mental health: Learning from return-to-work rehabilitation programs designed for workers with musculoskeletal disorders. *International Journal of Law and Psychiatry, 30*(4–5), 444–457.

Buist-Bouwman, M. A., de Graaf, R., Vollebergh, W. A., & Ormel, J. (2005). Comorbidity of physical and mental disorders and the effect on work-loss days. *Acta Psychiatrica Scandinavica, 111*(6), 436–443.

Burns, T., Catty, J., Becker, T., Drake, R. E., Fioritti, A., Knapp, M., et al. (2007). The effectiveness of supported employment for people with severe mental illness: A randomised controlled trial. *Lancet, 370*(9593), 1146–1152.

Burton, W. N., & Conti, D. J. (1998). Use of an integrated health data warehouse to measure the employer costs of five chronic disease states. *Disease Management, 1*(1), 17–26.

Bystritsky, A., Kerwin, L., Niv, N., Natoli, J. L., Abrahami, N., Klap, R., et al. (2010). Clinical and subthreshold panic disorder. *Depression and Anxiety, 27*(4), 381–389.

Campbell, K., Bond, G. R., Gervey, R., Pascaris, A., Tice, S., & Revell, G. (2007). Does type of provider organization affect fidelity to evidence-based supported employment? *Journal of Vocational Rehabilitation, 27*, 3–11.

Caveen, M., Dewa, C. S., & Goering, P. (2006). The influence of workplace factors on return to work outcomes. *Canadian Journal of Community Mental Health, 25*(2), 121–142.

Cherry, N. M., Chen, Y., & McDonald, J. C. (2006). Reported incidence and precipitating factors of work-related stress and mental ill-health in the United Kingdom (1996–2001). *Occupational Medicine (London), 56*(6), 414–421.

Cherry, N. M., & McDonald, J. C. (2002). The incidence of work-related disease reported by occupational physicians, 1996–2001. *Occupational Medicine (London), 52*(7), 407–411.

Clark, C., Pike, C., McManus, S., Harris, J., Bebbington, P., Brugha, T., et al. (2012). The contribution of work and non-work stressors to common mental disorders in the 2007 Adult Psychiatric Morbidity Survey. *Psychological Medicine, 42*(4), 829–842.

Clays, E., De Bacquer, D., Leynen, F., Kornitzer, M., Kittel, F., & De Backer, G. (2007). Job stress and depression symptoms in middle-aged workers–prospective results from the Belstress study. *Scandinavian Journal of Work, Environment and Health, 33*(4), 252–259.

Clumeck, N., Kempenaers, C., Godin, I., Dramaix, M., Kornitzer, M., Linkowski, P., et al. (2009). Working conditions predict incidence of long-term spells of sick leave due to depression: Results from the Belstress I prospective study. *Journal of Epidemiology and Community Health, 63*(4), 286–292.

Cohidon, C., Imbernon, E., & Gorldberg, M. (2009). Prevalence of common mental disorders and their work consequences in France, according to occupational category. *American Journal of Industrial Medicine, 52*(2), 141–152.

Comino, E. J., Harris, E., Chey, T., Manicavasagar, V., Penrose Wall, J., Powell Davies, G., et al. (2003). Relationship between mental health disorders and unemployment status in Australian adults. *The Australian and New Zealand Journal of Psychiatry, 37*(2), 230–235.

Conti, D. J., & Burton, W. N. (1994). The economic impact of depression in a workplace. *Journal of Occupational Medicine, 36*(9), 983–988.

Cook, J. A., Leff, H. S., Blyler, C. R., Gold, P. B., Goldberg, R. W., Mueser, K. T., et al. (2005). Results of a multisite randomized trial of supported employment interventions for individuals with severe mental illness. *Archives of General Psychiatry, 62*(5), 505–512.

Corbiere, M., Lanctot, N., Lecomte, T., Latimer, E., Goering, P., Kirsh, B., et al. (2010). A pan-Canadian evaluation of supported employment programs dedicated to people with severe mental disorders. *Community Mental Health Journal, 46*(1), 44–55.

Corey, D. T., Koepfler, L. E., Etlin, D., & Day, H. I. (1996). A limited functional restoration program for injured workers: A randomized trial. *Journal of Occupational Rehabilitation, 6*, 239–249.

Corrigan, P. W., Mueser, K. T., Bond, G. R., Drake, R. E., & Solomon, P. (2008). *Principles and practice of psychiatric rehabilitation: An empirical approach*. New York: The Guilford Press.

Crowther, R. E., Marshall, M., Bond, G. R., & Huxley, P. (2001). Helping people with severe mental illness to obtain work: Systematic review. *BMJ, 322*(7280), 204–208.

D'Souza, R. M., Strazdins, L., Clements, M. S., Broom, D. H., Parslow, R., & Rodgers, B. (2005). The health effects of jobs: Status, working conditions, or both? *Australian and New Zealand Journal of Public Health, 29*(3), 222–228.

D'Souza, R. M., Strazdins, L., Lim, L. L., Broom, D. H., & Rodgers, B. (2003). Work and health in a contemporary society: Demands, control, and insecurity. *Journal of Epidemiology and Community Health, 57*(11), 849–854.

de las Heras, C. G., Llerena, V., & Kielhofner, G. (2003). *The remotivation process: Model of human occupation clearinghouse*. Chicago: College of Applied Health Sciences, Department of Occupational Therapy.

Dersh, J., Gatchel, R. J., Polatin, P., & Mayer, T. (2002). Prevalence of psychiatric disorders in patients with chronic work-related musculoskeletal pain disability. *Journal of Occupational and Environmental Medicine/American College of Occupational and Environmental Medicine, 44*(5), 459–468.

Dewa, C. S., Burke, A., Hardaker, D., Caveen, M., & Baynton, M. A. (2006). Mental health training programs for managers: What do managers find valuable? *Canadian Journal of Community Mental Health, 25*(2), 221–239.

Dewa, C. S., Chau, N., & Dermer, S. (2009). Factors associated with short-term disability episodes. *Journal of Occupational and Environmental Medicine, 51*(12), 1394–1402.

Dewa, C. S., Chau, N., & Dermer, S. (2010). Examining the comparative incidence and costs of physical and mental health-related disabilities in an employed population. *Journal of Occupational and Environmental Medicine, 52*(7), 758–762.

Dewa, C. S., Chen, M. C., Chau, N., & Dermer, S. (2011). Examining factors associated with the length of short-term disability-free days among workers with previous short-term disability episodes. *Journal of Occupational and Environmental Medicine, 53*(6), 669–673.

Dewa, C. S., Dermer, S. W., Chau, N., Lowrey, S., Mawson, S., & Bell, J. (2009). Examination of factors associated with the mental health status of principals. *Work, 33*(4), 439–448.

Dewa, C. S., Goering, P., Lin, E., & Paterson, M. (2002). Depression-related short-term disability in an employed population. *Journal of Occupational and Environmental Medicine, 44*(7), 628–633.

Dewa, C. S., Hoch, J. S., Carmen, G., Guscott, R., & Anderson, C. (2009). Cost, effectiveness, and cost-effectiveness of a collaborative mental health care program for people receiving short-term disability benefits for psychiatric disorders. *Canadian Journal of Psychiatry, 54*(6), 379–388.

Dewa, C. S., Hoch, J. S., & Goering, P. (2008). Previous out-of-pocket drug expenditures and patterns of antidepressant use among workers receiving depression-related disability benefits. *Healthcare Policy, 4*(2), e149–e166.

Dewa, C. S., Hoch, J. S., Lin, E., Paterson, M., & Goering, P. (2003). Pattern of antidepressant use and duration of depression-related absence from work. *The British Journal of Psychiatry, 183*, 507–513.

Dewa, C. S., & Lin, E. (2000). Chronic physical illness, psychiatric disorder and disability in the workplace. *Social Science and Medicine, 51*(1), 41–50.

Dewa, C. S., Lin, E., Corbiere, M., & Shain, M. (2010). Examining the mental health of the working population: Organizations, individuals and haystacks. In D. Streiner & J. Cairney (Eds.), *Mental disorder in Canada: An epidemiological perspective*. Toronto: University of Toronto Press.

Dewa, C. S., Lin, E., Kooehoorn, M., & Goldner, E. (2007). Association of chronic work stress, psychiatric disorders, and chronic physical conditions with disability among workers. *Psychiatric Services, 58*(5), 652–658.

Dewa, C. S., McDaid, D., & Ettner, S. L. (2007). An international perspective on worker mental health problems: Who bears the burden and how are costs addressed? *Canadian Journal of Psychiatry, 52*(6), 346–356.

Dewa, C. S., Thompson, A. H., & Jacobs, P. (2011a). Relationships between job stress and worker perceived responsibilities and job characteristics. *International Journal of Occupational and Environmental Medicine, 2*(1), 37–46.

Dewa, C. S., Thompson, A. H., & Jacobs, P. (2011b). The association of treatment of major depressive episodes and work productivity. *Canadian Journal of Psychiatry, 56*(12), 743–750.

Drake, R. E., & Bond, G. R. (2008). Supported employment: 1998 to 2008. *Psychiatric Rehabilitation Journal, 31*(4), 274–276.

Druss, B. G., Rosenheck, R. A., & Sledge, W. H. (2000). Health and disability costs of depressive illness in a major U.S. corporation. *The American Journal of Psychiatry, 157*(8), 1274–1278.

Druss, B. G., Schlesinger, M., & Allen, H. M., Jr. (2001). Depressive symptoms, satisfaction with health care, and 2-year work outcomes in an employed population. *The American Journal of Psychiatry, 158*(5), 731–734.

Durand, M. J., & Briand, C. (2011). Interventions/programmes de retour au travail destinés aux travailleurs ayant un trouble mental transitoire. In M. Corbiere & M. J. Durand (Eds.), *Du trouble mental à l'incapacité au travail: Une perspective transdisciplinaire qui vise à mieux saisir cette problématique et à offrir des pistes d'interventions*. Québec: Presses de l'Université du Québec.

Durand, M. J., Corbiere, M., Briand, C., Coutu, M. F., St-Arnaud, L., & Charpentier, N. (2011). *Les facteurs reliés aux absences prolongées du travail en raison d'un trouble mental transitoire: Développement d'un outil de mesure*. Montréal: Institut de recherche Robert-Sauvé en santé et en sécurité du travail (IRSST).

Durand, M. J., Coutu, M. F., St-Arnaud, L., & Corbiere, M. (2009). Therapeutic return-to-work program: Can it be adapted for common mental health disorders? *Annual Canadian Congress for Research on Mental Health and Addiction in the Workplace, 4*.

Durand, M. J., & Loisel, P. (2001). La transformation de la réadaptation au travail d'une perspective parcellaire à une perspective systémique. *Perspectives interdisciplinaires sur le travail et la santé (PISTES), 3*.

Durand, M. J., Loisel, P., & Charpentier, N. (2004). *Le programme de Retour Thérapeutique au Travail (RTT): un programme de réadaption au travail basé sur les données probantes*. Longueuil: Centre de recherche clinique en réadaptation au travail PRÉVICAP.

Durand, M. J., Vachon, B., Hong, Q. N., Imbeau, D., Amick, B. C., 3rd, & Loisel, P. (2004). The cross-cultural adaptation of the Work Role Functioning Questionnaire in Canadian French. *International Journal of Rehabilitation Research, 27*(4), 261–268.

Durand, M. J., Vachon, B., Loisel, P., & Berthelette, D. (2003). Constructing the program impact theory for an evidence-based work rehabilitation program for workers with low back pain. *Work, 21*(3), 233–242.

Ettner, S. L., Frank, R. G., & Kessler, R. (1997). The impact of psychiatric disorders on labor market outcomes. *Industrial and Labor Relations Review, 51*(1), 64–81.

Ettner, S. L., & Grzywacz, J. G. (2001). Workers' perceptions of how jobs affect health: A social ecological perspective. *Journal of Occupational Health Psychology, 6*(2), 101–113.

Falardeau, M., & Durand, M. J. (2002). Negotiation-centred versus client-centred: Which approach should be used? *Canadian Journal of Occupational Therapy. Revue Canadienne d'ergotherapie, 69*(3), 135–142.

Faragher, E. B., Cass, M., & Cooper, C. L. (2005). The relationship between job satisfaction and health: A meta-analysis. *Occupational and Environmental Medicine, 62*(2), 105–112.

Farkas, M. D., Sullivan-Soydan, A., & Gagne, C. (2001). *An introduction to rehabilitation readiness*. Boston, MA: Boston University, Center for Psychiatric Rehabilitation.

Fougeyrollas, P., Noreau, L., Bergeron, H., Cloutier, R., Dion, S. A., & St-Michel, G. (1998). Social consequences of long term impairments and disabilities: Conceptual approach and assessment of handicap. *International Journal of Rehabilitation Research, 21*(2), 127–141.

Franche, R. L., Carnide, N., Hogg-Johnson, S., Cote, P., Breslin, F. C., Bultmann, U., et al. (2009). Course, diagnosis, and treatment of depressive symptomatology in workers following a workplace injury: A prospective cohort study. *Canadian Journal of Psychiatry. Revue Canadienne de Psychiatrie, 54*(8), 534–546.

Frone, M. R. (2000). Interpersonal conflict at work and psychological outcomes: Testing a model among young workers. *Journal of Occupational Health Psychology, 5*(2), 246–255.

Gatchel, R. J., & Okifuji, A. (2006). Evidence-based scientific data documenting the treatment and cost-effectiveness of comprehensive pain programs for chronic nonmalignant pain programs for chronic nonmalignant pain. *The Journal of Pain, 7*(11), 779–793.

Godin, I., Kornitzer, M., Clumeck, N., Linkowski, P., Valente, F., & Kittel, F. (2009). Gender specificity in the prediction of clinically diagnosed depression. Results of a large cohort of Belgian workers. *Social Psychiatry Psychiatric Epidemiology, 44*(7), 592–600.

Goldberg, R. J., & Steury, S. (2001). Depression in the workplace: Costs and barriers to treatment. *Psychiatric Services, 52*(12), 1639–1643.

Greenberg, P. E., Kessler, R. C., Birnbaum, H. G., Leong, S. A., Lowe, S. W., Berglund, P. A., et al. (2003). The economic burden of depression in the United States: How did it change between 1990 and 2000? *The Journal of Clinical Psychiatry, 64*(12), 1465–1475.

Greenberg, P. E., Stiglin, L. E., Finkelstein, S. N., & Berndt, E. R. (1993). The economic burden of depression in 1990. *The Journal of Clinical Psychiatry, 54*(11), 405–418.

Grzywacz, J. G., & Ettner, S. L. (2000). Lost time on the job: The effect of depression versus physical health conditions. *The Economics of Neuroscience, 2*(6), 41–46.

Guzman, J., Esmail, R., Karjalainen, K., Malmivaara, A., Irvin, E., & Bombardier, C. (2001). Multidisciplinary rehabilitation for chronic low back pain: Systematic review. *British Medical Journal, 322*, 1511–1516.

Health Insurance Association of America [HIAA]. (1995). *Disability claims for mental and nervous disorders*. Washington, DC: Health Insurance Association of America.

Hensel, J., Bender, A., Bacchiochi, J., Pelletier, M., & Dewa, C. S. (2010). A descriptive study of a specialized worker's psychological trauma program. *Occupational Medicine (London), 60*(8), 654–657.

Hildebrandt, J., Pfingsten, M., Saur, P., & Jansen, J. (1997). Prediction of success from a multidisciplinary treatment program for chronic low back pain. *Spine, 22*, 990–1001.

Hoch, J. S., & Dewa, C. S. (2008). Issues of kind of analysis and decision rule. In A. C. E. Tompa & R. Dolinschi (Eds.), *Economic evaluation of interventions for occupational health and safety: Developing good practice* (pp. 147–163). Oxford: Oxford University Press.

Hoffman, D. L., Dukes, E. M., & Wittchen, H. U. (2008). Human and economic burden of generalized anxiety disorder. *Depression and Anxiety, 25*(1), 72–90.

Holden, L., Scuffham, P. A., Hilton, M. F., Ware, R. S., Vecchio, N., & Whiteford, H. A. (2011). Health-related productivity losses increase when the health condition is co-morbid with psychological distress: Findings from a large cross-sectional sample of working Australians. *BMC Public Health, 11*, 417.

Ibrahim, S. A., Scott, F. E., Cole, D. C., Shannon, H. S., & Eyles, J. (2001). Job strain and self-reported health among working women and men: An analysis of the 1994/5 Canadian National Population Health Survey. *Women and Health, 33*(1–2), 105–124.

Jousset, N., Fanello, S., Bontoux, L., Dubus, V., Billabert, C., Vielle, B., et al. (2004). Effects of functional restoration versus 3 hours per week physical therapy: A randomized controlled study. *Spine, 29*(5), 487–493.

Judd, L. L., Schettler, P. J., Solomon, D. A., Maser, J. D., Coryell, W., Endicott, J., et al. (2008). Psychosocial disability and work role function compared across the long-term course of bipolar I, bipolar II and unipolar major depressive disorders. *Journal of Affective Disorders, 108*(1–2), 49–58.

Karasek, R., & Theorell, T. (1990). *Healthy work: Stress, productivity, and the reconstruction of working life* (pp. 89–103). New York: Basic Books.

Kendler, K. S., Gardner, C. O., & Prescott, C. A. (2002). Toward a comprehensive developmental model for major depression in women. *The American Journal of Psychiatry, 159*(7), 1133–1145.

Kessler, R. C., Akiskal, H. S., Ames, M., Birnbaum, H., Greenberg, P., Hirschfeld, R. M., et al. (2006). Prevalence and effects of mood disorders on work performance in a nationally representative sample of U.S. workers. *The American Journal of Psychiatry, 163*(9), 1561–1568.

Kessler, R. C., & Frank, R. G. (1997). The impact of psychiatric disorders on work loss days. *Psychological Medicine, 27*(4), 861–873.

Kessler, R. C., Ormel, J., Demler, O., & Stang, P. E. (2003). Comorbid mental disorders account for the role impairment of commonly occurring chronic physical disorders: Results from the National Comorbidity Survey. *Journal of Occupational and Environmental Medicine, 45*(12), 1257–1266.

Kielhofner, G. (2002). *A model of human occupation: Theory and application* (3rd ed.). Philadelphia: Lippincott, Williams & Wilkins.

Kilian, S., & Becker, T. (2007). FIPS—families with a mentally ill parent. *Psychiatrische Praxis, 34*(6), 310.

Kivimaki, M., Virtanen, M., Vartia, M., Elovainio, M., Vahtera, J., & Keltikangas-Jarvinen, L. (2003). Workplace bullying and the risk of cardiovascular disease and depression. *Occupational and Environmental Medicine, 60*(10), 779–783.

Korten, A., & Henderson, S. (2000). The Australian National Survey of Mental Health and Well-Being. Common psychological symptoms and disablement. *The British Journal of Psychiatry: The Journal of Mental Science, 177*, 325–330.

Laitinen-Krispijn, S., & Bijl, R. V. (2000). Mental disorders and employee sickness absence: The NEMESIS study. Netherlands Mental Health Survey and Incidence Study. *Social Psychiatry and Psychiatric Epidemiology, 35*(2), 71–77.

Latimer, E. A., Lecomte, T., Becker, D. R., Drake, R. E., Duclos, I., Piat, M., et al. (2006). Generalisability of the individual placement and support model of supported employment: Results of a Canadian randomised controlled trial. *The British Journal of Psychiatry: The Journal of Mental Science, 189*, 65–73.

Lerner, D., Adler, D. A., Chang, H., Berndt, E. R., Irish, J. T., Lapitsky, L., et al. (2004). The clinical and occupational correlates of work productivity loss among employed patients with depression. *Journal of Occupational and Environmental Medicine, 46*(6 Suppl), S46–S55.

Lerner, D., Amick, B. C., 3rd, Lee, J. C., Rooney, T., Rogers, W. H., Chang, H., et al. (2003). Relationship of employee-reported work limitations to work productivity. *Medical Care, 41*(5), 649–659.

Lerner, D., & Henke, R. M. (2008). What does research tell us about depression, job performance, and work productivity? *Journal of Occupational and Environmental Medicine, 50*(4), 401–410.

Lim, D., Sanderson, K., & Andrews, G. (2000). Lost productivity among full-time workers with mental disorders. *The Journal of Mental Health Policy and Economics, 3*(3), 139–146.

Lim, K. L., Jacobs, P., Ohinmaa, A., Schopflocher, D., & Dewa, C. S. (2008). A new population-based measure of the economic burden of mental illness in Canada. *Chronic Diseases in Canada, 28*(3), 92–98.

Lindstrom, M. (2005). Psychosocial work conditions, unemployment and self-reported psychological health: A population-based study. *Occupational Medicine (London), 55*(7), 568–571.

Loisel, P., Abenhaim, L., Durand, P., Esdaile, J. M., Suissa, S., Gosselin, L., et al. (1997). A population-based, randomized clinical trial on back pain management. *Spine, 22*(24), 2911–2918.

Loisel, P., & Corbiere, M. (2011). Compétences requises de l'intervenant qui facilite le retour ou la réintégration au travail de personnes à risque d'une incapacité prolongée. In M. Corbiere & M. J. Durand (Eds.), *Du trouble mental à l'incapacité au travail: Une perspective transdisciplinaire qui vise à mieux saisir cette problématique et à offrir des pistes d'intervention* (pp. 253–277). Quebec: Presses de l'Université du Québec.

Loisel, P., Durand, M. J., Berthelette, D., Vezina, N., Baril, R., Gagnon, D., et al. (2001). Disability prevention: New paradigm for the management of occupational back pain. *Disease Management and Health Outcomes, 9*(7), 351–360.

Loisel, P., Lemaire, J., Poitras, S., Durand, M. J., Champagne, F., Stock, S., et al. (2002). Cost-benefit and cost-effectiveness analysis of a disability prevention model for back pain management: A six year follow up study. *Occupational and Environmental Medicine, 59*(12), 807–815.

Lotters, F., Hogg-Johnson, S., & Burdorf, A. (2005). Health status, its perceptions, and effect on return to work and recurrent sick leave. *Spine, 30*(9), 1086–1092.

Maier, R., Egger, A., Barth, A., Winker, R., Osterode, W., Kundi, M., et al. (2006). Effects of short- and long-term unemployment on physical work capacity and on serum cortisol. *International Archives of Occupational and Environmental Health, 79*(3), 193–198.

Marcotte, D. E., Wilcox-Gok, V., & Redmon, D. P. (2000). The labor market effects of mental illness the case of affective disorders. In D. S. Salkavers & A. Sorkin (Eds.), *The Economics of Disability (Research in human capital and development, Volume 13, pp 181–210)*. Greenwich: JAI Press.

Marcotte, D. E., Wilcox-Gok, V., & Redmon, P. D. (1999). Prevalence and patterns of major depressive disorder in the United States labor force. *The Journal of Mental Health Policy and Economics, 2*(3), 123–131.

Marshall, T., Rapp, C. A., Becker, D. R., & Bond, G. R. (2008). Key factors for implementing supported employment. *Psychiatric Services, 59*(8), 886–892.

Marwaha, S., & Johnson, S. (2004). Schizophrenia and employment: A review. *Social Psychiatry and Psychiatric Epidemiology, 39*(5), 337–349.

Mayer, T. G., Gatchel, R. J., Mayer, H., Kishino, N. D., Keeley, J., & Mooney, V. A. (1987). A prospective two-year study of functional restoration in industrial low back injury. *Journal of the American Medical Association, 258*(13), 1763–1767.

Mayer, T. G., & Gatchel, R. J. (1988). *Functional restoration for spinal disorders: The sports medicine approach*. Philadelphia: Lea & Febiger.

McAlpine, D. D., & Warner, L. (2001). Barriers to employment among persons with mental illness: A review of the literature, *Institute for Health, Health Care Policy, and Aging Research*: Rutgers University.

McFarlane, A. C., & Bryant, R. A. (2007). Post-traumatic stress disorder in occupational settings: Anticipating and managing the risk. *Occupational Medicine (London), 57*(6), 404–410.

Mechanic, D., Bilder, S., & McAlpine, D. D. (2002). Employing persons with serious mental illness. *Health Affairs, 21*(5), 242–253.

Meichenbaum, D. H. (1993). Stress inoculation training: A twenty year update. In R. L. Woolfolk & P. M. Lehrer (Eds.), *Principles and practice of stress management*. New York: Guilford Press.

Mowbray, C. T., Holter, M. C., Teague, G. B., & Bybee, D. (2003). Fidelity criteria: Development, measurement, and validation. *American Journal of Evaluation, 24*(3), 315–339.

Muschalla, B., & Linden, M. (2009). Workplace phobia–a first explorative study on its relation to established anxiety disorders, sick leave, and work-directed treatment. *Psychology, Health and Medicine, 14*(5), 591–605.

New Freedom Commission on Mental Health. (2003). Achieving the promise: Transforming mental health care in America. Retrieved August 22, 2011 from http://www.nami.org/Content/NavigationMenu/Inform_Yourself/About_Public_Policy/New_Freedom_Commission/Default1169.htm.

Nicholas, G. (1998). Workplace effects on the stigmatization of depression. *Journal of Occupational and Environmental Medicine, 40*(9), 793–800.

Nieuwenhuijsen, K., Verbeek, J. H., de Boer, A. G., Blonk, R. W., & van Dijk, F. J. (2006). Predicting the duration of sickness absence for patients with common mental disorders in occupational health care. *Scandinavian Journal of Work, Environment and Health, 32*(1), 67–74.

Noordik, E., van Dijk, F. J., Nieuwenhuijsen, K., & van der Klink, J. J. (2009). Effectiveness and cost-effectiveness of an exposure-based return-to-work programme for patients on sick leave due to common mental disorders: Design of a cluster-randomized controlled trial. *BMC Public Health, 9*, 140.

Parent-Thirion, A., Fernández Macías, E., Hurley, J., & Vermeylen, G. (2007). *Fourth European working conditions survey*. Dublin: Fondation européenne pour l'amélioration des conditions de vie et de travail.

Patel, A., Knapp, M., Henderson, J., & Baldwin, D. (2002). The economic consequences of social phobia. *Journal of Affective Disorders, 68*(2–3), 221–233.

Pomaki, G., Franche, R. L., Khushrushahi, N., Murray, E., Lampinen, T., & Mah, P. (2010). *Best practices for return-to-work/stay-at-work interventions for workers with mental health conditions*. Vancouver: Occupational Health and Safety Agency for HealthCare in BC.

Rapp, C. A., Etzel-Wise, D., Marty, D., Coffman, M., Carlson, L., Asher, D., et al. (2010). Barriers to evidence-based practice implementation: Results of a qualitative study. *Community Mental Health Journal, 46*(2), 112–118.

Rinaldi, M., Miller, L., & Perkins, R. (2010). Implementing the individual placement and support (IPS) approach for people with mental health conditions in England. *International Review of Psychiatry, 22*(2), 163–172.

Romanov, K., Appelberg, K., Honkasalo, M. L., & Koskenvuo, M. (1996). Recent interpersonal conflict at work and psychiatric morbidity: A prospective study of 15,530 employees aged 24-64. *Journal of Psychosomatic Research, 40*(2), 169–176.

Romanow, R. J. (2002). *Building on values: The Future of Health Care in Canada—Final Report*. Ottawa: Government of Canada.

Rugulies, R., Bultmann, U., Aust, B., & Burr, H. (2006). Psychosocial work environment and incidence of severe depressive symptoms: Prospective findings from a 5-year follow-up of the Danish work environment cohort study. *American Journal of Epidemiology, 163*(10), 877–887.

Rytsala, H. J., Melartin, T. K., Leskela, U. S., Sokero, T. P., Lestela-Mielonen, P. S., & Isometsa, E. T. (2005). Functional and work disability in major depressive disorder. *The Journal of Nervous and Mental Disease, 193*(3), 189–195.

Rytsala, H. J., Melartin, T. K., Leskela, U. S., Sokero, T. P., Lestela-Mielonen, P. S., & Isometsa, E. T. (2007). Predictors of long-term work disability in Major Depressive Disorder: A prospective study. *Acta Psychiatrica Scandinavica, 115*(3), 206–213.

Sairanen, S., Matzanki, D., & Smeall, D. (2011). The business case: Collaborating to help employees maintain their mental well-being. *Healthcare Papers, 11*(Sp), 78–84.

Sanderson, K., & Andrews, G. (2006). Common mental disorders in the workforce: Recent findings from descriptive and social epidemiology. *Canadian Journal of Psychiatry. Revue Canadienne de Psychiatrie, 51*(2), 63–75.

Saunders, T., Driskell, J. E., Johnston, J. H., & Salas, E. (1996). The effect of stress inoculation training on anxiety and performance. *Journal of Occupational Health Psychology, 1*(2), 170–186.

Scheid, T. L. (1999). Employment of individuals with mental disabilities: Business response to the ADA's challenge. *Behavioral Sciences and the Law, 17*(1), 73–91.

Schmitz, N., Wang, J., Malla, A., & Lesage, A. (2007). Joint effect of depression and chronic conditions on disability: Results from a population-based study. *Psychosomatic Medicine, 69*(4), 332–338.

Schulze, B., & Angermeyer, M. C. (2003). Subjective experiences of stigma. A focus group study of schizophrenic patients, their relatives and mental health professionals. *Social Science and Medicine, 56*(2), 299–312.

Sherring, J., Robson, E., Morris, A., Frost, B., & Tirupati, S. (2010). A working reality: Evaluating enhanced intersectoral links in supported employment for people with psychiatric disabilities. *Australian Occupational Therapy Journal, 57*(4), 261–267.

Shields, M. (1999). Long working hours and health. *Health Rep, 11*(2), 33–48 (Eng); 37-55(Fre).

Shields, M. (2006). Stress and depression in the employed population. *Health reports/Statistics Canada, Canadian Centre for Health Information = Rapports sur la sante/Statistique Canada, Centre canadien d'information sur la sante, 17*(4), 11–29.

Shirado, O., Ito, T., Kikumoto, T., Takeda, N., Minami, A., & Strax, T. E. (2005). A novel back school using a multidisciplinary team approach featuring quantitative functional evaluation and therapeutic exercises for patients with chronic low back pain. *Spine, 30*, 1219–1225.

Siegrist, J. (2008). Chronic psychosocial stress at work and risk of depression: Evidence from prospective studies. *European Archives of Psychiatry and Clinical Neuroscience, 258*(Suppl 5), 115–119.

Simon, G. E., Ludman, E. J., Unutzer, J., Operskalski, B. H., & Bauer, M. S. (2008). Severity of mood symptoms and work productivity in people treated for bipolar disorder. *Bipolar Disorders, 10*(6), 718–725.

Smith, J. L., Rost, K. M., Nutting, P. A., Libby, A. M., Elliott, C. E., & Pyne, J. M. (2002). Impact of primary care depression intervention on employment and workplace conflict outcomes: Is value added? *The Journal of Mental Health Policy and Economics, 5*(1), 43–49.

Sroujian, C. (2003). Mental health is the number one cause of disability in Canada. *The Insurance Journal, 2003*, 8.

St-Arnaud, L., Saint-Jean, M., & Rhéaume, J. (2003). De la désinsertion à la réinsertion professionnelle à la suite d'un arrêt de travail pour un problème de santé mentale. *Santé Mentale au Québec, 28*(1), 193–211.

Stansfeld, S., & Candy, B. (2006). Psychosocial work environment and mental health–a meta-analytic review. *Scandinavian Journal of Work, Environment and Health, 32*(6), 443–462.

Stansfeld, S. A., Fuhrer, R., Shipley, M. J., & Marmot, M. G. (1999). Work characteristics predict psychiatric disorder: Prospective results from the Whitehall II Study. *Occupational and Environmental Medicine, 56*(5), 302–307.

Stephens, T., & Joubert, N. (2001). The economic burden of mental health problems in Canada. *Chronic Diseases in Canada, 22*(1), 18–23.

Stewart, W. F., Ricci, J. A., Chee, E., Hahn, S. R., & Morganstein, D. (2003). Cost of lost productive work time among US workers with depression. *JAMA: The Journal of the American Medical Association, 289*(23), 3135–3144.

Swain, K., Whitley, R., McHugo, G. J., & Drake, R. E. (2010). The sustainability of evidence-based practices in routine mental health agencies. *Community Mental Health Journal, 46*(2), 119–129.

The Australian Human Rights Commission. (2010). *Workers with mental illness: A practical guide for managers*. Sydney: The Australian Human Rights Commission.

The Standing Senate Committee on Social Affairs, Science and Technology. (2006). *Out of the shadows at last transforming mental health, Mental Illness and Addiction Services in Canada*. Ottawa: The Senate.

Torrey, W. C., Bond, G. R., McHugo, G. J., & Swain, K. (2012). Evidence-based practice implementation in community mental health settings: The relative importance of key domains of implementation activity. Administration and policy in mental health, 39(5), 353–364

Turk, D. C., & Swanson, K. (2007). Efficacy and cost-effectiveness treatment of chronic pain: An analysis and evidence-based synthesis. In M. E. Schatman & A. Campbell (Eds.), *Chronic pain management: Guidelines for multidisciplinary program development*. New York: Informa Healthcare.

United Nations. (1948). Universal Declaration of Human Rights. Retrieved August 22, 2011 from http://www.un.org/en/documents/udhr/index.shtml#a23.

United Nations. (1966). International Covenant on Economic, Social and Cultural Rights. Retrieved August 21, 2011 from http://www2.ohchr.org/english/law/cescr.htm.

van der Klink, J. J., Blonk, R. W., Schene, A. H., & van Dijk, F. J. (2003). Reducing long term sickness absence by an activating intervention in adjustment disorders: A cluster randomised controlled design. *Occupational and Environmental Medicine, 60*(6), 429–437.

van der Klink, J. J., & van Dijk, F. J. (2003). Dutch practice guidelines for managing adjustment disorders in occupational and primary health care. *Scandinavian Journal of Work, Environment and Health, 29*(6), 478–487.

van Oostrom, S. H., Anema, J. R., Terluin, B., Venema, A., de Vet, H. C., & van Mechelen, W. (2007). Development of a workplace intervention for sick-listed employees with stress-related mental disorders: Intervention Mapping as a useful tool. *BMC Health Services Research, 7*, 127.

van Oostrom, S. H., Heymans, M. W., de Vet, H. C., van Tulder, M. W., van Mechelen, W., & Anema, J. R. (2010). Economic evaluation of a workplace intervention for sick-listed employees with distress. *Occupational and Environmental Medicine, 67*(9), 603–610.

van Oostrom, S. H., van Mechelen, W., Terluin, B., de Vet, H. C., & Anema, J. R. (2009). A participatory workplace intervention for employees with distress and lost time: A feasibility evaluation within a randomized controlled trial. *Journal of Occupational Rehabilitation, 19*(2), 212–222.

van Oostrom, S. H., van Mechelen, W., Terluin, B., de Vet, H. C., Knol, D. L., & Anema, J. R. (2010). A workplace intervention for sick-listed employees with distress: Results of a randomised controlled trial. *Occupational and Environmental Medicine, 67*(9), 596–602.

Waghorn, G., & Lloyd, C. (2005). The employment of people with Mental Illness. *Australian e-Journal for the Advancement of Mental Health, 4*(2 Suppl), 1–43.

Wang, J., Adair, C. E., & Patten, S. B. (2006). Mental health and related disability among workers: A population-based study. *American Journal of Industrial Medicine, 49*(7), 514–522.

Wang, J., Schmitz, N., Dewa, C., & Stansfeld, S. (2009). Changes in perceived job strain and the risk of major depression: Results from a population-based longitudinal study. *American Journal of Epidemiology, 169*(9), 1085–1091.

Wang, P. S., Beck, A. L., Berglund, P., McKenas, D. K., Pronk, N. P., Simon, G. E., et al. (2004). Effects of major depression on moment-in-time work performance. *The American Journal of Psychiatry, 161*(10), 1885–1891.

Wong, K. K., Chiu, R., Tang, B., Mark, D., Liu, J., & Chiu, S. N. (2008). A randomized controlled trial of a supported employment program for persons with long-term mental illness in Hong Kong. *Psychiatric Services, 59*(1), 84–90.

World Health Organization. (2005). *Mental health action plan for Europe. Facing the challenges, building solutions*. Copenhagen: World Health Organization.

Cancer Survivors and Work

Michal C. Moskowitz, Briana L. Todd, and Michael Feuerstein

The opinions and assertions contained herein are the private views of the authors and are not to be construed as being official or as reflecting the views of the Uniformed Services University of the Health Sciences or the Department of Defense.

Introduction

To begin, as of 2007, it was estimated that there are 11.7 million individuals with a history of cancer living in the United States (American Cancer Society, 2011). This figure reflects a steady increase in cancer survival, which is largely credited to improvements in detection and treatment. Additional improvements in medical technology and therapy, increased exposure to risk factors, and the growing population are expected to increase the prevalence of cancer over the next 20 years. In fact, the 1.6 million new cancer cases estimated in 2010 in the US is expected to climb to 2.3 million new cancer cases in 2030 (Smith, Smith, Hurria, Hortobagyi, & Buchholz, 2009). The number of individuals who desire to remain in the workforce, which includes cancer survivors, is also increasing. Therefore, with more cancer survivors in the workplace, occupational health providers will need to become more aware of the problems and associated factors that cancer survivors experience related to work. Indeed, in order to better understand the nature of workplace problems, and to allow for more effective interventions, we will review the current state of cancer survivors in the workplace. First, we discuss the current and projected rates of cancer incidence, note trends in the age of the working population, and describe how and why work matters for many cancer survivors. Next, we discuss trends in return-to-work, work sustainability, and unemployment among cancer survivors. We present schematic figures, which depict difficulties faced by cancer survivors as they transition back to, and remain at, work. Here we include

M. Feuerstein, Ph.D., M.P.H. (✉)
Department of Medical and Clinical Psychology and Preventive Medicine and Biometrics,
Uniformed Services University of the Health Sciences,
4301 Jones Bridge Road, Bethesda, MD 20814, USA
e-mail: michael.feuerstein@usuhs.edu

M.C. Moskowitz, M.S. • B.L. Todd, M.A., M.S.
Department of Medical and Clinical Psychology,
Uniformed Services University of the Health Sciences,
4301 Jones Bridge Road, 20814, Bethesda, MD, USA
e-mail: Michal.moskowitz@usuhs.edu; briana.todd@usuhs.edu

a depiction of the temporal course of work capacity, designed to illustrate the unique circumstances of individual cancer survivors as they relate to work. The Chapter then reviews the growing literature on the demographic, medical, intrapersonal, and workplace factors associated with workplace challenges for cancer survivors. The identification of these factors and further research targeting modifiable relationships should help develop new approaches to facilitate return-to-work and improve the cancer survivor's work experience, when needed. Finally, we review the limited evidence basis for interventions related to cancer survivors and limited work outcomes. There is a tremendous need for additional advances in both research and practice, and we will discuss some promising future directions.

Background

Epidemiology

The most common cancer diagnoses among cancer survivors in the US are breast cancer (22% of all cancer survivors), prostate cancer (20%), colorectal cancer (9%), and gynecologic cancer (8%) (Altekruse et al., 2010). In the years of 1975–1979, the 5-year survival rate of all cancer sites was 49%. However, in the year 2003, this figure increased to 67% (Altekruse et al.). Cancer survival rates are largely dependent on cancer type. While prostate cancer's 5-year survival rate has escalated from 69% (1975–1979) to 99% (2003), the 5-year survival rate of lung and bronchus cancer has increased only slightly (i.e., from 13% in 1975–1979 to 16% in 2003). Differences in the invasiveness of the tumor, ability to detect the cancer, and availability of effective treatments are likely to affect these differing survival rates.

The incidence of cancer is projected to increase by 45% between the years of 2010 and 2030, from 1.6 to 2.3 million annual cases (Smith et al., 2009). Diagnoses in older adults and minorities will account for the largest percent increase. Population growth and changes in risk factors will also contribute to the increase of cancer incidence (Bray & Moller, 2006). It is important that readers recognize these are simply projections. Some researchers question the certainty of these figures because they are based on predictions of birth and death rates, which vary (Bray & Moller). However, when interpreted with caution, they do support the exacerbation of a current challenge we face as more cancer survivors are in the workplace. Knowledge of future cancer incidence allows health care providers and public health specialists to proactively plan for cancer control programs and resources that cancer patients and survivors will need in future years (Bray & Moller).

Increasing Age of the Working Population

Approximately 40% of cancer survivors are between 20 and 65 years old, within the age range of the working population (Altekruse et al., 2010). Yet, even cancer survivors who are older than 65 may wish or need to work as well. The employment status of workers ages 65 and older rose by 101% between the years 1977 and 2007 (Bureau of Labor Statistics, 2008). The percent increase of males engaged in work was 75%, whereas the percent increase of females engaged in work was 147%. This trend began in the late 1990s and has continued. The aging of the baby-boom generation does not solely account for this increase. The majority of employed older Americans ages 65 and up are now engaged in full-time work. In the past, a larger proportion of older American workers were employed part-time. Between the years of 2006 and 2016, the Bureau of Labor Statistics expects that the overall workforce will rise another 8.5%. The largest increase is projected for workers ages 65 and older. Older individuals are more likely than younger individuals to develop cancer (American Cancer Society, 2011). The projected increase in cancer prevalence, coupled with the rising age of the workforce, suggests that there will be a growing population of workers with a history of cancer.

The current economic climate has negatively affected the labor force and may have complicated return-to-work and work sustainability for cancer survivors. The unemployment rate in the US has escalated from 4% in 2000 to 9.6% in 2010, and it is even higher for some groups (e.g., 16.0% for African Americans) (Bureau of Labor Statistics, 2011). The number of available jobs has decreased, making it a more competitive job market. Cancer survivors will need to remain competitive in this type of environment. Their work performance will need to meet the demands of the modern workplace.

Meaning of Work

Many affected by cancer have a distinct set of problems at work compared to their peers with no history of cancer. These problems can make it difficult to return-to-work, function at work, and remain at work following cancer diagnosis and treatment. Qualitative studies highlight that cancer patients and survivors desire to remain employed after a diagnosis of cancer in spite of these factors. Work provides an individual with a sense of purpose, daily structure, identity, and financial support (Peteet, 2000; Rasmussen & Elverdam, 2008). In a discussion of the meaning of work, Peteet describes how the ability of a cancer survivor to provide for his or her family is central to that individual's identity. When work challenges this ability, there can be a loss of one's identity. Depressive and anxious symptoms may result. Returning to work following cancer also allows a cancer survivor to socially reintegrate. Work provides a social role for an individual where he or she can contribute knowledge and services to society (Peteet). Work also provides an opportunity to engage socially with other individuals (Kennedy, Haslam, Munir, & Pryce, 2007). These factors allow work to provide a normalcy in cancer patients' and survivors' lives that they strive to achieve.

Rasmussen & Elverdam (2008) conducted an ethnographic study consisting of observations and interviews with cancer survivors following a stay in a Denmark cancer rehabilitation center and 18 months later. The heterogeneous group of cancer survivors ($n=23$) consisted of males and females between the ages of 28 and 67. The process of returning to work was illustrated by three main themes: (1) work and working life disruption; (2) the reestablishment of work and working life; and (3) daily life without work and working life. These themes were largely consistent with Peteet's (2000) earlier research. Work structured a cancer survivor's life, providing a regular order and routine. Cancer survivors expressed that working after cancer allowed them to identify themselves as "ordinary." When they were unable to return to or remain at work, their identity was challenged. Cancer survivors expressed that returning to full-time work was a goal following cancer. Being a paid employee was analogous with being "normal" and "healthy." When the physical and emotional impact of cancer interfered with cancer survivors' ability to work, they were left needing to create a new structure for their daily life and redefine how they identified themselves.

The financial burden of cancer also extends into cancer survivorship. The National Cancer Institute divides cancer costs into three periods: (1) the initial phase (time after diagnosis); (2) the last year of life; and (3) the continuing or monitoring phase (time between the initial phase and the final year of life) (National Cancer Institute, 2010). Cancers with longer survival rates often incur greater financial expenditures for cancer care during the continuing phase. Financial strain is a motivating factor to return-to-work following cancer (Kennedy et al., 2007). Work is a necessary source of income and a source of health insurance, especially in the United States. Many individuals do not consider the financial impact of cancer at the time of diagnosis (Amir, Wilson, Hennings, & Young, 2011). However, some cancer patients or survivors report returning to work prematurely because they need to pay the mortgage and cancer-related expenses not included under their insurance policy, support their children, and cover other expenses. Cancer patients also worry that extended sick leave may negatively impact their job status (Amir et al). Financial pressure and the inability to financially provide for one's family can exacerbate poor emotional health related to cancer.

Overall Patters of Work and Cancer Survivors

Return-to-Work

A subset of cancer patients continue to work after a cancer diagnosis. However, the number of hours at work can vary. In a heterogeneous sample of Detroit cancer survivors employed at time of diagnosis ($n=141$), most (67%) were employed 5–7 years after diagnosis. Over half of the sample (54.5%) reduced their work schedule on at least one occasion due to cancer treatment, but the majority of those (86%) did eventually return to their pre-cancer work schedule within 5–7 years after diagnosis (Bradley & Bednarek, 2002). Roelen, Koopmans, Groothoff, van der Klink, & Bultmann (2010) examined 5,074 Dutch employees (ages 18–60) 2 years after diagnosis, who held a paid job at time of cancer diagnosis, and whose occupational physician documented sickness absence related to cancer. Of this sample, 73% returned to work (with pay equivalent to pre-cancer time) 2 years post-diagnosis. Within the sample, receiving a disability pension (13%) and quitting due to sickness absence (6%) were causes of unemployment. Breast cancer diagnoses had the highest rate of sickness absence. Seventy four percent of breast cancer survivors were absent from work for more than 6 months, and 46% did not return-to-work for more than 12 months. Return-to-work was independent of gender for all cancer types except for blood malignancies, where women's time to return-to-work was longer. Return-to-work did differ by type of cancer. For instance, at 2-years post-diagnosis, only 45% of lung cancer patients (204 out of 448) returned to work, whereas 88% of genital cancer survivors returned to work.

A systematic review of the early literature (1985–1999) noted that the mean rate of return-to-work after any cancer type was 62% (Spelten, Sprangers, & Verbeek, 2002). Another recent systematic review of the literature from January 2000 to November 2009 examined employment among heterogeneous cancer survivors and found a similar rate of return-to-work (Mehnert, 2011). On average, 63.5% of cancer survivors returned to work after an average of 151 days being absent from work. However, the percentage of cancer survivors returning to work largely differed by study (range=24–94%). Studies varied in cancer type, study design (e.g., cross-sectional vs. longitudinal), gender, and mean age of participants. This study indicated that, as time from diagnosis increased, a larger percentage of cancer survivors returned to work. An average of 40% of cancer patients either continued to work after diagnosis or returned to work at 6 months, with a mean of 62% at 12 months, a mean of 73% by 18 months, and a mean of 89% at 24 months.

Changes in return-to-work percentages have also been observed across time. A recent study conducted in the Netherlands examined an occupational health service register (Roelen, Koopmans, Groothoff, van der Klink, & Bultmann, 2011). Patterns of return-to-work were investigated for employees in whom a diagnosis of any cancer type was made in 2002, 2005, and 2008. Both partial return-to-work (returning to work and earning 50% of salary for a minimum of 28 consecutive days) and full return-to-work (returning to work and earning 100% of salary for a minimum of 28 consecutive days) decreased across time in this heterogeneous sample of cancer survivors (i.e., breast cancer, genital cancer, gastrointestinal cancer, lung cancer, skin cancer, and blood malignancies). The estimates of partial return-to-work decreased from 85% in among those diagnosed 2002, to 80% in 2005, and to 69% in 2008 in cancer survivors 2-years after diagnosis. Two years post-diagnosis, the estimates of full return-to-work decreased from 80% among those diagnosed in 2002, to 74% in 2005, and to 68% in 2008. The amount of time, measured in days, until cancer survivors had partial or full return-to-work all increased over the years. While not investigated in the study, the authors propose that alterations in disability policy instituted in 2004 may partially account for the decrease in return-to-work and increase in time to return-to-work. Difficulties at work that necessitate workplace accommodations, along with the economic decline during the years studied, may also have impacted return-to-work.

Work Sustainability

Although the majority of cancer survivors return-to-work after a cancer diagnosis or treatment, some cancer survivors have difficulty remaining at work. In a heterogeneous group of cancer survivors ($n=1,433$) 4 years after cancer diagnosis, 13% left the workforce due to unspecified "cancer-related reasons" (Short, Vasey, & Tuceli, 2005). However, the statistics on work sustainability differ across studies. In a sample of breast cancer survivors ($n=416$), 80% of survivors had returned to work at 12 months post-diagnosis (Bouknight, Bradley, & Luo, 2006). Of these breast cancer survivors, 7.6% were not working at 18 months post-diagnosis. In another sample of cancer survivors, 67% of those working at their initial diagnosis were employed 5–7 years later (Bradley & Bednarek, 2002). The majority of these cancer survivors (75.4%) reported full-time employment (type of work unspecified), and many worked in excess of a 40-h workweek. Other studies, though, found that cancer patients and survivors reduce their hours after a diagnosis of cancer, primarily during active treatment (Mehnert, 2011). After cancer survivors return-to-work, and even after several years back at work, they report greater perceived work limitations and reduced work ability as compared to individuals with no history of cancer (Calvio, Peugeot, Bruns, Todd, & Feuerstein, 2009; Hansen, Feuerstein, Calvio, & Olsen, 2008; Taskila, Martikainen, Hietanen, & Lindbohm, 2007). Cancer survivors attribute cancer as negatively impacting their physical and mental work ability (Taskila et al.), which may impact employment changes. Some cancer survivors indicate that they have made workplace changes (e.g., reduction in work hours) or even had to find a new place of employment (Mehnert, 2011).

Unemployment

A meta-analysis examining employment post-cancer found an increased risk of unemployment for cancer survivors (relative risk=1.37, 95% CI: 1.21–1.55) (de Boer, Taskila, Ojajarvi, van Dijk, & Verbeek, 2009). The systematic search of the literature (1966—June 2008) included 20,366 cancer survivors and 157,603 healthy control participants. A higher percentage of cancer survivors were unemployed in comparison to individuals with no history of cancer (33.8% of cancer survivors, 15.2% of noncancer controls). Breast cancer (relative risk=1.28, 95% CI: 1.11–1.49) and gastrointestinal cancer survivors (relative risk=1.44, 95% CI: 1.02–2.05) had the highest risk compared to control participants. Cancer survivors reported that retirement, health problems interfering in work, business closures, and quitting work were all reasons for unemployment after cancer (Bradley & Bednarek, 2002).

Work Disability

Cancer survivors can experience work limitations or work disability even years after diagnosis and treatment for cancer. A multi-state study of over 1,700 cancer survivors in the US, who were working at time of diagnosis, found that approximately one in five women (21%) and one in six men (16%) reported cancer-related work limitations or disability 1–5 years after diagnosis (Short et al., 2005).

Discrimination

Discrimination in the workplace is a concern for cancer survivors. A study of claims filed under the Americans with Disability Act found that, compared to all other illness groups, cancer survivors were more likely to file claims reporting disputes with termination and terms of employment (Feuerstein,

Luff, Harrington, & Olsen, 2007). An independent study of workplace discrimination among cancer survivors also used the same administrative data from the US Department of Justice. This study reported consistent results. However, this latter study also examined the resolution of claims and found that, compared to the general disability population, claims filed by cancer survivors were more likely to be found to be meritorious (i.e., claims indicated presence of discrimination as per administrative law judge) (McKenna, Fabian, Hurley, McMahon, & West, 2007). The consistency of findings on similar data from two separate groups not aware of the others' work was reassuring, and the positive adjudication decisions among the cancer survivor group, relative to other claimants, suggest the claims had merit.

Individual Variation in Work Patterns

Individuals vary widely in their patterns of employment following cancer (e.g., time to return-to-work, level of workload during and after cancer treatment, and work sustainability). For the occupational health provider, it is important not just to consider overall averages and ranges in work outcomes, but also the varied paths of individuals. The schematic diagram in Fig. 7.1 depicts six distinct work trajectories of cancer survivors. It is intended to help occupational health professionals visualize the unique paths of individuals, and to help identify individuals who are most at risk for adverse employment outcomes or who are most in need of assistance. Each graph depicts changes in the level of work performed by the cancer survivor (Y axis) over time (X axis), from diagnosis, through treatment, and over the short- and long-term periods following treatment.

Graph A shows a 26 year old female thyroid cancer survivor who continued working during treatment, albeit at a reduced capacity, and returned to full level of work as a fourth grade teacher following the completion of treatment. Graph B shows a 32 year old male melanoma survivor who stopped working during treatment, but who is also able to resume full work responsibilities as a software developer shortly after completing treatment. Survivors A and B do not demonstrate any problems resuming full work responsibilities following cancer, and they are unlikely to need any intervention.

Graph C shows a 52 year old male colorectal cancer survivor who stopped working during treatment and then returned to work as a delivery truck driver only at a reduced level following treatment. He is experiencing symptoms of fatigue and pain that interfere with his physical function at work. Graph D shows a 43 year old uterine cancer survivor who stopped working during treatment and then returned to full work responsibilities gradually during a long period after completion of treatment. She was experiencing low energy, subclinical depression, and feelings of anxiety, which led her to feel overwhelmed in her job as a sales associate. Because these cancer survivors were not able to immediately resume full work responsibilities, their success reintegrating into the workplace is contingent on establishing open communication and clear expectations with employers, and perhaps addressing some of the symptom burden experienced. Supervisors, human resource professionals, and/or occupational health providers must work with these cancer survivors to establish expectations regarding workplace adjustments (e.g., workload, hours, physical demands, time off, and control over work). In these examples, Survivor C was able to negotiate a reduced work schedule and retrained in tasks that were less physically demanding. Survivor D worked with her supervisor to develop a gradual return-to-work plan, which also involved reducing her sales targets.

Graph E depicts a 47 year old breast cancer survivor who initially returned to full levels of work as a program manager at a large consulting firm following cancer, but whose work level then declined. Immediately following treatment, she was eager to return-to-work and received high levels of support from her colleagues. However, within a month, that support waned, and she was expected to resume her original work demands. She has been experiencing fatigue and cognitive problems (slower processing speed and problems with working memory and executive function) that make it difficult for

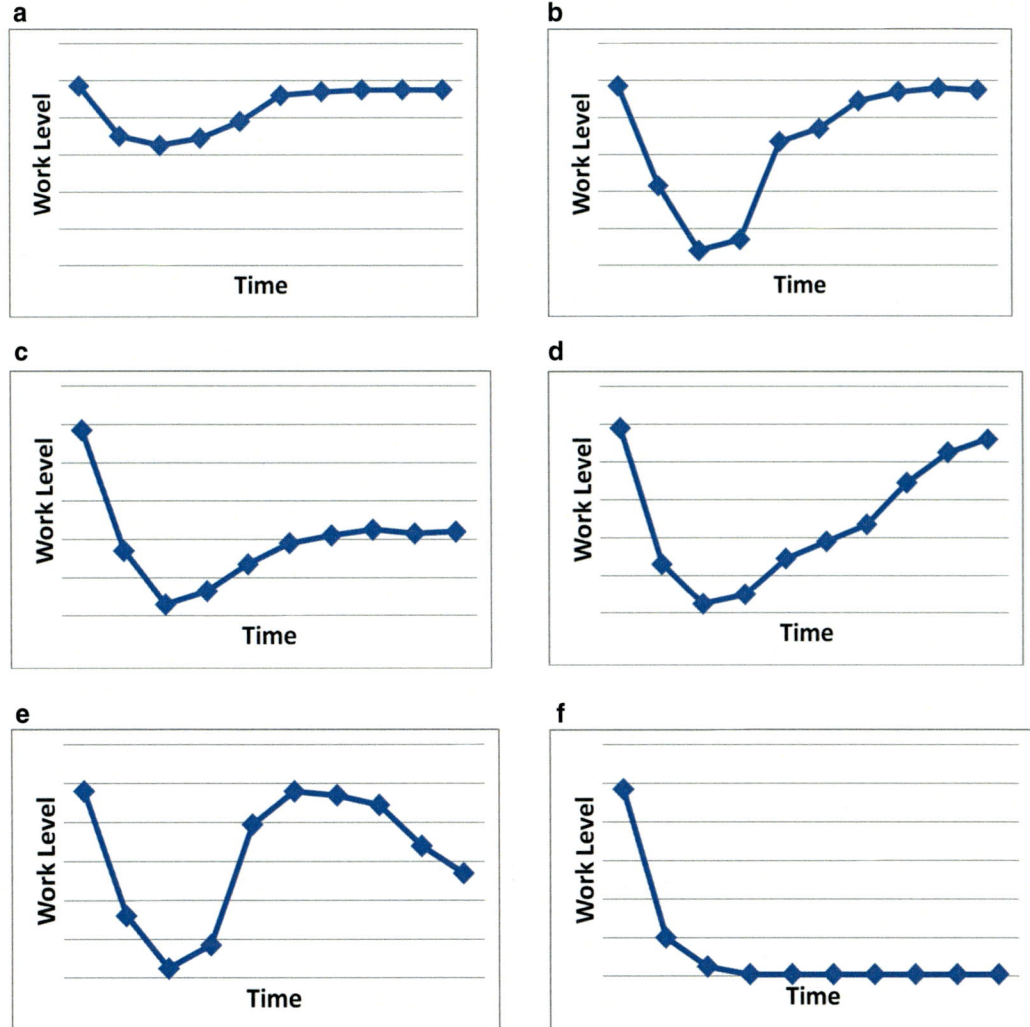

Fig. 7.1 Individual trajectories of work level after cancer. (**a**) Depicts a person who continued working during treatment, albeit at a reduced level, and returned to full work level after treatment. (**b**) Depicts a person who stopped working entirely during treatment, but returned to original work levels after treatment. (**c**) Depicts a person who stopped working during treatment and then returned to partial, but not full, work level. (**d**) Depicts a person who stopped working during treatment and gradually increased work until returning to the original level. (**e**) Depicts a person who initially returned to full levels of work but then began declining. (**f**) Depicts a person who stopped working during treatment and did not return

her to multi-task and meet deadlines. Her work performance has been declining, but she is afraid to approach her supervisor to ask about work accommodations. An occupational health provider who is in contact with her oncologist could work with Survivor E to help manage her symptoms. Human resource professionals could assist her in developing work adjustments.

Graph F depicts a 38 year old female central nervous system cancer survivor who stopped working during treatment and never returned to work as a litigation attorney. She is experiencing cognitive problems as a result of treatment, including impaired word-finding, poor concentration, difficulty with short-term memory, and attention to detail. Prior to her cancer diagnosis, she had been working 60 h per week at a high-pressure law firm. She felt that her employer would not be able to adjust her work demands enough for her to function well at work. However, she wants to be able to work to help

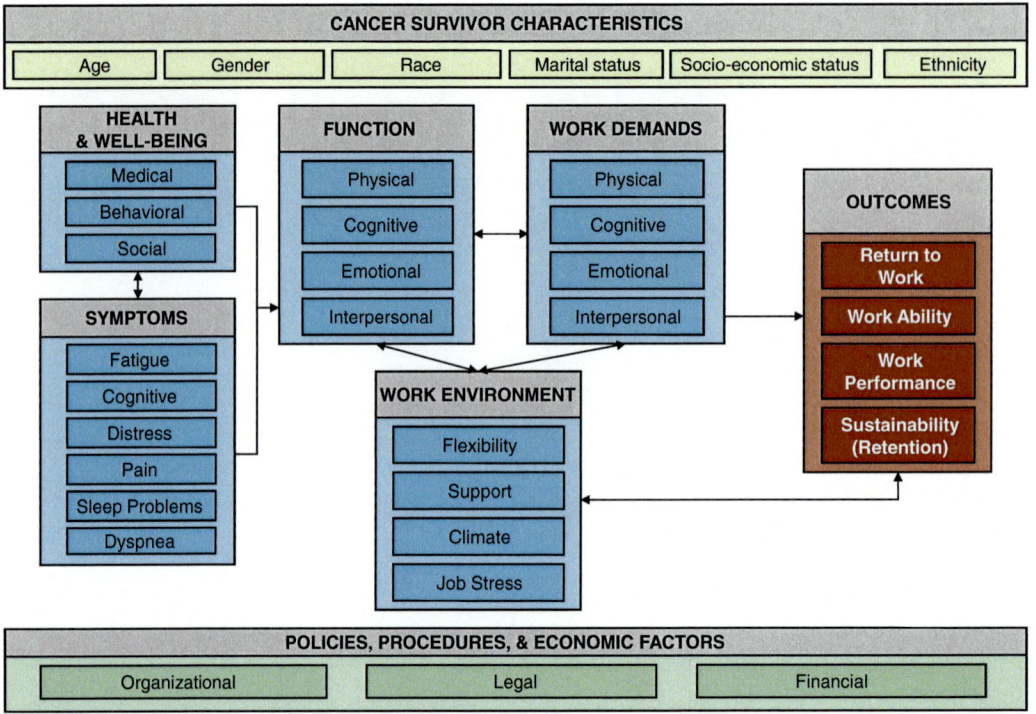

Fig. 7.2 Model of work and cancer (reprinted with permission from (Feuerstein et al., 2010) by Springer Science+Business Media, LLC.)

support her young children. She would be interested in exploring other occupational opportunities, but is discouraged about the difficulties in entering a new line of work.

These six examples illustrate various occupational paths of cancer survivors after diagnosis and treatment. Variables that have been related to work outcomes in cancer survivors will be discussed in the next section.

Model of Work and Cancer

Several variables enter into a cancer survivor's ability to return-to-work and decisions about whether to return-to-work, when to return-to-work, and which work-related changes to make (e.g., change in hours, amount of work, role, and employer). In order to illustrate the multidimensional factors that can potentially influence various work outcomes among cancer survivors, Feuerstein et al. (2010) developed a model of work and cancer. This model (Fig. 7.2) provides a conceptualization of cancer survivorship and work that is designed to help guide the evaluation, prevention, and management of work-related problems in cancer survivors. The model provides a framework for future research and practice, if evidence supports this, in the area of work and cancer survivorship (Feuerstein et al.).

On the left side of the figure are factors that describe the individual's health from a World Health Organization perspective (World Health Organization, 1946). These include the survivor's medical, behavioral, and social health and well-being, as well as symptoms (long-term and late effects), all of which can affect the survivor's ability to function physically, cognitively, emotionally, and interpersonally. Following these elements, it is proposed that the interaction between the cancer survivor's function (physical, cognitive, emotional, and interpersonal), work demands, and work environment, at some point in time, represent the second area of focus. The nexus between these three factors is a critical area for consideration by occupational health providers, human resource professionals, employers, and the individual cancer survivor. Various work outcomes (depicted on the right) are possible, and are proposed to be dependent upon an optimal match between the worker's functional ability and the work demands: If demands are below the worker's current level of function, the individual will likely be bored; if demands are too high for the person's level of function, job overload, or specific difficulties in completing certain job tasks can be experienced (Feuerstein et al., 2010). The work environment can be important in establishing the match between function and demand. For example, if a worker has flexibility in controlling the amount or pace of work, he/she can ensure that demands do not exceed functional ability. Social support from colleagues and supervisors can also be helpful to ensure that survivors take on work demands that are appropriate for the survivor's work abilities, or to support the accommodations that may be required to complete essential job demands. These elements are consistent with aspects of other models of work and health (Mehnert, 2011); however, they will need specific evidence in the context of cancer and work.

The top of this model depicts the cancer survivor's socio-demographic characteristics, while the bottom of the model shows the larger organizational, legal, and financial context in which the cancer survivor and his/her workplace are embedded. These variables, which are difficult to measure and change, are not necessarily direct targets for intervention for a given individual; however, they should still be considered by occupational health providers, human resource professionals, researchers, and those involved in generating policy related to work and cancer. This model represents several hypotheses that need to be supported by data. Several reviews (Amir & Brocky, 2009; Spelten et al., 2002; Taskila & Lindbohm, 2007) have discussed which variables are related to work outcomes in cancer survivors. Below is a review of the literature that addresses some of the most well-supported elements of the model.

Cancer Survivor Characteristics

Age
A review found that older age is associated with lower rates of return-to-work following cancer treatment (Taskila & Lindbohm, 2007). One study, however, found that older survivors were more likely to report work disability, but were not more likely to have quit working (Short et al., 2005).

Education and Income
Low education and low income are associated with lower return-to-work (Amir & Brocky, 2009; Taskila & Lindbohm, 2007). For example, one study of heterogeneous cancer survivors found that those with a postgraduate education are the least likely to quit working for a cancer-related reason (Short et al., 2005). A study of breast cancer survivors found that lower income and having less than a high school education was predictive of not returning to work at 12 months post-diagnosis, whereas having a college degree was associated with higher rates of return-to-work at 12 months (Bouknight et al., 2006). Similarly, a study of survivors of lung and colorectal cancer found that lower education and income were associated with lower rates of return-to-work (Earle et al., 2010). A study of breast cancer survivors 3 years after diagnosis found that a lower income at baseline was associated with not working at 3-year follow-up (Drolet et al., 2005). Reviews have noted the relationship between low education, low income, and physically demanding jobs: namely, that jobs involving physical labor are often lower paying and require a lower level of education (Amir & Brocky, 2009). Because cancer generally lowers a person's physical work capacity (Taskila & Lindbohm, 2007), low-wage blue collar workers with a low education level are less likely to be able to return-to-work compared to higher income, higher educated workers in white collar professions.

Health and Well-Being

Cancer Site

Considering the variability in treatment exposures, side effects, long-term symptoms, recurrence rates of tumors, incidence of new primary tumors, and overall prognosis across different types of cancers, it is not surprising that cancer site is an important variable related to work outcomes. Among women, work disability is most common in women with cancers of the central nervous system (OR = 5.765, 95% CI: 1.629–20.400), blood (OR = 5.303, 95% CI: 1.706–16.487), and head and neck (OR = 3.392, 95% CI: 1.018–11.299), whereas work disability is least common in women with history of uterine (OR = 0.583, 95% CI: 0.184–1.850), breast (OR = 0.621, 95% CI: 0.249–1.552), thyroid cancer (OR = 0.752, 95% CI: 0.242–2.337), or melanoma (OR = 0.623, 95% CI: 0.155–2.509) (Short et al., 2005). In men, work disability is most common in those with a history of central nervous system (OR = 3.574, 95% CI: 0.922–13.861) and blood cancers (OR = 2.181, 95% CI: 0.645–7.576), and least common in men who had prostate (OR = 0.107, 95% CI: 0.031–0.365) or head and neck cancers (OR = 0.197, 95% CI: 0.046–0.833) (Short et al.).

Similarly, the odds of quitting work is highest in survivors of lung cancer (OR = 1.218, 95% CI: 0.473–3.139), blood cancers (OR = 3.030, 95% CI: 1.238–7.416), and central nervous system cancers (OR = 2.202, 95% CI: 0.785–6.179), and is lowest in survivors of breast (OR = 0.440, 95% CI: 0.203–0.952), uterine (OR = 0.377, 95% CI: 0.117–1.212), or prostate cancer (OR = 0.485, 95% CI: 0.181–1.300) (Short et al., 2005). One review (Taskila & Lindbohm, 2007) noted that return-to-work rates are lowest in lung cancer because of the short life expectancy, and in central nervous system cancer survivors probably because of the high recurrence and the side effects of treatment (e.g., neurologic, cognitive, sensory, or other effects) (Taskila & Lindbohm). Central nervous system tumors are also characterized by a high mortality rate (Altekruse et al., 2010). One review noted that the sites with the highest rates of return-to-work are the cancer sites associated with younger age (e.g., testis and thyroid) (Mehnert, 2011).

Stage at Diagnosis

As one would expect, more advanced stage of disease at diagnosis is associated with negative work outcomes, including greater work disability in men (OR = 2.473, 95% CI: 1.052–5.815) and women (OR = 2.982, 95% CI: 1.765–5.040) (Short et al., 2005), higher likelihood of quitting work for cancer-related reasons (OR = 2.444, 95% CI: 1.487–4.019) (Short et al.), higher odds of unemployment in lung and colorectal cancer survivors (OR = 6.1, 95% CI: 2.8–13.2) (Earle et al., 2010), and lower odds of return-to-work at 12 months in breast cancer survivors (OR = 0.23, 95% CI: 0.08–0.65) (Bouknight et al., 2006).

Treatment Type

A review of cancer and work ability found that, compared with other treatments, chemotherapy has been consistently associated with worse work ability (self-reported current work ability assessed in relation to one's personal best work ability) in working cancer patients or survivors (Munir, Yarker, & McDermott, 2009). Cancer survivors who have undergone chemotherapy and/or radiation have lower rates of return-to-work (de Boer et al., 2008; Fantoni et al., 2010) and longer work absences (in breast cancer survivors) (Balak, Roelen, Koopmans, Ten Berge, & Groothoff, 2008; Fantoni et al., 2010), compared to those treated with surgery alone. For example, in a study of heterogeneous cancer survivors, those who had been treated with chemotherapy (either alone or together with other treatment types) had a 2.4 times greater risk of not returning to work compared to patients who received surgery alone, after correction for age and work ability.

General Health

Fair or poor health status in breast cancer survivors is associated with lower rates of return-to-work at 12 and 18 months (Bouknight et al., 2006). Cancer survivors who have a comorbid chronic illness (e.g., diabetes, chronic lung disease, heart problems, stroke, and arthritis) tend to have greater work disability and are more likely to quit work for cancer-related reasons (Short et al., 2005).

Symptoms

Many of the long-term and late effects of cancer, which are prevalent in a subset of cancer survivors (often 20–30%, but it may be over 50% depending on the symptom, cancer site, and time since diagnosis), are related to delayed or lower rates of return-to-work in cancer survivors. These effects include physical symptoms (Spelten et al., 2003; Steiner, Cavender, Main, & Bradley, 2004), depression (Spelten et al.), and functional limitations (Steiner et al.) in mixed cancer samples, and lymphedema in breast cancer survivors (Fantoni et al., 2010; Peugniez et al., 2010). Psychological symptoms, such as symptoms of depression, anxiety, or boredom, are associated with reduction in work hours (Steiner et al., 2008). Fatigue is one of the most commonly studied symptoms as it relates to work. Taskila, de Boer, van Dijk, & Verbeek (2010) found that, in a mixed sample of cancer survivors at 6 months after diagnosis, higher fatigue is related to greater work pressure, higher physical workload, and lower levels of work accommodations. Steiner et al. (2008) found that, in a cross-sectional study of 100 heterogeneous cancer survivors interviewed an average of 2 years after diagnosis, low energy was associated with a reduction in work hours.

In a longitudinal study of heterogeneous Dutch cancer survivors, de Boer et al. (2008) found that fatigue at 6 months post-diagnosis was a predictor of time taken to return-to-work. However, fatigue was correlated with perceived work ability and, when both were included in multivariate analyses, work ability was a better predictor (de Boer et al.). Likewise, Spelten et al. (2003) found that, in a prospective cohort study of Dutch heterogeneous cancer survivors, fatigue measured an average of 6 months after the first day of sick leave was associated with increased time to return-to-work, but that it was highly correlated with other symptoms. Another study found that fatigue was not related to duration of work absence before returning to work in Dutch breast cancer survivors (Balak et al., 2008). Methodological differences may in part account for these discrepant findings. For example, in the study of Dutch breast cancer survivors, fatigue was categorized as being present or absent based on its appearance in the medical file; the low incidence of fatigue in the study (nine patients or 13%) could be due to patients' neglecting to mention fatigue or physicians failing to document it (Balak et al.).

Cognitive/Emotional Factors

Personal Preferences

In some cases, the decision of how much to work following treatment of cancer is a personal one, driven in large part by cognitive and emotional factors. For some, a diagnosis of cancer leads to a change in priorities; a survivor may reduce his/her emphasis on work in favor of putting greater emphasis on spending time with friends and family or pursuing other interests (Spelten et al., 2002). After cancer diagnosis, work may lose some of its meaning and importance, which may lead a cancer survivor to work fewer hours or exert less effort at work (Johnsson, Fornander, Rutqvist, & Olsson, 2010). A longitudinal study of Canadian breast cancer survivors who were employed at baseline found that, 3 years after diagnosis, survivors were more likely than a comparison group to report that they valued work less now compared to 3 years ago (42 vs. 26%), although only 21% of the survivors were no longer working at 3 years post-diagnosis (Maunsell et al., 2004). The authors of that study found that attaching less value to work at baseline was associated with not working at 3 year follow-up (Drolet et al., 2005).

Perceptions of Work Ability

Return-to-work also appears to be influenced by the cancer survivor's perception of his/her work ability. As mentioned above, a longitudinal study of mixed cancer survivors by de Boer et al. (2008) found that perceived work ability at 6 months after diagnosis was a stronger predictor of subsequent rates of return-to-work than fatigue. These findings regarding perceptions of the value of work in one's life, as well as perceptions of the ability to work, highlight the importance of evaluating the individual's overall perspective on work following such a major life event.

Work Demands

Physical and Psychological Demands

Multiple reviews have found that cancer survivors who worked in blue collar jobs and/or physically demanding jobs are less likely to return-to-work (Amir & Brocky, 2009; Taskila & Lindbohm, 2007). One study found that, although survivors who work at physically demanding jobs are more likely to report higher levels of work disability, they are not more likely to quit work for cancer-related reasons (Short et al., 2005). A study of breast cancer survivors found that perceived physical and psychological constraints of the job were related to reduced rates of return-to-work (Fantoni et al., 2010), and a longitudinal study of a heterogeneous cancer sample found that physical workload was one of the strongest predictors of time to return-to-work (Spelten et al., 2003).

Work Environment

Flexibility

Workplace accommodations and benefits can play an important role in positive work outcomes. In qualitative studies, survivors reported that employers enabled them to reduce work hours or make other work adjustments immediately upon returning to work after cancer-related absence (Yarker, Munir, Bains, Kalawsky, & Haslam, 2010). They reported that flexibility in number of hours (Kennedy et al., 2007), ability to control the pace of the workday (Kennedy et al.), adjustments in the physical demands of the job itself (Main, Nowels, Cavender, Etschmaier, & Steiner, 2005), and reduced work-related travel (Main et al.) can greatly aid in the transition to resuming work. In contrast, breast cancer survivors reported that a lack of support from employers and inflexibility in work demands made it impossible for survivors to return-to-work (Taskila et al., 2010).

A review of employment outcomes in cancer survivors found that perceived employer accommodations are a consistent, strong predictor of return-to-work in cancer survivors (Mehnert, 2011). In a prospective study of breast cancer survivors, Bouknight et al. (2006) found that being provided with sick leave was positively associated with return-to-work at 12 months after diagnosis, and perceived employer accommodation for cancer illness and treatment needs was positively associated with return-to-work at 12 and 18 months post-diagnosis. A cross-sectional study of 328 heterogeneous cancer survivors in the UK found that having opportunities to work flexibly and paid time off for all medical appointments were associated with continuing to work during cancer treatment (Pryce, Munir, & Haslam, 2007), and a review found that control over number of hours and amount of work is related to return-to-work (Spelten et al., 2002). After treatment, cancer survivors who were offered a return-to-work meeting with their employer were more likely to return-to-work (Pryce et al., 2007).

Discrimination

Evidence regarding the presence of discrimination against cancer survivors was reviewed earlier. One study of breast cancer survivors found that perceived employer discrimination was associated with not returning to work at 12 months post-diagnosis (Bouknight et al., 2006).

Support and Environment

Several studies have noted how positive work outcomes appear to be tied closely to the social environment at work, whether it is characterized as a positive coworker attitude (Spelten et al., 2002), social support at work (Taskila et al., 2006), support from colleagues at the end of treatment (Fantoni et al., 2010) or a good social climate (Taskila et al., 2007). In contrast, a lower level of social support is associated with a higher proportion of wages lost due to cancer (Lauzier et al., 2008). Qualitative studies also provide a richer understanding of why social support matters, and how it changes over time from cancer-related absence, through the cancer survivor's initial transition back to work, and during the longer term period of work sustainability (Amir, Neary, & Luker, 2008; Johnsson et al., 2010; Kennedy et al., 2007; Main et al., 2005; Yarker et al., 2010). Cancer survivors interviewed in these studies described a similar trend: Participants who returned to work received a high level of support from coworkers and supervisors during their absence while undergoing treatment, and also received a high degree of support and understanding upon their initial return-to-work (Amir et al.; Johnsson et al.; Kennedy et al.; Main et al.; Yarker et al.). However, the cancer survivors who reported initial high levels of empathy, support, and flexibility said that these waned over time. Cancer survivors felt that, within a few weeks or months of their return-to-work, coworkers and supervisors expected them to resume their normal level of work performance (Amir et al.; Kennedy et al.; Yarker et al.). Cancer survivors reported difficulty in meeting these expectations because they were experiencing distressing and disabling persistent effects of cancer and its treatment, such as fatigue and cognitive difficulties, which made it difficult to resume normal work performance (Amir et al.; Kennedy et al.; Yarker et al.). Cancer survivors reported that they were not offered help or support in dealing with late effects, but they perceived that this was largely due to lack of colleagues' knowledge about late effects (Yarker et al.).

Employer Perspective

The attitudes and actions of employers play an important role in the return and retention of cancer survivors in the workplace. However, relatively few studies have examined the employer's perspective regarding the management and treatment of employees with cancer. Some of the literature on employers' perspectives regarding workers with disabilities or chronic illness reveals potential conflicts, such as beliefs that line managers are reluctant to accommodate disabled workers' needs, concerns that workers with disabilities would be less productive, and beliefs that coworkers would resent special accommodations that workers with disabilities receive (Fraser et al., 2010). In the UK, a survey of 252 employer representatives (primarily human resource professionals, as well as some occupational health professionals) assessed the availability of return-to-work services, as well as beliefs about successful work outcomes for cancer survivors (Grunfeld, Rixon, Eaton, & Cooper, 2008). Most organizations (81%) were large, with over 1,000 employees. The organizations most commonly provided return-to-work assistance to employees after an absence of 3–4 weeks or 5–6 weeks. At nearly all of respondent organizations (at least 95%), return-to-work services included phased returns (e.g., gradual reintroduction of duties), change in work duties (e.g., reducing physical workload or meetings with clients), workplace adjustments (e.g., changed hours or increased breaks), and physical environment changes (e.g., equipment).

Respondents also rated factors that they believed were related to successful work outcomes in employees who had cancer. The most common factors rated as "very important" were: employee's attitude toward work (95%); emotional ability to perform the job (94%); agreement between employee and employer over changes to hours/duties (91%); returning to work too soon (79%); ability to perform the job physically (78%); ability to keep the position open for the employee to return (74%); and other employees' attitudes towards the person returning to work (72%). In another paper (Grunfeld, Low, & Cooper, 2010) that was part of the same larger study, the authors surveyed those 252 employer representatives, as well as 194 recent cancer survivors (survivors within 4 weeks of completing treatment) who had not yet returned to work, and asked both groups about their expectations of how cancer survivors would function at work. Compared to the cancer survivors, employers had more negative expectations. Specifically, employers were less likely to say that an employee would have control over the effects and symptoms of cancer at work, and less likely to say that the effects and impact of cancer would be understood by coworkers. They were more likely to say that employees with cancer would experience symptoms at work, that cancer treatment would impair their ability to work, that employees' work-life would be adversely affected by cancer, that an employee would be affected emotionally at work, and that cancer would affect the employee for a long time. The authors suggested that the results demonstrated that recent cancer survivors may be overly optimistic about their ability to resume normal duties at work, and that there may be a mismatch between expectations and work ability upon returning to work.

Another study (Amir et al., 2010) surveyed 370 line managers in the UK, mostly from large organizations (500–900 employees). The authors conducted a factor analysis, which revealed five types of beliefs of line managers: (1) Fearful or negative attitudes about people with cancer and doubts about their ability to fulfill their work roles; (2) supportive or positive attitudes toward people with cancer in the workplace; (3) line managers' burden, or concern with the additional demands on line managers who oversee employees with cancer; (4) maintaining normality, or encouragement of employees with cancer to maintain sense of normalcy in their continued work roles; and (5) financial benefits, or belief that people with cancer should be provided financial benefits by staying home so that they do not need to work. The authors found that compared to male managers, female managers had less negative attitudes, believed more in employees with cancer maintaining normality, and were less concerned about line manager burden. The authors noted that the survey responses regarding line manager burden indicated that line managers had difficulty managing people with cancer, and they lacked support or guidance from senior management regarding how to handle these challenges (Amir et al.).

Occupational Health and Recommendations for Return-to-Work

In general, recommendations to facilitate return-to-work include decreased workload, a gradual return-to-work, accommodations at the workplace, and rehabilitation with occupational physicians (Krause, Dasinger, & Neuhauser, 1998; Verbeek, Spelten, Kammeijer, & Sprangers, 2003). Appointments with occupational health physicians typically do not occur until the end of treatment, at which time the cancer patient has a greater concern about the resumption of work (Verbeek, de Boer, & Taskila, 2009). Occupational health physicians and nurses can help cancer patients and survivors with the process of returning to work and rehabilitation, if needed. In large corporations, occupational physicians can have direct contact with the workplace. This connection can help to facilitate workplace accommodations. However, occupational physicians are generally removed from the team that treats the cancer patient (Wynn, 2009). Therefore, their ability to intervene as effective providers may be compromised. Occupational health physicians' limited knowledge about cancer and work also may restrict their ability to intervene for the cancer survivor. Some occupational physicians (19%) in the UK indicate not having enough information about how cancer affects work (Amir, Wynn, Whitaker, & Luker, 2009). Likewise, only 48% of occupational health physicians sampled expressed that their training provided them with knowledge about cancer, its prognosis, and functional outcomes.

A Survivorship Care Plan is a comprehensive history of tumor characteristics, treatment history, surveillance timeline, and potential health and functional problems (Hewitt, Greenfield, & Stovall, 2005). The individualized plan includes recommendations for short-term and long-term follow-up needs, including workplace difficulties. Currently, the use of these plans is limited (Stricker et al., 2011). However, these plans may allow for increased communication between the oncology team and the occupational health physician. Potentially, an occupational health physician could receive the Survivorship Care Plan to aid in the rehabilitation of the cancer survivor at work. An occupational health physician, along with primary care physicians, also may treat symptoms interfering with work. The effectiveness of these plans on work outcomes will need to be evaluated. In certain countries, such as the Netherlands, a cancer patient/survivor must see an occupational health physician to obtain a sickness absence and to return-to-work, and introducing such organized information for the survivor might improve work outcomes. Published research related to occupational health providers and cancer survivors returning to work is limited (Verbeek et al., 2009). This research has mainly been conducted in the Netherlands (Verbeek et al., 2003) and the UK (Amir et al., 2009).

While there are more limited recommendations concerning occupational health and cancer, perhaps we can gain information from other models of chronic illness. Young et al. (2005) proposed four phases of return-to-work for employees with an illness and injury. Phase 1, or "Off Work," is when the employee is not working due to the illness or injury. During "Re-Entry," or Phase 2, the employee resumes work at his/her pre-illness workplace or a new workplace. The manner and amount of work to be completed is discussed between all parties. Continuous monitoring of the work and the return-to-work goal takes place until the employee achieves the goal. This dynamic model highlights the need to find an appropriate match between employee capabilities and job requirements. Consideration of workplace accommodations and job modifications may be necessary. Phase 3, "Maintenance," involves maintaining the goal status and consideration into advancement at the workplace. In this sustainability phase, the employee aims at achieving goal productivity while he or she psychosocially reintegrates into the workplace. Phase 4, "Advancement," includes promotions and increased responsibility at the workplace. The problems that cancer survivors experience at work may be specific to the cancer-related medical history. The long-term and late effects of cancer do not always occur with other chronic illnesses. At this point, we do not know the extent of the utility that generic chronic illness recommendations have for cancer survivors. However, we can use them to generate hypotheses that then need to be validated with empirical research.

An example of such application is found in a paper by Verbeek et al. (2009). They did draw from other chronic diseases for recommendations. Verbeek et al. suggest that potential work problems should be approached following diagnosis and the creation of a treatment plan. At this point, factors such as occupation, employer–employee relations, health insurance, and social security (in the Netherlands, disability pension) can be considered. While some cancer patients may not think about returning to work at the time of diagnosis, other cancer patients express an interest in their physicians providing information on how cancer will affect their job (Frazier et al., 2009). A qualitative study of breast cancer survivors indicated that only some health care personnel discussed return-to-work with them (Nilsson, Olsson, Wennman-Larsen, Petersson, & Alexanderson, 2011). These breast cancer survivors expressed a desire for this discussion about topics, including barriers to returning to work to take place.

Table 7.1 Review of interventions for return-to-work [adapted from (de Boer et al., 2011)]

Type of intervention	Examples	Number of studies found	Level of evidence
Psychological	Patient education, individual counseling, and/or group discussion	5	Low
Physical	Walking program	1	Very low
Medical	Function-conserving cancer treatment vs. radical cancer treatment	9	Low
Multidisciplinary	Combination of psychological, vocational, and physical components	3	Moderate

Interventions

A limited number of studies have examined interventions targeted at employment in cancer survivors. De Boer et al. (2011) conducted a systematic review of interventions designed to enhance return-to-work in cancer survivors. Interventions were categorized as psychological, vocational, physical, medical or pharmacological, and multidisciplinary (a combination of any of these types). The authors identified 14 articles describing 14 randomized controlled trials (RCTs) and 4 controlled before–after studies (CBAs), for a total of 18 studies. The results are summarized in Table 7.1. They found five psychological interventions (patient education, individual counseling, and/or group discussion), one physical intervention (a walking program), nine medical interventions (chemotherapy, endocrine therapy, different types of surgery, and other treatments), and three multidisciplinary interventions which combined psychological, vocational, and physical components. Sixteen of the studies were conducted in the hospital, one took place in the community, and one did not report the setting. Methodological review of the studies found that there is low quality evidence of similar return-to-work rates for psychological interventions compared to care as usual. There is low quality evidence for medical interventions, showing that function-conserving approaches led to similar return-to-work rates as more radical cancer treatments. The authors found moderate evidence for multidisciplinary interventions with physical, psychological, and vocational elements resulting in greater return-to-work, and concluded that future intervention studies should contain multiple elements. They noted that the vocational element of interventions should focus on the work environment (e.g., work adjustments and supervisors) in addition to the individual survivor.

Another recent review article identified 23 articles describing 19 interventions, although most of them (15 of 19) were primarily focused on improving general functioning or quality of life rather than work outcomes (Tamminga, de Boer, Verbeek, & Frings-Dresen, 2010). Most of the interventions (68%) included person-directed work interventions, such as offering encouragement, education, or counseling about work. Most of the interventions (63%) did not involve the workplace, employer, or occupational physician in the intervention. Only 21% of interventions included vocational training, and 11% included work accommodations; these included rehabilitation and change of job, gradual return-to-work with limited work hours, sending letters from the treating physician to the occupational physician to increase communication, and calling or visiting the employer of patients. Only one of four controlled studies produced significant improvement in return-to-work. The authors advocated a shared model of cancer survivorship care, in which the treating physician communicates with the occupational physician or primary care physician to facilitate continuity of care. However, they only found one intervention that fit the shared care model of care.

Conclusions

This Chapter provided a perspective on cancer and work that has integrated the emerging research in this area. Despite the fact that the rate of publications on this topic has increased significantly over the past decade, we are just scratching the surface in terms of our identification of variables that are actual risk factors for work outcomes in cancer survivors. While we do have some idea from this research and other work in the area of work disability of the variables that are associated with various work outcomes, we have no knowledge of the mechanism of various factors that are associated with work outcomes in cancer survivors. For example, while we have evidence that fatigue and cognitive challenges are related to work limitations or perceived work ability, we do not have a clear idea of the specific impact of these symptoms on actual work tasks. We also know little about the short and longer term reactions of supervisors and coworkers, and their impact on work processes and work outcomes. Workplace-based studies can potentially inform us in a number of areas and represent one of the next steps in this area. This research should help us refine our understanding and development of interventions directed at specific work processes and outcomes.

As it relates to interventions, the literature clearly indicates that there is a major need for more robust evidence-based approaches that will improve outcomes through change in better documented risk factors. Such interventions should take into account these risk factors' mechanism of action that operates on the relationship between processes in the workplace and outcomes. If it is possible to empirically document the elements and their relationships [for example, in the model presented in Fig. 7.2 or any model of work and cancer outcomes, e.g., Steiner et al. (2004)], we should be able to develop more effective and specific interventions that would focus on correcting or changing these influences on various outcomes. This would not only make interventions more targeted to observed problems (e.g., cognitive challenges from chemotherapy or radiation exposure) but also accommodations at the workplace as well. Of course, the ultimate prevention of these symptoms might be some type of medication at the time of chemotherapy or radiation exposure that would result in the mitigation of symptoms such as fatigue, cognitive limitation, and pain. These drugs are being worked on, and it is hoped that the next edition of this text will not even need a chapter on cancer and work. However, as the model in Fig. 7.2 illustrates, there are many more potential factors other than symptoms that are associated with various work outcomes in cancer survivors. While this model of work and cancer bears many similarities to more generic work disability models, there may be areas that differ in subtle ways in one illness over another. For example, when we consider many work-related injuries or illnesses that are sources of work disability, it is important to emphasize that many of these cases, despite the experience of pain and limitations in areas of function, receive very little support at the onset of their work absence or work problems, and are often challenged as to the veracity of their claim that the injury or illness is work related. In contrast, the cancer survivor's cancer is generally not caused by toxic exposures at work. There is often a distinct difference in terms of initial reactions/support on the part of the employer and coworkers in these very different health problems in the context of work.

As described earlier, the support for the cancer survivor at work is often very active in the initial phase of work post diagnosis or during treatment but, as time goes on, there is less support and perhaps intolerance for a cancer survivor at work despite symptoms or late effects. In contrast, the worker with a work-related injury or illness typically receives very little support from the employer or coworkers at first, which declines even further over time. This difference might have some impact on work outcomes. We cannot assume a priori that the factors are identical or that all medical conditions influence work outcomes in a totally similar manner. Given the limited evidence on interventions in the area of cancer and work to date, the research in the last decade has not generated very many solutions. It is more accurate to say this research has helped raise awareness that, in some cancer survivors who desire or must work, not all is well when it comes to work. If one of our goals is to help those who experienced the trauma of a cancer diagnosis, treatment exposure, long-term and late effects and potential recurrence or new primary tumor, return to as normal a life as possible including work, we have much more to do. For those who want or need to return-to-work, let us continue to research and practice opportunities to mitigate or eliminate this stressor.

References

Altekruse, S. F., Kosary, C. L., Krapcho, M., Neyman, N., Aminou, R., Waldron, W., et al. (2010). *SEER cancer statistics review, 1975–2007*. Bethesda, MD: National Cancer Institute. Retrieved 21 September 2011, from http://seer.cancer.gov/csr/1975_2007/, based on November 2009 SEER data submission.

American Cancer Society. (2011). Cancer Facts & Figures 2011. Retrieved 21 September 2011, from http://www.cancer.org/acs/groups/content/…/documents/…/acspc-029771.pdf

Amir, Z., & Brocky, J. (2009). Cancer survivorship and employment: Epidemiology. *Occupational Medicine, 59*(6), 373–377.

Amir, Z., Neary, D., & Luker, K. (2008). Cancer survivors' views of work 3 years post diagnosis: A UK perspective. *European Journal of Oncology Nursing, 12*(3), 190–197.

Amir, Z., Wynn, P., Chan, F., Strauser, D., Whitaker, S., & Luker, K. (2010). Return-to-work after cancer in the UK: Attitudes and experiences of line managers. *Journal of Occupational Rehabilitation, 20*(4), 435–442.

Amir, Z., Wynn, P., Whitaker, S., & Luker, K. (2009). Cancer survivorship and return-to-work: UK occupational physician experience. *Occupational Medicine, 59*, 390–396.

Amir, Z., Wilson, K., Hennings, J., & Young, A. (2011). The meaning of cancer: Implications for family finances and consequent impact on lifestyle, activities, roles and relationships. *Psycho-Oncology.* The DOI is: 10.1002/pon.2021.

Balak, F., Roelen, C. A., Koopmans, P. C., Ten Berge, E. E., & Groothoff, J. W. (2008). Return-to-work after early-stage breast cancer: A cohort study into the effects of treatment and cancer-related symptoms. *Journal of Occupational Rehabilitation, 18*(3), 267–272.

Bouknight, R. R., Bradley, C. J., & Luo, Z. (2006). Correlates of return-to-work for breast cancer survivors. *Journal of Clinical Oncology, 24*(3), 345–353.

Bradley, C. J., & Bednarek, H. L. (2002). Employment patterns of long-term cancer survivors. *Psycho-Oncology, 11*, 188–198.

Bray, F., & Moller, B. (2006). Predicting the future burden of cancer. *Nature Reviews Cancer, 6*, 63–74.

Bureau of Labor Statistics. (2008). *Older workers. BLS Spotlight on Statistics*. Retrieved January 20, 2009, from http://www.bls.gov/spotlight

Bureau of Labor Statistics. (2011). *Local Area Unemployment Statistics*. Retrieved October 10, 2011, from http://www.bls.gov/lau/

Calvio, L., Peugeot, M., Bruns, G. L., Todd, B. L., & Feuerstein, M. (2009). Measures of cognitive function and work in occupationally active breast cancer survivors. *Journal of Occupational and Environmental Medicine, 52*(2), 219–227.

de Boer, A. G., Taskila, T., Tamminga, S. J., Frings-Dresen, M. H., Feuerstein, M., & Verbeek, J. H. (2011). Interventions to enhance return-to-work for cancer patients. *Cochrane database of systematic reviews*, (2), 1-64, CD007569 DOI is: 10.1002/14651858.CD007569.pub2.

de Boer, A. G. E. M., Taskila, T., Ojajarvi, A., van Dijk, F. J. H., & Verbeek, J. H. A. M. (2009). Cancer survivors and unemployment: A meta-analysis and meta-regression. *Journal of the American Medical Association, 301*(7), 753–762.

de Boer, A. G., Verbeek, J. H., Spelten, E. R., Uitterhoeve, A. L., Ansink, A. C., de Reijke, T. M., et al. (2008). Work ability and return-to-work in cancer patients. *British Journal of Cancer, 98*(8), 1342–1347.

Drolet, M., Maunsell, E., Brisson, J., Brisson, C., Masse, B., & Deschenes, L. (2005). Not working 3 years after breast cancer: Predictors in a population-based study. *Journal of Clinical Oncology, 23*(33), 8305–8312.

Earle, C. C., Chretien, Y., Morris, C., Ayanian, J. Z., Keating, N. L., Polgreen, L. A., et al. (2010). Employment among survivors of lung cancer and colorectal cancer. *Journal of Clinical Oncology, 28*(10), 1700–1705.

Fantoni, S. Q., Peugniez, C., Duhamel, A., Skrzypczak, J., Frimat, P., & Leroyer, A. (2010). Factors related to return-to-work by women with breast cancer in northern France. *Journal of Occupational Rehabilitation, 20*(1), 49–58.

Feuerstein, M., Luff, G. M., Harrington, C. B., & Olsen, C. H. (2007). Pattern of workplace disputes in cancer survivors: A population study of ADA claims. *Journal of Cancer Survivorship, 1*(3), 185–192.

Feuerstein, M., Todd, B. L., Moskowitz, M. C., Bruns, G. L., Stoler, M. R., Nassif, T., et al. (2010). Work in cancer survivors: A model for practice and research. *Journal of Cancer Survivorship: Research and Practice, 4*(4), 415–437.

Fraser, R. T., Johnson, K., Hebert, J., Ajzen, I., Copeland, J., Brown, P., et al. (2010). Understanding employers' hiring intentions in relation to qualified workers with disabilities: Preliminary findings. *Journal of Occupational Rehabilitation, 20*(4), 420–426.

Frazier, L. M., Miller, V. A., Miller, B. E., Horbelt, D. V., Delmore, J. E., & Ahlers-Schmidt, C. R. (2009). Cancer-related tasks involving employment: Opportunities for clinical assistance. *Journal of Supportive Oncology, 7*(6), 229–236.

Grunfeld, E. A., Low, E., & Cooper, A. F. (2010). Cancer survivors' and employers' perceptions of working following cancer treatment. *Occupational Medicine, 60*(8), 611–617.

Grunfeld, E. A., Rixon, L., Eaton, E., & Cooper, A. F. (2008). The organisational perspective on the return-to-work of employees following treatment for cancer. *Journal of Occupational Rehabilitation, 18*(4), 381–388.

Hansen, J. A., Feuerstein, M., Calvio, L., & Olsen, C. H. (2008). Breast cancer survivors at work. *Journal of Occupational and Environmental Medicine, 50*, 777–784.

Hewitt, M., Greenfield, S., & Stovall, E. (2005). *From cancer patient to cancer survivor: Lost in transition*. Washington DC: National Academic Press.

Johnsson, A., Fornander, T., Rutqvist, L. E., & Olsson, M. (2010). Factors influencing return-to-work: A narrative study of women treated for breast cancer. *European Journal of Cancer Care, 19*(3), 317–323.

Kennedy, F., Haslam, C., Munir, F., & Pryce, J. (2007). Returning to work following cancer: A qualitative exploratory study into the experience of returning to work following cancer. *European Journal of Cancer Care, 16*(1), 17–25.

Krause, N., Dasinger, L. K., & Neuhauser, F. (1998). Modified work and return-to-work: A review of the literature. *Journal of Occupational Rehabilitation, 8*(2), 113–139.

Lauzier, S., Maunsell, E., Drolet, M., Coyle, D., Hebert-Croteau, N., Brisson, J., et al. (2008). Wage losses in the year after breast cancer: Extent and determinants among Canadian women. *Journal of the National Cancer Institute, 100*(5), 321–332.

Main, D. S., Nowels, C. T., Cavender, T. A., Etschmaier, M., & Steiner, J. F. (2005). A qualitative study of work and work return in cancer survivors. *Psycho-Oncology, 14*(11), 992–1004.

Maunsell, E., Drolet, M., Brisson, J., Brisson, C., Masse, B., & Deschenes, L. (2004). Work situation after breast cancer: Results from a population-based study. *Journal of the National Cancer Institute, 96*(24), 1813–1822.

McKenna, M. A., Fabian, E., Hurley, J. E., McMahon, B. T., & West, S. L. (2007). Workplace discrimination and cancer. *Work, 29*(4), 313–322.

Mehnert, A. (2011). Employment and work-related issues in cancer survivors. *Critical Reviews in Oncology/Hematology, 77*, 109–130.

Munir, F., Yarker, J., & McDermott, H. (2009). Employment and the common cancers: Correlates of work ability during or following cancer treatment. *Occupational Medicine, 59*(6), 381–389.

National Cancer Institute. (2010). *Cancer trends progress report—2009/2010 update—costs of cancer care*. Bethesda: National Cancer Institute, US National Institutes of Health.

Nilsson, M., Olsson, M., Wennman-Larsen, A., Petersson, L.-M., & Alexanderson, K. (2011). Return-to-work after breast cancer: Women's experiences of encounters with different stakeholders. *European Journal of Oncology Nursing, 15*, 267–274.

Peteet, J. R. (2000). Cancer and the meaning of work. *General Hospital Psychiatry, 22*, 200–205.

Peugniez, C., Fantoni, S., Leroyer, A., Skrzypczak, J., Duprey, M., & Bonneterre, J. (2010). Return-to-work after treatment for breast cancer: Single-center experience in a cohort of 273 patients. *Annals of Oncology, 21*(10), 2124–2125.

Pryce, J., Munir, F., & Haslam, C. (2007). Cancer survivorship and work: Symptoms, supervisor response, co-worker disclosure and work adjustment. *Journal of Occupational Rehabilitation, 17*(1), 83–92.

Rasmussen, D. M., & Elverdam, B. (2008). The meaning of work and working life after cancer: An interview study. *Psycho-Oncology, 17*, 1232–1238.

Roelen, C. A., Koopmans, P. C., Groothoff, J. W., van der Klink, J. J., & Bultmann, U. (2010). Sickness absence and full return-to-work after cancer: 2-year follow-up of register data for different cancer sites. *Psycho-Oncology, 20*(9), 1001–1006.

Roelen, C. A. M., Koopmans, P. C., Groothoff, J. W., van der Klink, J. J. L., & Bultmann, U. (2011). Return-to-work after cancer diagnosed in 2002, 2005 and 2008. *Journal of Occupational Rehabilitation, 21*, 335–341.

Short, P., Vasey, J., & Tuceli, K. (2005). Employment pathways in a large cohort of adult cancer survivors. *Cancer, 103*, 1292–1301.

Smith, B., Smith, G. L., Hurria, A., Hortobagyi, G. N., & Buchholz, T. A. (2009). Future of cancer incidence in the United States: Burdens upon an aging, changing nation. *Journal of Clinical Oncology, 27*(17), 2758–2765.

Spelten, E. R., Sprangers, M. A. G., & Verbeek, J. H. A. M. (2002). Factors reported to influence the return-to-work of cancer survivors: A literature review. *Psycho-Oncology, 11*, 124–131.

Spelten, E. R., Verbeek, J. H., Uitterhoeve, A. L., Ansink, A. C., van der Lelie, J., de Reijke, T. M., et al. (2003). Cancer, fatigue and the return of patients to work-a prospective cohort study. *European Journal of Cancer, 39*(11), 1562–1567.

Steiner, J. F., Cavender, T. A., Main, D. S., & Bradley, C. J. (2004). Assessing the impact of cancer on work outcomes: What are the research needs? *Cancer, 101*(8), 1703–1711.

Steiner, J. F., Cavender, T. A., Nowels, C. T., Beaty, B. L., Bradley, C. J., Fairclough, D. L., et al. (2008). The impact of physical and psychosocial factors on work characteristics after cancer. *Psycho-Oncology, 17*(2), 138–147.

Stricker, C., Jacobs, L., Risendal, B., Jones, A., Panzer, S., Ganz, P., et al. (2011). *Survivorship care planning after the Institute of Medicine recommendations: How are we faring?* Epub ahead of print: Journal of Cancer Survivorship.

Tamminga, S. J., de Boer, A. G., Verbeek, J. H., & Frings-Dresen, M. H. (2010). Return-to-work interventions integrated into cancer care: A systematic review. *Occupational and Environmental Medicine, 67*(9), 639–648.

Taskila, T., de Boer, A. G., van Dijk, F. J., & Verbeek, J. H. (2010). Fatigue and its correlates in cancer patients who had returned to work-a cohort study. *Psycho-Oncology, 20*(11), 1236–1241.

Taskila, T., & Lindbohm, M. L. (2007). Factors affecting cancer survivors' employment and work ability. *Acta Oncologica, 46*(4), 446–451.

Taskila, T., Lindbohm, M. L., Martikainen, R., Lehto, U. S., Hakanen, J., & Hietanen, P. (2006). Cancer survivors' received and needed social support from their work place and the occupational health services. *Supportive Care in Cancer, 14*(5), 427–435.

Taskila, T., Martikainen, R., Hietanen, P., & Lindbohm, M.-L. (2007). Comparative study of work ability between cancer survivors and their referents. *European Journal of Cancer, 43*, 914–920.

Verbeek, J., de Boer, A., & Taskila, T. (2009). Primary and occupational health care providers. In M. Feuerstein (Ed.), *Work and cancer survivors*. New York: Springer.

Verbeek, J., Spelten, E., Kammeijer, M., & Sprangers, M. (2003). Return-to-work of cancer survivors: A prospective cohort study into the quality of rehabilitation by occupational physicians. *Journal of Occupational and Environmental Medicine, 60*, 352–357.

World Health Organization (1946). *Preamble to the Constitution of the World Health Organization as adopted by the International Health Conference*. U.S. Government Printing Office, Washington DC.

Wynn, P. (2009). Employment and the common cancers: Overview. *Occupational Medicine, 59*, 369–372.

Yarker, J., Munir, F., Bains, M., Kalawsky, K., & Haslam, C. (2010). The role of communication and support in return-to-work following cancer-related absence. *Psycho-Oncology, 19*(10), 1078–1085.

Young, A. E., Roessler, R. T., Wasiak, R., McPherson, K. M., van Poppel, M. N. M., & Anema, J. R. (2005). A developmental conceptualization of return-to-work. *Journal of Occupational Rehabilitation, 15*(4), 557–568.

The Problem of Absenteeism and Presenteeism in the Workplace

Krista J. Howard, Jeffrey T. Howard, and Alessa F. Smyth

Overview

It is common knowledge that the cost of health care for employees and their dependents is an important consideration for employees, employers, and insurance providers. Much is focused on the expenditures often referred to as "direct costs," such as those related to premiums, disability, physician appointments, specialists, prescriptions, and emergency care. However, within the work environment, there are hidden costs related with poor health. Commonly termed "indirect costs," these costs are most often associated with worker absenteeism and presenteeism. *Absenteeism* refers to the absence of a worker due to illness (either a personal illness or as a caretaker for a sick dependent). When employees are absent from work, it often creates a burden on the company not only for lost productivity but also for those who are responsible for the sick employee's neglected work. *Presenteeism*, on the other hand, refers to employees who are legitimately ill but continue to come to work. There are inherent problems with presentees: (1) if they are contagious, they put other employees at risk of becoming ill and (2) being ill often reduces the level of productivity and the quality of work. Indeed, in an analysis of the costs associated with both direct and indirect health-related issues, Hemp (2004) identified that, on average, medical and pharmaceutical costs (direct costs) only account for 24 % of the total health-related costs for employers. An examination of the indirect costs showed that 1 % was allotted for long-term disability, 6 % for short-term disability, and 6 % for absenteeism. Strikingly, 63 % of the health-care costs were attributed to presenteeism.

K.J. Howard, Ph.D. (✉) • A.F. Smyth, M.A.
Department of Psychology, Texas State University—San Marcos,
Psy 214C, 601 University Drive, San Marcos, TX 78666, USA
e-mail: krista.howard@txstate.edu

J.T. Howard, M.A.
Department of Demography, The University of Texas—San Antonio,
501 W. Cesar Chavez Blvd., San Antonio, TX 78207, USA

The aim of this chapter is to take a systematic approach to identifying the problems with absenteeism and presenteeism in the workplace. The first part of this chapter provides an overview of the methods used to measure and quantify the costs and productivity impacts of absenteeism and presenteeism. The second part of the chapter focuses on the various illnesses, injuries, health behaviors, and occupational factors that contribute to absenteeism and presenteeism. Lastly, the prevention and intervention strategies that various employers have developed and implemented are discussed to highlight the proactive efforts put forth to reduce absenteeism and presenteeism in the workplace.

Quantitative Measurement Approaches to Assess the Effects of Absenteeism and Presenteeism in the Workplace

The concepts of absenteeism and presenteeism are easily defined, such that absenteeism is simply the absence of a worker due to personal illness or the illness of a dependent. Presenteeism occurs when a worker is ill but continues to work and often results in a loss of productivity, which is noted as the amount of work performed within a given timeframe, as well as a loss in work quality. Ultimately, absenteeism and presenteeism are important not only because of the direct impact they have on worker health and well-being but also because they represent the two sources of productivity losses that are directly attributable to worker illness. From an economic perspective, the productivity losses related to absenteeism and presenteeism contribute both to lost revenue for employers and also potentially to lost wages and decreased earning potential for workers. This is especially true in cases where the employer provides either limited or no sick leave (Samuel & Wilson, 2007).

These concepts of absenteeism and presenteeism are easy to understand. However, in order to study the topic scientifically, they need to be operationally defined in a way that allows them to be measured quantitatively. This means that absenteeism and presenteeism must be measured in a way that can be expressed by numeric values, such as the number of hours of work missed due to absence within a given period of time, or the number of hours of decreased productivity due to working while ill. In addition to measuring the amount of work missed due to absence or the amount of productivity lost due to presenteeism, there is also much interest in translating these overall productivity losses into monetary terms. This section provides a general overview of the methods used to measure absenteeism and presenteeism quantitatively, and reviews a variety of common approaches to assessing their economic impact.

Measuring Absenteeism and Presenteeism

Many approaches to the measurement of absenteeism and presenteeism have been developed over the last few decades. Typically, these concepts are measured using self-report survey instruments, which ask workers a series of questions regarding their recent work performance, the number of days missed due to illness, their ability to meet various performance and productivity standards and so on. Aside from questionnaires, both concepts can be measured from actual employee records of attendance and job productivity. Of course, many employers do not have sufficient processes set up to capture all of the relevant information related to absenteeism and presenteeism. While most employers have the ability to track employee absence, many do not have adequate systems in place to measure all of the relevant aspects of productivity that could be affected by presenteeism. Likewise, most employers do not capture information about specific health conditions that ultimately result in absence and/or productivity loss due to presenteeism. The remainder of this section focuses specifically on the various self-report questionnaires that are used to measure absenteeism and presenteeism, which are followed by an overview of the various methods for assessing their economic impact.

General Instruments

Currently, there are six commonly used measurement instruments for evaluating the effects of illness on absenteeism and presenteeism in general: (1) the Work Productivity and Activity Impairment Questionnaire (WPAI), (2) the Work Limitations Questionnaire (WLQ), (3) the Health and Work Performance Questionnaire (HPQ), (4) the Health and Work Questionnaire (HWQ), (5) the Endicott Work Productivity Scale (EWPS), and (6) the Health and Labor Questionnaire (HLQ) (Lofland, Pizzi, & Frick, 2004; Prasad, Wahlquist, Shikiar, & Shih, 2004; Schultz & Edington, 2007). Each of these instruments asks workers to respond to a number of questions regarding their ability to effectively operate at home, work, school, and social settings in relation to their current health status (Prasad et al., 2004). Based on the responses to these questions, researchers are then able to estimate the extent of impairment at work for each worker.

In 1993, Reilly Associates, a health, life quality, and economic research and consulting firm, developed the *Work Productivity and Activity Impairment Questionnaire* (WPAI) to measure the effect of health on productivity at work and outside of work (Lofland et al., 2004; Prasad et al., 2004; Reilly, Zbrozek, & Dukes, 1993; Schultz & Edington, 2007). Several versions of the WPAI exist, including disease-specific versions, which are covered later in this section. The general version, typically referred to as WPAI-GH, has six questions and measures effects of both absenteeism and presenteeism. The first question verifies the employment status of the respondent, followed by three questions regarding the hours missed due to health problems, hours missed due to other reasons and total hours worked in the last 7 days. The remaining two questions ask the respondent to indicate the extent to which health problems have impacted their ability to do work and other daily activities outside of work in the past 7 days on a 11-point scale, where 0 is "no impact" and 10 is "completely prevented the respondent from working." Given the few number of questions in the survey, it is easy to administer and requires very little time to complete. A number of studies have established the validity and reliability of the WPAI (Prasad et al., 2004). The strengths of the WPAI are its (1) simplicity and low burden of administration, (2) high degree of validity and reliability, (3) versatility in extending to specific diseases, and (4) applicability to economic assessment.

The *Work Limitations Questionnaire* (WLQ) was initially developed based on patients with a variety of chronic illnesses, including asthma, Crohn's disease, liver disease, depression, and anxiety (Lerner et al., 2001; Lofland et al., 2004; Prasad et al., 2004). It has since been tested on additional illness populations, and found to be a valid and reliable instrument for measuring absenteeism and presenteeism. The WLQ consists of 25 items covering four job demand categories: (1) Time Management, (2) Physical Requirements, (3) Mental/Interpersonal, and (4) Output. Respondents are asked to rate each of the 25 items in relation to the extent to which their health condition has limited their ability to perform their job in either the last 2 weeks or the last 4 weeks. All items are asked on a 5-point Likert scale, where 1 = "Limited None of the Time" and 5 = "Limited All of the Time." A key strength of the WLQ is that it measures impacts to specific job performance skill areas, whereas most instruments measure only overall job performance.

The *Health and Work Performance Questionnaire* (HPQ) was first published in 2003 by researchers at Harvard Medical School, in collaboration with the World Health Organization (WHO) (Kessler et al., 2004; Prasad et al., 2004). The HPQ contains 24 items relating to hours missed from work, workplace accidents, diminished productivity, usual productivity and productivity of other workers within the last 4 weeks, as well as basic demographic information. Each item is measured on an 11-point Likert scale, where 0 = "Worst Performance" and 10 = "Top Performance." The HPQ has been tested within a number of occupational populations, including airline reservation agents, telecommunication customer service representatives, railroad engineers and automobile manufacturing executives, and has been found to have a high degree of validity and reliability in measuring absenteeism and presenteeism across many health conditions (Kessler et al., 2004). The strengths of the HPQ are (1) its relatively high validity, reliability, and generalizability and (2) its applicability to assessing economic impacts. The potential limitations of this instrument, however, are that (1) it may not predict white-collar job productivity particularly well and (2) it does not distinguish between different aspects of productivity (Prasad et al., 2004).

The *Health and Work Questionnaire* (HWQ) assesses 24 items, measured on a 10-point Likert scale, relating to the employees' perception of their own view of their work, coworker's view of their work and their supervisor's view of their work (Shikiar, Halpern, Rentz, & Khan, 2004). Specific work-related dimensions include the following: amount of work, work efficiency, work quality, restlessness at work, boredom at work, concentration at work, exhaustion at work, and work/environment satisfaction, among others. The HWQ has been tested within a population of airline reservation agents to assess the impact of smoking on productivity and absence in which the researchers compared results from the questionnaire to objective measures of absence and productivity supplied by the employer. The results of this study showed that the HWQ was successful primarily in predicting absenteeism, but not worker productivity (Prasad et al., 2004; Shikiar et al., 2004).

The *Endicott Work Productivity Scale* (EWPS) instrument was designed to measure both absenteeism and presenteeism related to any disease or disorder (Endicott & Nee, 1997; Lofland et al., 2004; Prasad et al., 2004). The questionnaire consists of 25 items, with each item measured on a Likert scale from 1 = "Never Affected" to 5 = "Almost Always Affected." The items ask the respondents to indicate to what extent their condition has affected their work productivity within the last week. The EWPS has been tested for validity and reliability, but only for the condition of depression. However, with respect to depression, the EWPS has been shown to have a high degree of validity and reliability.

Similar to the WLQ, the *Health and Labor Questionnaire* (HLQ) measures four modules of activity, including (1) work absenteeism, (2) work presenteeism, (3) household activity, and (4) impediments to work and household productivity (Prasad et al., 2004; van Roijen, Essink-Bot, Koopmanschap, Bonsel, & Rutten, 1996). Each module asks the respondents to provide an estimate of the number of hours that are missed from work (absenteeism), needed to make up for decreased productivity (presenteeism) and those spent on household activities, within the past 2 weeks. In order to determine the degree of work productivity loss, respondents with illness are compared to either the general population or a control group of non-ill respondents with respect to the hours associated with each of the three modules. The fourth module asks respondents to rate the degree to which their health condition limits their ability to complete work or household activities. The impediment rating is measured on a 3-point scale, where 0 = No Impediment, 1 = Some Impediment, and 2 = A lot of Impediment. The HLQ has been tested for validity and feasibility with a sample of the general population, as well as four different health condition samples, including migraine, spinal cord injury, knee replacement, and hip replacement (Prasad et al., 2004; van Roijen et al., 1996). Findings suggest that there is a high degree of feasibility, meaning the questionnaire is relatively easy to administer and takes only about 10 min to complete, that there is a high degree of validity for modules 1, 3, and 4 (van Roijen et al., 1996). However, the developers of the HLQ have recommended that more research be conducted on module two before utilizing the instrument for assessment of presenteeism (van Roijen et al., 1996).

National Health Inventory Survey

Each year, the National Center for Health Statistics, an agency of the Center for Disease Control and Prevention, conducts a nationwide survey focused on multiple factors, such as general health, health behaviors, occupational factors, etc. (CDC, 2010). Table 8.1 depicts the rates of absenteeism by industry, which is measured as workdays missed in the past 365 days, for all respondents and for those who missed at least 1 day of work in the past year. Also included in Table 8.1 is the percentage of respondents in each industry who report having paid sick leave.

Table 8.1 Rates of absenteeism by industry

Industry	Percent of respondents with paid sick leave	All respondents, $N=17,461$, days absent/year		Absentees[a], $N=7,114$, days absent/year	
		Mean	Standard deviation	Mean	Standard deviation
Accommodation and Food Services	17.1	3.3	16.4	8.2	22.3
Agriculture, Forestry, Fishing	16.3	3.7	18.7	11.0	27.1
Armed Forces	76.0	2.6	9.2	9.7	14.9
Arts, Entertainment, Recreation	34.9	2.9	13.7	9.6	25.3
Construction	24.4	4.0	18.0	11.6	29.8
Education Services	75.2	3.9	18.9	7.5	22.4
Finance and Insurance	74.5	3.0	9.0	6.8	14.9
Health Care and Social Assistance	61.1	4.2	16.3	9.2	23.0
Information Industries	66.9	5.0	20.9	8.7	22.7
Management of Companies and Enterprises	72.2	4.1	14.1	16.5	29.0
Manufacturing	56.0	3.5	14.2	9.9	23.0
Mining	59.2	1.5	3.7	5.0	5.9
Other Services (excluding Public Administration)	17.1	2.9	12.1	8.1	19.1
Professional, Scientific, Technical Services	60.4	3.3	13.2	7.8	21.1
Public Administration	85.3	5.3	18.2	11.4	29.3
Real Estate/Rental	40.3	4.2	26.8	13.1	46.7
Retail Trade	42.0	4.0	17.0	9.8	24.8
Transportation and Warehouse	57.9	5.8	25.3	13.3	29.6
Utilities	89.1	5.5	18.4	10.4	26.0
Waste Management and Remediation Services	28.2	2.8	14.5	9.2	28.7
Wholesale Trade	63.1	3.0	12.4	8.1	20.1

National Health Inventory Survey—2010
Center for Disease Control and Prevention—National Center for Health Statistics
http://www.cdc.gov/nchs/nhis.htm
[a]Absentees are a subset of all respondents who reported a minimum of one absence within the last 365 days

Disease-Specific Instruments

There are several instruments that have been developed for measuring absenteeism and presenteeism for specific disease conditions. The *Work Productivity and Activity Impairment Questionnaire* (WPAI) has been modified into four different disease-specific versions, including (1) the WPAI-Special Health Problem survey, (2) the WPAI-Allergic Rhinitis survey, (3) the WPAI-Gastro-Esophageal Reflux survey, and (4) the WPAI-Chronic Hand Dermatitis survey (Prasad et al., 2004). The WPAI-Special Health Problem survey can be easily modified to address any specific condition by simply replacing generic terms in the survey questions with terms specific to the disease of interest (e.g., diabetes, hypertension, arthritis, etc.). A number of specific studies have been conducted for each of these WPAI disease-specific surveys, the findings of which have provided statistical support for the validity and reliability of each version in measuring workplace productivity loss associated with allergic rhinitis, GERD and chronic hand dermatitis respectively (Reilly, Lavin, Kahler, & Pariser, 2003; Reilly, Tanner, & Meltzer, 1996; Wahlquist, Carlsson, Stalhammar, & Wiklund, 2002). In addition to the disease-specific versions of the WPAI, there are also two questionnaires that have been developed specifically for assessing the impact of migraine headache on productivity, both workplace and household activities. The Migraine Disability Assessment (MIDAS) is a questionnaire with seven questions that assesses the impact of migraine on work, household and daily activities (Prasad et al., 2004; Stewart, Lipton, Kolodner, Liberman, & Sawyer, 1999; Stewart et al., 2000). The MIDAS survey asks respondents questions about the frequency and severity of headache, the amount of time missed from work/school, household and other activities and the number of days in which productivity was reduced by half or more for work/school and household activities.

Subsequent psychometric studies have found that MIDAS does provide a high degree of validity and reliability, especially in measuring frequency and severity of headache episodes and in establishing the relationship between migraine headache incidence and increased absenteeism and presenteeism (Stewart et al., 1999). However, the researchers also found that recall of headache episodes seemed to be much more accurate than recall of work productivity loss episodes. The explanation of this finding is that headache episodes occur more frequently than the amount of work missed, which makes them more memorable. Another possible explanation for the more accurate recall of headache episodes is that they are, by definition, very painful, and therefore may be more memorable due to the experience of increased physical and emotional distress as compared to the relatively mundane experience of day-to-day work routines. Of course, both of these mechanisms, frequency of occurrence and experience of pain, could be present. Whatever the underlying cause of differences in recall, the researchers concluded that more research into recall bias was needed, as well as possible modifications to the questionnaire (Stewart et al., 2000).

The *Migraine Work and Productivity Loss Questionnaire* (MWPLQ) is an instrument that asks respondents a series of 29 questions, most of which consist of items about the difficulty of various types of work tasks, but also asks about the number of hours of work missed, the amount of impairment at work, and several questions about migraine therapies and recent attacks (Lerner et al., 1999; Prasad et al., 2004). There are seven areas, or domains, of work for which questions are asked: (1) time management, (2) quality, (3) quantity, (4) bodily effort, (5) interpersonal demands, (6) mental effort, and (7) environmental factors. The questions are presented on a 6-point Likert scale, ranging from "No Difficulty" to "So Much Difficulty, Couldn't Do At All." A follow-up study found significant evidence that the MWPLQ has a high degree of validity and reliability in measuring the impact of migraine on work productivity (Davies, Santanello, Gerth, Lerner, & Block, 1999). No problems of episode recall, like those found in the MIDAS questionnaire, were reported. However, there was a low correlation between MWPLQ items and the SF-36 Health survey, which is another general health status questionnaire used in the assessment of a variety of health conditions, but not an instrument designed to measure absenteeism and presenteeism.

A recent measure, the Absenteeism Screening Questionnaire, has been developed to assess and predict long-term absenteeism for patients with low back pain (Truchon et al., 2012). This screening device shows strong psychometric capabilities for identifying individuals with acute back pain who may benefit from primary interventions to increase likelihood of return-to-work.

While many measures are specifically designed to assess absenteeism and presenteeism, other well-established measures that evaluate other aspects of health have also been shown to be good indicators of increased sick leave and lost productivity. The Patient Health Questionnaire (PHQ) is a well-validated self-report instrument used to evaluate Axis I psychopathology, including somatization, depression, anxiety, panic, and other clinical disorders (Spitzer et al., 1999). A subset of the PHQ that focuses on somatoform disorders (PHQ-15) was recently assessed to determine an association with somatization and increased sick leave (de Vroege, Hoedeman, Nuyen, Sijtsma, & van der Felz-Cornelis, 2012). This study used a receiving operator characteristic (ROC) analysis to derive a cutoff score of ≥ 9 points on the PHQ-15 that would indicate higher likelihood of frequent sick leave.

Another example is the Fear-Avoidance Beliefs Questionnaire (FABQ), was originally developed to assess maladaptive behaviors related to pain conditions (Waddell, Newton, Henderson, Somerville, & Main, 2007). Inrig, Amey, Borthwick, and Beaton (2012) recently evaluated using the FABQ to assess work return following leave associated with upper extremity injuries. The findings showed that workers exhibiting higher levels of fear-avoidance were less likely to return to work.

Cost Models for Assessing the Economic Impact of Productivity Loss

From an economic standpoint, it is essential to quantify the impact of these indirect costs associated with poor health, by translating the lost time and productivity into dollar amounts. Several models have been developed that attempt to capture the true costs of worker absenteeism and presenteeism. This section highlights each of the models developed for quantifying indirect costs of illness. First, the Human Capital Approach is a straightforward calculation of production loss that simply multiplies the time lost by the absent or impaired employee's wage (Johannesson, 1996). One inherent problem identified with using the Human Capital Approach is that the total calculation can be seen as an overestimation if worker replacement is not considered. For individuals with long-term absences, this estimation for lost productivity is seen to be very high using the Human Capital Approach. Another concern about using the Human Capital Approach questions the assumption that an individual's wage is an appropriate measure of the total value of productivity (Brouwer, van Exel, Koopmanschap, & Rutten, 2002). In the case where the absent or impaired worker is part of a team, his/her absence can have a cascading effect on the productivity of other team members (Koopmanschap et al., 2005).

The second model developed to quantify worker absenteeism and presenteeism is the Friction Cost Method (Koopmanschap, Rutten, van Ineveld, & van Roijen, 1995). The premise of the Friction Cost Method is that after an initial adaptation period, termed the "friction period," the absent worker would be replaced, and the lost hours from an impaired employee could also be overcome by replacement or through working extra hours. From this perspective, the emphasis for the calculation is based on the "value added" by a productive employee/replacement rather than focusing directly on the wages paid. By using the Friction Cost Method, the estimates of productivity loss due to illness are much lower as compared to the Human Capital Approach (Johannesson & Karlsson, 1997). Finally, a third approach for quantifying productivity costs shifts away from assigning dollar amounts to lost time, and redirects focus on the individual's quality of life. This method was put forth by the US Panel charged with evaluating cost-effectiveness related to health care (Gold, Siegel, Russell, & Weinstein, 1996; Koopmanschap et al., 2005). The panel recognizes that the quality of life of individuals who are ill or injured has a direct impact on their finances, specifically through their decrease of income.

By using an approach focusing on quality of life as part of the health assessment, this method should, theoretically, include the quantitative productivity losses measured by other approaches. While the theory behind assessing quality of life is acknowledged as being reasonable, there is still a large debate as to whether this method accurately quantifies lost productivity due to illness or injury (Brouwer et al., 2002).

Both the Human Capital Approach and the Friction Cost Method were specifically developed to assess the costs of productivity loss due to worker absence. While there is much debate over the best mathematical formula for quantifying indirect costs due to worker absences, it is considerably more difficult to assess the costs of productivity losses for presentees. That being said, the Human Capital and Friction Cost methods have both been extended to provide estimates of costs associated with presenteeism in some studies (Lofland et al., 2004). However, the calculations for estimating costs of presenteeism are not as straightforward as absenteeism. There are a number of reasons that make assessing the costs of presenteeism difficult. For instance, many individuals remain at work while sick, and presenteeism can often occur prior to and immediately following an absence related to illness (Brouwer et al., 2002). Furthermore, the specific type of illness can have a direct effect on the degree of productivity loss while present at work. Many studies have been published regarding specific dollar amounts associated with specific illnesses (see Sect. "Factors Related to Absenteeism and Presenteeism in the Workplace" of this chapter). Because of these difficulties, economists are currently developing new models to help better quantify productivity costs associated with presenteeism.

Factors Related to Absenteeism and Presenteeism in the Workplace

Many studies have evaluated factors related to absenteeism and presenteeism in the workplace. Most of these studies have focused on specific illnesses, injuries, health behaviors, and occupational factors that have been shown to increase the rates of absenteeism and presenteeism in various fields of work. This section provides an overview of the current research specific to acute illnesses, chronic illnesses, health behaviors, such as obesity, smoking, and alcoholism, and psychosocial factors, and examines the prevalence of absenteeism and presenteeism along with the estimated direct and indirect costs. Additionally, research specific to how occupational factors, such as stress and burnout, work type, demand, scheduling, and job satisfaction, relate to absenteeism and presenteeism is presented.

Acute Illness

Acute illnesses are oftentimes the most thought about as regards to absenteeism and presenteeism. These types of illnesses can include, but are not limited to, allergies, colds, flu, acute low back pain, gastrointestinal distress, etc. In contrast to chronic illnesses, acute illnesses are episodic and are usually remedied within a few days. This section assesses various types of common acute illnesses that have been linked to absenteeism and presenteeism in the workplace.

Allergies
Allergic reactions occur when the immune system responds abnormally to the presence of a foreign substance. While some reactions are more severe, such as those caused by certain foods or insect bites, most individuals suffer from seasonal allergies resulting from exposure to various types of pollen. The prevalence of individuals in the USA reporting seasonal allergies with symptoms lasting more than 6 days within 1-year duration was estimated at 30 % (Nathan et al., 2008). Based on a large-scale survey by Loeppke et al. (2007), the most prevalent health condition reported by employees was

allergies. In fact, medical and drug costs estimated for treating allergies were found to be approximately one-third the accumulated costs associated with increased rates of absenteeism and presenteeism related to allergy symptoms. Another evaluation of the effects of allergies on worker productivity showed that for employees in the manufacturing industry, as allergy symptoms increased to moderate and severe levels, productivity losses also increased (Bunn et al., 2003). As part of a wellness screening, Lamb et al. (2006) identified that individuals experiencing allergic symptoms worked, on average, 2.3 fewer hours per day as compared to employees not experiences allergy symptoms. In an evaluation of the impact of medical conditions on worker productivity for Lockheed Martin employees, allergies or sinus problems were found to be highly prevalent (59.8 % of personnel), and accounted for 4.1 % average productivity loss (Hemp, 2004).

An examination of the relationship between pollen counts and worker productivity showed that, as pollen counts increased, untreated allergies resulted in greater absenteeism and lower productivity as compared to treated allergies (Burton, Conti, Chen, Schultz, & Edington, 2001). Sullivan, Navaratnam, Lorber, and Shekar (2010) conducted a study on the cost-effectiveness of a non-sedating H1-antagonist (*desloratadine*) for patients with persistent allergic rhinitis. The findings support that the treatment provided significant cost-savings in relation to work productivity, that is, individuals receiving the medication were shown to exhibit significantly greater worker productivity as compared to those who received a placebo. While it is not plausible for individuals to avoid exposure to environmental allergens, these studies presented support the need for adequate treatment for individuals with allergies in order to reduce the negative effects of increased absenteeism and presenteeism.

Influenza

Influenza, an acute respiratory virus that spreads rapidly, can affect up to 20 % of any given population (CDC, 2008). The economic burden of an influenza pandemic is considerable. Based on 2003 data, direct costs associated with medical care in the US were estimated over $10 billion annually. Moreover, the costs associated with earnings lost due to illness or death approximated $16 billion annually. It is estimated that the total economic burden of influenza, including medical care and productivity losses, equates to over $87 billion annually (Molinari, Ortega-Sanchez, & Messonnier, 2007). Of these total societal costs for the influenza pandemic, more than 80 % are attributed to absenteeism or presenteeism (Szucs, 1999). Based on a comprehensive review of the literature on lab-reported, physician-diagnosed, and self-diagnosed influenza, the average length of absence from work ranged between 3 and 7 days (Keech & Beardsworth, 2008). A consideration to be made when evaluating the effects on worker productivity in relation to influenza is to distinguish rates of absenteeism based on the individual's illness from the time missed due to taking care of an ill dependent. Palmer, Rousculp, Johnston, Mahadevia, and Nichol (2009) surveyed employees with children to assess the days missed and hours of presenteeism for personal influenza illness, household influenza illness, and a combination of both personal and household influenza illness. Employees with personal influenza illnesses reported more than twice the number of days missed from work as compared to employees without influenza illnesses. Findings also showed that employees missed more days of work caring for household influenza illnesses, relative to the days missed for caring for household acute respiratory illnesses. In fact, 17.7 % of employee absences were attributed to household influenza illness. With respect to presenteeism, employees with acute respiratory illnesses reported being less productive for 1.8 h each day they worked with symptoms; however, employees with influenza-like illness reported being less productive for 4.8 h each day worked with symptoms. Likewise, employees with household influenza illness reported significantly less productive work time as compared to employees with other wintertime respiratory illnesses.

In a study on influenza-based absenteeism and presenteeism, Ablah et al. (2008) surveyed individuals with varying types of occupations regarding whether or not they have left work early or if they have ever remained at work with symptoms of an influenza-like illness. Between 70 and 80 % of workers stated that they have left work because of influenza symptoms. When asked if they have ever continued working with influenza symptoms, roughly 60 % stated they have. This included employees working in health-care (59 %) and school systems (57 %). Interestingly, only 27 % of employees who work in health education reported that they have continued to work while experiencing influenza symptoms. While influenza is highly contractible within families, schools and workplaces, many strategies have been studied to prevent the spread of the virus. By educating individuals about hand washing and covering sneezes, and by offering easy access to vaccinations, employers can proactively help their employees reduce their risk of developing influenza-like illnesses (later in this chapter, a description of interventions aimed at influenza prevention is presented).

Acute Gastrointestinal Illness
Several studies have evaluated the effects of gastrointestinal illnesses on employees' rates of absenteeism and reduced productivity at work. Two common gastrointestinal disorders that have been evaluated extensively are functional dyspepsia and gastroesophageal reflux disease (GERD). Functional dyspepsia is characterized by upper-abdominal pain and discomfort for which there is no identifiable cause. In a recent study conducted by Brook et al. (2010), use of sick days for employees with functional dyspepsia was significantly greater compared to those without functional dyspepsia; however, there were no significant differences in rates of short-term or long-term disability. Presenteeism for employees with functional dyspepsia was more pronounced. The work productivity for employees with functional dyspepsia was 12 % less than the control group.

Gastroesophageal reflux disease (GERD) is a condition for which gastric acid from the stomach enters the esophagus, resulting in pain (heartburn), regurgitation, and other symptoms such as coughing, asthma, and hoarseness (Brook et al., 2007). Although GERD is not generally life threatening, there is an economic burden associated with medical treatments and indirect costs. In a comparison of direct to indirect costs for GERD, the costs associated with absenteeism and presenteeism amounted to more than three times the costs associated with medical care and treatments (Loeppke et al., 2007). In a study on presenteeism associated with GERD, Gisbert et al. (2009) observed a decrease of 26 % in productivity for employees diagnosed with GERD. In a study at Lockheed Martin, 15 % of the employees were diagnosed with GERD. The analysis showed that average productivity loss associated with GERD was 5.2 % which accounted for $582,660 in aggregate losses (Hemp, 2004). As with many acute illnesses, appropriate medical assessment and treatment is imperative to reduce negative consequences, such as absenteeism and lost productivity. While gastrointestinal disorders, such as functional dyspepsia and GERD, are very prevalent, these conditions are often preventable and manageable with the appropriate medical treatment.

Acute Pain Conditions
Pain conditions affect everyone at some point in their lives. However, individual differences in the intensity and duration of the pain are highly variable. When evaluating the effects of pain conditions on work-related absenteeism and presenteeism, most studies have focused on specific pain sources. This section is focused on how acute or episodic pain conditions such as migraine and premenstrual syndrome affect absenteeism and lost productivity at work.

Migraine. Migraine headache is an episodic condition, but can become persistent for many who suffer from this painful disorder. Although the medical treatment for migraine is relatively inexpensive, the costs associated with absenteeism and lost production are high. Hu, Markson, and Lipton (1999) estimated that, of the total costs associated with migraine, approximately 93 % are attributed to indirect costs (both absenteeism and presenteeism). In fact, the majority of the indirect costs due to migraine disorders involve presenteeism (Levin-Epstein, 2005). The prevalence of migraine disorder is highest between the ages of 22 and 55, which are noted as "peak employment years" (Berry, 2007), but rates are most pronounced between 30 and 49 years of age (Hazard, Munakata, Bigal, Rupnow, & Lipton, 2009). Typically, females are more likely to be diagnosed with migraine disorder, which is commonly attributed to hormonal fluctuations (Berry, 2007; Hazard et al., 2009). A general problem for individuals with migraine disorders is that they often attempt to treat their own symptoms with over-the-counter medications and remedies rather than seeking treatment from a medical provider (Berry, 2007; Linde & Dahlof, 2004). As part of the American Migraine Study (1998), of the individuals not seeking medical treatment for their migraines, 61 % reported severe to very severe pain, and 67 % reported severe disability (Lipton & Stewart, 1998). The 2004 AMPP study identified that only 12 % of individuals with migraine disorder were taking prophylactic medication to prevent the occurrence of migraines (Lipton, Bigal, & Diamond, 2007). From an employer's perspective, two steps can be made to help employees with migraine disorders. First, employers can identify employees who regularly suffer from migraine headaches and recommend that the employees seek medical treatment rather than self-medicating for persistent migraine. Second, the employers can proactively identify and regulate migraine triggers that can occur in the workplace, such as lighting intensity or unusual smells (perfumes, candles, secondhand smoke, etc.) (Berry, 2007).

Premenstrual Disorders. Current research has shown how women with premenstrual disorders, such as premenstrual syndrome and premenstrual dysphoric disorder, exhibit high rates of absenteeism and lost productivity in the workplace (Heinemann, Minh, Filonenko, & Uhl-Hochgraber, 2010). In this international study, women reporting as having either mild or no PMS/PMDD symptoms were compared to those with moderate-to-severe symptoms. When evaluating absenteeism, those with moderate-to-severe symptoms were 2.4 times more likely to miss at least 1 day of work per month, compared to those with mild or no PMS/PMDD symptoms. Rates of worker productivity losses were also much higher for the moderate-to-severe PMS/PMDD group, such that 69.4 % of those with moderate-to-severe symptoms, as compared to 23.4 % of those with mild or no symptoms reported moderate reductions in productivity and efficiency.

Chronic Illness

Classifying chronic illnesses leads to a much wider range in intensity and duration of the illness symptoms. The following section highlights research on various chronic health conditions as they relate to decreased worker productivity and increased absenteeism.

Pulmonary Diseases

Pulmonary diseases, such as uncontrolled asthma and chronic obstructive pulmonary disease (COPD), are found to have an impact on absenteeism and worker productivity. Based on 2007 data from the American Lung Association, costs associated with asthma approximated $20 billion, which included medical care (physician visits, hospital care, prescriptions), mortality and morbidity (including costs attributed to productivity losses) (ALA, 2009). Parents of children with asthma are oftentimes absent from work due to dependent care. Yet, only about 8 % of the costs associated with asthma are in relation to absenteeism. In fact, it is estimated that presenteeism for individuals with asthma decreases productivity by more than one-third (Hoppin, Stillman, & Jacobs, 2010). In a large-scale survey assessing rates of absenteeism and quality of life for both individuals with asthma and those who are caregivers for individuals with asthma, the findings show that uncontrolled asthma has a much greater impact on worker productivity and absenteeism as compared to those with asthma that is better controlled (Dean, Calimim, Kindermann, Khandker, & Tinkelman, 2009). In fact, 43 % of adults with uncontrolled asthma reported missing days from work, relative to only 23 % of adults with controlled asthma. Of those who are caretakers of dependents with asthma, 31 % reported missing work due to care of dependents with uncontrolled asthma, as compared to 16 % of the caretakers of dependents with controlled asthma. This delineation between controlled and uncontrolled asthma is an important one. In order to reduce the negative symptoms and poor impact on worker productivity associated with uncontrolled asthma, appropriate assessment and treatment for asthma conditions is imperative.

As a leading researcher on pulmonary diseases, Dr. William Bunn provides insight into how chronic obstructive pulmonary disease (COPD) affects workplace productivity (Vogenberg, 2009). While the prevalence of smoking overall is on the decline, blue-collar workers who smoke represent twice the number of white-collar workers who smoke. Medical costs and costs related to short-term disability (absenteeism) are approximately three times greater for employees with COPD, as compared to the medical and absentee costs for employees without this disease. A key message provided by Dr. Bunn is that because smoking is a major risk factor for the development of COPD, employers who provide cessation programs for their employees can drastically reduce medical and absentee costs in conjunction with the occurrence of this disease.

Chronic Pain Illnesses

Many individuals suffer from chronic pain conditions that are more organic in nature, as opposed to being the result of an injury. Researchers have studied the socioeconomic burden of chronic pain conditions such as arthritis, osteoarthritis and fibromyalgia. Needless to say, individuals with these chronic pain conditions exhibit high levels of absenteeism and reduced productivity in the workplace.

Arthritis. Arthritis is a chronic pain condition associated with breakdown or inflammation of the joint, causing swelling, stiffness and limited movements. The leading cause of worker disability is attributed to arthritis (Escorpizo et al., 2007). In fact, more than half of all individuals who suffer from arthritis have reported work disability (Dunlop, Manheim, Yelin, Song, & Chang, 2003), and those with arthritis are less likely to be employed because of their debilitating condition (Jantti, Aho, Kaarela, & Kautiainen, 1999). Loeppke et al. (2007) projected the costs for absenteeism and presenteeism for individuals with arthritis to more than triple the costs associated with medical care and treatment of the chronic pain condition. Burton et al. (2008) estimated that in a company with 10,000 employees, the costs of rheumatoid-arthritis absenteeism amounted to $1.55 million annually. In the study on employees at Lockheed Martin, the prevalence rate of arthritis was 19.7 %, and the rate of worker productivity loss associated with arthritis was 5.9 % (Hemp, 2004). As part of a nationwide study, employees with arthritis reported an average of 4.5 h of lost productivity per week due to pain (Stewart, Ricci, Chee, Morganstein, & Lipton, 2003).

Osteoarthritis. Osteoarthritis is a chronic pain condition that predominately affects weight-bearing joints, such as the hip and the knee. It is estimated that up to 27 million adults in the USA are affected by osteoarthritis, and over half of all cases are reported in individuals 65 years or older (Kotlarz, Gunnarsson, Fang, & Rizzo, 2010; Lozada et al., 2011). A recent study evaluating the aggregate absenteeism costs attributed to individuals with osteoarthritis reported annual costs to approximate $10.3 billion in the USA (Kotlarz et al., 2010). Sadosky, Bushmakin, Cappelleri, and Lionberger (2010) conducted a cost analysis on lost productivity based on the level of severity of osteoarthritis. Costs associated with patients with mild levels of severity of osteoarthritis averaged $6,096 per year, whereas those with moderate levels averaged $13,251 per year. Patients reporting severe levels of osteoarthritis averaged $17,214 per year in productivity losses.

Fibromyalgia. Fibromyalgia is a chronic pain condition for which the patient experiences widespread muscle pain without any etiological source. Accounting for <5 % of the general population, fibromyalgia is more likely to affect females with increasing age (Wolfe, Ross, Anderson, Russell, & Hebert, 1995). Annual medical care costs, including office visits to primary care and rheumatology specialists and hospital coverage, is found to be significantly greater for individuals with fibromyalgia

($7,286) compared to those without fibromyalgia ($3,915). Annual costs related to disability and absenteeism are also greater for individuals with fibromyalgia ($2,913) relative to those without fibromyalgia ($1,359) (White et al., 2008). Furthermore, White et al. (2008) also evaluated rates of absenteeism for individuals with fibromyalgia and found that, on average, fibromyalgia employees miss almost three times as many workdays due to disability and medically related issues, as compared to employees without fibromyalgia. Kleinman et al. (2009) evaluated the levels of lost productivity for individuals with fibromyalgia and, based on both self-report and objective-based criterion, individuals with fibromyalgia exhibited significantly lower rates of worker productivity as compared to those without fibromyalgia.

Multiple Sclerosis. Multiple sclerosis is a debilitating degenerative disorder of the central nervous system that restricts physical activity and causes problems with walking, balance, and other impairments. It is estimated that between 70 and 80 % of individuals diagnosed with multiple sclerosis are not able to work (Roessler et al., 2003). For those who continue to work, research has shown that the cost burdens for employers are primarily due to short and long-term disability and general absenteeism. Ivanova et al. (2009) conducted a cost analysis comparing employees with multiple sclerosis to a matched control group. The average annual costs of medical expenses for employees with multiple sclerosis were $15,277, compared to $3,948 for the control group. Indirect costs associated with disability, and medically related absenteeism was reported to be $5,769 annually for employees with multiple sclerosis, whereas expenses for those in the matched control group were $1,417 annually. Naci, Fleurence, Birt, and Duhig (2010) conducted a comprehensive literature review on the indirect costs associated with employees with multiple sclerosis. To date, there are no studies available assessing costs attributed to presenteeism and reduced productivity for employees with multiple sclerosis.

Chronic Pain: Musculoskeletal Injuries

Chronic occupational musculoskeletal disorders are highly prevalent in the working community and, not only can these injuries be debilitating to the individual, but they can also be very costly for the employer and insurance companies. It is estimated that approximately $70 billion are spent annually on health-care utilization and work productivity losses due to patients with chronic pain conditions (Gatchel, 2004). The majority of workplace injuries related to musculoskeletal disorders can occur either gradually or suddenly, as in the case of an accident. Sprains, strain or tearing of the back muscles, overexertion, and falls were the most commonly reported events causing workplace injuries. Upper-extremity injuries of the shoulder and wrist were more likely caused by overexertion or repetitive motions, and falls and overexertion were the most reported causes of lower-extremity injuries (Courtney & Webster, 2001). While overexertion was the source reported for 75.6 % of all musculoskeletal disorders in 2007 (Bureau of Labor Statistics, 2007), disorders caused by falls in general were identified to be the most disabling of all musculoskeletal injuries (Courtney & Webster, 2001).

Occupational injuries are routinely reported by incidence rates and by duration of absence from work. According to the Bureau of Labor Statistics, in 2007, the overall rate of nonfatal occupational musculoskeletal injuries requiring time away from work was reported to be 35 per 10,000 full-time employees. The median days of work absence was 9, and 27.9 % of injured employees were absent from work more than 30 days. Based on specific body region affected by the occupational musculoskeletal injury, 48 % were back injuries, 14.5 % were upper-extremity injuries, 1.6 % were cervical injuries, 8.1 % were lower-extremity injuries, and 4.7 % affected multiple body regions. Based on the nature of the injury, 75.3 % of musculoskeletal injuries were reported as sprains or strains, 13.7 % were reported as soreness or pain, and 3.6 % were identified as carpel tunnel syndrome (Bureau of Labor Statistics, 2007).

The prevalence rates of musculoskeletal injuries are typically reported for specific occupations and industries. For musculoskeletal injuries of the neck, back, and upper-extremity regions, the top five industries cited for the highest percentages of workers' compensation claims were air transportation, foundation and building contractors, couriers, nursing home facilities, and general freight trucking companies (Bonauto, Silverstein, Adams, & Foley, 2006). In 2007, nursing aides, attendants, and orderlies reported the highest rate of injury or illness at 465 per 10,000 full-time workers; while transportation and material movers with musculoskeletal injuries accounted for the greatest duration of work absence, with a median of 11 days and 31.7 % absent more than 30 days (Bureau of Labor Statistics, 2007).

Evaluating the costs associated with musculoskeletal disorders, Loeppke et al. (2007) estimated that the total costs, both direct and indirect, for back and neck pain equated to the total costs for arthritis and to surpass the total costs of all other chronic pain conditions. Interestingly though, while the direct costs associated with arthritis is about 10 % of the total costs, costs for medical care and treatments for back, neck, and other chronic pain conditions surpass the costs associated with absenteeism and presenteeism. In a study on back pain exacerbations for US workers, Ricci et al. (2006) identified the prevalence of individuals with back pain to be 15.1 %. Within this cohort, 42 % reported back pain exacerbations within the prior 2 weeks. In a cost analysis of employees with back pain, it is estimated that total costs for employers approximates $7.4 billion annually. Moreover, it is estimated that 71.6 % of this total cost is attributed to workers with exacerbated back pain.

Health Behaviors

Various poor health behaviors such as smoking, alcoholism, and obesity have been evaluated to understand the relationship among these factors with absentee rates and reduced worker productivity. Burton et al. (2005) conducted a study to determine the effects of health risk factors on worker productivity. In this study, the various factors considered included lifestyle factors (smoking, physical inactivity, seatbelt use, alcohol use, and use of relaxation medication), perception factors (life dissatisfaction, poor physical health, job dissatisfaction, and high stress), and biological factors (high blood pressure, high cholesterol, and obesity). The estimated loss of productivity increased with each additional risk factor. Individuals reporting only one risk factor were identified to exhibit 1.9 % lost productivity. The addition of each risk factor was attributed to an additional 2.4 % estimated excess loss of productivity.

Alcoholism/Smoking

A few studies have evaluated the effects of alcohol use and smoking on worker absenteeism and reduction in worker productivity. These studies have found a positive relationship between alcohol use and smoking with increased absences and reduced productivity. For example, in an evaluation on the effects of alcoholism on absenteeism, Roche, Pidd, Berry, and Harrison (2008) examined the rates of employee absences during a 3 month duration. The average percentage of employees who missed work due to alcohol use was 3.5 % overall. This percentage was much higher for the younger age groups (8.8 % for the 14–19-year-old group, and 7.5 % for the 20–29-year-old group). Based on occupation type, 4.1 % of blue-collar workers missed at least 1 day due to alcohol use, compared to 2.9 % of professionals. Further analyses were conducted based on four levels of alcohol consumption: abstinence, low risk, short-term risky, and high-risk levels. Individuals considered to be short-term risky (high number of drinks in a given setting, but a low weekly average) were found to be 12 times more likely to miss work relative to those who abstain from drinking. Individuals in the high-risk group (averaging more than 28 drinks per week for males or 14 drinks per week for females) were found to be 22-times more likely to miss work compared to the abstinence group.

In an evaluation on risk factors associated with absenteeism and presenteeism, Goetzel et al. (2009) found that women with alcohol use/smoking reported an average of 2.3 unproductive days annually, whereas men with alcohol use/smoking reported 1.93 annual unproductive days. Stewart et al. (2003) compared rates of presenteeism for smokers, and found that 29.7 % of employees who smoke at lease a pack a day reported more than 2 h of lost productivity time per week, as compared to only 17.4 % of nonsmokers. In a comprehensive multivariate analysis of psychosocial factors associated with the likelihood of sickness absences, women who smoked regularly were 1.4 times more likely to exhibit absenteeism, and men who used alcohol as a sedative were 2.1 times more likely to report sickness absences (Voss, Floderus, & Diderichsen, 2004).

Obesity/Physical Activity
The prevalence of obesity in US adult populations is approximately 34 %, and the estimates of overweight and obesity combined is 68 % (Flegal, Carroll, Ogden, & Curtin, 2010). Both obesity and overweight individuals are at a higher risk for certain health consequences, such as coronary heart disease, type 2 diabetes, cancers, hypertension, dyslipidemia (high cholesterol and high triglycerides), stroke, liver and gallbladder disease, sleep apnea and respiratory problems, osteoarthritis and gynecological problems (NIH, 1998). Obesity is also related to high rates of absenteeism and presenteeism in the workplace, thus contributing to an increasing amount of direct and indirect health-care costs. Several studies have evaluated the rates of absenteeism and productivity losses in relation to obese employees. Individuals with a body mass index (BMI) greater than 29 had 1.5 % more productivity losses compared to employees in the normal or overweight ranges (Burton et al., 2005). Goetzel et al. (2010) evaluated the direct and indirect cost burden of overweight and obese workers based on doctors visits, emergency room visits, hospitalizations, absenteeism and presenteeism. The study showed that obese employees had 20 % more doctors' visits and 26 % more emergency room visits compared to non-obese employees. Furthermore, evaluations of presenteeism showed that overweight employees were 10 % less productive, and obese employees were 12 % less productive, relative to normal weight workers. Gates, Succop, Brehm, Gillespie, and Sommers (2008) assessed presenteeism for individuals who were moderately to severely obese (BMI > 34) and found that these employees showed 4.2 % loss in productivity, as compared to only 1.2 % of all other employees. Indirect costs of absenteeism and presenteeism for obese workers amounted to approximately ten times that of the general medical expenditures (Loeppke et al., 2007). In light of these data, many employers have taken an initiative to help their employees lose weight by becoming more physically active. In a study by van Strien and Koenders (2010), physical activity, sports and dietary restrictions were evaluated in relation to absenteeism rates for overweight employees. The findings showed that increased physical activity was a moderator for decreased absenteeism. Dietary restrictions, on the other hand, were found to moderate the effects of obesity on increased absenteeism. Carson, Baumgartner, Matthews, and Tsouloupas (2010) examined the effects of both workplace and leisure physical activity in relation to emotional exhaustion, absenteeism and turnover. Poor physical activity was found to mediate the effects of emotional exhaustion on absenteeism and turnover.

Psychological Factors

Psychosocial distress is highly prevalent in the general population, and not only is found to exacerbate other comorbid health conditions but has also been shown to play a considerable role in absenteeism and decreased worker productivity. This section highlights current research on both anxiety and depression and how these types of psychological distress affect employee costs associated with medical expenditures and lost productivity.

Anxiety

Anxiety disorder affects approximately 18 % of US adults, with 22 % of these cases are classified as "severe." Common symptoms include feeling fearful with worry and uncertainty (Kessler, Chiu, Demler, & Walters, 2005). Successful treatment of anxiety disorders typically includes medication, psychotherapy or a combination of both (Hyman & Rudorfer, 2000). Several studies have evaluated the effects of anxiety disorder on health-care expenditures and indirect costs. For example, Caverly, Cunningham, and MacGregor (2007) developed a study that classified employees as having either high or low absenteeism and either high or low presenteeism. Within this study, 20.3 % of the employees with both high absenteeism and presenteeism reported anxiety, while 18.6 % of those with low absenteeism and high presenteeism reported anxiety. However, only 8 % of employees with high levels of absenteeism and low levels of presenteeism reported anxiety disorders. This supports the hypothesis that anxiety is more associated with reduced work productivity than being absent from work. In a cost analysis comparing direct to indirect costs associated with anxiety disorder, Loeppke et al. (2007) reported that the medical and pharmaceutical costs for treating anxiety were approximately 12 % of the costs associated with absenteeism and presenteeism. Based on a multi-study analysis on how psychosocial distress affects absenteeism, the average days of work missed within a 4-week duration due to anxiety disorders ranged from 0.6 to 3.8 days (Hilton, Sheridan, Cleary, & Whiteford, 2009).

Depression

Mood disorders include bipolar disorder, dysthymic disorder and major depressive disorder. The 12-month prevalence of any mood disorder in US adults is 9.5 %, with 45 % of these cases being classified as "severe." The 12-month prevalence rate for US adults with major depressive disorder is 6.7 % (Kessler, Chiu, Demler, & Walters, 2009). Of all health-care expenditures in the USA, 6.2 % are allotted for mental health care (Mark et al., 2005). Greenberg et al. (2003) estimated the total costs for depression to approximate $83 billion, with 62 % of this total applied to absenteeism and reduced productivity. Several studies have also focused on the indirect costs associated with employees with depression disorder and depressive symptoms. In epidemiological-based studies, comparisons were made evaluating absenteeism and presenteeism related to common mental health disorders. For depressive disorders, the estimates based on the prior 30 days showed a range of 0.5–3.1 days missed, and a range of 2.8–8.2 days of reduced productivity (Hilton et al., 2009; Sanderson & Andrews, 2006; Sanderson, Tilse, Nicholson, Oldenburg, & Graves, 2007). In the Caverly et al. (2007) study, comparing employees with high and low levels of absenteeism and presenteeism, the findings showed that 21 % of employees with high presenteeism reported depressive conditions, regardless of the level of absenteeism.

In a comparison of the top ten health conditions by cost, Loeppke et al. (2007) identified depression as having the highest overall total costs, with the majority related to absenteeism and presenteeism. Indeed, mental health conditions are strongly related to other comorbid health conditions such that psychological distress can develop in conjunction with the presence of a health condition, and likewise depression can exacerbate the physical health disorder. The key to reducing expenditures associated with depression involves both accurate and timely assessment of the condition along with appropriate treatment and compliance (Birnbaum et al., 2010).

Occupational Factors

While both physical health and mental health are strongly correlated with absenteeism and presenteeism in the workplace, occupational factors have also been shown to be very costly to employers.

Occupational factors related to job satisfaction and occupational commitment have both been found to be inversely related to absenteeism and presenteeism. This section highlights the research that has been conducted on various occupational factors such as job stress, job characteristics, and job satisfaction that are associated with increased absenteeism and reduced worker productivity.

Job Stress

Burnout is a common work factor for employees with consistently high stress levels. Occupational stress can be either physical or psychosocial, and it has been shown to have a strong negative effect on general health, health behaviors, worker productivity and quality of life. Several studies have evaluated the effects of occupational stress as it relates to increased absenteeism and presenteeism in the workplace. In one study comparing employees with either high or low rates of absenteeism and presenteeism, Caverly et al. (2007) identified stress to be a more prevalent factor for individuals with high rates of presenteeism, as compared to those with high rates of absenteeism. When the employees in this study were asked about their reasons for presenteeism, the top two responses were: (1) others depend on them (i.e., no back-up or coverage from other employees) and (2) the workload is too high. In a study predicting absenteeism and presenteeism, Gilmour and Patten (2007) found that employees with high self-perceived work stress were 1.4 times more likely to exhibit reduced productivity, and were also 1.8 times more likely to be absent from work within a 2-week period. Burton et al. (2005) estimated a 4.1 % reduction in productivity due to perceived high stress at work.

Job Type, Demand and Schedules

Other occupational factors associated with the job type, level of job demand, level of job control and shift schedules have been taken into consideration as predictors of increased absenteeism and decreased worker productivity. In a comparison of employees who reported either experiencing presenteeism or not during the prior 2 weeks, it was found that the level of work experience was a significant factor. In fact, employees with greater levels of work experience were less likely to exhibit reduced productivity (Rantanen & Tuominen, 2011). Type of work was also found to be associated with both absenteeism and presenteeism. Gilmour and Patten (2007) found that white-collar workers were 30 % less likely to exhibit presenteeism as compared to sales, service and blue-collar workers. Additionally, sales and service employees were 30 % less likely to be absent from work compared to white-collar and blue-collar employees. Shift work is also related to higher rates of absenteeism. Nurses who work 12-h shifts or evenings, nights or mixed shift types are more likely to be absent from work as compared to nurses on 8-h day shifts (Rajbhandary & Basu, 2010).

When evaluating the level of demand and the amount of control an employee has in his/her position in relation to presenteeism, more than 40 % of those with low demand and high control reported at least 2 h of reduced productivity in the past week, compared to 23 % of those with high demand and low control positions (Stewart et al., 2003). Work factors such as work overload and effort-reward imbalance were also seen to be associated with increased rates of absenteeism (Rajbhandary & Basu, 2010).

Job Satisfaction

Job satisfaction is a self-report item that explains how satisfied or dissatisfied an employee is at his/her current job. Various occupational components can affect this assessment of job satisfaction, such as job security, opportunity for career advancement, organizational trust, supervisor trust, peer support, etc. Job satisfaction is an important variable to consider because it not only is correlated with absenteeism and reduced productivity but also is indicative of turnover. Several studies have evaluated factors related to job satisfaction and their effects on rates of absenteeism and presenteeism. Caverly et al. (2007) assessed the correlations between various occupational factors and absenteeism/

presenteeism. While job security and job satisfaction were the variables most correlated with absenteeism, stronger correlations were found for presenteeism: job security, career opportunities, trust and supervisor support. Burton et al. (2005) reported a 3 % reduction in worker productivity for employees reporting high levels of job dissatisfaction. In a comparison of employees who reported presenteeism behaviors in the prior 4 weeks, Rantanen and Tuominen (2011) showed a significant difference in levels of job satisfaction between those with and without reduced productivity. Those not reporting presenteeism showed approximately 20 % higher rates of job satisfaction as compared to those who were considered as presentees.

Current Intervention Strategies to Prevent or Reduce the Effects of Absenteeism and Presenteeism in the Workplace

Intervention and prevention programs, such as corporate wellness, smoking cessation and healthy lifestyle programs, offer many benefits to employers, including improved morale, less stress, and greater focus among employees, lower insurance premiums, reduced employee absenteeism and increased productivity (Mulligan, 2010). For the employees themselves, these interventions aim to make them happier and healthier. Due to escalating health-care costs and profits lost to absenteeism and presenteeism, employers have begun to use intervention strategies to address and improve employee health. The Association for Worksite Health Promotion (Mercer, 1999) reported the same findings, citing improved employee health, increased morale, and the lessening of health-care costs as the impetus for employers to provide disease-prevention and health promotion programs. When employees are emotionally and physically able to work, and also have the desire to work, employers witness less absenteeism and presenteeism (O'Donnell, 2000).

Illness Prevention Strategies

As the earlier literature review demonstrated, there are several significant issues with illness related presenteeism, including decreased productivity, increased health-care costs, and increased risk of the spread of communicable diseases. In a recent review article, Samuel and Wilson (2007) suggest that all companies should evaluate their rates of presenteeism, especially "customer-facing" businesses because customers do not want to be assisted by ill employees. Likewise, allowing healthy employees to be exposed to their sick coworkers increases the risk that they too will become sick, which only exacerbates the problems lost productivity and costs. In the same article the authors outline the problem of presenteeism as well as several employer and legislative solutions.

Stay at Home
Perhaps one of the most basic illness prevention strategies available to employers is simply allowing sick employees to stay at home while ill. One barrier to stay at home is a lack of recognition of the problems associated with illness related presenteeism. As Samuel and Wilson (2007) point out, managers need to be educated about the issue of presenteeism so that they will encourage sick employees to stay home. In addition to educating managers, ensuring that employees are informed about the importance of their health and reminding them that it benefits, not only themselves but their company and coworkers as well. Another barrier to the stay at home solution is that not all employers offer paid sick time. However, given the high costs of presenteeism associated with lost productivity and the risk of the spread of disease, those employers who do not offer paid sick leave may wish to reconsider their policies. Employers who recognize the problems with presenteeism and seek to encourage employees

to stay at home when ill will find it much easier to convince them if they offer paid sick leave. The combined approach of education and paid sick leave will most likely serve the company's long-term financial interests.

Samuel and Wilson (2007) also discuss government policies on providing paid sick leave, which addresses some of the problems with presenteeism. In some states, the Family and Medical Leave Act (FMLA) has been passed, which is a leave statute that ensures employers will allow time off for covered employees, even if the time is unpaid. Several states have Temporary Disability Insurance (TDI) programs to provide employees with paid short- and long-term leave for injuries and/or illnesses that are not work-related. In February 2007, San Francisco passed a groundbreaking Sick Leave Ordinance that entitled all employees of the county to paid, accrued, hourly sick leave. This time off work can be used for illness, injury, diagnosis, treatment, medical care, and to care for family members. Although there is a 30-h cap on accrued sick leave, employees can keep their unused leave from year-to-year. Other cities and states such as Madison, WI, and the states of Washington, Massachusetts, and Vermont have proposed similar bills for mandated sick leave. At the time of publication none of these measures have passed; however, citizen and government support for these new laws are growing.

One of the most common methods of prophylaxis used in the prevention of disease is vaccination. In the USA, vaccinations are routinely given to prevent a wide range of childhood diseases, such as polio, rubella, measles, mumps, diphtheria, tetanus, and chicken pox. In adulthood, vaccination efforts are typically focused on influenza, due to the enormous health and economic consequences discussed earlier in this chapter. In response to the threat of influenza pandemic, many private and public health clinics, government and public health departments, as well as many private employers now offer access to inexpensive influenza vaccinations. Although many employers have on-site influenza vaccinations, the majority of employees do not take advantage of this convenience. Nowalk et al. (2010) aimed to increase employee vaccination rates by offering two options: an intranasal (LAIV) vaccine and an injectable (TIV) influenza vaccine. They also offered an incentive to employees and increased awareness of the vaccination clinic. Fifty-three companies with vaccine clinics, totaling 1,222 participants, were included in this study. Most of these companies served as controls, while "Choice" sites were given both the LAIV and TIV vaccines and advertised only the choice between vaccines. "Choice Plus" sites also offered both types of vaccinations, but increased advertising as well as highlighted the choice of vaccines, and offered a monetary incentive to employees. The LAIV vaccination was 6.5 % higher in Choice sites and 9.9 % higher for Choice Plus sites. The TIV vaccination resulted in a 15.9 % higher participation from employees aged 50 or older in the Choice Plus sites, but no increase in TIV vaccination was found in either the Choice or Choice Plus sites for employees ages 18–49.

Health Behaviors and Interventions

Companies have seen double-digit growth rates in health-care costs, which has piqued employers' interest in worksite health promotion programs (Nyman, Barleen, & Abraham, 2010). Many studies have been published that evaluate individual corporate wellness programs, reporting the overall effectiveness of managing diseases and risk factors in terms of absenteeism and presenteeism. The University of Minnesota's wellness program includes both lifestyle management (LM) and disease management (DM). The DM program included employees with diabetes, asthma, coronary artery disease, congestive heart failure, arthritis, depression, osteoporosis, musculoskeletal diseases, low-back pain, migraines, gastrointestinal disorder, as well as other health issues. The LM program included employees with obesity, tobacco and alcohol use, hypoglycemia, chronic pain, osteoporosis, pregnancy, and other conditions. Significant results were found in reducing absenteeism by approximately 4 h per employee per year in the DM program, but the LM program was shown to not be effective in the reduction of absenteeism. The only factor of the LM program that affected significant reduction in absenteeism was the fatigue program.

Pelletier, Boles, and Lynch (2004) conducted a study on 500 employees who participated in a health promotion program at a large national company. All participants belonged to the corporate-sponsored fitness centers, and had access to a multitude of wellness programs and services through the employee benefits department. These employees completed the *Health Risk Assessment* (HRA) pre- and post-study, answering 20 questions regarding smoking, exercise, diet, chronic conditions, health status, demographics, and biometric measures. Risk scores were calculated for coronary heart disease, based on 11 risk factors: poor diet, unhealthy body mass index (BMI), high cholesterol, physical inactivity, stress, lack of preventive health-care visits, lack of emotional fulfillment, high blood pressure, tobacco use, diabetes, and alcohol use. Participants also completed the *Work Productivity and Activity Impairment Questionnaire* (General Health) (WPAI-GH) to measure the amount of work missed (absenteeism), work impairment (presenteeism), and impaired activity all due to health issues. At the time of the first surveys, employees with an unhealthy body-mass index (BMI), lack of physical activity, lack of emotional fulfillment, diabetes, and high blood pressure had a significantly greater amount of absenteeism and presenteeism. Results of the wellness program showed a significant risk reduction in employees who improved their diet, cholesterol, stress, and engaged in preventative health-care visits. Forty-nine percent of participants reduced their number of health risks, with 19 % reducing two or more, and 30 % reducing one risk factor. Employees who improved their diet and emotional fulfillment had significant improvements in presenteeism; however, no specific health factor was found to reduce absenteeism.

Wendt, Tsai, Bhojani, and Cameron (2010) evaluated the effect of Shell's Disability Management Program on absenteeism over the course of 5 years. From 1996 to 2002, absenteeism rates among Shell employees increased by 54 %, leading to the development of an in-house disability management program. In 2002, 13,000 employees were managed by two full-time case managers, and site nurses and administrative staff devoted 20 % of their time toward the program. In 2008, 17,500 employees were supported by four full-time case managers, three administrative staff, and 5–10 % of work time from a physician-manager and multiple site nurses. Shell's Disability Management Program also began to include "transitional duty," benefits staff, and human resources. Transitional duty allowed employees to return to work in a part-time or restricted capacity, which enabled them to come back to work sooner than if they had waited for fully recovery from illness or injury. After an employee had missed work for four consecutive days, a letter from a doctor was required, and a case manager was assigned to the employee. The case manager coordinated communication between the employer, health-care provider, human resources, benefits, etc. in order to ensure the employee received proper treatment and accommodations. Then, the appropriateness of transitional duty was assessed and, when the employee was ready to return to work, an evaluation of fitness was performed. Results revealed that, overall, hourly employee absences per year decreased by 31 %, while staff absences increased by 3.4 %. Similarly, the researchers found a 30 % decrease in illness days per year among hourly workers, but there was no statistically significant change in illness days among staff employees. However, this trend was not consistent through the course of the study. From 2002 to 2004, there was an overall decrease in absenteeism equating to 1.2 days per year per employee (a decrease from 5.4 to 4.2 days). From 2004 to 2006, there was an increase in absences of 0.8 days per year (an increase to 5.0 days), and this number reversed itself during the 2006–2008 time frame, bringing absenteeism back to the 2004 average rate of 4.2 days per employee per year, which was solely due to decreased absenteeism in hourly workers. Decreases in absenteeism for specific conditions were also reported. Days lost due to circulatory system disorders decreased by 34 % from 2002 to 2008. Absences in the digestive system diagnostic category decreased by 46 %, the genitourinary system by 47 %, injuries by 34 %, the musculoskeletal system by 23 %, pregnancy by 37 %, and absences due to respiratory system issues decreased by 42 %. Shell saved a total of 34,731 days over this 5-year period and had an estimated total savings of $9,740,000, which equates to a 2.4:1 return on investment.

Depression

Major Depressive Disorder is a debilitating chronic condition that affects 15.7 % of employees during their lifetime, and 8.6 % of employees in a 12-month period (Marcotte, Wilcox-Gok, & Redmon, 1999; McIntyre, Liauw, & Taylor, 2011). It is projected that depression will be the second leading cause of disability by the year 2020 (Murray & Lopez, 1997; Wells et al., 1989). Depression and related stress conditions cause the most workforce impairment (Birnbaum et al., 2010), and the lack of effective response to depression accounts for a disproportionate amount of work lost due to presenteeism and absenteeism (Wang et al., 2007). McIntyre et al. (2011) reported that chronic medical conditions associated with depression, such as obesity, diabetes mellitus, cardiovascular disease, pain disorders, dementing disorders, and other chronic stress-sensitive disorders, interact with depression to cause workforce dysfunction. In a comprehensive review on the effects of depression in the workplace, McIntyre et al. (2011) reported the efficacy of many different intervention strategies. Stress management programs in the workforce that emphasized adequate sleep, exercise, muscle relaxation, the importance of interpersonal relationships, and the challenging of anxiety provoking and depressogenic thoughts have shown to be effective in reducing employees' depressive symptoms (Mino, Babzono, Tsuda, & Yasuda, 2006). Wang et al. (2007) conducted a research study on approximately 150,000 employees of several large national companies. They evaluated the effects of depression screening, outreach, and care management of depressed workers through a telephone program. The need for treatment was assessed, appropriate individuals were referred to in-person treatment, and the researchers encouraged and monitored treatment adherence and provided therapeutic interventions by telephone. Depression was measured with the *Quick Inventory for Depressive Symptoms Self-Report* (QIDS-SR), and the *WHO Health and Productivity Questionnaire* (HPQ) was used to assess work performance. Employees were randomly assigned to the usual care group or the telephone intervention group, and completed these assessments at baseline, 6 and 12 months. QIDS-SR scores at 6 and 12 months were significantly lower for the intervention group than the usual care group, and there was also significantly higher job retention, as well as more hours worked among employees in the intervention cohort.

A Canadian study found that workers who were compliant with antidepressant medication were significantly more likely to return to work instead of claiming long-term disability or leaving their employment (Dewa, Hoch, Lin, Paterson, & Goering, 2003). The researchers also found a 3-week reduction in the length of disability among depressed employees who had early interventions. Laxman, Lovibond, and Hassan (2008) suggest that workplace interventions need to de-stigmatize mental illness and to improve access to services through employment assistance programs in order to adequately treat mood disorders in employees. The researchers emphasize the need for these programs to have open communication between the employee, employer, and the health-care provider.

Smoking and Alcohol Cessation

A study conducted in Long Island, New York mailed surveys to 524 companies to evaluate the effectiveness of their wellness programs (Mulligan & Rosenberg, 2004). Ninety-three companies indicated they provided wellness programs to their employees, and the most prevalent type of intervention was smoking cessation. The 2004 study also showed that these smoking cessation programs benefited employers most in terms of lowered health-care costs. To examine this issue more carefully, Mulligan (2010) sent abbreviated surveys to these same 524 companies, only asking for information concerning smoking cessation programs. One-hundred seven out of 115 employer respondents indicated the presence of a smoking cessation program. Survey results showed that 85 % of companies provided nicotine replacement therapies, and 52 % provided coverage for Zyban, an antidepressant shown to assist cessation (Mulligan, 2010). Telephone counseling was a part of 42 % of the programs, 32 % had group behavioral activities, 10 % offered financial incentives, and 8 % charged smokers more for health insurance compared to their nonsmoking counterparts. Ninety-eight percent of these companies reported that their smoking cessation program caused lower health-care costs.

Quanbeck, Lang, Enami, and Brown (2010) studied the cost–benefit of interventions for employees who had issues with alcohol, with the cost of absenteeism and impaired presenteeism taken into account. The researchers estimated the cost of problem drinking among employees for a theoretical Wisconsin company without a treatment program, and also developed a model to estimate the cost of implementing a program that included screening, brief intervention, and referral to treatment (SBIRT). They concluded that SBIRT was cost-beneficial to employers, and when absenteeism and presenteeism were included in the analysis, the theoretical firm would save $771 per employee by using this treatment program.

Obesity/Physical Activity

Employers and researchers have studied and implemented health-based interventions targeting overweight, obesity, lack of exercise, and poor nutrition in relation to absenteeism and presenteeism. A behavioral change model called *A Lifestyle Intervention Via Email* (Alive!) was tested on a group of 787 employees of Kaiser Permanente of Northern California (Block et al., 2008). These employees were randomly assigned to the intervention group or the wait-list control group. The participants in the intervention group chose between increasing their physical activity, increasing their dietary intake of fruits and vegetables, or decreasing their consumption of added sugars, as well as saturated fats and trans fats. The Alive! model elicited and maintained healthy behaviors by assessing the individual and providing feedback, goals, tips, and reminders, as well as weekly goal-setting and the promotion of social support. Participants' health-related quality of life, presenteeism, self-efficacy, and stage of change were assessed at the beginning and end of the program by the SF-8 Health Survey Short Form (Block et al., 2008). Presenteeism was measured by self-assessed "reduction in difficulty accomplishing work tasks because of physical and emotional problems," and participants in the intervention group were 1.47 times more likely to report a reduction than the control group. This study also found a statistically significant improvement in mental health, health status, self-efficacy for changing one's diet, and stage of change for physical activity and the consumptions of more produce and less fats.

In a study of overweight and obese employees, Oberlinner et al. (2007) reported that, due to the prevalence of overweight and obesity and their associated medical issues, The Commission of the European Community supports health promotion and disease prevention in the workplace. In Germany, the BASF Chemical Company began a health promotion campaign called "Trim Down the Pounds—Losing Weight Without Losing Your Mind." Out of 34,000 employees at the BASF site in Ludwigshafen, 1,313 participants entered this program, agreeing to lose at least 2 body-mass index (BMI) points, or to reduce their weight to a BMI of <25 over the course of 9 months. Physicians who assessed any obesity-related diseases monitored all participants, and normal-weight coworkers acted as weight-loss helpers. At the conclusion of the study, 658 participants had lost weight, 440 of which had lost more than 2 BMI points. Medical benefits were found, including the reduction of obesity-related diseases. The researchers suggest it is possible to prevent overweight and obesity by encouraging healthy eating habits and physical exercise in the workplace. This benefits both the employee in terms of health, and benefits the employer in terms of cost in improved employee productivity.

Jenny Craig has partnered with corporations to promote workplace weight-loss through diet and exercise (Martin, Talamini, Johnson, Hymel, & Khavjou, 2010). They have established a Rewards Program that focuses on personalized treatment, goal setting, motivational interviewing, and providing discounts based on length of participation. Out of 81,505 members of Jenny Craig's Rewards Program who enrolled in 2005, 2,418 enrolled through their employer. Retention was significantly higher in Rewards Corporate members at 25.9 weeks than Rewards Noncorporate members, who averaged 21.9 weeks of participation. Due to longer retention periods, the average percentage of weight loss was also higher among Rewards Corporate members at 7.16 %, while Rewards Noncorporate participants showed a mean of 6.20 % of body weight lost. A major strength of this study is that it illustrates how the findings of clinical trials translate to "real world" experiences.

Occupational Injury Prevention

It is widely accepted that occupational musculoskeletal injuries are caused by a multitude of factors, including physical biomechanics and the stresses placed upon specific body regions, ergonomics and workplace structure, and psychosocial and cognitive components. Numerous interventions have been put into place in occupational settings that are aimed at reducing occupational musculoskeletal injuries and limiting the duration of disability following an injury. The most successful interventions have been tailored to specific occupational settings, rather than "blanketed" to all areas involving a certain type of injury (i.e., low back, upper-extremity, etc.). Interventions geared at reducing occupational musculoskeletal injuries can incorporate a global initiative or many specific components depending on the needs of the individuals within the organization. In a systematic review of interventions designed to prevent upper-extremity and neck injuries in the workplace, some of the workstation interventions that were found to be successful included having appropriate lighting, enhanced keyboards, a specialized computer mouse designed to eliminate neuropathic wrist pain, and workstation adjustment based on the ergonomic needs of the individual, such as adjustable chairs and tools that lessen vibration (Boocock et al., 2007).

Other intervention strategies aimed at preventing neck and upper-extremity injuries include various forms of exercise. For example, Waling, Javholm, and Sundelin (2002) found that administrative workers assigned to one of four training programs (strength training, endurance, coordination, or stress reduction) all reported a significant decrease in the intensity and frequency of upper-extremity pain. Ludewig and Borstad (2003) developed an intervention to reduce shoulder pain in construction workers with shoulder impingement syndrome. Through a stretching and strength training program that participants were asked to complete at home, self-reported reductions in shoulder pain and increased satisfaction in shoulder function were obtained. In a study comparing short and long bouts of exercise within a fibromyalgia population, Schachter, Busch, and Peloso (2003) found positive effects for both duration types for reduction of the severity of the disease and in improved self-efficacy. Furthermore, the group with extended exercise durations also showed improvements in physical function and psychological distress. Several interventions involving exercise for reducing the incidence of occupational musculoskeletal injuries have been evaluated and shown to have positive effects on the reduction of injuries and an increase in function (Boocock et al., 2007). Furthermore, many interventions have been implemented specifically to lessen the risk of low back injury in occupations involving lifting (Hefti et al., 2003; Kim, Hayden, & Mior, 2004; Schenk, Doran, & Stachura, 1996).

Another key factor for prevention and intervention of occupational musculoskeletal injuries is involving the employees in the decision-making processes. Education is an essential component in prevention and intervention programs, such that employees will learn not only how poor ergonomic workplace environments contribute to musculoskeletal distress but also how other factors, such as sedentary work style, repetitive movements, and psychosocial stress play a part in the occurrence of workplace injuries (Carrivick, Lee, & Yau, 2002; Kashima, 2003; Pehkonen et al., 2009; Robertson et al., 2009). Identifying potential risks is also essential in preventing occupational musculoskeletal injuries. However, appropriate steps must be taken in order to reduce such risks. Depending on the demand of the given occupation, appropriate ergonomic principles must be established and followed to ensure employee safety. Many methods of intervention have been identified regarding reduction of injury, but the main concepts that should be considered are the following: identifying areas of risk; educating the employees and supervisors of those risk factors; and creating a work environment that is conducive to eliminating such risks. Encouraging physical activity for sedentary workers and customizing workstations to accommodate the needs of individual employees are proactive measures that contribute to the prevention of injury. Including employees as active members of the intervention team, and allowing their input in decision-making processes aimed at prevention of injuries, has been shown to be directly related to increased safety precautions. Occupational musculoskeletal injury prevention affects both the employee and the employer. By proactively keeping the employees safe, employer costs for medical care, productivity loss, and absenteeism can be substantially reduced (Gatty, Turner, Buitendorp, & Batman, 2003; Martin, Irvine, Fluharty, & Gatty, 2003; Morgan & Chow, 2007; Tompa, Dolinschi, de Oliveira, & Irvin, 2009).

Conclusions

It is general knowledge that costs associated with illnesses, injuries and health behaviors are very high, especially considering the costs of health-care premiums, doctor visits, treatments, and medications. These costs are commonly referred to as direct costs. Moreover, there are hidden, indirect costs that far surpass the direct health-care costs of illnesses and injuries. These indirect costs are tied to lost production due to absenteeism and presenteeism, and have been shown to be a dire economic problem in the workplace. As a result, many researchers and economists have attempted to identify the sources and evaluate the effects of absenteeism and presenteeism in the workplace. As we have reviewed, there are many tools that have been developed to assess the frequency and duration of absenteeism and presenteeism in multiple workplace settings, as related to lost production. Furthermore, several models have been created to quantify the total cost attributed to lost productivity. Yet, to date, there is no direct measure that accurately accounts for all production losses associated with illness and injuries for workers.

Most of the research available on the effects of absenteeism and presenteeism has focused on specific diseases, injuries, and health behaviors. As also reviewed in this chapter, there are considerable data available on the costs and effects of absenteeism and presenteeism specific to each type of illness, injury, or health behavior, in addition to occupational factors. Through this comprehensive review of the effects of absenteeism and presenteeism specific to each illness, injury, and health behavior, we have shown how the indirect costs associated with production losses are significantly greater than direct health-care costs. Understanding how absenteeism and presenteeism affect production loss, many employers have taken proactive approaches to helping their employees stay healthy. We have outlined several precautionary measures that employers have utilized to reduce the incidence of illness, injury, and poor health behaviors by offering a venue of interventional regimes to their employees. By adopting this model of prevention, employers will find that rates of absenteeism and presenteeism related to illness, injury and health behaviors can decrease dramatically, thereby reducing the degree of indirect costs associated with production losses.

References

American Lung Association, Epidemiology and Statistics Unit. (ALA, 2009). Trends in asthma morbidity and mortality. Chapel Hill, NC: http://www.lung.org/finding-cures/our-research/epidemiology-and-statistics-rpts.html

CDC (2008). *Key facts about influenza and the influenza vaccine*. Centers for Disease Control and Prvention. National Center for Health Statistics. Atlanta, GA: http://www.cdc.gov/flu/protect/keyfacts.htm

Hoppin, P., Stillman, L., & Jacobs, M. (2010). Asthma: A business case for employers and health care purchasers. Lowell Center for Sustainable Production, Asthma Regional Council. Lowell, MA: www.asthmaregionalcouncil.org/uploads/.../hria_asthma_report.pdf

Lozada, C.J., Diamond, H.S., Agnew, S., Bal, B.S., Basu, P.A., Chansky, H.A., et al. (2011). Osteoarthritis. Medscape Reference: Drugs, Diseases & Procedures. http://emedicine.medscape.com/article/330487-overview.

Mercer, & AfWHP. (1999). *National Worksite Health Promotion Survey.* Northbrook, IL: Mercer/AfWHP.

NIH, N. O. E. I. (1998). *Clinical guidelines on the identification, evaluation and treatment of overweight and obesity in adults.* NIH Publication, 98-4083.

Ablah, E., Konda, K., Tinius, A., Long, A., Vermie, G., & Burbach, C. (2008). Influenza vaccine coverage and presenteeism in Sedgwick County, Kansas. *American Journal of Infect Control, 36,* 588–591.

Berry, P. A. (2007). Migraine disorder. *American Association of Occupational Health Nurses Journal, 55*(2), 51–56.

Birnbaum, H. G., Ben-Hamadi, R., Kelley, D., Hsieh, M., Seal, B., Kantor, E., et al. (2010). Assessing the relationship between compliance with antidepressant therapy and employer costs among employees in the United States. *Journal of Occupational and Environmental Medicine, 52*(2), 115–124.

Block, G., Sternfeld, B., Block, C. H., Block, T. J., Norris, J., Hopkins, D., et al. (2008). Development of Alive! (A Lifestyle Intervention Via Email), and its effect on health-related quality of life, presenteeism, and other behavioral outcomes: Randomized controlled trial. *Journal of Medical Internet Research, 10,* e43.

Bonauto, D., Silverstein, B., Adams, D., & Foley, M. (2006). Prioritizing industries for occupational injury and illness prevention and research, Washington State workers' compensation claims, 1999–2003. *Journal of Occupational and Environmental Medicine, 48,* 840–851.

Boocock, M. G., McNair, P. J., Larmer, P. J., Armstrong, B., Collier, J., Simmonds, M., et al. (2007). Interventions for the prevention and management of neck/upper extremity musculoskeletal conditions: A systematic review. *Occupational Environmental Medicine, 64,* 291–303.

Brook, R. A., Kleinman, N. L., Choung, R. S., Melkonian, A., Smeeding, J. E., & Talley, N. J. (2010). Functional dyspepsia impacts absenteeism and direct and indirect costs. *Clinical Gastroenterology and Hepatology, 8,* 498–503.

Brook, R. A., Wahlquist, P., Kleinman, N. L., Wallanders, M. A., Campbell, S. M., & Smeeding, J. E. (2007). Cost of gastro-oesophageal reflux disease to the employer: A perspective from the United States. *Alimentary Pharmacology and Therapeutics, 26,* 889–898.

Brouwer, W. B. F., van Exel, N. J. A., Koopmanschap, M. A., & Rutten, F. F. H. (2002). Productivity costs before and after absence from work: As important as common? *Health Policy, 61,* 173–187.

Bunn, W. B., Pikelny, D. B., Paralkar, S., Slavin, T., Borden, S., & Allen, H. M. (2003). The burden of allergies—And the capacity of medications to reduce this burden—In a heavy manufacturing environment. *Journal of Occupational and Environmental Medicine, 45,* 941–955.

Bureau of Labor Statistics. (2007). *Occupational injury and illness report.* http://www.bls.gov/IIF

Burton, W. N., Chen, C. Y., Conti, D. J., Schultz, A. B., Pransky, G. S., & Edington, D. W. (2005). The association of health risks with on-the-job productivity. *Journal of Occupational and Environmental Medicine, 47*(8), 769–777.

Burton, W., Conti, D. J., Chen, C., Schultz, A. B., & Edington, D. W. (2001). The impact of allergies and allergy treatment on worker productivity. *Journal of Occupational and Environmental Medicine, 43,* 64–71.

Burton, W., Morrison, A., Yuan, Y., Li, T., Marioni, R. E., & Maclean, R. (2008). Productivity cost model of the treatment of rheumatoid arthritis with abatacept. *Journal of Medical Economics, 11,* 3–21.

Carrivick, P. J. W., Lee, A. H., & Yau, K. K. W. (2002). Effectiveness of a participatory workplace risk assessment team in reducing the risk and severity of musculoskeletal injury. *Journal of Occupational Health, 44,* 221–225.

Carson, R. L., Baumgartner, J. J., Matthews, R. A., & Tsouloupas, C. N. (2010). Emotional exhaustion, absenteeism, and turnover intentions in childcare teachers: Examining the impact of physical activity behaviors. *Journal of Health Psychology, 15*(6), 905–914.

Caverly, N., Cunningham, J. B., & MacGregor, J. N. (2007). Sickness presenteeism, sickness absenteeism, and health following restructuring in a public service organization. *Journal of Management Studies, 44*(2), 304–319.

CDC. (2010). *National Health Interview Survey.* Publication no. from http://www.cdc.gov/nchs/nhis.htm

Courtney, T. K., & Webster, B. S. (2001). Antecedent factors and disabling occupational morbidity—Insights from the new BLS data. *American Industrial Hygiene Association Journal, 62,* 622–632.

Davies, G., Santanello, N., Gerth, W., Lerner, D., & Block, G. (1999). Validation of a migraine work and productivity loss questionnaire for use in migraine studies. *Cephalagia, 19*(5), 497–502.

de Vroege, L., Hoedeman, R., Nuyen, J., Sijtsma, K., & van der Felz-Cornelis, C. (2012). Validation of the PHQ-15 for somatoform disorder in the occupational health care setting. *Journal of Occupational Rehabilitation, 22*(1), 51–58.

Dean, B. B., Calimim, B. M., Kindermann, S. L., Khandker, R. K., & Tinkelman, D. (2009). The impact of uncontrolled asthma on absenteeism and health-related quality of life. *Journal of Asthma, 16,* 861–866.

Dewa, C. S., Hoch, J. S., Lin, E., Paterson, M., & Goering, P. (2003). Pattern of antidepressant use and duration of depression-related absence from work. *The British Journal of Psychiatry, 183,* 507–513.

Dunlop, D. D., Manheim, L. M., Yelin, E. H., Song, J., & Chang, R. W. (2003). The costs of arthritis. *Arthritis and Rheumatism, 49,* 101–113.

Endicott, J., & Nee, J. (1997). Endicott Work Productivity Scale (EWPS): A new measure to assess treatment effects. *Psychopharmacological Bulletin, 33*(1), 6–13.

Escorpizo, R., Bombardier, C., Boonen, A., Hazes, J. M. W., Lacaille, D., Strand, V., et al. (2007). Worker productivity outcome measures in arthritis. *The Journal of Rheumatology, 34*(6), 1372–1380.

Flegal, K. M., Carroll, M. D., Ogden, C. L., & Curtin, L. R. (2010). Prevalence and trends in obesity among US adults, 1999–2008. *JAMA, 303*(3), 235–241.

Gatchel, R. J. (2004). Comorbidity of chronic mental and physical health disorders: The biopsychosocial perspective. *American Psychologist, 59*, 792–805.

Gates, D. M., Succop, P., Brehm, B. J., Gillespie, G. L., & Sommers, B. D. (2008). Obesity and presenteeism: The impact of body mass index on workplace productivity. *Journal of Occupational and Environmental Medicine, 50*(1), 39–45.

Gatty, C. M., Turner, M., Buitendorp, D. J., & Batman, H. (2003). The effectiveness of back pain and injury prevention programs in the workplace. *Work, 20*, 257–266.

Gilmour, H., & Patten, S. B. (2007). Depression and work impairment. *Health Reports, 18*(1), 9–22.

Gisbert, J. P., Cooper, A., Karagiannis, D., Hatlebakk, J., Agreus, L., Jablonowski, H., et al. (2009). Impact of gastroesophageal reflux disease on work absenteeism, presenteeism and productivity in daily life: A European observational study. *Health and Quality of Life Outcomes, 7*(90).

Goetzel, R. Z., Gibson, T. B., Short, M. E., Chu, B., Waddell, J., Bowen, J., et al. (2010). A multi-worksite analysis of the relationships among body mass index, medical utilization, and worker productivity. *Journal of Occupational and Environmental Medicine, 52*(1), S52–S58.

Goetzel, R. Z., Smith Carls, G., Wang, S., Kelly, E., Mauceri, E., Columbus, D., et al. (2009). The relationship between modifiable health risk factors and medical expenditures, absenteeism, short-term disability, and presenteeism among employees at Novartis. *Journal of Occupational and Environmental Medicine, 51*(4), 487–499.

Gold, M. R., Siegel, J. E., Russell, L. B., & Weinstein, M. C. (1996). *Cost-effectiveness in health and medicine.* New York, NY: Oxford University Press.

Greenberg, P.E., Kessler, R.C., Birnbaum, H.G., Leong, S.A., Lowe, S.W., Berglund, P.A., et al. (2003). The economic burden of depression in the United States: How did it change between 1990 and 2000? *Journal of Clinical Psychiatry*, 64(12), 1465–1475.

Hazard, E., Munakata, J., Bigal, M. E., Rupnow, M. F. T., & Lipton, R. B. (2009). The burden of migraine in the United States: Current and emerging perspectives on disease management and economic analysis. *International Society for Pharmacoeconomics and Outcomes Research, 12*(1), 55–64.

Hefti, K. S., Farnham, R. J., Docken, L., Bentaas, R., Bossman, S., & Schaefer, J. (2003). Back injury prevention. *American Association of Occupational Health Nurses Journal, 51*(6), 246–251.

Heinemann, L. A., Minh, T. D., Filonenko, A., & Uhl-Hochgraber, K. (2010). Exploration evaluation of the impact of severe premenstrual disorders on work absenteeism and productivity. *Women's Health, 20*, 58–65.

Hemp, P. (2004). Presenteeism: At work—But out of it. *Harvard Business Review, 82*, 49–58.

Hilton, M. F., Sheridan, J., Cleary, C. M., & Whiteford, H. A. (2009). Employee absenteeism measures reflecting current work practices may be instrumental in a re-evaluation of the relationship between psychological distress/mental health and absenteeism. *International Journal of Methods in Psychiatric Research, 18*(1), 37–47.

Hu, X. H., Markson, L. E., & Lipton, R. B. (1999). Burden of migraine in the United States: Disability and economic costs. *Archives of Internal Medicine, 159*, 813–818.

Hyman, S. E., & Rudorfer, M. V. (2000). Anxiety disorders. In D. C. Dale & D. D. Federman (Eds.), *Scientific America medicine* (Vol. 3). New York, NY: Healtheon/WebMD Corp.

Inrig, T., Amey, B., Borthwick, C., & Beaton, D. (2012). Validity and reliability of the Fear-Avoidance Beliefs Questionnaire (FABQ) in workers with upper extremity injuries. *Journal of Occupational Rehabilitation, 22*, 59–70.

Ivanova, J. I., Birnbaum, H. G., Samuels, S., Davis, M., Phillips, A. L., & Meletiche, D. (2009). The cost of disability and medically related absenteeism among employees with multiple sclerosis in the US. *Pharmacoeconomics, 27*(8), 681–691.

Jantti, J., Aho, K., Kaarela, K., & Kautiainen, H. (1999). Work disability in an inception cohort of patients with seropositive rheumatoid arthritis: A 20-year study. *Rheumatology, 38*, 1138–1141.

Johannesson, M. (1996). The willingness to pay for health changes, the human-capital approach and the external costs. *Health Policy, 36*, 231–244.

Johannesson, M., & Karlsson, G. (1997). The friction cost method: A comment. *Journal of Health Economics, 16*, 249–255.

Kashima, S. R. (2003). A petroleum company's experience in implementing a comprehensive medical fitness for duty program for professional truck drivers. *Journal of Occupational and Environmental Medicine, 45*(2), 185–196.

Keech, M., & Beardsworth, P. (2008). The impact of influenza on working days lost. A review of the literature. *Pharmacoeconomics, 26*(11), 911–924.

Kessler, R. C., Ames, M., Hymel, P., Loeppke, R., McKenas, D. K., Richling, D. E., et al. (2004). Using the World Health Organization Health and Work Performance Questionnaire (HPQ) to evaluate the indirect workplace costs of illness. *Journal of Occupational and Environmental Medicine, 46*(6), S23–S37.

Kessler, R. C., Chiu, W. T., Demler, O., & Walters, E. E. (2005). Prevalence, severity, and comorbidity of twelve-month DSM-IV disorders in the National Comorbidity Survey Replication (NCS-R). *Archives of General Psychiatry, 62*(6), 617–627.

Kessler, R. C., Chiu, W. T., Demler, O., & Walters, E. E. (2009). Prevalence, severity and comorbidity of 12-month DSM-IV disorders in the national comorbidity survey replication. *Archives of General Psychiatry, 62*, 617–627.

Kim, P., Hayden, J. A., & Mior, S. A. (2004). The cost-effectiveness of a back education program for firefighters: A case study. *Journal of Canadian Chiropractic Association, 48*(1), 13–19.

Kleinman, N., Harnett, J., Melkonian, A., Lynch, W., Kaplan-Machlis, B., & Silverman, S. (2009). Burden of fibromyalgia and comparisons with osteoarthritis in the workforce. *Journal of Occupational and Environmental Medicine, 51*(12), 1384–1393.

Koopmanschap, M. A., Burdorf, A., Jacob, K., Meerding, W. J., Brouwer, W. B. F., & Severens, H. (2005). Measuring productivity changes in economic evaluation. *Pharmacoeconomics, 23*(1), 47–54.

Koopmanschap, M. A., Rutten, F. F. H., van Ineveld, B. M., & van Roijen, L. (1995). The friction cost method for measuring indirect costs of disease. *Journal of Health Economics, 14*, 171–189.

Kotlarz, H., Gunnarsson, C. L., Fang, H., & Rizzo, J. A. (2010). Osteoarthritis and absenteeism costs: Evidence from US national survey data. *Journal of Occupational and Environmental Medicine, 52*(3), 263–268.

Lamb, C. E., Ratner, P. H., Johnson, C. E., Ambegaonkar, A., Joshi, A. V., Day, D., et al. (2006). Economic impact of workplace productivity losses due to allergic rhinitis compared with select medical conditions in the United States from an employer perspective. *Current Medical Research and Opinion, 22*, 1203–1210.

Laxman, K. E., Lovibond, K. S., & Hassan, M. K. (2008). Impact of bipolar disorder in employed populations. *American Journal of Managed Care, 14*, 757–764.

Lerner, D., Amick, B., Malspeis, S., Rogers, W., Santanello, N., Gerth, W., et al. (1999). The migraine work and productivity loss questionnaire: Concepts and design. *Quality of Life Research, 8*(8), 699–710.

Lerner, D., Amick, B., III, Rogers, W., Malspeis, S., Bungay, K., & Cynn, D. (2001). The work limitations questionnaire. *Medical Care, 39*(1), 72–85.

Levin-Epstein (2005). *Presenteeism and paid sick days*. Center for Law and Social Policy. Washington, DC: www.clasp.org/publications/presenteeism.pdf

Linde, M., & Dahlof, C. (2004). Attitudes and burden of disease among self-considered migraineurs: A nation-wide population-based survey in Sweden. *Cephalalgia, 24*(6), 455–465.

Lipton, R. B., Bigal, M. E., & Diamond, M. (2007). Migraine prevalence disease burden, and the need for preventative therapy. *Neurology, 68*, 343–349.

Lipton, R. B., & Stewart, W. F. (1998). Medical consultation for migraine: Results from the American Migraine Study. *Headache, 38*, 87–96.

Loeppke, R., Taitel, M., Richling, D., Parry, T., Kessler, R. C., Hymel, P., et al. (2007). Health and productivity as a business strategy. *Journal of Occupational and Environmental Medicine, 49*(7), 712–721.

Lofland, J. H., Pizzi, L., & Frick, K. D. (2004). A review of health-related workplace productivity loss instruments. *Pharmacoeconomics, 22*(3), 165–184.

Ludewig, P. M., & Borstad, J. D. (2003). Effects of a home exercise programme on shoulder pain and functional status in construction workers. *Occupational Environmental Medicine, 60*, 841–849.

Marcotte, D. E., Wilcox-Gok, V., & Redmon, P. D. (1999). Prevalence and patterns of major depressive disorder in the United States labor force. *The Journal of Mental Health Policy and Economics, 2*, 123–131.

Mark, T., Coffey, R. M., McKusick, D., Harwood, H., King, E., Bouchery, E., et al. (2005). *National expenditures for mental health services and substance abuse treatment 1991–2001*. DHHS Publication US Department of Health and Human Services, No. SMA 05-3999.

Martin, S. A., Irvine, J. L., Fluharty, K., & Gatty, C. M. (2003). A comprehensive work injury prevention program with clerical and office workers: Phase I. *Work, 21*, 185–196.

Martin, C. K., Talamini, L., Johnson, A., Hymel, A. M., & Khavjou, O. (2010). Weight loss and retention in a commercial weight-loss programs and the effect of corporate partnership. *International Journal of Obesity, 34*, 742–750.

McIntyre, R. S., Liauw, S., & Taylor, V. H. (2011). Depression in the workforce: The intermediary effect of medical comorbidity. *Journal of Affective Disorders, 128*(Suppl. 1), S29–S36.

Mino, Y., Babzono, A., Tsuda, T., & Yasuda, N. (2006). Can stress management at the workplace prevent depression? A randomized controlled trial. *Psychotherapy and Psychosomatics, 75*, 177–182.

Molinari, N. A. M., Ortega-Sanchez, I. R., & Messonnier, M. L. (2007). The annual impact of seasonal influenza in the US: Measuring disease burden and costs. *Vaccine, 25*(27), 5086–5096.

Morgan, A., & Chow, S. (2007). The economic impact of implementing an ergonomic plan. *Nursing Economics, 25*(3), 150–156.

Mulligan, P. (2010). Corporate smoking cessation on long island. *Health Promotion Practice, 11*(2), 182–187.

Mulligan, P., & Rosenberg, S. (2004). *The impact of corporate wellness programs on Long Island*. Philadelphia, PA: Northeast Decision Sciences Institute.

Murray, C. J., & Lopez, A. D. (1997). Global mortality, disability, and the contribution of risk factors: Global burden of disease study. *Lancet, 349*(7), 1436–1442.

Naci, H., Fleurence, R., Birt, J., & Duhig, A. (2010). Economic burden of multiple sclerosis. *Pharmacoeconomics, 28*(5), 363–379.

Nathan, R. A., Meltzer, E. O., Derebery, J., Campbell, U. B., Stang, P. E., Corrao, M. A., et al. (2008). The prevalence of nasal symptoms attributed to allergies in the United States: Findings from the burden of rhinitis in an America survey. *Allergy Asthma Proceedings, 29*, 600–608.

Nowalk, M. P., Lin, C. J., Toback, S. L., Rousculp, M. D., Eby, C., Raymund, M., et al. (2010). Improving influenza vaccination rates in the workplace: A randomized trial. *American Journal of Preventive Medicine, 38*, 237–246.

Nyman, J. A., Barleen, N. A., & Abraham, J. M. (2010). The effectiveness of health promotion at the University of Minnesota: Expenditures, absenteeism, and participation in specific programs. *Journal of Occupational and Environmental Medicine, 52*(3), 269–280.

O'Donnell, M. P. (2000). Health and productivity management: The concept, impact, and opportunity. Commentary to Goetzel and Ozmindowski. *American Journal of Health Promotion, 14*, 215–217.

Oberlinner, C., Lang, S., Germann, C., Traugh, B., Eberle, F., Pluto, R., et al. (2007). Prevention of overweight and obesity in the workplace BASF-health promotion campaign "trim down the pounds–losing weight without losing your mind". *Gesundheitswesen (Bundesverband Der Ärzte Des Öffentlichen Gesundheitsdienstes (Germany)), 69*(7), 385–392.

Palmer, L. A., Rousculp, M. D., Johnston, S. S., Mahadevia, P. J., & Nichol, K. L. (2009). Effect of influenza-like illness and other wintertime respiratory illnesses on worker productivity: The child and household influenza-illness and employee function (CHIEF) study. *Vaccine, 28*, 5049–5056.

Pehkonen, I., Takala, E., Ketola, R., Viikari-Juntura, E. R. A., Leino-Arjas, P., Hopsu, L., et al. (2009). Evaluation of a participatory ergonomic intervention process in kitchen work. *Applied Ergonomics, 40*, 115–123.

Pelletier, B., Boles, M., & Lynch, W. (2004). Change in health risks and work productivity over time. *Journal of Occupational and Environmental Medicine, 46*, 746–754.

Prasad, M., Wahlquist, P., Shikiar, R., & Shih, Y. T. (2004). A review of self-report instruments measuring health-related work productivity. *Pharmacoeconomics, 22*(4), 226–243.

Quanbeck, A., Lang, K., Enami, K., & Brown, R. L. (2010). A cost-benefit analysis of Wisconsin's Screening, Brief Intervention and Referral to Treatment Program: Adding the employer's perspective. *Wisconsin Medical Journal, 109*, 9–14.

Rajbhandary, S., & Basu, K. (2010). Working conditions of nurses and absenteeism: Is there a relationship? An empirical analysis using National Survey of the Work and Health of Nurses. *Health Policy, 97*, 152–159.

Rantanen, I., & Tuominen, R. (2011). Relative magnitude of presenteeism and absenteeism and work-related factors affecting them among health care professionals. *International Archives of Occupational Environmental Health, 84*, 225–230.

Reilly, M., Lavin, P., Kahler, K., & Pariser, D. (2003). Validation of the dermatology life quality index and the work productivity and activity impairment-chronic hand dermatitis questionnaire in chronic hand dermatitis. *Journal of the American Academy of Dermatology, 48*(1), 128–130.

Reilly, M., Tanner, A., & Meltzer, E. (1996). Work, classroom, and activity impairment instruments: Validation studies in allergic rhinitis. *Clinical Drug Investigation, 11*(5), 278–288.

Reilly, M., Zbrozek, A., & Dukes, E. (1993). The validity and reproducibility of a work productivity and activity impairment instrument. *Pharmacoeconomics, 4*(5), 353–365.

Ricci, J. A., Stewart, W. F., Chee, E., Leotta, C., Foley, K., & Hochberg, M. C. (2006). Back pain exacerbations and lost productive time costs in United States workers. *Spine, 31*(26), 3052–3060.

Robertson, M., Amick, B. C., DeRango, K., Rooney, T., Bazzani, L., Harrist, R., et al. (2009). The effects of an office ergonomics training and chair intervention on worker knowledge, behavior and musculoskeletal risk. *Applied Ergonomics, 40*, 124–135.

Roche, A. M., Pidd, K., Berry, J. G., & Harrison, J. E. (2008). Workers' drinking patterns: The impact on absenteeism in the Australian work-place. *Addiction, 103*, 738–748.

Roessler, R., & Rumrill, P. (2003). Multiple sclerosis and employment barriers: A systematic perspective on diagnosis and intervention. *Work, 21*, 71–23.

Sadosky, A. B., Bushmakin, A. G., Cappelleri, J. C., & Lionberger, D. R. (2010). Relationship between patient-reported disease severity in osteoarthritis and self-reported pain, function and work productivity. *Arthritis Research and Therapy, 12*, R162.

Samuel, R. J., & Wilson, L. M. (2007). Is presenteeism hurting your workforce? *Employee Benefit Plan Review, 61*, 5–7.

Sanderson, K., & Andrews, G. (2006). Common mental disorders in the workplace: Recent findings from descriptive and social epidemiology. *The Canadian Journal of Psychiatry, 51*(2), 63–74.

Sanderson, K., Tilse, E., Nicholson, J., Oldenburg, B., & Graves, N. (2007). Which presenteeism measures are more sensitive to depression and anxiety? *Journal of Affective Disorders, 101*, 65–74.

Schachter, C. L., Busch, A. J., & Peloso, P. M. (2003). Effects of short versus long bouts of aerobic exercise in sedentary women with fibromyalgia: A randomized controlled trial. *Physical Therapy, 83*, 340–358.

Schenk, R. J., Doran, R. L., & Stachura, J. J. (1996). Learning effects of a back education program. *Spine, 21*(19), 2183–2188.

Schultz, A. B., & Edington, D. W. (2007). Employee health and presenteeism: A systematic review. *Journal of Occupational Rehabilitation, 17*, 547–579.

Shikiar, R., Halpern, M., Rentz, A., & Khan, Z. (2004). Development of the Health and Work Questionnaire (HWQ): An instrument for assessing productivity in relation to worker health. *Work, 22*, 219–229.

Spitzer, R.L., Kroenke, K., & Williams, J.B., (1999). Validation and utility of a self-report version of PRIME-MD: The PHQ Primary Care Study. *JAMA, 282*(18), 1737–1744

Stewart, W., Lipton, R., Kolodner, K., Liberman, J., & Sawyer, J. (1999). Reliability of the migraine disability assessment score in a population-based sample of headache sufferers. *Cephalagia, 19*(2), 107–114.

Stewart, W., Lipton, R., Kolodner, K., Sawyer, J., Lee, C., & Liberman, J. (2000). Validity of the Migraine Disability Assessment (MIDAS) score in comparison to a diary-based measure in a population sample of migraine sufferers. *Pain, 88*(1), 41–52.

Stewart, W. F., Ricci, J. A., Chee, E., Morganstein, D., & Lipton, R. B. (2003). Lost productive time and cost due to common pain conditions in the US workforce. *JAMA, 290*(18), 2443–2454.

Sullivan, P. W., Navaratnam, P., Lorber, R., & Shekar, T. (2010). The cost-effectiveness of treatment with desloratadine in patients with persistent allergic rhinitis. *Current Medical Research and Opinion, 26*(6), 1389–1397.

Szucs, T. (1999). The socio-economic burden of influenza. *Journal of Antimicrob Chemother, 44*, 11–15.

Tompa, E., Dolinschi, R., de Oliveira, C., & Irvin, E. (2009). A systematic review of occupational health and safety interventions with economic analyses. *Journal of Occupational and Environmental Medicine, 51*, 1004–1023.

Truchon, M., Schmouth, M. E., Cote, D., Fillion, L., Rossignol, M., & Durand, M. (2012). Absenteeism Screening Questionnaire (ASQ): A new tool for predicting long-term absenteeism among workers with low back pain. *Journal of Occupational Rehabilitation, 22*(1), 27–50.

van Roijen, L., Essink-Bot, M., Koopmanschap, M., Bonsel, G., & Rutten, F. F. H. (1996). Labor and health status in economic evaluation of health care: The health and labor questionnaire. *International Journal of Technology Assessment in Health Care, 12*(3), 405–415.

van Strien, T., & Koenders, P. (2010). How do physical activity, sports and dietary restraint related to overweight-associated absenteeism? *Journal of Occupational and Environmental Medicine, 52*(9), 858–864.

Vogenberg, F. R. (2009). The economic burden of COPD in the workplace; Interview with William B. Bunn, III, MD, JD, MPH. *American Health and Drug Benefits, 2*(4), 198–199.

Voss, M., Floderus, B., & Diderichsen, F. (2004). How do job characteristics, family situation, domestic work, and lifestyle factors relate to sickness absence? A study based on Sweden Post. *Journal of Occupational and Environmental Medicine, 46*(11), 1134–1143.

Waddell, G., Newton, M., Henderson, I., Somerville, D., & Main, C. J. (2007). Fear-Avoidance Beliefs Questionnaire. *Clinical Journal of Pain, 23*(8), 720–725.

Wahlquist, P., Carlsson, J., Stalhammar, N., & Wiklund, I. (2002). Validity of a work productivity and activity impairment questionnaire for patients with symptoms of gastro-esophageal reflux disease (WPAI-GERD): Results from a cross-sectional study. *Value Health, 5*(2), 106–113.

Waling, K., Javholm, B., & Sundelin, G. (2002). Effects of training on female trapezius myalgia: An intervention study with a 3-year follow-up period. *Spine, 27*, 789–796.

Wang, P. S., Simon, G. E., Avorn, J., Azocar, F., Ludman, E. J., McCulloch, J., et al. (2007). Telephone screening, outreach, and care management for depressed workers and impact on clinical and work productivity outcomes: A randomized controlled trial. *The Journal of the American Medical Association, 298*, 1401–1411.

Wells, K. B., Stewart, A., Hays, R. D., Burnam, M. A., Rogers, W., Daniels, M., et al. (1989). The functioning and well-being of depressed patients: Results from the Medical Outcomes Study *The Journal of the American Medical Association, 262*, 914–919.

Wendt, J. K., Tsai, S. P., Bhojani, F. A., & Cameron, D. L. (2010). The Shell Disability Management Program: A five-year evaluation of the impact on absenteeism and return-on-investment. *Journal of Occupational and Environmental Medicine, 52*(5), 544–550.

White, L. A., Birnbaum, H. G., Kaltenboeck, A., Tang, J., Mallett, D., & Robinson, R. L. (2008). Employees with fibromyalgia: Medical comorbidity, healthcare costs and work loss. *Journal of Occupational and Environmental Medicine, 50*(1), 13–24.

Wolfe, F., Ross, K., Anderson, J., Russell, I. J., & Hebert, L. (1995). The prevalence and characteristics of fibromyalgia in the general population. *Arthritis and Rheumatism, 38*(1), 19–28.

Occupational Burnout

Cindy A. McGeary and Donald D. McGeary

Introduction

Burnout is a relatively new concept (coined with its contemporary intent in 1975), although interest in this topic has significantly increased over the last 40 years. Most who have studied burnout agree that it is a multifaceted construct, including (but not limited to) domains like work-supportive energy (i.e., exhaustion and fatigue), perception of work meaningfulness, work-directed concentration and focus, and extent of work engagement. Although definitions vary, the most widely accepted model of burnout has been developed by Dr. Christina Maslach, Professor of Psychology at the University of California at Berkley, who conceptualized it as a tripartite construct comprised of emotional exhaustion, depersonalization, and personal accomplishment. Although many agree with the validity of the Maslach model, there has been some debate on the relative value of its components. Exhaustion has received the greatest attention throughout the burnout research literature, with some suggesting that it is a primary or singularly necessary criterion for burnout (Maslach, Schaufeli, & Leiter, 2001; Shirom, 1989; cf. Pines & Aronson, 1988). Maslach and colleagues argue that one factor is not enough to fully define the complex process of occupational burnout. They note, "…the fact that exhaustion is a necessary criterion for burnout does not mean it is sufficient. If one were to look at burnout out of context, and simply focus on the individual exhaustion component, one would lose sight of the phenomenon entirely" (p. 403).

Occupational burnout can be a significant concern for workers and employers alike. There are reasonable data to suggest that employees experiencing burnout exhibit significant decrements in the

C.A. McGeary, Ph.D.
Department of Psychology, The University of Texas at Arlington,
501 S. Nedderman Dr., Box 19528, Arlington, TX 76019, USA
e-mail: doncindymcgeary@yahoo.com

D.D. McGeary, Ph.D., A.B.P.P. (✉)
Department of Psychiatry, The University of Texas Health Science Center San Antonio,
7703 Floyd Curl Drive, San Antonio, TX 78229, USA
e-mail: McGeary@uthscsa.edu

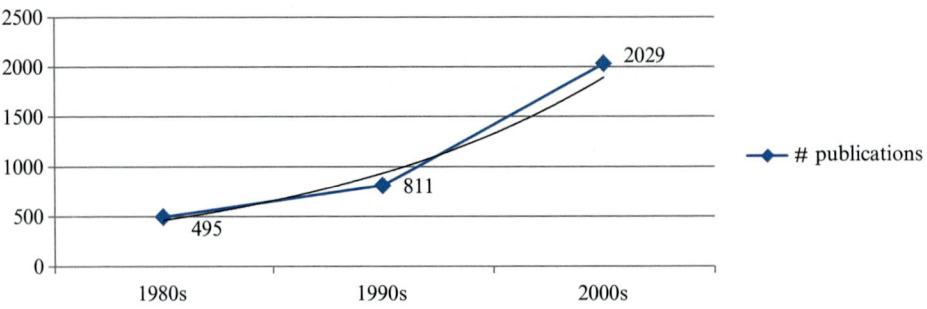

Fig. 9.1 Number of burnout PSYCHINFO publications

quality and quantity of their work output (Firth & Britton, 1989), increased rates of absenteeism and thoughts of leaving their jobs (Chambers, 1993), degraded indices of physical health and immune functioning (Armon, Melamed, Shirom, & Shapira, 2010; Mommersteeg, Heijnen, Kavelaars, & van Doornen, 2006; Shirom et al., 2006), decreased career satisfaction and quality of life (Demerouti, Bakker, Nachreiner, & Schaufeli, 2000; Evans et al., 2006; Sprang, Clark, & Whitt-Woosley, 2007), and even changes in risk for suicidal ideation (Dyrbye et al., 2008). The purpose of this chapter is to provide the reader with an historical context for the evolution of burnout research, to examine what is currently known about models of burnout, to review mediating and moderating variables linked to burnout development and maintenance, to introduce various assessment options for burnout treatment and research, and to direct the reader to resources for burnout interventions. Finally, although our understanding of the burnout concept has grown tremendously since the term was coined in the mid-1970s, there are still numerous gaps in the research that should be addressed. We hope to orient the reader to these gaps and provide directions for future research.

The History of Burnout

Burnout has been a subject of speculation, consternation, and concern since the formal development of work concepts thousands of years ago (cf. Donkin, 2010). Scientific investigation of the occupational burnout construct, however, likely started in the latter part of the twentieth century as greater attention was paid to the personal toll of work on workers. Subsequent research has firmly established a scientific basis for burnout, and burnout research has significantly grown in the extant research literature as a result. A rudimentary OvidSP search of PSYCHINFO for burnout (termed as "(burnout.ti OR burnout.ab) limit to peer reviewed journal") reveals over 3,800 published studies dating back to 1975. The number of burnout papers recorded in each decade since the 1980s reveals an exponentially increasing trend providing clear evidence of the growth in burnout research interest. As work on burnout continues, it is clear that studies of burnout will proliferate well into the near future. For example, the first three decades of burnout research revealed publication increases of 64% from the 1980s to the 1990s and 150% from the 1990s to the 2000s. Over 500 burnout papers were published over the first 2 years of the 2010s decade which, when prorated over the rest of the decade, would result in over 2,500 publications between 2010 and 2020 representing an increase of 23% (Fig. 9.1).

Maslach et al. (2001) offer one of the best overviews of how burnout research has developed since its formal inception in the 1970s. They note that the concept of burnout, although initially well-intended as a way of helping others understand the relationship between workers and their work, was poorly received by the scientific community as a representation of "pop psychology." As a result, few academic researchers were willing to critically examine the topic, and scientific submissions covering burnout research had a poor chance at publication. Maslach et al. (2001) posit, however, that research on burnout began to grow beginning with a "Pioneering Phase," during which the concept was originally introduced and defined by pioneers like Herbert Freudenberger (1975) and Christina Maslach (1976). It is clear from their accounts that these early concepts were based not only on their research at the time but also on personal experience with loss of energy and motivation in their own work environments. Unfortunately, burnout was originally considered a social rather than research concern, and was not treated with significant scientific rigor until the 1980s, when changes in the organization of social services and the individualization of modern work resulted in increased burnout among American workers (Cherniss, 1980; Maslach & Schaufeli, 1993). As burnout proliferated, social scientists and behavioral health researchers began to recognize the importance of addressing this concern.

The "Empirical Phase" of burnout research, during which the concept has been scientifically examined through empirical research and more substantively defined, began in the 1980s and has extended to the present. Maslach and Schaufeli (1993) note that early burnout research seemed to be relegated to clinical rather than academic investigation. Only 10% of studies reviewed by Perlman and Hartman in 1982 presented empirical data on burnout, and the majority of "scientific" submissions in the early 1980s provided anecdotal or clinical accounts of burnout symptoms in patients. Maslach and Jackson (1984), based upon their attempt to publish the initial psychometric details about the Maslach Burnout Inventory, expressed their concern that some academics may not embrace the empirical study of burnout. They suggested that the scientific community had (erroneously) deemed burnout a "pseudoscientific" or "fad" concept, thereby attributing a low priority to burnout research. However, research rapidly grew with the dissemination of the first theories and self-report measures of burnout, suggesting that the scientific community may have been waiting for a clear operational definition of the construct before testing it.

Examining burnout research proliferation year-by-year shows a clear jump in burnout research from 1981 to 1982, coinciding with the first publication of Maslach's influential burnout inventory. It must also be noted, however, that this "jump" also coincides with the re-categorization of burnout in the NCBI Medical Subject Headings (MeSH) from "Stress, Psychological" (introduced in 1973) to "Burnout, Professional" (subsumed as a separate category under "Stress, Psychological" in 1982). Although likely not a cause for the increased prevalence of burnout research, this change in MeSH structure may make "burnout" research artificially easier to find after 1982 and, therefore, more scientifically obvious or prominent. Regardless, the scientific importance of burnout is growing and there is much work to be done in order to expand on the existing theories. The new millennium brought about significant growth in burnout research, though factors attributable to this rise are unclear. Although the ongoing conflicts in Iraq and Afghanistan may play a role in the growth of burnout research (occupational burnout among military personnel and their health-care providers is a concern during wartime), a PSYCINFO search combining burnout (burnout.ti or burnout.ab) and military (military.mp or combat.mp or war.mp) terms limited to publication between 2002 and 2011 returns only 40 publications. Obviously, the rapid increase in burnout research over the last decade is motivated by more than the ongoing war effort (Fig. 9.2).

Models of Burnout

Maslach Burnout Model

The most commonly referenced definition of burnout was initially reported by Maslach in 1982. At first, Maslach's model of burnout characterized burnout as a syndrome that mainly affected people

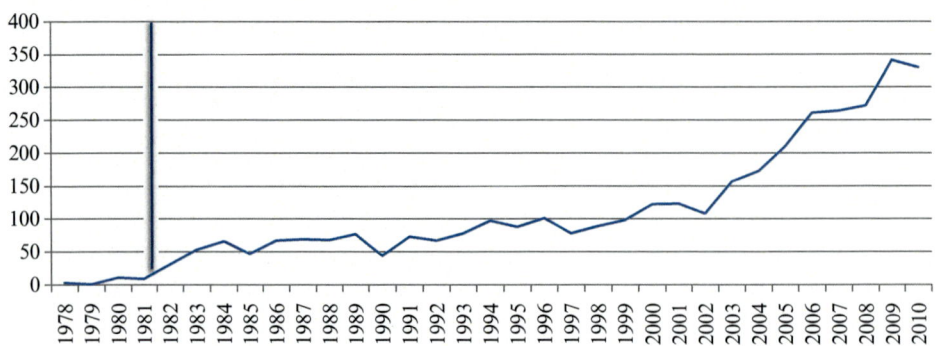

Fig. 9.2 Number of "burnout" publications, per year

who work in human resources and health care (primarily jobs that require the direct care of others), but it is now believed that burnout can emerge in any occupation, including management and technology (Leiter & Schaufeli, 1996; Maslach & Schaufeli, 1993). As a result, Maslach's model has now expanded to include all professions, further contributing to the growth in burnout research and interest. Although proposed burnout mechanisms vary, Maslach and Leiter (1997) proposed that burnout occurs when there are mismatches between professionals and their job contexts. They defined an occupational mismatch as a situation in which working relationships change in a way that is unacceptable to the worker. For example, workers who find themselves saddled with an unwanted, increased workload are vulnerable to burnout. Occupational mismatch appears to contribute to burnout not only categorically (e.g., present=risk for burnout; absence=no risk) but also linearly. Leiter and Maslach (2000) found that greater job–worker mismatches result in linear increases in the likelihood of burnout.

In Maslach's multidimensional model, burnout consists of three primary dimensions: emotional exhaustion, depersonalization (cynicism), and reduced personal accomplishment. Emotional exhaustion occurs when an individual feels overextended and exhausted by the many emotional demands at work (Maslach & Goldberg, 1998). The most common sources of emotional exhaustion include work overload and personal conflict at work. When exhausted, workers lack the needed energy to complete their assigned tasks and feel unable to muster the energy to deal effectively with others. They also lack the ability or resources to replenish their energy. Depersonalization occurs when an employee is detached and cynical toward the individuals receiving a service or care. Depersonalization represents a negative or excessively detached response to other people (Maslach & Goldberg, 1998), likely resulting from an overload of emotional exhaustion. Initially, depersonalization may be self-protective. It allows an employee to become detached from his/her work and provides emotional protection from the work environment. However, it may also lead to dehumanization, which can lead to deterioration in the quality of care or service that is provided (Maslach & Jackson, 1981). Reduced personal accomplishment occurs when an employee appraises him/herself as ineffective in fulfilling one's job responsibilities (Maslach, Jackson, & Leiter, 1996). This personal accomplishment component is a self-evaluative dimension of burnout (Maslach & Goldberg, 1998). It includes a decline in productivity and a decrease in feelings of competence. Individuals experience a growing sense of inadequacy about their ability to help others, which may lead to a sense of failure.

In the Maslach model, it is believed that emotional exhaustion appears first (Maslach & Goldberg, 1998), leading to depersonalization. In other words, lack of energy makes it difficult to focus on job demands and the needs of others, leading to detachment at work. Research suggests that reduced personal accomplishment develops separately from exhaustion and depersonalization. Recently, research has identified another factor that seems to play a significant role in burnout: work engagement. High levels of work engagement (described as a state of high energy, instead of exhaustion, strong involvement, rather than detachment, and a high sense of self-efficacy, instead of decreased personal accomplishment) seem to predict burnout, though the relationship between burnout and work engagement seems to be more than purely antipodal. Indeed, engagement is seen as a positive trait rather than a negative one (Maslach & Goldberg, 1998) and is a predictor of job satisfaction rather than an indicator of burnout.

Job–Person Fit Model

The Job–Person Fit Model of burnout is a causal explanatory model that focuses on the role of subjective employee assessment of self and the work situation, which may or may not accurately represent objective, real relationships. The basic premise of this model is that stress results from a poor fit between the individual and the job (French & Kahn, 1962). When applied to burnout, greater mismatches between job and employee are believed to contribute to and increased likelihood for burnout to occur (Maslach & Goldberg, 1998). Maslach and Leiter (1997) identified six areas where a mismatch can occur. In each of the six areas, a mismatch between person and job results in burnout symptoms as defined by the Maslach model (emotional exhaustion, cynicism, and a decrease in personal efficacy). This approach differs from other burnout models because it focuses on the relationship between the employee and the job, rather than on either factor alone, which can be beneficial because it allows multiple avenues for burnout prevention.

According to Maslach and Leiter (1997), the first and most common mismatch relates to work overload. Employees have too much to do and not enough resources available to complete tasks. It becomes difficult to keep up with the pace of work, and the individual falls further behind. If the situation becomes chronic and the employee is not given the opportunity for needed rest and recuperation, burnout sets in. This can lead to decreased work quality and a disintegration of work relationships. Another job mismatch occurs when employees lack control over the work they are expected to complete (Maslach & Leiter, 1997). Lack of control is evident when an employee is not given a voice in decision-making or feels as though they are being micromanaged. Often, employees want their opinions and thoughts to impact the work setting. However, if people feel they are not heard or valued, it often leads to feelings of work-related ineffectiveness that can potentiate burnout.

Another proposed mechanism of burnout through Job–Person Fit Model involves perceptions of insufficient awards resulting from work (Maslach & Leiter, 1997). This job mismatch focuses on the negative consequences of a perceived lack of meaningful rewards for work completed by an employee. These rewards can be both internal and external. Internal rewards can include praise and feelings of pride in a job well done which lead to feeling effective in their job (or ineffective when absent). External rewards include the obvious, such as pay and benefits. If a worker feels as though the rewards of work are incongruent with effort, burnout can result. A fourth job–person mismatch occurs when an employee loses a sense of connection with coworkers, called breakdown of community (Maslach & Leiter, 1997). Individuals often work best in situations where others provide positive social support for one another. This allows employees to "weather the storm" together when work conditions become difficult; however, if there is not a sense of community in one's workplace, conflict may result. Unresolved conflict produces negative feelings, frustration, and decreases the likelihood of positive social support.

Absence of fairness in the workplace is also considered a characteristic of job mismatch (Maslach & Leiter, 1997). Fairness allows employees to feel respected and gives them a sense of what to expect in the workplace. Unfairness can occur in a number of ways. It may occur when the workload is not equally shared, or when salaries and promotions are not based on work performance. Feelings of unfairness may be propagated if there is not a grievance policy in place to allow employees to discuss frustrations. Finally, the last area of job mismatch involves value conflict (Maslach & Leiter, 1997). This occurs in situations where there is a mismatch between employees' personal values and the requirements to carry out the job. This can be seen in jobs where employees are not allowed to be forthcoming with all information or may even be asked to lie. It can also be seen when an individual's values do not align with the overall organization's goals (i.e., in the military).

Job Demands–Resources Model

The central tenet of the Job Demands–Resources Model (JD-R) is that work characteristics invoke two different processes: consideration of job demands weighed against perceived job resources. This process occurs regardless of the occupation being examined, and both of these two processes have the ability to explain the complex relationship between burnout and work engagement (Bakker, Hakanen, Demerouti, & Xanthopoulou, 2007; Schaufeli & Bakker, 2004). The first process (consideration of job demands) states that high levels of perceived demands associated with work may lead to depletion in energy, which then leads to exhaustion and health problems that are characteristic of occupational burnout (Demerouti et al., 2000; Lee & Ashworth, 1996). Job demands are physical, social, and organizational aspects of the job that expend both physical and mental effort, and are associated with psychosocial costs such as exhaustion (Crawford, LePine, & Rich, 2010). Factors like workload, time pressures, and the work environment can contribute to perceived job demands. The increased stress from responding to job demands may eventually leave an employee feeling drained, ultimately leading to burnout. Job resources represent the other side of the Job Demands Resources Model, and can motivate an individual to persist with work resulting in improved work engagement. Job resources include aspects of an occupation that enable employees to achieve work goals, stimulate personal growth, and help manage job demands. This could include anything that enables an employee to get the job done, reduce job demands on a psychosocial (stress) or physical (strain) level, and stimulate personal growth and development (Demerouti, Bakker, Janssen, & Schaufeli, 2001; Demerouti, Bakker, Nachreiner, & Schaufeli, 2001). Job resources can include job control, participation in decision-making, receiving constructive feedback about work, and the presence of social support.

When job resources are not available and job demands begin to predominate, workers may begin to experience frustration that may lead to work disengagement. Disengagement is characterized by low motivation, lack of interest in work, and a weakening loyalty to the organization. Disengagement from work may be a self-protective mechanism, whereby a frustrated worker avoids the frustration of not meeting work-related goals by interrupting effort or simply not caring about goal completion (Peterson et al., 2008). In jobs with both high demands and limited job resources, it is assumed that employees will experience both exhaustion and disengagement. Employees experience stressful work conditions that are not mediated by positive factors that encourage engagement in the work environment. Various models of occupational burnout tout exhaustion and disengagement as the primary causal components. In these models, exhaustion, cynicism, and a decreased efficacy within the workplace all contribute to burnout (Demerouti, Bakker, Janssen, et al., 2001; Demerouti, Bakker, Nachreiner, et al., 2001; Maslach et al., 1996).

Crawford et al. (2010) introduced a differentiated Job Demands-Resources Model. This updated model demonstrates the variable role of job demands across different occupations by incorporating components of the transactional theory of stress. According to the *Transactional Theory of Stress*, individuals evaluate stress situations in terms of the impact of these situations on the individual's well-being, especially when stressors are perceived as being either challenging or threatening (Lazarus & Folkman, 1984). This can further be divided into two factors: challenge stressors and hindrance stressors (Cavanaugh, Boswell, Roehling, & Boudreau, 2000). Challenges tend to be seen as stressful job demands that promote job mastery, personal growth, or future gains (Crawford et al., 2010). Challenge demands may include things such as high workload, time pressure, or increased levels of job responsibility. Some employees see these challenges in a positive light as opportunities for personal growth and feel that their increased efforts will be rewarded (i.e., pay raise, praise, or promotion). Because these types of job demand generally elicit positive emotions, they can often lead to improved work performance vis-à-vis engagement and active problem-focused coping styles. Despite the increase in positive feelings and engagement, however, job challenges can deplete energy resources and increase strain which, in turn, result in increases in probability of developing burnout. Hindrances, on the other hand, are stressful job demands that have the potential to prevent personal growth, learning, and goal attainment (Crawford et al., 2010). Employees tend to appraise hindrances as stressful demands that deter progress toward goal attainment and personal rewards, such as pay raise, promotion, or recognition. Hindrances include anything that employees feels needlessly obstructs them from goal acquisition, such as job politics, job role conflicts, and daily hassles. They generally elicit negative emotions and employees disengage from work because they do not feel as though they have the coping skills to effectively deal with the stressors leading to burnout. Therefore, for this model, job characteristics can be categorized in terms of challenge and hindrance demands instead of merely as job demands. Job resources remain the same in both models. Job resources are still viewed as negatively related to burnout in Crawford's model because an individual with plentiful work resources is more easily able to meet job demands (Crawford et al., 2010). Job resources are also positively associated with engagement because individuals who have the available resources to successfully meet job demands are likely to feel their needs for autonomy, growth and development, and competence are being met, thereby allowing them to become more willing to become engaged in the work environment.

Conservation of Resources Theory

Conservation of Resources Theory (CRT) provides yet another comprehensive lens used to explain burnout (Hobfoll & Shirom, 1993). In the CRT model, burnout is viewed as the psychosocial strain that results from depletion of personal coping resources in the workplace. This psychosocial strain is most likely to occur in situations where there is either an actual or perceived loss of resources. Ultimately, individuals are motivated to acquire and protect resources, which can include anything individuals' find personally valuable in their work environment. These resources typically fall into four different categories: object, conditions, personal, or energy (Wright & Hobfoll, 2004). Object resources are usually tangible items, such as a home or automobile that a worker uses to facilitate work activity. Condition resources are less tangible, often described as status in the community or organization. Personal resources describe subjective work-related experiences, such as feelings of achievement and self-efficacy, that help motivate an individual to work. And finally, energy resources can include various resources that may be expended in service to work completion, like time or money. Resources are believed to function in a personal economy whereby, once resources are acquired, an individual invests them to obtain additional resources (Hobfoll, 2001). For example, an individual may develop skills at work, which are then transferred into improved work performance in the hopes of acquiring more resources (such as increased pay or promotion; Halbesleben, Harvey, & Bolino, 2009). If resources are threatened, lost, or if demands exceed resources, individuals are likely to experience negative consequences and distress leading to emotional exhaustion, the key component of burnout (Harris, Harvey, & Kacmar, 2009). Once employees become emotionally exhausted, they are less likely to reinvest their limited resources and instead become defensive to protect remaining resources (Hobfoll, 2001). It is likely that, once an employee experiences a loss in resources, the quality of their work declines because they become focused on only engaging in the most necessary of tasks or parts of their jobs that have typically provided the best return in the past (Baltes, 1997).

Psychosocial Inventories

The following is a brief discussion of the most commonly researched psychosocial inventories measuring burnout. This partial list includes the Maslach Burnout Inventory, the Burnout Measure, the Shirom-Melamed Burnout Questionnaire, The Oldenburg Burnout Inventory, and the Copenhagen Burnout Inventory. This list is not meant to be exhaustive, as there are other less commonly used measures of burnout available.

Maslach Burnout Inventory

A number of self-report instruments have been developed to measure the construct of burnout, but the most popular by far is the Maslach Burnout Inventory (MBI; Maslach et al., 1996) which has three versions available—the MBI Human Services Survey, the MBI Educators Survey and the MBI General Survey (for all occupations). The inventory is self-administered, and takes approximately 10–15 min to complete. The original MBI consists of 22 items, divided into three subscales (emotional exhaustion, depersonalization, and personal accomplishment), which have been confirmed in factor analyses (Maslach et al., 1996). Statements are written in the form of personal feelings or attitudes. Participants use a 0–6 Likert-type scale to indicate frequency of experiencing a particular feeling regarding work from "never" to "daily." Higher scores on depersonalization (score range 0–48) and emotional exhaustion (score range 0–54) indicate higher levels of burnout. The personal accomplishment (score range 0–48) subscale is scored in the opposite direction, with lower scores indicating higher levels of burnout. This instrument has been shown to have sufficient validity, reliability, and internal consistency (Maslach & Jackson, 1981; Pines & Maslach, 1978).

Burnout Measure

Another commonly used instrument to assess burnout is the *Burnout Measure* (BM; Pines & Aronson, 1988). The BM is a 21-item self-report instrument (rated on a 7-point frequency scale; ranging from "never" to "always") that assesses an individual's level of physical, emotional and mental exhaustion. The BM assesses burnout using a total score. Prior to the construction of the MBI's alternate forms, the BM was commonly used because (unlike the original MBI) it had the ability to be used outside the human service professions (Schaufeli & Van Dierendonck, 1993). The BM is conceived as a one-dimensional measure of burnout. Internal consistency of the BM ranges from 0.91 to 0.93 (Pines & Aronson, 1981). This measure correlates highly with the MBI's dimensions of exhaustion and depersonalization, and moderately with personal accomplishment (Schaufeli, Enzmann, & Girault, 1993). The BM has also shown a 1-month test–retest reliability of 0.89 (Pines, 1988).

Shirom-Melamed Burnout Questionnaire

The *Shirom-Melamed Burnout Questionnaire* (SMBQ) is a 22-item measure of burnout (Melamed et al., 1992; Shirom, 1989). This measure consists of an emotional exhaustion and physical fatigue subscale, a tension and listlessness subscale, and a cognitive weariness subscale. Each item is scored on a 7-point Likert-type scale, ranging from 1 ("almost never") to 7 ("almost always"). Use of this measure was found to be positively associated with episodic stress (Shirom, 1989) and chronic work stress (Kushnir & Melamed, 1992). The SMBQ has demonstrated satisfactory validity (Lindstrom, Aman, & Norberg, 2011).

Oldenburg Burnout Inventory

A more recent measure of burnout is the *Oldenburg Burnout Inventory* (OLBI; Demerouti, Bakker, Janssen, et al., 2001; Demerouti, Bakker, Nachreiner, et al., 2001). This inventory incorporates both positively and negatively worded items to assess two core dimensions of burnout: exhaustion and disengagement from work. Exhaustion is defined as the consequences of intense physical, affective, and cognitive strain. Exhaustion is due to the long-term, prolonged exposure to work demands. The items on the exhaustion subscale refer to feelings of emptiness, being overtaxed from work, having a strong need for rest, and experiencing physical exhaustion. Disengagement is the distancing of oneself from work in general (Demerouti, Mostert, & Bakker, 2010) due to prolonged work demands. Disengagement also encompasses experiencing negative attitudes toward work. Each subscale consists of eight items (four are positively worded; four are negatively worded). Each item has four responses ranging from 1 ("totally disagree") to 4 ("totally agree"). The OLBI has been shown to have factorial validity and convergent validity with the MBI-General Survey (Demerouti, Bakker, deJonge, Janssen, & Schaufeli, 2003).

Copenhagen Burnout Inventory

The *Copenhagen Burnout Inventory* (CBI; Kristensen, Borritz, Villadsen, & Christensen, 2005) is a measure of burnout consisting of 19-items and three scales that measure different dimensions of burnout. These dimensions include personal burnout, work-related burnout, and client-related burnout. The first scale (personal burnout) is a measure of the degree of physical and psychosocial fatigue and exhaustion experienced by a person regardless of their participation in the workforce. The work-related burnout scale measures physical and psychosocial fatigue as it relates to work. The client-related burnout scale measures physical and psychosocial fatigue related to working with clients. A higher score on the measure indicates a higher level of burnout. The three scales have shown good criterion-related validity and reliability in studies with Danish and Australian samples (Kristensen et al., 2005; Winwood & Wincfield, 2004).

Utrecht Work Engagement Scale (UWES)

The *Utrecht Work Engagement Scale* (Schaufeli, Salanova, Gonzalez-Roma, & Bakker, 2002) is one of the most widely used measures of work engagement in the World, and is comprised of items that are divided between two scales: vigor and dedication. All UWES items are scored on a 7-point Likert-type scale assessing the frequency, with which the respondent experiences each symptom (0 = "never" and 6 = "always"). Vigor subscale items include statements assessing the frequency with which an individual experiences high levels of energy at work. Dedication subscale items assess the frequency of feelings of meaningfulness or fulfillment at work. The original version of the UWES included 24 items, most of which were positively transformed versions of items from the MBI (Schaufeli & Bakker, 2003). The measure was eventually distilled down to 15 items through multiple psychometric evaluations (Demerouti, Bakker, Janssen, et al., 2001; Demerouti, Bakker, Nachreiner, et al., 2001; Schaufeli, Salanova, Gonzalez-Roma, & Bakker, 2002), and has been thoroughly validated in its shorter form. The resulting measure has demonstrated strong factor validity and internal consistency (ranging from 0.80 to 0.90 across scales), with surprising cross-national invariance and stability over time (Schaufeli & Bakker, 2003). Multiple studies have confirmed the content and construct validity of the measure. In 2006, the UWES was shortened further to nine items (UWES-9), and continued to demonstrate solid psychometrics (Schaufeli, Bakker, & Salanova, 2006).

Predictors of Burnout

Understanding occupational burnout can be vital for those concerned about both the retention of workers and the enhancement of work-related output. A number of studies have illuminated the various deleterious impacts of burnout on work performance. Maslach and Leiter (2008) offer a particularly elegant summary wherein they briefly outline the research on job performance and burnout across a number of occupations. Overall, burnout contributes to absenteeism and presenteeism from work, impaired job performance, decreased job satisfaction, intention to quit, and job loss. There is also some evidence to suggest that burnout shares common etiological pathways with depression (suggesting that depression could present as a risk factor for burnout; Iacovides, Fountoulakis, Moysidou, & Ierodiakonou, 1999), although a brief review of the existing literature on depression and burnout appears to be equivocal (cf. Leiter & Durup, 1994). Based on the findings to date, the first step in intervention for occupational burnout may be to develop a more comprehensive understanding of the panoply of factors that contribute to burnout and burnout-related occupational outcomes.

Although Maslach (1982a, 1982b) offers one of the most widely agreed-upon models of occupational burnout, there has been varied consensus on how multiple extraneous variables mediate or moderate the relationship between Maslach's three dimensions (emotional exhaustion, depersonalization, and personal accomplishment) and the ultimate outcomes of burnout. Lee and Ashworth (1996) made an early attempt to address this issue through a comprehensive meta-analysis of studies addressing burnout moderation through the lens of conservation of resources theory. Their review of 66 relevant studies confirmed the 3-factor burnout model reported by Maslach and Jackson in 1986, but further elaborated that the personal accomplishment dimension was discretely determined from both emotional exhaustion and depersonalization. When examined in the context of *Conservation of Resources Theory*, Maslach's definition of occupational burnout showed more sensitivity to work demands than available resources. This finding suggests that increased work stressors may be more determinant of ultimate burnout (using this model) than deprivation of resources, which Lee and Ashworth (1996) explain on the balance of loss and gain. They note that work stress could be perceived as a loss to beleaguered workers because of the resources (i.e., gains) they must invest or sacrifice to manage the increased demands. Because job stresses (i.e., losses) are weighed more heavily in the research than job resources (i.e., gains), increased stress will ultimately lead to burnout even in the context of increased resources. Rubino, Luksyte, Perry, and Volpone (2009) have expanded on these findings somewhat after they examined burnout in the context of stress–strain theoretical models, hypothesizing that work-related motivation may play a valuable mediating role between work-related stress and burnout.

Ballenger-Browning et al. (2011) undertook a more recent evaluation of burnout predictors in a study of military mental health providers. Using Maslach's model of burnout, the investigators sought to explore the demographic and work-related variables that contribute to burnout. With the increased burden of mental health problems associated with ongoing US military involvement in Iraq and Afghanistan, the investigators hypothesized increased risk of occupational burnout in this sample attributable to increased workload, demographic factors, and deployment-related experiences. Interestingly, in a sample of 97 military mental health providers, they found burnout levels comparable to those of civilian providers, and lower than the normative sample used to develop the Maslach Burnout Inventory. In a subsequent review of 26 additional burnout studies, Ballenger-Browning and colleagues confirmed that levels of burnout on two of Maslach's three subscales for the military sample fell into the lowest quartile of all mental health provider studies. Part of this discrepancy may have been attributable to a heterogeneous sample comprised of case managers, social workers, psychologists, psychiatrists, psychiatry residents, and technical staff, all of whom likely face unique challenges that contribute to work stress. Indeed, the authors noted that psychiatrists were at greater risk for burnout compared to psychologists, and were significantly more likely to work long hours than the other professions. It must be noted, however, that lower military burnout rates (at least among mental health providers) may also be attributable to military-specific contextual factors that protect these treatment providers against burnout (e.g., high levels of social support, personal sense of accomplishment, etc.). After examining burnout contributing factors, the authors found that longer work hours, female gender, and more complex work tasks (i.e., working with more complicated patients) were predictive of increased burnout risk. Conversely, high levels of peer support and greater work experience were associated with lower burnout risk.

Although there have been great strides in the research to identify factors contributing to burnout risk, there has been relatively little research on positive, protective factors. Bakker, Schaufeli, Leiter, and Taris (2008) aptly note that burnout-related research has begun to shed light on a few protective factors, with the greatest amount of support generated for work engagement. Work engagement has been conceptually defined as the diametric opposite of Maslach's burnout dimensions (Maslach & Leiter, 1997). Whereas burnout is characterized by decreased energy and cynicism, work engagement encompasses increased energy and task involvement. Similarly, the lack of personal effectiveness experienced by a burned out worker is replaced by increased efficacy associated with high work engagement. Some suggest that work engagement is cultivated through a worker's identification with his or her work and ability to focus energy onto work tasks (i.e., attention and concentration; Bakker et al., 2008; Kahn, 1990; Rothbard, 2001), and there is ample evidence to suggest that enhancing job resources (colleagues, positive feedback, autonomy, etc.) results in improved work engagement (Bakker et al., 2008).

The exact relationship between burnout and positive constructs like work engagement has yet to be fully defined, although Bakker and colleagues explore some theories suggesting that work engagement is completely separate from burnout, but with a strongly negative reciprocal relationship. Thus, workers with little work engagement are at increased risk for burnout, and vice versa. Gonzalez-Roma, Schaufeli, Bakker, and Lloret (2006) used a nonparametric Mokken scaling method to definitively test the relationship between burnout (exhaustion and cynicism) and work engagement (vigor and dedication). Their analysis revealed that the two constructs do interact in an antipodal manner, and are representative of opposite ends of bipolar dimensions describing energy and identification with work. It has been argued, however, that diametric opposition between burnout and work engagement does not necessarily mean that engagement can be inferred by a lack of burnout (i.e., low scores on a burnout scale do not indicate high levels of work engagement; Schaufeli & Bakker, 2003). So, both it may be necessary to thoroughly assess both burnout and work engagement to truly understand an individual's adjustment to work.

Maslach and Leiter (2008) examined a large sample ($n_{T1}=992$, $n_{T2}=812$) of North American workers in order to identify early predictors of burnout and work engagement. They hypothesized that burnout characteristics would be consistent over time (through mutual maintenance of exhaustion and cynicism), that this consistency in burnout traits would result in less change in burnout and engagement over time (compared to those with less consistency—early warning burnout patterns—who would demonstrate more change), and that incongruities in various domains of worklife (workload, control, fairness, reward, community, and values) would contribute to burnout over time. Maslach and Leiter determined that it was possible to identify individuals at risk for later burnout, with incongruities in worklife fairness and inconsistent (i.e., unstable) burnout characteristics serving as the most telling early risk factors. However, the authors were quick to caution that the particular relevance of fairness as a risk factor in this study may have been attributable to particular problems of fairness within the organization they examined. As a result, other worklife domains may account for greater variance in organizations where those domains are more problematic. Based on these findings, and Maslach and Leiter's expectations that organizational problems are likely to be clustered within suborganizations (units, divisions, etc.), the authors recommend addressing widespread burnout using organizational (rather than individually tailored) interventions, including ongoing assessment of burnout risk and organizational intervention targeting a worklife domain "tipping point" toward burnout. Interestingly, the investigators found that worklife domain incongruities do not seem to contribute to any change in work engagement. In other words, changes in worklife predict burnout, but not work engagement. Maslach and Leiter concluded that work engagement may actually be a normative response to work, whereas occupational burnout represents a departure from normal.

Burnout and Special Populations

Several populations have come to the forefront when addressing burnout concerns, resulting in a specialized body of research examining the nature and outcomes of burnout in special occupations with high burnout risk. These professions tend to include jobs in which workers are expected to work long hours working for and with other people (i.e., service occupations). These service-oriented professions include mental health, health care, teachers, and law enforcement (McVicar, 2003).

Burnout and Mental Health

Research has found that mental health providers represent a population of workers with the highest risk of burnout (Snibbe, Radcliffe, Weisberger, Richards, & Kelly, 1989; Thomsen, Soares, Nolan, Dallender, & Arnetz, 1999). This is likely due to the intensive nature and degree of involvement necessary to provide successful mental health treatment. Burnout among mental health providers can lead to decreased effectiveness of the providers, leading ultimately to poorer treatment outcomes and prolonged suffering of their patients (Priebe et al., 2004). A qualitative study of mental health professionals (Reid, Johnson, & Morant, 1999) indicated that administrative demands, lack of resources, work overload, relapsing patients, and responsibility for patients were the top sources of stress for mental health providers. These stressors, and severe distress in the workplace, have been linked with staff absenteeism, poor staff retention, and reduced job performance (AlbuAlRub & Al-Zaru, 2008).

Studies have also shown that psychiatry, in particular, tends to be a high burnout profession (Kumar, 2007). This is likely due to external factors (such as work environment), internal factors (such as personality and appraisal styles), and mediating factors (such as social support). Emotional exhaustion is the most common burnout symptom reported by psychiatrists (Prosser et al., 1996). Although most psychiatrists work fewer hours than other physicians or surgeons, they report more depression and burnout related to workload (Deary, Agius, & Sadler, 1996). This may be due to psychiatrists dealing with extremely distressed and ill individuals on a daily basis, which may put them at risk for inheriting some of their patients' emotional distress (a phenomenon commonly referred to as "emotional contagion"). Burnout is a frequent outcome of the chronic exposure to emotional and interpersonal stressors that psychiatrists confront on a daily basis (Benbow, 1998; FarberFarber, 1983). Protective factors for this profession, such as lifestyle factors and focusing on one's nonprofessional life, may be important to discourage burnout (Kumar, 2007).

A segment of providers in the mental health field face the unique challenge of working with patients and being active duty military. This population may be doubly at risk for burnout, dealing with both the stress of working with patients and the ever-increasing demands of serving in the military during wartime. Mental health providers in the military not only treat patients but also must meet the daily demands of military life (which include deployments and frequent change of duty stations). All this must be accomplished while the active duty mental health force decreases due to individuals getting out of the military leaving an undermanned workforce (Pueschel, 2011). In recent years, due to Operation Enduring Freedom/Operation Iraqi Freedom, an increasing number of military members are suffering from mental health disorders, with a higher prevalence of the disorders being traumatic stress disorders (Ballenger-Browning et al., 2011). Furthermore, military mental health providers themselves may also be exposed to combat trauma during deployments. These unique stressors of working with trauma patients and amplified workload due to the increases in mental health problems in the military population along with a decreasing workforce, is a recipe for burnout. While research (Ballenger-Balling et al., 2011) has found that providers in the military score significantly better on two of three of the subscales on the MBI when compared to civilian mental health providers, indicating lower levels of burnout, there are still areas of concern. In the military, being female, working longer hours, treating more patients with personality disorders, being a psychiatrist, and treating more patients per week were indicators of higher rates of burnout. Alternately, employment as a psychologist, having a greater number of patients with traumatic brain injury (TBI), having social contacts at work, and more clinical experience were predictors of lower burnout scores on the MBI. For a thorough list of recommendations for the prevention of burnout among military mental health providers before, after, and during deployment please see Linnerooth et al. (2011).

Burnout and Health-care Workers

Individuals who work in the health-care services (medical students, physicians, and nurses) often experience workplace stressors that have the potential to lead to burnout. Nurses report inadequate staffing, problems with coworkers, emotional needs of patients, shift work, and lack of reward and social support as common sources of stress (AlbuAlRub & Al-Zaru, 2008; McVicar, 2003). Dyrbye et al. (2010) found that medical students with burnout were more likely to engage in cheating or dishonest clinical behaviors. Medical students suffering from burnout were also less likely to hold altruistic views regarding physicians' responsibility toward society. This suggests that burnout may alter physicians' views on their responsibility to promote public health and advocate for patients. Agius, Blenkin, Deary, Zealley, and Wood (1996) found that burned out medical professionals experience higher rates of suicide, early retirement, increased substance use, and marital problems. Peterson (2008) also found that health-care workers suffering from burnout were more likely to experience sleep problems.

Burnout and Teachers

In the USA, up to 25% of beginning teachers leave the teaching field before their third year, and almost 40% leave the profession within the first 5 years of teaching (Milner & Woolfolk Hoy, 2003). Teachers routinely face stressors related to improving standardized test scores, peer violence, behavior problems, uninvolved parents, work overload, poor career structure, and low salaries (Grayson & Alvarez, 2007; Schonfeld, 2001). McGuire (1979) first warned that public school teachers were experiencing a significant degree of burnout. Teachers experience emotional exhaustion when they are unable to physically or emotionally provide for students due to extreme fatigue and stress (Maslach et al., 1996). This exhaustion develops over time as one's emotional resources are drained. Teachers experience depersonalization as cynical attitudes toward students, parents, coworkers, and the workplace. Diminished feelings of personal accomplishment are found as teachers begin to feel they are no longer adding to students' development (Maslach et al., 1996). These symptoms of burnout lead to low self-esteem, decreased self-confidence, and depression (Schonfeld, 2001). Teachers who feel ineffective report low job satisfaction, along with resentment, frustration, boredom, irritability, anger, and hopelessness (Blasé, 1982). This impacts the school system due to increased teacher absenteeism, high turnover, mental health and medical claims, deteriorating performance, and early retirement (Burke, Greenglass, & Schwarzer, 1996; Leithwood, Menzies, Jantzi, & Leithwood, 1999). These teachers may also have reduced tolerance for classroom behavior problems (Grayson & Alvarez, 2007), and less flexibility and acceptance to various student needs (Capel, 1991).

The risk of burnout in teachers is increased when teachers have unmet or unrealistic goals and lack professional accomplishment (Evers, Tomic, & Brouwers, 2004). Some research has found teachers between the ages of 20 and 30 years old experience higher levels of burnout (Friedman & Farber, 1992). However, findings regarding age as a predictor of burnout have not been consistent across the literature. Some studies found no evidence for ages as a predictor of teacher burnout (Zabel & Zabel, 2001). Research has also found mixed results in terms of gender and teacher burnout (Chang, 2009).

Burnout and Law Enforcement

Those serving in law enforcement often face stressful situations daily. Negative aspects of the job include lack of respect, excessive paperwork, confrontational and negative public contact, shift work, threats of violence, and sometimes boredom (Greller & Parsons, 1988; Jermier, Gaines, & McIntosh, 1989; Stotland & Pendleton, 1989). Work-setting characteristics may also increase stress among law enforcement. These include low quality supervision, unmet expectations, and constraints within the organizational environment (Burke, 1994). Due to an accumulation of these stressors, burnout may occur. Police officers reporting higher levels of burnout were found to be more likely to display anger, spend time away from family, and have poor marriages. Burnout can lead to deteriorating work performance, absenteeism, low-morale, emotional problems, and physical conditions, such as headaches and ulcers among law enforcement (Kroes, 1976). Research has also shown that burnout influences how police officers interact with the public, as well as their attitudes toward violence (Kop, Euweman, & Schaufeli, 1999).

Engagement, as well as burnout, has been examined with police officers. Research has found that job resources, in terms of social support from supervisors and coworkers, were related to engagement (Richardson, Burke, & Martinussen, 2006). Cynicism was found to be associated with increased health complaints and reduced commitment and efficacy. Engagement in law enforcement was found to be associated with fewer health complaints and increased commitment and efficacy.

Burnout Prevention

The available research has not shown efficacy in treating burnout once it has set in (Kumar, 2007). Therefore, it is best to take a preventative approach to dealing with burnout. Prevention research has focused on prevention techniques focused on the individual (person-centered approaches) and at the organizational level (situation-centered approaches). Maslach and Goldberg (1998) recommend three steps prior to developing a burnout prevention model. First, one should have a clear definition of the construct (burnout) that is being treated. Secondly, one must examine the intended outcome (improved physical health or job performance). Lastly, one must have a method to assess burnout so that it can be determined whether the intervention had the intended effect (decreasing burnout). Some person-centered approaches focus on changing the person's relationship to the job, and others focus on increasing an individual's coping skills so that job stressors are better managed (Maslach & Goldberg, 1998). More research has been conducted in this area of decreasing burnout. This is likely due to the fact that it is often cheaper for an individual to make lifestyle changes or increase coping skills rather than making global organizational changes. However, it can be argued that an individual also has more control in these areas to make changes on the individual level rather than raging a battle with their employer. It is likely that an individual will see noticeable changes sooner when using person-centered approaches, increasing their sense of self-efficacy and control.

Person-Centered Approaches

Engaging in relaxing activities may help to prevent burnout and offset the stress response (Maslach & Goldberg, 1998). Relaxing activities can include activities that require little effort, such as deep breathing, mindfulness training, or meditation. Relaxing activities can also be more involved, such as taking a vacation. A vacation allows employees to take a break from the daily stressors associated to work that can lead to burnout. Lounsbury and Hoopes (1986) found that satisfaction with vacation was related to improved satisfaction with life and work. Etzion, Eden, and Lapidot (1998) found that employees who took vacations were less likely to suffer from burnout when compared to their coworkers who did not take vacations. However, the employee must perceive his/her vacation as satisfying and, preferably, not have any contact from work (i.e., phone calls, e-mail, etc.) to fully benefit from the respite experience.

An individual may decide to change his/her work pattern (Maslach & Goldberg, 1998). A relatively easy solution to decrease burnout is to decrease the number of hours that one works. However, this is not always as simple as it seems. Many individuals are not financially secure enough to reduce their work hours. In some situations, an employer may not allow a decrease in employee's work hours. In these situations, it may be helpful to take more breaks or avoid working overtime. Research has suggested that it is not necessarily the amount of work that causes burnout, but an imbalance between work and the rest of one's life (Grosch & Olsen, 1995; Riordan & Saltzer, 1992). Therefore, improving the areas of life outside of work may prove beneficial in decreasing overall burnout.

In addition, an employee may decide to work to improve her/his coping skills (Maslach & Goldberg, 1998). The goal is not to remove the work stressors, but to change how the employee responds to the work stressors. This often includes the use of cognitive-restructuring. Cognitive-restructuring allows an individual to look at situations differently, to monitor their own thoughts regarding their job, and reduce work expectations. It also allows an employee to take a "step back" and evaluate others behaviors before becoming reactive to the situation. More behaviorally focused coping skills include the use of time management techniques, improving communication skills, learning problem-solving techniques, and increasing social support.

Social support can also help to prevent burnout (Maslach & Goldberg, 1998). It is very easy to isolate one's self when experiencing job stress. Accessing support from friends, family, professionals, and coworkers allows for a sounding board in difficult situations. It is not uncommon for an individual to engage in psychotherapy due to work stressors. A professional can serve as a safe confidant while examining distorted thoughts that may discourage healthy coping. Increased social support and social activities can also serve as a distractor when experiencing stressful times at work. Physical exercise may help to offset stress and allow an individual to blow off steam while encouraging a healthy lifestyle. Consistent physical exercise encourages better sleep, decreases muscle tension, and improves mood. If one engages in physical exercise with someone else, it also increases social support.

Situation-Centered Approaches

There is much less research available when examining situation-centered approaches to the prevention of burnout. Most that is available focuses on enhancing the job experience (Maslach & Goldberg, 1998). Some strategies focus on increasing employees' sense of control and self-efficacy by allowing them to have a voice in the organizational decision-making. Another strategy involves training employees in other areas of their job to allow for greater personal development. Organizations may be able to increase an individual's self-esteem by openly praising workers who deserve it. In turn, increasing an individual's positive feelings toward work may be helpful (Grayson & Alvarez, 2007). Organizations that work primarily with people may want to initiate training on the prevention of burnout, provide occupational orientation to novice providers, and find ways for older members of the profession to mentor newer members so that socialization to the profession can occur (Gustavsson, Lennart, & Rudman, 2010). These strategies may decrease the likelihood of burnout amongst employees.

Organizations may also focus on encouraging employees' feelings of engagement regarding work. Sirota, Mischkin, and Meltzer (2005) recommend equity or fair treatment within organizations. Fair treatment, which includes justice at work, job security, fair pay and respect, results in engaged employees. Schaufeli and Salanova (2006) also make recommendations to encourage engagement at the organizational level among employees. These include assessing and evaluating employees to ensure people are placed in the most appropriate job for their skillset. They also include finding ways to decrease work stressors while enhancing job resources available to employees. It is recommended that leadership set a positive socioemotional climate and provide training and career development to build employee self-efficacy.

Conclusions and Directions for Future Research

Although great progress has been made in burnout research, some have observed that our understanding of burnout is still incomplete and in need of continued investigation (Maslach & Schaufeli, 1993). Because of its symptomatic similarity to other conditions, like depression and anxiety, additional work is required to examine how burnout can/should be distinguished from other conditions. Additionally, more may need to be done to illuminate how burnout relates to similar concepts like job stress (cf. Lee & Ashworth, 1996; Maslach, 2003; Maslach & Schaufeli, 1993). Ultimately, one can reasonably conclude that occupational burnout is a complex phenomenon, impacted by multiple factors contributing to the relationship between a worker and his or her work environment. Although relatively new, this concept has garnered increased attention throughout the years, and will continue to grow in importance as we unlock more knowledge about the impact of burnout on workers and their work output. Everyone reading this chapter is encouraged to contribute to this endeavor by critically evaluating the possible role of burnout mechanisms in their own interactions with patients. These hypothesized mechanisms can be evaluated at micro (single-subject design) and macro (comprehensive randomized trials) levels, the results of which can help us to continue to recognize not only how burnout occurs but also how it can be mitigated (or even replaced with work engagement).

References

Agius, R. M., Blenkin, H., Deary, I. J., Zealley, H. E., & Wood, R. A. (1996). Survey of perceived stress and work demands of consultant doctors. *Occupational and Environmental Medicine, 53*(4), 217–224.

AlbuAlRub, R. F., & Al-Zaru, I. M. (2008). Job stress, recognition, job performance and intention to stay at work among Jordanian hospital nurses. *Journal of Nurse Management, 16*(3), 227–236.

Armon, G., Melamed, S., Shirom, A., & Shapira, I. (2010). Elevated burnout predicts the onset of musculoskeletal pain among apparently healthy employees. *Journal of Occupational Health Psychology, 15*, 399–408.

Bakker, A. B., Hakanen, J. J., Demerouti, E., & Xanthopoulou, D. (2007). Job resources boost work engagement, particularly when job demands are high. *Journal of Educational Psychology, 99*, 274–284.

Bakker, A. B., Schaufeli, W. B., Leiter, M. P., & Taris, T. W. (2008). Work engagement: An emerging concept in occupational health psychology. *Work & Stress, 22*, 187–200.

Ballenger-Browning, K. K., Schmitz, K. J., Rothacker, J. A., Hammer, P. S., Webb-Murphy, J. A., & Johnson, D. C. (2011). Predictors of burnout among military mental health providers. *Military Medicine, 176*(3), 253–260.

Baltes, P. B. (1997). On the incomplete architecture of human ontogeny: Selection, optimization, and compensation as foundation of development theory. *American Psychologist, 52*, 366–380.

Benbow, S. (1998). Burnout: Current knowledge and relevance to old age psychiatry. *International Journal of Geriatric Psychiatry, 13*, 520–526.

Blasé, J. J. (1982). A social-psychological grounded theory of teacher stress and burnout. *Educational Administration Quarterly, 18*, 93–113.

Burke, R. J. (1994). Stressful events, work-family conflict, coping, psychological burnout, and well-being among police officers. *Psychological Reports, 75*, 787–800.

Burke, R. J., Greenglass, E. R., & Schwarzer, R. (1996). Predicting teacher burnout over time: Effects of work stress, social support, and self-doubts on burnout and its consequences. *Anxiety, Stress and Coping, 9*, 261–275.

Capel, S. A. (1991). A longitudinal study of burnout in teachers. *British Journal of Educational Psychology, 61*, 36–45.

Cavanaugh, M. A., Boswell, W. R., Roehling, M. V., & Boudreau, J. W. (2000). An empirical examination of self-reported work stress among U.S. Managers. *Journal of Applied Psychology, 85*, 65–74.

Chambers, R. (1993). Avoiding burnout in general practice. *The British Journal of General Practice, 43*, 442–443.

Chang, M. (2009). An appraisal perspective of teacher burnout: Examining the emotional work of teachers. *Educational Psychology Review, 21*, 193–218.

Cherniss, C. (1980). *Professional burnout in the human service organizations*. New York, NY: Praeger.

Crawford, E. R., LePine, J. A., & Rich, B. L. (2010). Linking job demands and resources to employee engagement and burnout: A theoretical extension and meta-analytic test. *Journal of Applied Psychology, 95*(5), 834–848.

Deary, I. J., Agius, R. M., & Sadler, A. (1996). Personality and stress in consulting psychiatrists. *International Journal of Social Psychiatry, 42*, 112–123.

Demerouti, E., Bakker, A. B., deJonge, J., Janssen, P. P. M., & Schaufeli, W. B. (2003). The convergent validity of two burnout instruments: A multitrait-multimethod analysis. *European Journal of Psychological Assessment, 19*(1), 12–23.

Demerouti, E., Bakker, A. B., Janssen, P. P. M., & Schaufeli, W. B. (2001). Burnout and engagement at work as a function of demands and control. *Scandinavian Journal of Work, Environment & Health, 27*, 279–286.

Demerouti, E., Bakker, A. B., Nachreiner, F., & Schaufeli, W. B. (2000). A model of burnout and life satisfaction amongst nurses. *Journal of Advanced Nursing, 32*(2), 454–464.

Demerouti, E., Bakker, A. B., Nachreiner, F., & Schaufeli, W. B. (2001). The job demands resources model of burnout. *Journal of Applied Psychology, 86*(3), 499–512.

Demerouti, E., Mostert, K., & Bakker, A. B. (2010). Burnout and work engagement: A thorough investigation of the independency of both constructs. *Journal of Occupational Health Psychology, 15*(3), 209–222.

Donkin, R. (2010). *The history of work*. Great Britain: Palgrave Macmillan.

Dyrbye, L. N., Thomas, M. R., Massie, S., et al. (2008). Burnout and suicidal ideation among U.S. medical students. *Annals of Internal Medicine, 149*, 334–341.

Dyrbye, L. N., Massie, S., Eacker, A., Harper, W., Power, D., Durning, S. J., et al. (2010). Relationship between burnout and professional conduct and attitudes among US medical students. *Journal of the American Medical Association, 304*(11), 1173–1180.

Etzion, D., Eden, D., & Lapidot, Y. (1998). Relief from job stressors and burnout: Reserve service as a respite. *Journal of Applied Psychology, 83*(4), 577–585.

Evans, S., Huxley, P., Gately, C., Webber, M., Mears, A., Pajak, S., et al. (2006). Mental health, burnout, and job satisfaction among mental health social workers in England and Wales. *The British Journal of Psychiatry, 188*, 75–80.

Evers, W. J. G., Tomic, W., & Brouwers, A. (2004). Burnout among teachers: Students' and teachers' perceptions compared. *School Psychology International, 25*, 131–148.

Farber, B.A. (1983). Introduction: A critical perspective on burnout. In B. A. Farber (Ed.), *Stress and burnout in the human services professions* (pp. 1–20). New York: Pergamon Press.

Firth, H., & Britton, P. (1989). "Burnout", absence, and turnover among British nursing staff. *Journal of Occupational Psychology, 62*, 55–59.

French, J. R. P., Jr., & Kahn, R. L. (1962). A programmatic approach to studying the industrial environment and mental health. *Journal of Social Issues, 18*(3), 1–47.

Freudenberger, H. (1975). The staff burn-out syndrome in alternative institutions. *Psychotherapy: Theory, Research & Practice, 12*(1), 73–82.

Friedman, I. A., & Farber, B. A. (1992). Professional self-concept as a predictor of teacher burnout. *Journal of Educational Research, 86*(1), 28.

Gonzalez-Roma, V., Schaufeli, W. B., Bakker, A. B., & Lloret, S. (2006). Burnout and work engagement: Independent factors or opposite poles? *Journal of Vocational Behavior, 68*, 165–174.

Grayson, J. L., & Alvarez, H. K. (2007). School climate factors relating to teacher burnout: A mediator model. *Teaching and Teacher Education, 24*, 1349–1363.

Greller, M., & Parsons, C. K. (1988). Psychosomatic complaints scale of stress: Measure development and psychometric properties. *Educational and Psychological Measurement, 48*, 1051–1065.

Grosch, W. N., & Olsen, D. C. (1995). Prevention: Avoiding burnout. In M. B. Sussman (Ed.), *A perilous calling: The hazards of psychotherapy practice* (pp. 275–287). New York, NY: Wiley.

Gustavsson, J. P., Lennart, H., & Rudman, A. (2010). Early career burnout among nurses: Modeling a hypothesized process using an item response approach. *International Journal of Nursing Studies, 47*, 864–875.

Halbesleben, J. R. B., Harvey, J., & Bolino, M. (2009). Too engaged? A conversation of resources view of the relationship between work engagement and work interference with family. *Journal of Applied Psychology, 94*(6), 1452–1465.

Harris, K. J., Harvey, P., & Kacmar, K. M. (2009). Do social stressors impact everyone equally? An examination of the moderating impact of core self-evaluations. *Journal of Business Psychology, 24*, 153–164.

Hobfoll, S. E. (2001). The influence of culture, community, and the nested self in the stress process: Advancing conservation of resources theory. *Applied Psychology: An International Review, 50*, 337–370.

Hobfoll, S. E., & Shirom, A. (1993). Stress and burnout in the workplace: Conservation of resources. In R. T. Golembiewski (Ed.), *Handbook of organization behavior* (pp. 41–46). New York, NY: Marcel Dekker.

Iacovides, A., Fountoulakis, K. N., Moysidou, C., & Ierodiakonou, C. (1999). Burnout is nursing staff: Is there a relationship between depression and burnout? *International Journal of Psychiatry in Medicine, 29*, 421–433.

Jermier, J. M., Gaines, J., & McIntosh, N. J. (1989). Reactions to physically dangerous work: A conceptual and empirical analysis. *Journal of Organizational Behavior, 10*, 15–23.

Kahn, W. A. (1990). Psychological conditions of personal engagement and disengagement at work. *Academy of Management Journal, 33*, 692–724.

Kop, N., Euweman, M., & Schaufeli, W. (1999). Burnout, job stress, and violent behavior among Dutch police officers. *Work & Stress, 13*, 326–340.

Kristensen, T. S., Borritz, M., Villadsen, E., & Christensen, K. B. (2005). The Copenhagen Burnout Inventory: A new tool for assessment of burnout. *Work & Stress, 19*, 192–207.

Kroes, W. H. (1976). *Society's victim-the policeman: An analysis of job stress in policing*. Springfield, IL: Thomas.

Kumar, S. (2007). Burnout in psychiatrists. *World Psychiatry, 6*, 186–189.

Kushnir, T., & Melamed, S. (1992). The Gulf War and its impact on burnout and well-being of working civilians. *Psychology Medicine, 22*, 987–995.

Lazarus, R. S., & Folkman, S. (1984). *Stress, appraisal, and coping*. New York, NY: Springer.

Lee, R. T., & Ashworth, B. E. (1996). A meta-analytic examination of the correlates of the three dimensions of job burnout. *Journal of Applied Psychology, 81*, 123–133.

Leiter, M. P., & Durup, J. (1994). The discriminant validity of burnout and depression: A confirmatory factor analytic study. *Anxiety, Stress, and Coping, 7*, 357–373.

Leiter, M. P., & Maslach, C. (2000). *Preventing burnout and building engagement: A complete program for organizational review*. San Francisco, CA: Jossey-Bass.

Leiter, M. P., & Schaufeli, W. B. (1996). Consistency of the burnout construct across occupations. *Anxiety, Stress, and Coping, 9*, 229–243.

Leithwood, K. A., Menzies, T., Jantzi, D., & Leithwood, J. (1999). Teacher burnout: A critical challenge for leaders of restructuring schools. In R. Vandenberghe & A. M. Huberman (Eds.), *Understanding and preventing teacher burnout: A sourcebook of international research and practice* (pp. 1–13). New York, NY: Cambridge University Press.

Lindstrom, C., Aman, J., & Norberg, A. L. (2011). Parental burnout in relation to sociodemographic factors as well as disease duration and glycaemic control in children with Type 1 diabetes mellitus. *Acta Paediatrica, 100*(7), 1011–1017.

Linnerooth, P., Mrdjenovich, A., & Moore, B. (2011). Professional burnout in clinical military psychologists: Recommendations before, during, and after deployment. *Professional Psychology: Research and Practice, 42*(1), 87–93.

Lounsbury, J. W., & Hoopes, L. L. (1986). A vacation from work: Changes in work and nonwork outcomes. *Journal of Applied Psychology, 71*, 392–401.

Maslach, C. (1976). Burned-out. *Human Behavior, 5*(9), 16–22.

Maslach, C. (1982a). Understanding burnout: Definitional issues in analyzing a complex phenomenon. In W. S. Paine (Ed.), *Job stress and burnout* (pp. 29–40). Beverly Hills, CA: Sage.

Maslach, C. (1982b). *Burnout: The cost of caring*. Englewood Cliffs, NJ: Prentice Hall.

Maslach, C. (2003). Job burnout: New directions in research and intervention. *Current Directions in Psychological Science, 12*, 189–192.

Maslach, C., & Goldberg, J. (1998). Prevention of burnout: New perspectives. *Applied and Preventive Psychology, 7*, 63–74.

Maslach, C., & Jackson, S. E. (1981). The measurement of experienced burnout. *Journal of Occupational Behavior, 2*, 15.

Maslach, C., & Jackson, S. (1984). Burnout in organizational settings. *Applied Social Psychology Annual, 5*, 133–153.

Maslach, C., & Jackson, S. E. (1986). *Maslach Burnout Inventory manual* (2nd ed.). Palo Alto, CA: Consulting Psychologist Press.

Maslach, C., Jackson, S. E., & Leiter, M. P. (1996). *Burnout inventory manual* (3rd ed.). Palo Alto, CA: Consulting Psychologist Press.

Maslach, C., & Leiter, M. P. (1997). *The truth about burnout: How organizations cause personal stress and what to do about it*. San Francisco, CA: Jossey-Bass.

Maslach, C., & Leiter, M. P. (2008). Early predictors of job burnout and engagement. *Journal of Applied Psychology, 93*, 498–512.

Maslach, C., & Schaufeli, W. B. (1993). Historical and conceptual development of burnout. In W. B. Schaufeli, C. Maslach, & T. Marek (Eds.), *Professional burnout: Recent developments in theory and research*. Philadelphia, PA: Taylor & Francis.

Maslach, C., Schaufeli, W. B., & Leiter, M. P. (2001). Job burnout. *Annual Review of Psychology, 52*, 397–422.

McGuire, W. H. (1979). Teacher burnout. *Today's Education, 68*, 5.

McVicar, A. (2003). Workplace stress in nursing: A literature review. *Journal of Advanced Nursing, 44*(6), 633–642.

Melamed, S., Kushnir, T., & Shirom, A. (1992). Burnout and risk factors for cardiovascular diseases. *Behavioral Medicine, 18*(2), 53–60.

Milner, H. R., & Woolfolk Hoy, A. (2003). Teacher self-efficacy and retaining talented teachers: A case study of an African-American teacher. *Teaching and Teacher Education, 19*, 263–276.

Mommersteeg, P. M. C., Heijnen, C. J., Kavelaars, A., & van Doornen, L. J. P. (2006). Immune and endocrine function in burnout syndrome. *Psychosomatic Medicine, 68*, 879–886.

Perlman, B., & Hartman, E. (1982). Burnout: Summary and future research. *Human Relations, 35*, 283–305.

Peterson, U., Demerouti, E., Bergstrom, G., Samuelsson, M., Asberg, M., & Nygren, A. (2008). Burnout and physical and mental health among Swedish healthcare workers. *Journal of Advanced Nursing, 62*(1), 84–95.

Pines, A. (1988). On burnout and buffering effects of social support. In B. Farber (Ed.), *Stress and burnout in the human services professions* (pp. 155–174). New York, NY: Pergamon.

Pines, A., & Aronson, E. (1981). *Burnout: From tedium to personal growth*. New York, NY: Free Press.

Pines, A., & Aronson, E. (1988). *Career burnout: Causes and cures*. New York, NY: Free Press.

Pines, A., & Maslach, C. (1978). Characteristics of staff burnout in mental health settings. *Hospital Community Psychiatry, 29*(4), 233–237.

Priebe, S., Fakhoury, W., White, I., Watts, J., Bebbington, P., & Billings, J. (2004). Characteristics of teams, staff and patients: Associations with outcomes of patients in assertive outreach. *British Journal of Psychiatry, 185*, 306–311.

Prosser, D., Johnson, S., Kulpers, E., Szmukler, G., Bebbington, P., & Thornicroft, G. (1996). Mental health, "burnout" and job satisfaction among hospital and community-based mental health staff. *British Journal of Psychiatry, 169*, 334–337.

Pueschel, M. *PHS, DoD partnering to provide mental health care in MTFs*. http://home.fhpr.osd.mil/press-newsroom/fhpr-news/current_news/11-08-03/PHS_DoD_Partnering_to_Provide_Mental_Health_Care_in_MTFs.aspx. Accessed 20 October 2012.

Reid, Y., Johnson, S., & Morant, N. (1999). Explanations for stress and satisfaction in mental health professionals: A qualitative study. *Social Psychiatry and Psychiatric Epidemiology, 34*, 301–308.

Richardson, A. M., Burke, R. J., & Martinussen, M. (2006). Work and health outcomes among police officers: The mediating role of police cynicism and engagement. *International Journal of Stress Management, 13*(4), 555–574.

Riordan, R. J., & Saltzer, S. K. (1992). Burnout prevention among health care workers working with the terminally ill: A literature review. *Omega, 25*, 17–24.

Rothbard, N. P. (2001). Enriching or depleting? The dynamics of engagement in work and family roles. *Administrative Science Quarterly, 46*, 655–684.

Rubino, C., Luksyte, A., Perry, S. J., & Volpone, S. D. (2009). How do stressors lead to burnout? The mediating role of motivation. *Journal of Occupational Health Psychology, 14*(3), 289–304.

Schaufeli, W., & Bakker, A. (2003). *Utrecht Work Engagement Scale: Preliminary Manual (Version 1)*. Utrecht University.

Schaufeli, W. B., & Bakker, A. B. (2004). Job demands, job resources, and their relationship with burnout and engagement: A multi-sample study. *Journal of Organizational Behavior, 25*, 293–315.

Schaufeli, W. B., Bakker, A. B., & Salanova, M. (2006). The measurement of work engagement with a short questionnaire: A cross-national study. *Educational and Psychological Measurement, 66*, 701–716.

Schaufeli, W. B., Enzmann, D., & Girault, N. (1993). The measurement of burnout: A review. In W. B. Schaufeli, C. Maslach, & T. Marek (Eds.), *Professional burnout: Recent developments in theory and research* (pp. 199–215). Washington, DC: Taylor & Francis.

Schaufeli, W. B., & Salanova, M. (2006). Work engagement: An emerging psychological concept and its implications for organizations. In S. W. Gilliland, D. D. Steiner, & D. P. Skarlicki (Eds.), *Research in social issues in management (Vol. 5): Managing social and ethical issues in organizations*. Greenwich, CT: Information Ages Publishers.

Schaufeli, W. B., Salanova, M., Gonzalez-Roma, V., & Bakker, A. B. (2002). The measurement of engagement and burnout: A confirmatory analytic approach. *Journal of Happiness Studies, 3*, 71–92.

Schaufeli, W. B., & Van Dierendonck, D. (1993). The construct validity of two burnout measures. *Journal of Organizational Behavior, 14*, 631–647.

Schonfeld, I. S. (2001). Stress in first-year women teachers: The context of social support and coping. *Genetic, Social, and General Psychology Monographs, 127*, 7547–8756.

Shirom, A. (1989). Burnout in work organization. In C. L. Cooper & I. Robertson (Eds.), *International review of industrial and organizational psychology* (pp. 25–48). New York, NY: Wiley.

Shirom, A., Melamed, S., Toker, S., Berliner, S., & Shapira, I. (2006). Burnout and health review: Current knowledge and future directions. In G. P. Hdgkinson & J. K. Ford (Eds.), *International review of industrial and organizational psychology* (Vol. 20). Chichester: Wiley.

Sirota, D., Mischkin, L. A., & Meltzer, M. I. (2005). *The enthusiastic employee: How companies profit by giving workers what they want*. Philadelphia, PA: Wharton School Publishing.

Snibbe, J. R., Radcliffe, T., Weisberger, C., Richards, M., & Kelly, J. (1989). Burnout among primary care physicians and mental health professionals in a managed health care setting. *Psychological Reports, 65*, 775–780.

Sprang, G., Clark, J. J., & Whitt-Woosley, A. (2007). Compassion fatigue, compassion satisfaction, and burnout: Factors impacting a professional's quality of life. *Journal of Loss and Trauma, 12*, 259–280.

Stotland, E., & Pendleton, M. (1989). Workload, stress and strain among police officers. *Behavioral Medicine, 26*, 5–17.

Thomsen, S., Soares, J., Nolan, P., Dallender, J., & Arnetz, B. (1999). Feelings of professional fulfillment and exhaustion in mental health personnel: The importance of organizational and individual factors. *Psychotherapy and Psychosomatics, 68*, 157–164.

Winwood, P., & Winefield, A. H. (2004). Comparing two measures of burnout among dentists in Australia. *International Journal of Stress Management, 11*, 282–289.

Wright, T. A., & Hobfoll, S. E. (2004). Commitment, psychological well-being and job performance: An examination of conservation of resources (COR) theory and job burnout. *Journal of Business and Management, 9*, 389–406.

Zabel, R. H., & Zabel, M. K. (2001). Revisiting burnout among special education teachers: Do age, experience, and preparation still matter? *Teacher Education and Special Education, 24*(2), 128–139.

Self-medication and Illicit Drug Use in the Workplace

Fong Chan, Ebonee Johnson, Emma K. Hiatt, Chih Chin Chou, and Elizabeth da Silva Cardoso

Overview

Substance use has been observed throughout history and remains an urgent public health concern in many countries. In the United States alone, the cost of alcohol and other drug use is estimated to be greater than $240 billion per year (Martin, 2001). According to Janikowski, Cardoso, and Lee (2005), substance use is defined as experimental or casual consumption in which the individual exercises little control, whereas substance abuse is the maladaptive pattern of substance use, including excessive use, compulsions to use, and continued use despite negative consequences. Excessive and prolonged use of substances may result in addiction. Substance dependence is the compulsive use of a substance accompanied by increasing amounts needed to achieve the desired effect, despite negative consequences. Substance abuse and dependence are major national health crises with wide-ranging consequences (Benshoff & Janikowski, 2000; Janikowski et al., 2005). Substance abuse and addiction

F. Chan, Ph.D. (✉)
Department of Rehabilitation Psychology and Special Education, University of Wisconsin—Madison, 1000 Bascom Mall, Room 403, Madison, WI 53706-1326, USA
e-mail: chan@education.wisc.edu

E. Johnson, M.S. • E.K. Hiatt, M.A.
Department of Rehabilitation Psychology and Special Education, University of Wisconsin—Madison, 1000 Bascom Mall, Madison, WI 53706-1326, USA
e-mail: etjohnson6@wisc.edu; ekhiatt@wisc.edu

C.C. Chou, Ph.D.
Department of Disability and Psychoeducational Studies, University of Arizon, 1430 E. Second Street, P.O. Box 210069, Tuscon, AZ 85721, USA
e-mail: chouc@email.arizona.edu

E. da Silva Cardoso, Ph.D.
Department of Educational Foundations and Counseling Programs, Hunter College, City University of New York, 695 Park Ave, New York, NY 10065, USA
e-mail: ecardoso@hunter.cuny.edu

dominate the individual's life, creating problems across the spectrum of physical, psychological, and social functioning (Janikowski et al., 2005). The prevalence rates for illicit drug use, marijuana use, and nonmedical use of a psychotherapeutic drug in the United States are reported to be 8.7, 6.6, and 2.8% respectively (Substance Abuse and Mental Health Services Administration [SAMHSA], 2011).

Both in terms of the general population and people with co-occurring disabilities, substance use significantly impacts life functioning, including employment. Contrary to popular belief, most people who use alcohol or illicit drugs are employed. Illicit drug use (i.e., nonmedical use of cannabis, cocaine, heroin, hallucinogens, inhalants, or prescription medication) differs based on employment status. Of the estimated 19.3 million current illicit drug users, including adults aged 18 or older, 12.9 million (66.6%) are employed either full or part time. Alcohol use also differs based on employment status, such that adults employed full-time (63.9%) are more likely to use alcohol than unemployed adults (58.3%). Furthermore, among 57.4 million adult binge drinkers, 74.4% are employed either full or part time, and among the 16.6 million heavy drinkers in the USA, 74.9% are employed (SAMHSA, 2011).

While it is certainly conceivable that substance use affects workplace performance, the bidirectional relationship between the workplace factors and substance use points to the workplace as an environmental risk factor for substance use. Substance use impairs alertness and reflexes, interferes with accuracy and efficiency, raising the likelihood of serious accidents (Canadian Center for Occupational Health and Safety, 2008). Substance use may also increase absenteeism, affect job performance, and reduce overall productivity. Substance abuse and addiction pose significant treatment challenges for rehabilitation, public health, and occupational health professionals. Theories have been proposed to explain the occurrence and maintenance of addiction in the workplace in spite of its overwhelming negative outcomes. One theory that attempts to explain the phenomenon of substance use is the self-medication hypothesis of substance use (Khantzian, 1999; Khantzian, Mack, & Schatzberg, 1974), and it may be useful for understanding substance use in the workplace.

Self-medication Hypothesis of Alcohol or Illicit Drug Use

Self-medication is a term used to describe the self-soothing use of substances to treat untreated or undiagnosed mental distress, mental illnesses, and/or psychosocial trauma. Self-medication theory was initially based on research specific to heroin use (Khantzian et al., 1974), and was later used to examine properties of cocaine, alcohol, and other substances (Khantzian, 1985). Despite its early roots in psychodynamic theory, the self-medication hypothesis was further explored through the "lens" of behavior theory, with emphases on positive reinforcement and operant conditioning. In recent years, the original self-medication hypothesis has been updated to reflect a more integrated model of self-medication.

Psychodynamic Model

Originating from research conducted by Khantzian et al. (1974), the self-medication hypothesis asserts that substance abuse serves a compensatory function by modulating and soothing the self from unmanageable or distressful psychological states. From a psychodynamic perspective, Khantzian (1977) theorized that drug users compensate for deficient ego function through drug use, in which the drug or "ego solvent" acts on parts of the unconscious self that are blocked by defense mechanisms (Khantzian, 1997). It is hypothesized that drug users experience greater psychiatric distress than nonusers, and substance dependence evolves from the gradual incorporation of the drug effects into the defensive activities of the ego. An individual's choice of drug is based on the interaction of the psychopharmacological properties of the substance and the affective state from which the individual is seeking relief. Therefore, the drug's effects replace the maladaptive or nonexistent ego mechanisms of defense, and the choice of drugs is random (Khantzian, 1985).

Behaviorist Model

Despite its psychodynamic roots, the self-medication hypothesis was also interpreted using a behavioral paradigm proposed by Duncan (1975). Using the behavioral perspective, Duncan described the nature of positive reinforcement (e.g., presence of pleasant sensation), negative reinforcement (e.g., reduction in negative affective states), and avoidance of withdrawal symptoms as the underlying factors of problematic drug use. Duncan's interpretation of the *Self-medication Hypothesis* was a departure from previous behavioral theory in which drug dependence occurred through operant conditioning, and requires both positive and negative forms of reinforcement. Conversely, Duncan posited that only negative reinforcement was required for drug dependence in that drug dependence is an avoidance behavior providing temporary respite from a problem. Therefore, the use of a substance is an operant behavior generated through positive reinforcement (Duncan, 1974). The *Self-medication Hypothesis* demonstrated its adaptability to multiple levels of influence in Duncan's public health model of drug dependence, in which the agent (drug of choice) infects the host (drug user) through a vector (e.g., peers), while the environment supports the disease through stressors and lack of support (Duncan, 1975).

Integrated Model

In recent years, Khantzian revised the *Self-medication Hypothesis* (the Updated Theory) to consider the affective, behavioral, and cognitive components of self-medication (Khantzian & Albanese, 2008). Although concepts of dependence, tolerance, and withdrawal derived from biological models have greatly contributed to our understanding of addiction, biological models are unable to account for factors that lead to relapse after years of sobriety (Khantzian & Albanese, 2008). In updating the *Self-medication Hypothesis*, Khantzian and Albanese (2008) clarify that the self-medication hypothesis is intended only to complement current models of addiction, and it does not represent a substitute for biopsychosocial models of addiction (Khantzian, 1997). Again, the original *Self-medication Hypothesis* posits that an individual uses drugs or alcohol in order regulate emotional processes and achieve stability (Suh, Ruffins, Robins, Albanese, & Khantzian, 2008), whereas Khantzian's Updated Theory identifies the individual's *inability to cope with strong emotions* as the primary motivator for substance use (Hall & Queener, 2007). This updated *Self-medication Hypothesis* has two essential components related to the cause and specificity of addiction.
- The first component posits that addiction is caused by the impact of the drug of choice on alleviating psychological distress. Distress occurs because people are unable to regulate their emotions, sense of self-worth, relationships, or behavior (Khantzian, 1985, 1999; Khantzian & Albanese, 2008).
- The second component attests to the presence of specificity in the individual's drug of choice (Khantzian & Albanese, 2008). In other words, the selected drug of choice is not random, because the individual bases his or her selection on the impact of a certain drug on his or her affective state (Khantzian, 1985, 1999). Therefore, the individual's drug of choice represents an external mechanism for modifying his or her emotions (Hall & Queener, 2007; Khantzian, 1985; Suh et al., 2008). For example, alcohol and sedative drugs may relieve feelings of depression and anxiety (Khantzian, 1997), opiates are hypothesized to be used as a self-medication for aggression and

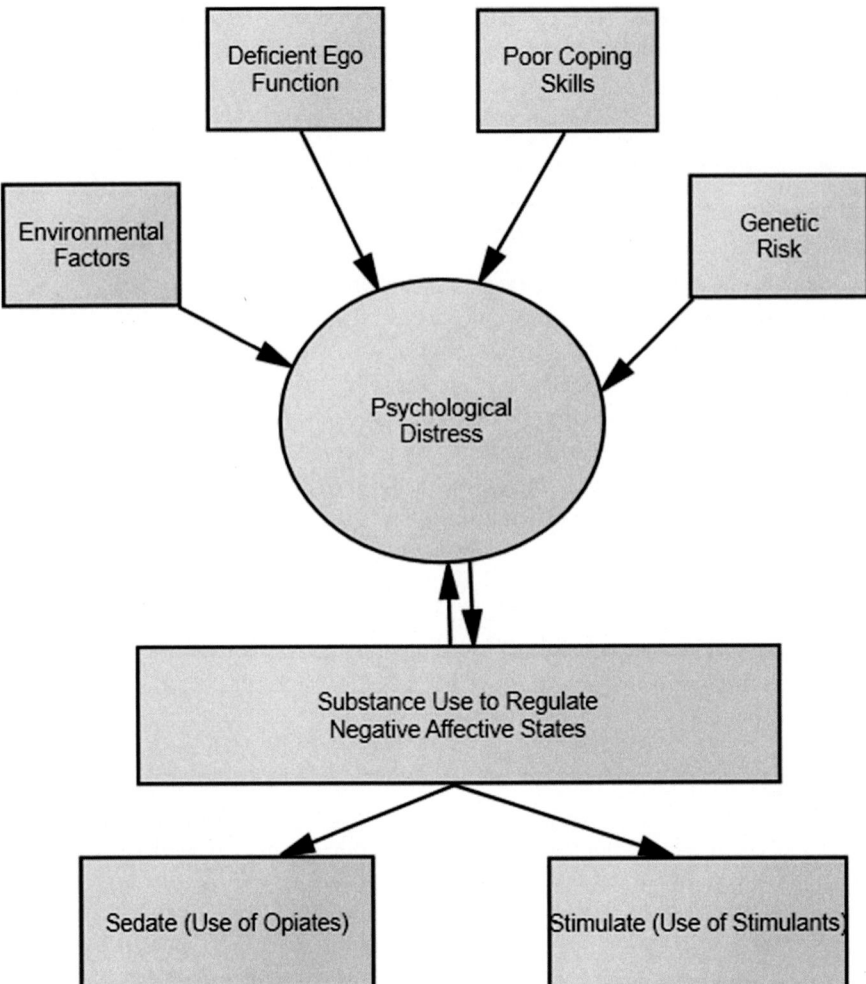

Fig. 10.1 A graphical depiction of the self-medication hypothesis

rage (Khantzian, 1999), and psychostimulants are used by individuals who experience depression in order to reduce anhedonia and increase self-esteem (Khantzian & Albanese, 2008).

Summarizing the integrative perspective, addiction allows an individual to manage his or her affective, behavioral, and cognitive states (Khantzian, 1985; Suh et al., 2008). Khantzian and Albanese (2008) state:

> ... while much has been written about how the widespread availability of addictive drugs, their pleasure-producing effects, and the human proclivity for self-destruction make addiction likely, our clinical experience convincingly demonstrates that the short-term ability of addictive substances to relieve, change or make more tolerable the distress associated with the problems of dysregulated emotions, self-worth, relationships, and behaviors powerfully reinforces dependence on the substance (p. 13).

Furthermore, the problem of using substances to regulate negative emotional states interacts with personal characteristics, genetic vulnerability, and the environment to facilitate addiction. Therefore, the process leading to addiction is not exclusively related to hedonism, pleasure seeking, or destructive tendencies, but are primarily a result of vulnerabilities in the human psyche (Khantzian & Albanese, 2008). Figure 10.1 provides a graphical depiction of the essential elements of the *Self-medication Hypothesis*.

Empirical Evidence

In order to test the *Self-medication Hypothesis*, mental health symptoms that pre-date the onset of substance-use disorders are considered evidence of self-medication. However, empirical evidence supporting the self-medication hypothesis in the clinical and epidemiological literature is less than unequivocal. Kessler et al. (1996) reported that 51% of the participants in the National Comorbidity Study who met criteria for a substance disorder at some time in their life also met criteria for a mental disorder at some point, and in the large majority of cases, individuals reported that the mental disorder preceded the substance disorder. Using a retrospective study design, Suh et al. (2008) used six *Minnesota Multiphasic Personality Inventory-2* (*MMPI-2*) special scales (Repression, Overcontrolled Hostility, Psychomotor Acceleration, Depression, Posttraumatic Stress Disorder, and Cynicism scales) as independent variables to predict drug use in a large sample of drug users and non-drug users ($N=402$). Logistic regression predicted three models defined by "drug of choice." Repression and, inversely, Depression scales significantly predicted the alcohol group. Psychomotor Acceleration was the only significant predictor of the cocaine group. Cynicism significantly predicted the heroin group. The results partially confirmed Khantzian's (1997) clinical observations and demonstrated the relationship between psychological traits and drug of choice. The clinical implications of the findings highlight the relevance of psychodynamic perspectives in understanding drug addiction. The authors note that, in advancing the constructs of the self-medication hypothesis, it will be important to develop assessment tools providing a valid measure of the affective experience specified by the self-medication theory (Suh et al., 2008). Bolton, Cox, Clara, and Sareen (2006) conducted a study of *Self-medication Hypothesis* using a nationally representative sample, and also reported that self-medication is a common occurrence amongst persons diagnosed with anxiety disorders.

Potvin, Sepehry, and Stip (2006) conducted a meta-analysis based on 11 studies ($k=11$; $N=1,135$) to test the self-medication hypothesis in patients with a dual diagnosis of schizophrenia and a substance-abuse disorder, predicated on the assumption that individuals with schizophrenia use psychoactive substances to seek relief from negative symptoms. These investigators found a moderate effect size (Hedges' $g=-0.47$, $p<0.001$), indicating that patients dually diagnosed with schizophrenia and a substance-use disorder experience fewer negative symptoms. The results suggest either substance abuse relieves the negative symptoms of schizophrenia, or patients with fewer negative symptoms would be more prone to substance-use disorders. However, a number of research design problems plagued the various retrospective studies. Specifically, these studies tended to use highly selected samples of patients with advanced substance-use disorders who may have had problems accurately recalling the temporal sequence of the onset of mental health symptoms and substance-use disorders.

More recently, Fergusson, Boden, and Horwood (2009) conducted a prospective study using a longitudinal birth cohort with three repeated measurements, at ages 18, 21, and 25 years, in order to examine causal links between alcohol abuse or dependence and major depression, using structural equation modeling as the method of analysis. These researchers controlled for confounding factors, and the results suggested three possibilities: (a) alcohol abuse caused depression; (b) depression caused alcohol abuse; or (c) alcohol abuse and depression share a reciprocal, causal relationship. However, the structural model with causal pathways leading from alcohol abuse to depression provided a better fit to the data than either alternative models (i.e., the depression led to alcohol abuse model or the reciprocal model). Therefore, Fergusson et al. concluded that while alcohol abuse played a causal role in increasing risks of depression, depression did not necessarily cause alcohol abuse. Similarly, Hall and Queener (2007) assessed anxiety, depression, hostility, and alexithymia levels in 70 methadone maintenance treatment patients to test Khantzian's Updated Theory, and they were unable to establish a causal link between negative affective states and substance use. They concluded that evidence does not support the hypothesized causal relationship between negative and ambiguous affective states and substance use.

Finally, Boden and Fergusson (2011) conducted a meta-analytic study to examine the associations between alcohol use disorders and major depression, and to also evaluate the evidence for the existence of a causal relationship between the disorders. Specifically, the study examined the potential causal relationships that may be present in the association between alcohol use disorders and major depression: (a) alcohol use disorders causes major depression; (b) major depression causes alcohol use disorders (i.e., the "self-medication" hypothesis); and (c) a reciprocal causal relationship exists between alcohol use disorders and major depression, such that each disorder increases the risk of the other disorder simultaneously. The authors found that the presence of either disorder doubled the risks of the second disorder, with pooled adjusted odds ratios ranging from 2.00 to 2.09. Importantly, the data supported a causal linkage between alcohol use disorders and major depression, such that increasing involvement with alcohol increases risk of depression and not vice versa. Because a number of studies have shown that treatment of alcohol use disorders results in a reduction of major depression symptoms, Boden and Fergusson recommend that treatment of major depression should include assessment and treatment of alcohol use disorders. Conversely, for individuals who reported using alcohol to self-medicate symptoms of depression, a combination of treatments for alcohol use disorders and major depression may be warranted.

The Work-Stress Paradigm of Self-medication

As mentioned earlier, substance use can affect the workplace. The *Self-medication Hypothesis* suggests that people use alcohol or illicit drugs to cope with untreated or undiagnosed mental distress and drug use behavior may continue into the workplace, thus affecting work performance. However, with globalization, business organizations are placing a strong emphasis on maximizing productivity and efficiency, reducing costs, and enhancing product quality to remain competitive in a global market, leading to increasingly stressful work environments (Noonan & Wagner, 2010). In the context of work, stress can be defined as physical and psychosocial response that occurs when the requirements and/or conditions of the workplace are not aligned with the worker's capabilities, resources, or needs (National Institute for Occupational Health and Safety, 1999). From the *Self-medication Hypothesis* perspective, a stressful workplace may cause psychosocial distress which, in turn, leads to alcohol or illicit drug use, particularly for individuals with problems regulating negative emotions.

Frone (1999) reviewed four basic work-stress paradigm models to examine the relationship between work stress and alcohol use, although these models may be adapted and applied to other substances as well. The models include the (a) simple cause–effect model, (b) meditation model, (c) moderation model, and (d) moderated mediation model. In the simple cause and effect model, there is a simple direct relationship between work stress and substance use, with mixed empirical findings. This model is limited because of the simple premise that work stressors may cause substance use without the influence of intervening variables.

In the mediation model, variables are proposed to link work stressors and substance use, including job dissatisfaction, negative affect, and coping strategies. This model is useful because it attempts to explain the underlying mechanism by which work stressors relate to substance use. According to Frone (1999), empirical support for this model of employee alcohol use indicated the relationship between certain work stressors and alcohol use, and that they are also mediated by anxiety level (Vasse, Nijhuis, & Kok, 1998), negative affect (Martin, Roman, & Blum, 1996), and job dissatisfaction (Greenberg & Grunberg, 1995).

In the moderation model, work stressors interact with other variables that inhibit or facilitate substance use among employees. In other words, the relationship between alcohol use and work stressors differs as a function of the moderating variable(s). Frone (1999) cites empirical evidence for the following moderators leading to increased alcohol use: (a) high psychological importance of work to self-definition (Frone, Russell, & Cooer, 1997), (b) alcohol use as a coping strategy to relax and forget about problems (Grunberg, Moore, Anderson-Connolly, & Greenberg, 1999), and (c) traditional gender-role attitudes for women and egalitarian gender-roles for men (Parker & Harford, 1992).

In the moderated meditation model, there is an explanation of how and when work stressors impact substance use. This model is based on the assumption that work stressors are positively related to job dissatisfaction, which is positively related to alcohol use in persons who are vulnerable to relapse (Cooper, Russell, & Frone, 1990; Grunberg, Moore, & Greenberg, 1998).

Frone (1999) proposed a conceptual model entitled the *Work-Stress Paradigm*, which theorized that risky health behavior, such as substance use, occurs because of aversive work conditions, heavy work load, job insecurity, alienation, interpersonal conflict with fellow employees and/or supervisors, and unfair processes regarding pay, benefits, and promotion. Importantly, work alienation, which has typically been studied as a paradigm apart from work stress (Trice & Sonnenstuhl, 1990), relates to work characteristics that lead to job dissatisfaction, including minimally skilled jobs and employees having little to no control in workplace decision making. Work-related stressors also occur when work-related demands interfere with other aspects of life, specifically work–family conflict (Frone, 1999).

In addition to the inability to manage work-related stress with appropriate regulation of negative emotions, lacking a repertoire of positive coping responses may also lead to alcohol or illicit drug use in the workplace. Bandura's (1969) coping deficits model of alcohol use proposed that persons consumed alcohol to reduce stress because alternative coping skills were not available (Colder, 2001). Considering the limitations of applying coping models in examining work stress and substance use among employees, Grunberg et al. (1998) present a modified model linking specific job stressors (changes in benefits, conditions, skills, and/or safety; work demands, job insecurity, criticism, support, and feeling stuck) to alcohol use (heavy drinking and negative consequences), while job satisfaction and coping reasons for drinking mediate the relationship. They found that coping reasons for drinking were significantly associated with heavy alcohol use ($r=0.29$) and negative consequences to drinking ($r=0.50$).

Another model related to adverse coping mechanisms in the workforce is the spillover or generalization model (Cooper, 1983; Martin, 1990; Martin, Blum, & Roman, 1992), which contends that "individuals do not or cannot compartmentalize their lives; that negative characteristics of jobs not only create stressful emotional, mental, and physical states within the worker, but also that such stressful conditions will extend beyond the workday into the individual's non-work life" and "negative or stressful job characteristics might result in both negative work and non-work outcomes" (Grunberg et al., 1998, p. 487). Rather than utilizing positive coping strategies (e.g., exercise, hobbies, etc.), substance use becomes the primary coping mechanism for stress. According to the *Self-medication Hypothesis*, people use alcohol or illicit drugs to self-soothe from unmanageable or distressful psychological states. However, these problems in self-regulation interact with personal characteristics, genetic vulnerability, and the environment to facilitate addiction.

Due to the workplace being the primary social atmosphere in which most employed people spend a large majority of time, understanding substance use within the context of the workplace is distinct and based on the boundaries the environment imposes via workplace rules and/or cultural norms (Ames & Grube, 1997). Within the cultural paradigm, these rules and/or cultural norms may either facilitate or inhibit substance use (Ames & Grube, 1997). With regard to alcohol consumption, workplace-drinking groups have served as a group response to certain job conditions such as repetitive tasks, overtime, and shift work (Ames & Grube, 1997). Furthermore, alcohol use may reflect union solidarity or serve as a celebratory function, such as payday, holiday weekends, or the ending of the workday and/or week (Ames & Grube, 1997).

Within the availability paradigm, social and physical factors of alcoholic substances may explain the difference in alcohol use among employees, as previous research identified availability as an overall correlate of alcohol consumption (Ames & Grube, 1997). However, few studies examine the role of social and physical availability on work-related alcohol use. Of the few studies focusing on availability, ethnographic studies reveal social and physical availability as a major influence in developing and maintaining patterns and networks in work-related alcohol consumption. The general availability theory suggests the social and physical availability of alcohol increases its use and problems associated with usage (Ames & Grube, 1997).

Physical availability is "the extent to which there is access to alcohol in a given environment and to the barriers or costs associated with obtaining it" (Ames & Grube, 1997, p. 383). Thus, in the work context, physical availability of alcohol can be defined as "the ease or difficulty with which an individual can obtain alcohol for work-related consumption" including "obtaining alcohol on or near the work premises and at work-related events, polices and rules against brining alcohol into a work setting or obtaining it at work, and the degree to which such policies can be enforced" (p. 384). Objective physical availability is defined as "the actual legal, or organizational and geographical factors that affect the costs of acquiring alcohol" (p. 383), and it relates to "the extent to which such elements actually exist in the workplace" (p. 383). Subjective physical availability is defined as "the belief about the ease or difficulty of obtaining alcohol" (p. 383). In the work context, subjective physical availability relates to "perceptions or beliefs about how difficult it is to obtain and consume alcohol in work-related contexts" (p. 384).

Social availability is defined as "the degree of normative support for drinking within one's social environments" (Ames & Grube, 1997, p. 383). In the work context, social availability refers to the "normative support for work-related drinking within one's work environment" including two dimensions: (a) frequency of use among friends and coworkers, and (b) (dis)approval by coworkers and superiors. Objective social availability is defined as the actual drinking and approval of drinking by family, friends, and others, while subjective social availability is defined as perceptions of drinking norms in a given environment (Ames & Grube). In the work context, objective social availability relates to "the actual presence of drinking and approval in the work environment" (p. 384); and subjective social availability relates to the "individual's perceptions of work-related drinking patterns of his or her coworkers and work friends, and perceptions of the extent to which friends, coworkers and supervisors approve or disapprove of his or her drinking" (p. 384). Therefore, within Frone's (1999) work-stress paradigm of self-medication in the workplace, the work culture may interact with work stress to affect illicit drug use in the workplace. The physical and social availability variables are therefore important moderator variables between stress and illicit drug use in the workplace. Table 10.1 provides a summary of the work-stress paradigm models discussed in this section.

Empirical Evidence

Wiesner, Windle, and Freeman (2005) conducted a cross-sectional study evaluating the relationship between work stress, alcohol and drug use, and depression in a sample of 583 young adult workers. Their findings de-emphasized direct relationships between work stress and drug/alcohol use, and instead emphasized the moderating relationships of job demands and gender. Young adult workers in low skilled variety jobs were 1.85 times more likely to experience depressive symptoms, and were also 2.07 times more likely to be heavy alcohol users (Wiesner et al., 2005). The explanation that the inability of young unskilled workers to regulate negative emotions resulting from the stress of monotonous job tasks, thereby leading to substance use, provides support for the work-stress paradigm of self-medication. In terms of moderating effects, there was a significant association between low skill

10 Self-medication and Illicit Drug Use in the Workplace

Table 10.1 Work-stress paradigms of self-medication

Model	Root cause of substance abuse
Simple cause–effect model	Work stressors
Mediation model	Underlying mechanisms (e.g., job dissatisfaction, negative effect, and coping skills) mediate work stressors effect on substance use
Moderation model	Work stressors interact with moderator variables (i.e., protective and/or vulnerability factors) that inhibit or facilitate substance use among employees
Moderated mediation model	Job dissatisfaction mediates the effect of work stressors while vulnerability factors moderate alcohol use in persons at risk
Work stress model	Work stressors and/or aversive work conditions (i.e., heavy work load) result in substance use
Coping deficits model	Substance use acts as a coping mechanism for stress, and may be accessed due to lack of knowledge of alternative coping skills
Spillover or generalization model	Substance use acts as a coping mechanism enabling the individual to manage the impact of work stressors on work and non-work activities (i.e., home life)
Cultural model	Workplace culture may facilitate or inhibit substance use
Availability model	Social availability (i.e., actual or perceived support of substance use) and physical availability (i.e., actual or perceived access to substances) increase likelihood of substance use

variety jobs and heavy alcohol use by gender such that men were at a 2.81 greater risk to be heavy alcohol users. When considering high workload, men were 6.1 times less likely to be heavy drug users. As a protective factor, persons with a high workload and low intrinsic work motivation were at a 0.61 lower risk for being heavy drug users.

Using interview data from 984 employees of a manufacturing plant, Ames and Grube (1997) tested a model that accounted for demographic variables and alcohol use outside of work, in which work-related alcohol consumption increased as a direct increase of (a) subjective physical availability of alcohol at work, (b) perceived approval of alcohol use by others, and (c) perceived alcohol use by others at work. Of the 984 employees, 23% reported drinking at work at least once, and 43% of those reported having two or more drinks. The model was able to predict drinking at work ($R^2=0.42$) and perceived work-related drinking by others ($R^2=0.29$). The model accounted for variance caused by several factors, such as (a) drinking before work (21%), (b) subjective physical availability (20%), (c) perceived approval of work-related drinking by others (36%), (d) belief about best friend's work-related drinking (15%), and the (e) combined demographics of age (younger), religiosity (less), and gender (male), such that younger, less religious men were 20% more likely to use alcohol in the workplace. Testing of the model revealed that the strongest predictor of work-related alcohol use was subjective social availability at work ($R^2=0.20$), specifically, beliefs about alcohol use among coworkers and other friends at work ($R^2=0.36$). Importantly, physical availability of alcohol was not significantly related to alcohol use in this study.

Substance-Abuse Interventions in the Workplace

Screening

The *Self-medication Hypothesis* offers several reasons for alcohol and illicit drug use in the workplace. People with difficulty regulating negative emotions use alcohol or illicit drugs to treat untreated or undiagnosed mental distress, and substance-use behavior may infiltrate the workplace. Similarly, individuals with severe mental illnesses, such as schizophrenia, use alcohol or illicit drugs to relieve psychiatric symptoms. Therefore, timely screening and treatment of mental health problems in the workplace may prevent the development of substance-use disorders, particularly among workers vulnerable to mental health problems because of poor ability to regulate negative emotions or a deficiency in positive coping resources and responses (Harris & Edlund, 2005).

Stress Reduction

Changes in the modern workplace and increasing globalization have led to greater job insecurity, causing the workplace to become an increasingly stressful place. Stress in the workplace can cause significant psychosocial distress, which may lead to alcohol or illicit drug use. Depression is responsible for the largest portions of short- and long-term disability claims (Noonan & Wagner, 2010). Employees receiving treatment for depression are twice as likely to use short-term disability, relative to coworkers who have never been treated for mental health issues. In addition, disability-related costs were $1,038 for workers receiving treatment for depression, but averaged a mere $325 per year for employees not diagnosed and being treated for depression (Birnbaum et al., 2010). Therefore, occupational stress management and accommodation for workers experiencing related mental health issues may be necessary in the prevention and management of alcohol and illicit drug use problems in the workplace.

Workplace stress is determined by multiple, interactive factors. Noonan and Wagner (2010) identified many major determinants of workplace stress—job control, job strain, job complexity, lack of variety in work, lack of use for employee skills, amount of control/decision latitude, physical work environment, workload and pace, role ambiguity, social support, hours of work, and shift-work. In addition, employees tend to experience high levels of strain when the organization goals are ambiguous and resources are inadequate and inappropriate to meet organization goals (Noonan & Wagner, 2010). Psychosocial adjustment in the workplace may be affected by interactive factors, such as the employees' tendency to react negatively to stress and the presence of job-specific and organizational level stressors.

According to Lazarus and Folkman's (1984) model of stress, appraisal, and coping, coping serves a mediating function between situational appraisals, the person-environmental relationship, and emotional response (Folkman & Lazarus, 1988). Appraisal represents a two-stage process that consists of primary and secondary appraisals (Lazarus & Folkman, 1984). Primary appraisals involve assessing the meaning of an event and determining what is at stake for the individual (Franks & Roesch, 2006); secondary appraisal involves determining the stressfulness of a situation in terms of the harm/loss, threat, or challenge the situation will produce. The coping process involves a primary appraisal (i.e., whether the event is harmful/loss, a threat, or a challenge), a secondary appraisal (i.e., generating potential responses), and the coping response. Two common dimensions to these models include emotion-focused coping, in which the coping is directed to a person, and problem-focused coping, in which coping is more situation-focused (Endler & Parker, 1990). Problem-solving coping has been reported to be particularly effective in reducing stress associated with role ambiguity, workload, and lack of resources (Noonan & Wagner, 2010), whereas emotional-coping was found to be a moderator between stress and alcohol use (Veenstra et al., 2007).

Noonan and Wagner (2010) recommended that stress management initiatives should be contextual, considering the needs and sources of stress-related problems at both the individual and organizational level. For example, if it is the work environment that contributes to significant psychosocial strain, then implementing changes to redesign tasks, altering the organizational structure, improving communication, or improving worker autonomy can reduce stress and improve organizational health and the well-being of employees. Health promotion and wellness efforts are directed at reducing the specific sources of stress within the context of the physical, social, and organizational environment (Noblet, 2003). At the individual level, the goals of stress management interventions can be to improve employee resilience, improve coping abilities, and empower the employee to take more personal control in managing workplace stress by providing employees with training in time management, coping, assertiveness, cognitive restructuring, relaxation, meditation, and physical fitness. Enhancing social support in the workplace is also an important stress-reduction strategy. Companies can help employees reduce occupational stress by helping them develop conflict resolution skills, identify supportive resources available, engage in team building activities, participate in formal and/or informal workplace support groups, and find a mentor can foster social support within the work setting. Stress reduction interventions may be particularly important for employees with characteristics of negative affectivity who are prone to experience psychological distress in a stressful work environment. Many of these approaches have been discussed in other chapters of this handbook.

Psychosocial Treatment

If negative affective states lead to alcohol and illicit drug use in the workplace, early screening and treating employees with mental health issues (such as depression and anxiety) may reduce substance-abuse problems in the workplace. There is strong evidence to support that the combined use of antidepressant medication and counseling/psychotherapy is superior in reducing depressive symptoms than either treatment alone (Scott, 2001; The Treatment for Adolescents with Depression Study Team, 2004). In a recent study, Zobel et al. (2011) examined the long-term benefits of combined pharmacological and psychotherapeutic depression treatment in 124 in-patients with a diagnosis of major depressive disorder. They randomly assigned the patients to a 5-week interpersonal psychotherapy plus pharmacotherapy (IPT) group, or a medication plus clinical management (CM) group. Results indicated that patients in both treatment groups significantly reduced depressive symptoms between baseline and 5-year follow-up, with a sharper reduction early in the follow-up phase. The rate and acceleration of change in depression was greater for patients in the combination therapy group. Also, 28% of the IPT patients showed a sustained remission compared with 11% of the CM patients ($p<0.05$). They concluded that, in the long-term, a combination of psycho- and pharmacotherapy was superior in terms of sustained remission rates, relative to standard psychiatric treatment. Early trauma was also found to be a moderator of the relationship between treatment and outcomes, and it should be assessed routinely in depressed patients.

The relationship between employee use of antidepressants and absenteeism has also been examined in employees diagnosed with clinical depression. Birnbaum and his associates (2010) studied the effect of antidepressant treatment between compliant and noncompliant comparison groups. While medical costs were similar between compliant and noncompliant patients, drug costs were higher for compliant patients due to the cost of antidepressants. However, costs associated with employee absenteeism were lower for those compliant with antidepressant use ($3,857 vs. $4,907, $p<0.05$), and absenteeism costs were also lower among depressed patients ($3,976 vs. $5,899, $p=0.047$). Conversely, presenteeism costs were greater for depressed patients whom were compliant with antidepressant use ($19,170 vs. $15,829, $p<0.05$). In summary, findings indicate an interaction between compliance and diagnosis of depression, such that increased compliance with antidepressants is significantly associated with reduced absenteeism costs in employees diagnosed with clinical depression.

Given the relationship between employee mental health and workplace productivity, Lerner et al. (2012) evaluated the efficacy of a work-focused intervention aimed at treating employees with depression. The intervention was comprised of three components, including (a) work coaching and modification interventions to accommodate specific job performance difficulties related to depression, (b) coordination of care between the employee and his or her primary care physician (PCP) or other prescribing professional to promote adherence to pharmacotherapy and the use of evidence-based depression treatment, and (c) cognitive-behavioral therapy strategies to facilitate behavioral change and modification of cognitive distortions that may interfere with functioning and job performance. Compared to the control group who did not receive the work-focused intervention, participants in the intervention group demonstrated significant improvement in all outcome measures, including subscale scores on the *Work Limitations Questionnaire* (time management, performance of physical tasks, performance of mental-interpersonal tasks, and performance of output tasks), productivity loss scores, a measure of work absence, and productivity loss due to absence. The unadjusted mean at-work productivity cost savings for the treatment group was $1,182.70 annually per participant, as compared to $96.10 annually for usual care. In terms of absences, the unadjusted mean savings was $2,395.90 annually per participant in the treatment group, whereas members of the control group averaged an annual cost increase of $3043.30. The total unadjusted mean productivity cost savings for the treatment group was $3,578.60 annually per participant, as compared to an annual cost increase of $2,947.20 per participant in usual care.

In summary, the above research concludes that factors of early screening and treatment, treatment adherence, interventions that combine psychotherapy and pharmacotherapy, job accommodation, and workplace support are most important to the effective treatment of mental health problems in the workplace.

Substance-Abuse Treatment

The *Self-medication Hypothesis* is intended to complement current models of addiction, and it does not represent a substitute for more comprehensive biopsychosocial models of addiction (Khantzian & Albanese, 2008). Therefore, treatment of substance abuse in the workplace must employ a multidimensional approach. Factors specific to the workplace environment, such as physical availability of substances and social acceptance of substance use, can contribute to alcohol or illicit drug use. For many work organizations, an important strategy for minimizing alcohol problems among employees is the establishment and enforcement of policies addressing alcohol use in the workplace. Workplace policies have the potential to alter the workplace culture or other social environments that support substance use in the workplace. At the individual level, several treatment modalities are widely employed to achieve rehabilitation, and new treatment programs are frequently being developed and modified to best meet client needs (Cardoso, Wolfe, & West, 2009). For instance, behavioral couple therapy is one approach to substance abuse that emphasizes the interaction between the person abusing substances and his or her partner as a key component of sobriety and abstinence (Longabaugh et al., 2005). Another treatment modality is alcohol behavioral couple therapy (ABCT), in which both parties, the alcohol-dependent patient and his or her partner, participate in therapy. ABCT derives its underlying theoretical framework from cognitive-behavioral theory, social–interpersonal systems, and social exchange models of intimate relationships. Therapy focuses on developing mutual awareness of high-risk situations, such as fighting with a significant other, that can lead to alcohol use.

Motivational interviewing (MI) addresses alcohol and substance use through directive client-centered counseling that is aimed at eliciting behavioral change by supporting clients in exploring the substance abuse, resolving ambivalence that a problem exists, and empowering the individual in accepting responsibility for change and avoiding confrontations that lead to negative outcomes (Bombardier, 2000; Mendel & Hipkins, 2002; Prochaska & Diclementi, 1986). There is evidence that patients receiving MI demonstrate greater participation in treatment and are more likely to reduce their substance use when compared to patients who do not receive MI (Hettema, Steele, & Miller, 2005). Motivational interviewing has also been examined as an intervention in group therapy settings (Santa Ana, Wulfert, & Nietert, 2007), and researchers have examined the outcomes of group MI (GMI) in work with patients who had coexisting diagnoses of substance abuse and psychiatric disability. Individuals with dual diagnoses tend to exhibit high rates of noncompliance and frequently fail to follow through with aftercare treatment following discharge from inpatient settings. Individuals with dual diagnoses of substance abuse and psychiatric disability are two times as likely to use illicit drugs when compared to persons without a dual diagnosis (Lemaire, Mallik, & Rever, 2004). When applied to individuals with coexisting substance abuse and psychiatric disability, research suggests that GMI results in greater treatment participation and reduced substance use when compared to patients who did not receive GMI.

Contingency management (CM) is an alternate treatment modality, and it has received considerable attention in recent years. Derived from behavioral theory, CM is a type of operant conditioning that uses reinforcement to reduce or eliminate drug use (Higgins et al., 1994), according to the assumption that behavior is controlled or shaped by the consequences of the behavior. Because substance use is heavily influenced by the context in which it occurs, alternative non-drug reinforcement tends to decrease substance use if the rewards are available and used in a manner not compatible with drug use. There are various types of CM, including voucher-based reinforcement therapy (VBRT), in which patients receive vouchers rewarding biological samples (e.g., urine, breath) negative for substances (indicating that the client has remained abstinent of substances). Once earned, vouchers may be exchanged for goods and services compatible with a drug-free lifestyle, and the value of vouchers may increase with continued abstinence and repeated negative findings in biological samples. Conversely, vouchers are withheld if the biological sample is not submitted, or if the sample yields a positive result, confirming the presence of substances in the bloodstream, indicative of recent substance use (Prendergast, Podus, Finney, Greenwell, & Roll, 2006). An alternate CM program employs variable-magnitude of reinforcement procedures. Similar to the voucher system, this system requires the patient to draw a random number corresponding to a reward. Patients who test positive for substances are not afforded the opportunity to draw a number, whereas patients who test negative for drug use are permitted to select a random number and obtain the corresponding reward. Rewards range in cash value; and the value of a draw increases as long as the person remains abstinent from all substances. In some cases, regular drug testing may represent a condition for treatment (Prendergast et al., 2006).

In their synthesis of the CM literature, Prendergast et al. (2006) conducted a meta-analysis of three CM approaches: (a) voucher-based programs, (b) draws, and (c) take-home doses of methadone or cash. Aggregate findings support the effectiveness of various CM techniques when used during standard treatment programs for dependence on alcohol, tobacco, or illicit drugs. The effect of CM decreases following removal of reinforcement, but the reduction in effect takes place over an extended period of time, allowing the person to continue treatment for longer periods of time while abstinent and motivated to function without drugs.

Another option for employees is self-help groups. Although self-help is not considered a professional treatment per se, self-help groups are ubiquitous and are frequently identified as an adjunctive component to substance-abuse treatment. Self-help groups often reflect the disease model of addiction and are coupled with the 12-steps of recovery, developed by the founding members of Alcoholics' Anonymous (AA). The success of AA has fostered the development of other self-help groups based on the 12-step program, including Narcotics Anonymous (NA) and Cocaine Anonymous (CA). The first step in the sequential process of recovery requires that the individual recognize that he or she is powerless over substances. Individuals complete the twelfth and final step upon recognition of a "spiritual awakening." According to the principles of AA, abstinence from substances is maintained long-term through sharing one's story of addiction and spreading this message to other alcoholics.

Another treatment option involves inpatient treatment programs that typically follow a disease model of addiction and emphasizes 12-steps to recovery (Budziack, 1993). Inpatient treatment may take place in a medical or community setting. Inpatient programs in the medical setting are housed in a hospital or medical center, and they provide continuous nursing care and direct physician supervision of treatment. Alternatively, inpatient or freestanding programs offer inpatient treatment in a community-based setting with lower levels of direct medical care. Community-based inpatient programs are more appropriate for clients without co-occurring medical conditions, and they can be treated less expensively in the community as opposed to the medical setting. One advantage of inpatient care is interruption of the pattern of use and removal of environmental triggers that tend to increase use. A challenge inherent to inpatient programs lies in generalizing treatment gains to the post-discharge environment, because patients often return to an environment with powerful triggers for drug use.

Similar to inpatient treatment, therapeutic communities require the patient's full-time residence on-site. Based on social learning theory, therapeutic communities emphasize prevention, skills training, self-help, client responsibility, in addition to two principles unique to therapeutic community philosophy: credible role models and community building (Wexler, Magura, Beardsley, & Josepher, 1994). Building on social skills and natural supports, cognitive-behavioral training is employed during self-help groups, and behavioral skills training is aimed at overcoming social anxieties, interpreting nonverbal cues, and anger management (Egelko & Galanter, 1993). The integrated, multimodal approach employed among therapeutic communities empowers members in the formation of one's self-help concept. Therapeutic communities have been shown to foster a sense of safety and structure in addition to a supportive environment. Research findings suggest that therapeutic communities foster confrontation during reality therapy, which may ultimately benefit reasoning and abstract thought (Bratter, Bratter, Radda, & Steiner, 1993).

Although intensive outpatient treatment programs do not require residence, sessions typically entail 4 h of treatment activities per day, 4 days per week for 4 weeks, and are also known as $4 \times 4 \times 4$ programs. Outpatient treatment tends to be more problem-focused and employs abbreviated versions of the treatment schedules used in inpatient programs. Importantly, intensive outpatient programs are less expensive than inpatient programs and are often reported to be less intrusive and less stigmatizing.

Conclusions and Future Directions

Both in terms of the general population and people with co-occurring disabilities, substance abuse and addiction create problems across the spectrum of physical, psychological, and social functioning, including employment (Janikowski et al., 2005), and the majority of individuals using substances are employed (SAMHSA, 2011). In the workplace setting, substance use impairs alertness and reflexes, interferes with accuracy and efficiency, and increases the likelihood of serious accidents (Canadian Center for Occupational Health and Safety, 2008). Moreover, substance use increases absenteeism, reduces productivity, and negatively affects job performance. Employing the integrative perspective, addiction allows an individual to manage his or her affective, behavioral, and cognitive states (Khantzian, 1985; Suh et al., 2008).

The Self-medication Hypothesis suggests that people use alcohol or illicit drugs in an attempt to treat mental distress, generally distress that has gone untreated or undiagnosed, and drug use behavior may continue into the workplace, thus affecting work performance. In addition, workplace stress may lead to psychosocial distress, resulting in alcohol or illicit drug use, particularly for individuals with problems regulating negative emotion (Khantzian, 1999, 1974). When the psychodynamic roots of the Self-medication Hypothesis were challenged by the onset of behaviorism and subsequent focus on reinforcement, Khantzian offered his Updated Theory in which addiction is caused by the impact of the drug of choice on alleviating psychological distress. Distress occurs because people are unable to regulate their emotions, sense of self-worth, relationships, or behavior (Khantzian, 1985, 1999; Khantzian & Albanese, 2008). The second component asserts the selected drug of choice is not random, and selection is based on the impact of a certain drug on his or her affective state (Khantzian, 1985, 1999). Therefore, the individual's drug of choice represents an external mechanism for modifying his or her emotions (Hall & Queener, 2007; Khantzian, 1985; Suh et al., 2008).

Empirical evidence supporting the self-medication hypothesis in the clinical and epidemiological literature is less than unequivocal. There is evidence to support the association between personality traits and drug-of-choice (Khantzian, 1997). Most importantly, in order to address substance abuse in the workplace, organizations must recognize the impact of environmental risk factors inherent in the work setting, such as a physical and social availability of substances.

Research on coping and the work-stress relationship find employee's coping abilities and response to work stress are associated with substance use. Environmental and personal variables interact to affect psychosocial adjustment in the workplace. For example, the employees' tendency to react negatively to stress, combined with the presence of job-specific and organizational level stressors may increase likelihood of substance use. In addition, individual coping style predicts stress-reduction, such that individuals who demonstrate problem-solving coping tend to be more effective in reducing stress associated with role ambiguity, workload, and lack of resources (Noonan & Wagner, 2010). Conversely, emotional-coping was found to moderate the relationship between stress and alcohol use (Veenstra et al., 2007).

Intervention methods vary widely, frequently hinging on a specific theoretical orientation of behavioral change. Programs of CM are based on behavioral principles of positive and negative reinforcement, whereas interactional theory guides couples therapy in examining patterns of use in the context of the relationship. Psychosocial treatment is distinct in its integrative, multimodal approach, particularly among the integrative, multimodal approaches of psychosocial treatment and therapeutic communities.

In recent years, the original self-medication hypothesis has been updated to reflect a more integrated model of self-medication, while remaining adaptable to the parameters of a variety of rehabilitation settings, including inpatient, intensive outpatient, and community-based programs. While, the outpatient treatment tends to be more problem-focused, employing abbreviated treatment schedules not unlike those of inpatient programs. Most importantly, treatment services must remain available and accessible to those with substance-use disorders, and given the lower expense when compared to inpatient programs, intensive outpatient programs have great potential for growth. Furthermore, integrative, multimodal approaches to treatment, such as intensive outpatient programs, are often reported to be less intrusive and less stigmatizing than inpatient programs.

Acknowledgments The contents of this chapter were developed with support through the Rehabilitation Research and Training Center on Effective Vocational Rehabilitation Service Delivery Practices established at both the University of Wisconsin-Madison and the University of Wisconsin-Stout under a grant from the Department of Education, National Institute on Disability and Rehabilitation Research (NIDRR) grant number PR# H133B100034. However, these contents do not necessarily represent the policy of the US Department of Education, and endorsement by the Federal Government should not be assumed.

References

Ames, G. M., & Grube, J. W. (1997). Alcohol availability and workplace drinking: Mixed method analyses. *Journal of Studies on Alcohol, 60*, 383–393.

Bandura, A. (1969). *Principles of behavior modification*. New York, NY: Holt, Rinehart, & Winston.

Benshoff, J. J., & Janikowski, T. P. (2000). *The rehabilitation model of substance abuse counseling*. Belmont, CA: Brooks/Cole.

Birnbaum, H. G., Ben-Hamadi, R., Kelley, D., Hsieh, M., Seal, B., Kantor, E. et al. (2010). Assessing the relationship between compliance with antidepressant therapy and employer costs among employees in the United States. *Journal of Occupation and Environmental Medicine, 52*, 115–124.

Boden, J. M., & Fergusson, D. M. (2011). Alcohol and depression. *Addiction, 106*, 906–914.

Bolton, J., Cox, B., Clara, I., & Sareen, J. (2006). Use of alcohol and drugs to self-medicate anxiety disorders in a nationally representative sample. *Journal of Nervous & Mental Disease, 194*(11), 818–826.

Bombardier, C. (2000). Addressing the needs of clients with traumatic injury and alcoholism. In A. Cohen (Ed.), *Directions in substance abuse counseling*. New York, NY: Hatherleigh.

Bratter, B. I., Bratter, T. E., Radda, H. T., & Steiner, K. M. (1993). The residential therapeutic caring community. Special issue: Psychotherapy for the addictions. *Psychotherapy, 30*(2), 299–304.

Budziack, T. J. (1993). Evaluating treatment services. In A. W. Heinemann (Ed.), *Substance abuse and physical disability* (pp. 239–255). Binghamton, NY: The Haworth Press.

Canadian Center for Occupational Health and Safety. (2008). *Substance abuse in the workplace*. Hamilton, Ontario, Canada: Author.

Cardoso, E., Wolf, A. W., & West, S. L. (2009). Substance abuse: Models, assessment, and interventions. In F. Chan, E. Cardoso, & J. Chronister (Eds.), *Psychosocial interventions for people with chronic illness and disability. A handbook for evidenced based rehabilitation health professionals* (pp. 399–434) New York: Springer Publishing Company.

Colder, C. R. (2001). Life stress, physiological and subjective indexes of negative emotionality, and coping reasons for drinking: Is there evidence for a self-medication model of alcohol use. *Psychology of Addictive Behaviors, 15*(3), 237–245.

Cooper, C. L. (1983). Identifying stressors at work: Recent research developments. *Journal of Psychosomatic Research, 27*, 369–376.

Cooper, M. L., Russell, M., & Frone, M. R. (1990). Work stress and alcohol effects: A test of stress-induced drinking. *Journal of Health & Social Behavior, 31*, 260–276.

Duncan, D. F. (1974). Reinforcement of drug abuse: Implications for prevention. *Clinical Toxicology Bulletin, 4*, 69–75.

Duncan, D. F. (1975). The acquisition, maintenance and treatment of polydrug dependence: A public health model. *Journal of Psychedelic Drugs, 7*, 209–213.

Egelko, S., & Galanter, M. (1993). Introducing cognitive-behavioral training into a self-help drug treatment program. Special issue. *Psychotherapy, 30*(2), 214–221.

Endler, N. S., & Parker, J. D. A. (1990). Multidimensional assessment of coping: A critical evaluation. *Journal of Personality and Social Psychology, 58*, 844–854.

Fergusson, D. M., Boden, J. M., & Horwood, J. J. (2009). Tests of causal links between alcohol abuse or dependence and major depression. *Archives of General Psychiatry, 66*, 260–266.

Folkman, S., & Lazarus, R. S. (1988). *Manual for the ways of coping questionnaire*. Palo Alto, CA: Consulting Psychologist Press.

Franks, H. M., & Roesch, S. C. (2006). Appraisals and coping in people living with cancer: A meta-analysis. *Psycho-Oncology, 15*, 1027–1037.

Frone, M. R. (1999). Work stress and alcohol use. *Alcohol Research & Health, 23*, 284–291.

Frone, M. R., Russell, M. R., & Cooer, M. L. (1997). Job stressors, job involvement, and employee health: A test of identity theory. *Journal of Occupational & Organizational Psychology, 68*, 1–11.

Greenberg, E. S., & Grunberg, L. (1995). Work alienation and problem alcohol behavior. *Journal of Health & Social Behavior, 36*, 83–102.

Grunberg, L., Moore, S., Anderson-Connolly, R., & Greenberg, E. (1999). Work stress and self-reported alcohol use: The moderation role of escapist reasons for drinking. *Journal of Occupational Health Psychology, 4*(1), 29–36.

Grunberg, L., Moore, S., & Greenberg, E. S. (1998). Work stress and problem alcohol behavior: A test of the spillover model. *Journal of Organizational Behavior, 19*(5), 487–502.

Hall, D., & Queener, J. E. (2007). Self-medication hypothesis of substance use: Testing Khantzian's Updated Theory. *Journal of Psychoactive Drugs, 39*(2), 151–158.

Harris, K. M., & Edlund, M. J. (2005). Self-medication of mental health problems: New evidence from a national survey. *Health Services Research, 40*, 117–134.

Hettema, J., Steele, J., & Miller, W. R. (2005). Motivational interviewing. *Annual Review of Clinical Psychology, 1*, 91–111.

Higgins, S. T., Budney, A. J., Bickel, W. K., Foerg, F. E., Donham, R., & Badger, G. J. (1994). Incentives improve outcome in outpatient behavioral treatment of cocaine dependence. *Archives of General Psychiatry, 51*, 568–576.

Janikowski, T. P., Cardoso, E., & Lee, G. K. (2005). Substance abuse, disability, and case management. In F. Chan, M. J. Leahy, & J. L. Saunders (Eds.), *Case management for rehabilitation health professionals* (Vol. 2, pp. 247–274). Osage Beach, MO: Aspen Professional Services.

Kessler, R. C., Nelson, C. B., McGonagle, K. A., Edlund, M. J., Frank, R. G., & Leaf, P. J. (1996). The epidemiology of co-occurring addictive and mental disorders: Implications for prevention and service utilization. *American Journal of Orthopsychiatry, 66*, 17–31.

Khantzian, E. J. (1985). The self-medication hypothesis of addictive disorders: Focus on heroin and cocaine dependence. *American Journal of Psychiatry, 142*(11), 1259–1264.

Khantzian, E. J. (1997). The self-medication hypothesis of substance use disorders: A reconsideration and recent applications. *Harvard Review of Psychiatry, 4*(5), 231–244.

Khantzian, E. J. (1999). Self-regulation and self-medication factors in alcoholism and the addictions: Similarities and differences. In J. Lilienfeld & J. Oxford (Eds.), *The languages of addiction* (pp. 43–68). New York, NY: St. Martin's Press.

Khantzian, E. J., & Albanese, M. J. (2008). *Understanding addiction as self-medication: Finding hope behind the pain.* New York, NY: Rowman & Littlefield Publishers, Inc.

Khantzian, E. J., Mack, J. F., & Schatzberg, A. F. (1974). Heroin use as an attempt to cope: Clinical observations. *American Journal of Psychiatry, 131*, 160–164.

Lazarus, R. S., & Folkman, S. (1984). *Stress, appraisal, and coping.* New York, NY: Springer.

Lemaire, G., Mallik, K., & Rever, K. (2004). Factors influencing community-based rehabilitation for persons with co-occurring psychiatric and substance abuse disorders. *Journal of Addictions Nursing, 15*, 15–22.

Lerner, D., Adler, D., Hermann, R. C., Chang, H., Ludman, E., et al. (2012). Impact of a work-focused intervention on the productivity and symptoms of employees with depression. *Journal of Occupational & Environmental Medicine, 54*, 128–135.

Longabaugh, R., Donovan, D. M., Karno, M. P., McCrady, B. S., Morgenstern, J. S., & Tonigan, J. (2005). Active ingredients: How and why evidence-based alcohol behavioral treatment interventions work. *Alcoholism: Clinical and Experimental Research, 29*(2), 235–247.

Martin, J. K. (1990). Jobs, occupations, and patterns of alcohol consumption: A review of the literature. In P. Roman (Ed.), *Alcohol problem intervention in the workplace* (pp. 45–65). Westport, CT: Quorum.

Martin, S. (2001). *Monitor on psychology: Special issue on substance abuse.* Washington, DC: American Psychological Association.

Martin, J. K., Blum, T. C., & Roman, P. M. (1992). Drinking to cope and self-medication: Characteristics of jobs in relations to workers' drinking behavior. *Journal of Organizational Behavior, 13*, 55–71.

Martin, J. K., Roman, P. M., & Blum, T. C. (1996). Job stress, drinking networks, and social support and work: A comprehensive model of employees' problem drinking. *Sociological Quarterly, 37*, 579–599.

Mendel, E., & Hipkins, J. (2002). Motivating learning disabled offenders with alcohol-related problems: A pilot study. *British Journal of Learning Disabilities, 30*, 153–158.

National Institute for Occupational Health and Safety. (1999). *Stress at work. DHHS (NIOSH) Publication No. 99-101.* Washington, DC: Author.

Noblet, A. (2003). Building health promoting work settings: Identifying the relationship between work characteristics and occupational stress in Australia. *Health Promotion International, 18*, 351–359.

Noonan, J., & Wagner, S. L. (2010). Workplace stress management: Theory and recommendations. *Vocational Evaluation and Work Adjustment Bulletin, 31*(1), 3–16.

Parker, D. A., & Harford, T. C. (1992). Gender-role attitudes, job competition, and alcohol consumption among women and men. *Alcoholism: Clinical & Experimental Research, 16*, 159–165.

Potvin, S., Sepehry, A. A., & Stip, E. (2006). A meta-analysis of negative symptoms in dual diagnosis schizophrenia. *Psychological Medicine, 36*, 431–440.

Prendergast, M., Podus, D., Finney, J., Greenwell, L., & Roll, J. (2006). Contingency management for treatment of substance use disorders. A meta-analysis. *Addiction, 101*, 1546–1560.

Prochaska, J., & DiClementi, C. (1986). Toward a comprehensive model of change. In W. Miller & N. Heather (Eds.), *Treating addictive behaviors: Process of change.* New York, NY: Plenum.

Santa Ana, E. J., Wulfert, E., & Nietert, P. (2007). Efficacy of group motivational interviewing (GMI) for psychiatric in patients with chemical dependency. *Consulting Clinical Psychiatry, 75*(5), 816–822.

Scott, J. (2001). Cognitive therapy for depression. *British Medical Bulletin, 57*, 101–113.

Substance Abuse and Mental Health Services Administration, & Center for Behavioral Health Statistics and Quality. (2011, May 26). *The TEDS report: Substance abuse treatment admissions that were labor force dropouts.* Rockville, MD

Suh, J. J., Ruffins, S., Robins, C. E., Albanese, M. J., & Khantzian, E. J. (2008). Self-medication hypothesis: Connecting affective experience and drug of choice. *Psychoanalytic Psychology, 25*(3), 518–532.

The Treatment for Adolescents with Depression Study Team. (2004). Fluoxetine, cognitive-behavioral therapy, and their combination for adolescents with depression. *Journal of American Medical Association, 292*, 807–820.

Trice, H. M., & Sonnenstuhl, W. J. (1990). On the construction of drinking norms in work organizations. *Journal of Studies on Alcohol, 51*, 201–220.

Vasse, R. M., Nijhuis, F. J. N., & Kok, G. (1998). Associations between work stress, alcohol consumption, and sickness absence. *Addiction, 93*, 231–241.

Veenstra, M. Y., Lemmens, P. H. H. M., Friesema, I. H. M., Tan, F. E. S., Garretsen, H. F. L., Knottnerus, J. A., et al. (2007). Coping style mediates impact of stress on alcohol use: A prospective population-based study. *Addiction, 102*, 1890–1898.

Wexler, H. K., Magura, S., Beardsley, M. M., & Josepher, H. (1994). An AIDS education and relapse prevention model for high-risk parolees. *Journal of the Addictions, 29*(3), 361–386.

Wiesner, M., Windle, M., & Freeman, A. (2005). Work stress, substance use, and depression among young adult workers: An examination of main and moderator effect models. *Journal of Occupational Health Psychology, 10*(2), 83–96.

Zobel, I., Kech, S., van Calker, D., Dykierek, P., Berger, M., Schneibel, R., et al. (2011). Long-term effect of combined interpersonal psychotherapy and pharmacotherapy in a randomized trial of depressed patients. *Acta Psychiatrica Scandinavica, 123*, 276–282.

Beyond the Playground: Bullying in the Workplace and Its Relation to Mental and Physical Health Outcomes

Madeline Rex-Lear, Jennifer M. Knack, and Lauri A. Jensen-Campbell

Bullying in the American workplace is not a new phenomenon. Much of the research has focused on specific factors of workplace hostility such as sexual harassment (Dougherty & Smythe, 2004), ethnicity, gender, and age discrimination (e.g., Schneider, Hitlan, & Radhakrishnan, 2000). However, the effects of destructive interpersonal relationships in the workplace on an individual's health and well-being have frequently been ignored or understated. In this chapter, we present a developmental approach to bullying but focus primarily on workplace bullying among adults and the negative consequences that this type of victimization has on physical and mental health correlates. We begin by presenting a biopsychosocial model that explores how being bullied affects mental and physical health. We then examine the construct of bullying, review existing research on bullying in schools (e.g., during childhood and adolescence), and draw parallels between research on workplace bullying and school bullying to bolster the importance of studying bullying across multiple age groups and situations. Next, we explore potential factors that may influence the link between being bullied in the workplace and mental and physical health. Finally, we consider the implications of research on workplace bullying.

Theoretical Model

This chapter proposes an empirically based biopsychosocial stress model that considers being bullied as a chronic social stressor. This biopsychosocial model mirrors the general format of many biobehavioral investigations of health and illness (e.g., Anderson, Kiecolt-Glaser, & Glaser, 1994; Dougall & Baum, 2001;

M. Rex-Lear, Ph.D. (✉) • L.A. Jensen-Campbell, Ph.D.
Department of Psychology, University of Texas at Arlington,
501 S. Nedderman Dr., Box 19528, Arlington, TX 76019, USA
e-mail: rexlear@uta.edu; lcampbell@uta.edu

J.M. Knack, Ph.D.
Department of Psychology, Clarkson University,
169 Science Center, PO Box 5825, Potsdam, NY 13699-5825, USA
e-mail: jknack@clarkson.edu

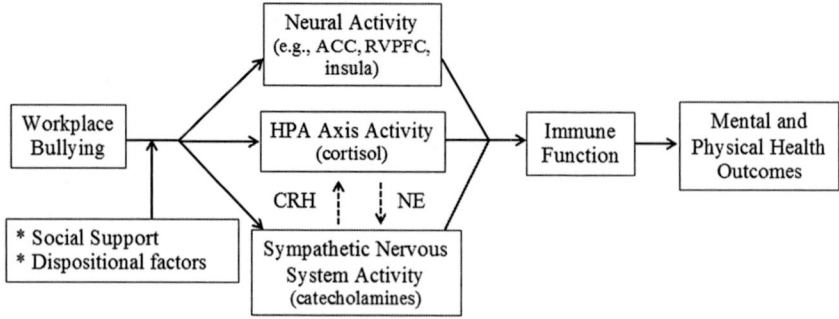

Fig. 11.1 Theoretical model of link between being bullied and mental and physical health outcomes

Gatchel, 2004; Knack, Gomez, & Jensen-Campbell, 2011a; Lazarus & Folkman, 1984; Rex-Lear, 2010). The model reinforces empirical research that posits stress as a mechanism by which a stressor, specifically being bullied, is associated with a series of biological, behavioral, and psychological changes that negatively influence physical and mental health outcomes (Barnet, Spence, Manuck, & Jennings, 1997; Ben-Eliyahu, Page, Yirmiya, & Shakhar, 1999; Knack, Jensen-Campbell, & Baum, 2011b) (see Fig. 11.1). In particular, cognition, brain function, HPA axis activity (e.g., cortisol production), sympathetic nervous system activity, and immune functioning can be compromised. We postulate that these systems are intricately interwoven and that the stress of being bullied alters how these systems function. However, this model notes that not all people who are bullied experience negative health consequences. Thus, the pathway linking being bullied in the workplace with mental and physical health consequences is also expected to be influenced by dispositional factors (e.g., personality, affect) and social support (see Fig. 11.1).

Defining Bullying

Being the target of bullying is frequently referred to as *peer victimization*. This chapter uses the terms being bullied and peer victimization interchangeably. Peer victimization is a stable phenomenon which often extends over multiple developmental periods. It can begin as early as preschool, peaks in early adolescence (Brendgen, Vitaro, Bukowski, Doyle, & Markiewicz, 2001; Nansel, Haynie, & Simons-Morton, 2003), and typically remains stable throughout high school (Williams & Guerra, 2007). Although bullying may peak in adolescence, there is ample evidence to suggest that it extends beyond the schoolyard into college, the workplace, and other social domains (Chapell et al., 2004; Straight, Harper, & Arias, 2003). Indeed, it is important to consider what is known about the effects of bullying during other developmental periods as the effects continue with age. For example, Smith, Singer, Hoel, & Cooper (2003) noted that people involved in bullying during school (both as bully victims and as bullies) were at higher risk for experiencing workplace bullying. Regardless of age or domain, peer victimization does not include an isolated episode of equal status peers arguing or fighting with one another, nor does it include individuals who are teasing each other in a good-natured manner. Bullying is a phenomenon in which frequent and repeated aggressive acts by one or more individuals are directed at another person with the intent to intimidate or harm the targeted person (e.g., Olweus, 1993; Rayner & Hoel, 1997; Smith, 1997). It is marked by a power differential in which the perpetrators(s) have more perceived power or higher status levels than the target individual(s) whether they are peers or supervisors. In turn, targeted individuals are typically perceived as being unable or unwilling to defend themselves (Smith, 1997).

Bullying in the American workplace has been given a variety of different names: workplace incivility (Andersson & Pearson, 1999; Cortina, Magley, Williams, & Langhout, 2001); social undermining (Duffy, Ganster, & Pagon, 2002); and interpersonal deviance (Bennett & Robinson, 2003). Other nations have employed terms including harassment (Brodsky, 1976), scapegoating (Thylefors, 1987), workplace trauma (Björkqvist, Österman, & Hjelt-Back, 1994), abusive behavior/emotional abuse (Keashly, 1998), bullying (Einarsen, 1996; Rayner, 1997), aggression (Kaukiainen et al., 2001), and mobbing (Leymann, 1990a, 1990b; Zapf, 1999) among others. They all seem to refer to variations of the same phenomenon—workplace victimization.

History of Workplace Bullying

Work related harassment and poor treatment of workers has manifested in some form or fashion since organized labor has dominated the western democracies. Many individuals were mistreated, underrepresented, and poorly managed on many levels. In the 1960s Swedish researcher Heinz Leymann recognized the long-term bullying that we are familiar with in schools, and in the 1980s he identified the same types of behaviors existed in the workplace. Leymann stated that the term bullying implied physical aggression traditionally associated with children and youth but found that this rarely occurred in the workplace. Rather, aggression in the workplace tended to favor more subtle, sophisticated behaviors (e.g., verbal or relational aggression); thus, he preferred the term mobbing for these types of behaviors. Collaboration with researchers from different nations eventually saw two main areas of study evolve—*bullying* in schools and *mobbing* in the workplace (Leymann, 1990a, 1990b).

Although American research distinguishes between types of bullying (e.g., relational versus physical bullying) it unifies all these behaviors under the main criteria of bullying as we defined above. Early work by Leymann and others identified poorly organized working environments including hospitals, schools, and religious organizations as environments where mobbing was likely to occur. These types of organizations with multiple hierarchies often had poor conflict management policies which were found to be a common factor in the development and proliferation of bullying practices (Leymann, 1990a, 1990b).

Much of the research on bullying in the workplace has evolved out of research conducted in Sweden, Norway, and Finland on victimization following Olweus' work on school bullying (Björkqvist et al., 1994; Einarsen, Raknes, & Matthiesen, 1994; Olweus, 2003). Workplace victimization can be assessed from different perspectives in which superiors (downward bullying) or colleagues (horizontal bullying) are the aggressor(s). Empirical findings clearly suggest that leaders can actively behave in destructive and counterproductive ways toward subordinates (Einarsen, Aasland, & Skogstad, 2007). According to Rayner and Hoel's (1997) review of the literature, bullying behaviors within the workplace can be classified into four categories including threat to personal standing, isolation, overwork, and destabilization. Rayner and Hoel noted that victims of workplace bullying feel harassed by superiors and that their work performance is usually impacted. In contrast, bullying in schools emphasizes that bullying occurs between *peers* rather than from teachers or other authority figures. Although the source (e.g., superiors versus colleagues) of bullying may be influential, we focus on the general effects of being the target of workplace bullying without differentiating the source. Bullying in the workplace is a significant issue for organizations, but interpretation can be difficult because of the many types of aggression and how they are employed. Thus, this chapter will discuss workplace aggression within the construct of bullying as defined above.

Bullying Styles and Prevalence

Peer victimization has been shown to be a stable phenomenon and is a prominent form of social rejection that cuts across age, race, gender, and socioeconomic status (Juvonen, Graham, & Schuster, 2003). It has been documented among preschool children in daycare centers (Perren & Alsaker, 2006) to retirees and elderly individuals in nursing homes and hospital settings (Rex-Lear, 2011; Rosen, Pillemer, & Lachs, 2008; Walker & Richardson, 1998). Bullying can occur through either overt (i.e., direct) or covert (i.e., indirect) means, and it is seen in several different forms including physical (e.g., hitting, pushing), verbal (e.g., taunting, name calling), relational/social (e.g., gossiping, excluding from peer group), or cyber (e.g., via e-mail, text messages) abuse. Although these forms of bullying are seen throughout the life span, physical forms of bullying are more common among younger children, whereas relational and verbal forms of bullying are common from mid- to late-adolescence and continue throughout late adulthood (Archer & Coyne, 2005; Björkqvist, Lagerspetz, & Kaukiainen, 1992; Crick & Bigbee, 1998; Crick & Nelson, 2002). In the workplace, bullying behaviors and negative incidents become more frequent and more serious the longer they occur, and the longer the bullying behaviors persist, the higher the number of people likely to become involved (Einarsen & Skogstad, 1996; Zapf & Gross, 2001). In 1999, Zapf found the average duration for being bullied by one person was 28 months; the duration increased to 36 months when 2–4 people were involved, and an average of 55 months when more than four people were involved.

Workplace bullying has been recorded in many work domains including hospitals and prisons (Vartia & Hyyti, 2002), academia (McKay, Arnold, Fratzl, & Thomas, 2008), as well as across a wide range of professions including restaurant workers, university employees, electricians, psychologists, and industrial workers (Einarsen, 1999; Einarsen & Skogstad, 1996). According to recent research, approximately 37 % of employees in the United States have been bullied (Zogby International, 2010). Zapf, Dormann, and Frese (1996) reported 5–10 % of employees are subjected to bullying at any one time, and almost 80 % of bullying cases involve superiors as the alleged bullies (Einarsen, Hoel, Zapf, & Cooper, 2003; Namie & Namie, 2000, 2006). Björkqvist et al. (1994) found that 30 % of men and 55 % of women reported being the recipient of some form of workplace bullying. These statistics are comparable with the estimated 10–30 % of youth who report being bullied (e.g., Nansel et al., 2001; Perry, Kusel, & Perry, 1988). These behaviors can cause severe social, psychological, and physical (psychosomatic) health problems for those exposed to such negative acts. Although this chapter focuses predominantly on the health correlates of workplace bullying it is noteworthy that along with deleterious physical and psychological consequences targets may also suffer negative economic consequences. They might experience long-term sick leave, layoffs, transfers, reassignments to lower-level tasks, and either forced termination or voluntary termination in order to avoid the bullying atmosphere (Leymann, 1990a, 1990b).

Being Bullied, Biological Functioning, and Health

Considering the amount of time individuals invest in working environments, it is unsettling to think that many individuals are experiencing detrimental health outcomes as a direct consequence of victimization at work. Much like the pattern of results that has emerged throughout the child and adolescent studies, poor interpersonal relations have significant effects on physical and mental well-being during adulthood. Consequently, both quantitative and qualitative studies have begun to document physical and mental health correlates associated with being the target of workplace bullying.

Physical and Psychological Health Outcomes

Research suggests that subtle aggressive acts, albeit indirect or direct (e.g., relational, verbal), are more prolific in the workplace than the traditional physical types of aggression associated with children (Einarsen, 1999; Keashly & Harvey, 2005; Zapf et al., 1996). Kaukiainen and colleagues (2001) found that covert or indirect aggression was the most frequently reported type of aggression used. For example, workplace bullying tactics often include humiliation, attacks on individual's self-esteem, attacking a coworker's private life (Moreno-Jiménez, Rodríguez-Muñoz, Pastor, Sanz-Vergel, & Garrosa, 2009), isolation, social exclusion, and emotional abuse (Escartín, Zapf, Arrieta, & Rodríguez-Carballeira, 2010; Yildirim & Yildirim, 2007). Many of the psychosocial health correlates associated with school-aged children and being bullied are also found in workplace bullying research.

While examining the relationship between different types of abuse and health outcomes Striegel-Moore, Dohm, Pike, Wilfley, & Fairburn (2002) assessed whether bullying by peers was associated with an increased risk for developing binge eating disorder in women. They interviewed women already diagnosed with binge eating disorder, a healthy group, and a psychiatric comparison group ($N=520$). Striegel-Moore and colleagues hypothesized that binge eating may well be a coping mechanism for individuals experiencing extreme environmental and/or personal stressors (Wilfley, Pike, Dohm, Striegel-Moore, & Fairburn, 2001). They found that women with binge eating disorder were significantly more likely than healthy comparison women to report a history of being bullied. This finding was consistent with previous findings of eating disorders and discrimination among children and adults (Puhl & Brownell, 2001). This study, although not conclusive, provides evidence that the experience of bullying can have far-reaching effects long after the immediate experience. In turn, this study lent support to the hypothesis that victimization experiences at one point in life do indeed have the capacity to affect physical health outcomes at a later life stage.

Other outcomes include depression, behavioral problems, and risky behaviors such as substance abuse and alcoholism (Archer & Coyne, 2005; Crick & Grotpeter, 1995; Dodge, 1989; Egan & Perry, 1998; Kupersmidt, Coie, & Dodge, 1990; McDougall, Hymel, Vaillancourt, & Mercer, 2001) and suicide ideation (Forero, McLellan, Rissel, & Bauman, 1999; Rigby, 2000; van der Wal, de Wit, & Hirasing, 2003). More specifically, workplace bullying behaviors have been linked with reduced self-confidence, low self-worth, suicidal thoughts, self-contempt, self-loathing, and symptoms of post-traumatic stress disorder (PTSD) (Einarsen, Raknes, & Matthiesen, 1994; Lewis, Coursol, & Wahl, 2002; Leymann & Gustafsson, 1996; Mikkelsen & Einarsen, 2002; Thylefors, 1987). Literature on PTSD has traditionally focused on factors such as life threatening situations, extreme traumas, and severity of incidents experienced. However, other research suggests that post traumatic stress symptoms can still develop in the absence of an acute, dramatic stressor (Scott & Stradling, 1994). Comparing post traumatic stress levels of bullied employees with victims of other traumatic incidences, Matthiesen and Einarsen (2004) established a strong relationship between the psychological stress of workplace bullying and PTSD symptomology among employees. Bullied individuals reported higher psychiatric stress levels than those in comparison groups. Matthiesen and Einarsen determined that because workplace bullying can take a chronic debilitating course it undermines bullied individual's abilities to effectively cope with stressors both in and out of the workplace. Rodríguez-Muñoz, Moreno-Jiménez, Vergel, and Hernández (2010) also found that nearly half of participants who reported workplace bullying met DSM-IV-TR criteria for PTSD and women who were bullied reported more PTSD symptoms than did bullied men. These findings point to the serious mental health effects that workplace bullying has on many individuals. Although some might argue a causal relationship between individual differences of victims of bullying and negative psychological outcomes the evidence is debatable as we discuss below.

In order to reduce the stress associated with being bullied, targeted employees often try to avoid the workplace bully. Similar to findings in adolescent bullying research, some targets of workplace bullying seem to attempt to cope by using absenteeism behaviors (Voss, Floderus, & Diderichsen, 2004). For example, hospital staff members who experienced workplace bullying were more frequently absent from work due to sickness, had a higher body mass, and had a higher prevalence of chronic disease than other hospital staff members who were not targets of workplace bullying (Kivim ki, Elovainio, & Vahtera, 2000); even early retirement has been linked with bullying in the workplace (Einarsen & Skogstad, 1996). It is still unclear whether employees are absent in an attempt to avoid facing workplace bullying or due to actual illness; some evidence (e.g., Kivim ki et al., 2000) has suggested that victims of workplace bullying may be missing work due to illness and psychosomatic symptoms. Indeed, there are clear associations between reports of being bullied and psychosomatic symptoms among employees (Mikkelsen & Einarsen, 2001). For example, Kaukiainen et al. (2001) examined employees' perceptions that their health and well-being were attributed to aggression in the workplace. Studying a cross-section of occupations across a wide age range of employees (20–60 years), they found that males' lack of well-being was positively correlated with all types of experienced aggression. Overall, employees who considered themselves to be frequently victimized reported experiencing more psychosocial and somatic problems than those who had been victimized to a lesser extent or not at all. Furthermore, the victimized group tended to attribute their psychosocial symptoms to being a target of workplace aggression more often than the less victimized group.

Other work has determined that being bullied was associated with both psychosocial and physical symptoms only months after bullying was experienced (Hallberg & Strandmark, 2006). Psychosomatic symptoms reported included headaches, inflammation, hypersensitivity to sounds, respiratory and cardiac complaints, hypertension, and general body pain. Although self-reported, these results suggest a dose-response pattern in that, over time, somatic complaints became chronic. In a qualitative study, Thomas (2005) interviewed ten support staff personnel in an educational institute who reported workplace bullying; the most commonly reported physical symptoms associated with workplace bullying included headaches, fatigue, stomach problems, and bowel problems. Of the few studies to consider biological characteristics, Kivimäki et al. (2004) completed a large prospective study of Finnish hospital workers ($N=4,791$). They prospectively examined the association between work stressors and the onset of fibromyalgia (a functional somatic syndrome with no known etiology characterized by multiple symptoms including widespread muscle pain, tenderness, and sleep disturbance; Kivimäki et al., 2002). In addition to considering high work load and low decision latitude in the workplace, Kivimäki and colleagues assessed the role of workplace bullying as a predictor for stress-related health symptoms (e.g., fibromyalgia, osteoarthritis, sciatica). They controlled for age, sex, income, smoking, comorbid psychiatric disorders, and body mass index. The strongest associations were found between workplace bullying and the incidence of fibromyalgia. Furthermore, the 234 respondents who reported being the target of workplace bullying were more than four times as likely as nonbullied employees to develop fibromyalgia. These findings suggest that prolonged stress from being bullied may affect immune system functioning that can result in chronic health conditions. It is feasible that this relationship is due to the characteristically low cortisol levels associated with fibromyalgia patients (see below for a discussion on cortisol).

These above findings also extend the work of researchers studying experiences of bullying in children and adolescents. For example, victimized children report more physical health complaints than non-victimized children, including more headaches, stomach pain, sore throats, and colds (e.g., Knack, et al., 2011a, b; Rigby, 1998; Williams, Chambers, Logan, & Robinson, 1996; Wolke, Woods, Bloomfield, & Karstadt, 2001). These health problems appear to persist over time. Victimized children continue to have poorer health outcomes than their nonvictimized peers three years after an initial assessment even after controlling for initial differences in health (Rigby & Slee, 1999). Similarly, Knack, Iyer, and Jensen-Campbell (2012) found that being the target of peer victimization predicted higher reports of severe health problems for college-age students (e.g., heart problems, bone/joint problems, chest pain, high blood pressure) and more general health problems over time.

Often the insidious nature of bullying in the workplace can create health problems that are not necessarily attributed to the immediate problem. As this phenomenon is still not widely recognized or acknowledged in the American workplace targets may be treated for symptoms without ever addressing the underlying causes of their health problems (Lewis et al., 2002). More longitudinal research would be pertinent to enable medical professionals, the legal system, and the bullied individual to recognize potential consequences of workplace victimization and be able to treat each issue accordingly.

Sex Differences in Bullying Experiences and Reporting

In general, men report greater deficits in physical health outcomes than women do (Zapf et al., 1996). Even among non-victimized individuals, men experience more *types* of physical impairment (life threatening diseases and physical impairment), whereas women generally report more *symptoms* (more frequent illness) over the life span (Verbrugge, 1985). It has also been suggested that women experience more psychosocial distress (e.g., anxiety, guilt) on a day-to-day basis across the life span than men do (Verbrugge, 1985). These gender differences in emotional processing and response may have direct consequences on the physical and emotional health of men and women exposed to bullying phenomenon. In a large British national study Hoel, Faragher, and Cooper (2004) assessed sex differences in the effects of observing or experiencing bullying on health in people working in public, private, and voluntary sector jobs. They found that self-reported bullying and health were significantly correlated with physical and mental well-being. The correlations between bullying and physical health outcomes were slightly higher for men than women (Rex-Lear, 2011; Zapf et al., 1996). This finding corroborates findings in the children's victimization literature where bullied boys tended to report more *physical* symptoms, such as cuts and bruises, than did bullied girls (e.g., Rigby, 1998). In addition, Hoel and colleagues found the effects of being a victim appeared to increase with age. They also determined that respondents who recalled being bullied in the past were less affected than recent targets.

The Whitehall studies (I and II) of British Civil servants are an excellent example of examining social determinants of health in both men and women in the workplace. These studies examined mortality rates among male and female civil servants aged 20–64 and emphasized a steep inverse association between social class and health outcomes (Marmot, Rose, Shipley, & Hamilton, 1978; Marmot et al., 1991). The Whitehall studies highlighted how lower social status in the workplace (which can include perceiving being bullied or feeling threatened in the workplace) and a lower sense of control were associated with risk factors of coronary heart disease such as obesity, smoking, higher blood pressure, less leisure time, and lower activity levels. Furthermore, self-perceived health status and symptoms were worse in participants in lower compared to higher status jobs. In light of these findings, more recent work with participants of the Whitehall II study cohort has implied that lower employment grades, work stress, and anticipation of work stress are associated with a larger cortisol awakening response in employees (especially women) (Kunz-Ebrecht, Kirschbaum, Marmot, & Steptoe, 2004). These fluctuations in cortisol regulation due to chronic stress may act as a mechanism that potentially disrupts immune system functioning, leaving the body less able to prevent cardiovascular and other chronic health disorders.

Bullying and Neuroendocrine Function

When a stressor is detected, two key hormonal systems, namely the sympathetic nervous system (SNS) and the hypothalamic pituitary adrenal (HPA) axis, are activated by the hypothalamus, signaling the release of corticotrophin releasing hormone (CRH). The SNS's main role is to mobilize the body's nervous system "fight or flight response" to deal with acute stressors. More recent attention has been paid to the role that the HPA axis' production of cortisol has on the immune system and endocrine function (Dickerson & Kemeny, 2004; Eisenberger, Taylor, Gable, Hilmert, & Lieberman, 2007; Purvis & Cross, 2006). Within the HPA axis, the release of CRH triggers a cascade of events resulting in the release of cortisol (McEwen, 1998). Cortisol inhibits immune functioning and, together with other systems (e.g., sympathetic nervous system), regulates physiological responses to allow the body to more effectively respond to a stressor. This increased level of cortisol in the face of an acute stressor is beneficial in the short term, but the extended response associated with chronic exposure to stressors can place individuals at risk for adverse psychosocial and physical outcomes (e.g., long-term immune suppression) (Cicchetti & Tucker, 1994).

Surprisingly, there is little research examining the association between being bullied and cortisol levels during an acute stressor. Although Hamilton, Newman, Delville, and Delville (2008) did not find differential cortisol levels in bullied versus non-bullied college students during a modified version of the Tier Social Stress Test, other researchers have found that people who are bullied do have different patterns of cortisol in response to an acute stressor relative to people who are not bullied. Knack, et al. (2011b) found that adolescents who were bullied had a *decrease* in cortisol over the 30 min period after delivering a speech; adolescents who were not bullied showed an increase in cortisol during this period of time. Ouellet-Morin et al. (2011) found a similar blunted cortisol response during an acute stressor using a monozygotic twin design. Together, these results suggest that people who are bullied react differently to stressors than people who are not bullied. Interestingly, daily hassles predict health complaints more strongly than major life events/stressors (e.g., DeLongis, Coyne, Dakof, Folkman, & Lazarus, 1982; DeLongis, Folkman, & Lazarus, 1988). It follows that reducing the frequency of incidents of workplace bullying would predict better health among employees.

Recent research has demonstrated that, contrary to expectations, children and adolescents who report being bullied have *lower* levels of cortisol throughout the day than their non-victimized counterparts (Kliewer, 2006; Knack, et al., 2011a and b; Vaillancourt et al., 2008). Moreover, these lower levels of cortisol, especially in the morning, may mediate the relationship between peer victimization and poor physical health outcomes (Knack, et al., 2011a and b). In the few studies that have examined the relationship between workplace bullying and cortisol levels, a similar association has been documented. Hansen et al. (2006) and Hansen, Hogh, and Persson (2011) found that lower levels of cortisol were associated with frequently being bullied at work. Monteleone et al. (2009) also found lower salivary cortisol levels in the morning among adults who experienced workplace bullying compared to non-bullied adults. The duration and seriousness of the bullying may be important in understanding how peer victimization influences biological functioning. The plasticity of the neuroendocrine system and its ability to adjust to reach a new level of homeostasis may be particularly important in understanding the long-term ramifications of being the recipient of chronic peer victimization. For example, dealing with an on-going stressor has been found to lead to diminished coping resources and slower recovery following exposure to an acute stressor (i.e., greater sensitization; Gump & Matthews, 1999). Knack and Vaillancourt (2012) reviewed research suggesting that similar patterns of cortisol levels (both diurnal and reactivity levels) are found among people who experience social stress in other social relationships, namely intimate partner violence and child maltreatment. Additional research is certainly needed to better understand this relationship and to examine whether differences in cortisol levels due to workplace bullying are associated with physical health differences.

Bullying and Immune Functioning

A major contribution of stress research has been the recognition that the human brain's plasticity allows it to adapt to environmental change. It is possible that environmental stressors tax the plasticity of biological systems and alter an individual's normal course of development and endocrine function (Cicchetti & Tucker, 1994). The plasticity of the neuroendocrine system is particularly important in understanding the long-term costs of being victimized within the workplace; these alterations may render individuals more vulnerable to future negative experiences (Dersh, Polatin, & Gatchel, 2002). It should also be pointed out that endocrine, nervous, and immune systems share a common biochemical language (e.g., hormones, cytokines, and neurotransmitters). As such, the disruption of homeostasis in the endocrine system can modulate the functioning of the nervous and immune systems (Padgett et al., 2002). Chronic stress from workplace bullying may alter the balance in the functioning of the endocrine system which, in turn, should lead to greater immune dysregulation and increased inflammatory responses. Elevated proinflammatory cytokines and C-reactive proteins, in turn, increase the risk for developing serious chronic health problems such as coronary heart disease (Kendall-Tackett, 2009). Stress from social traumas is thought to prime inflammatory responses leading to more rapid inflammatory responses with each subsequent social stressor which, in turn, increases the likelihood that a chronic illness will develop (Kendall-Tackett, 2009; Kunz-Ebrecht et al., 2004).

Bullying and Cognitive Functioning

In addition to altering neuroendocrine and immune functioning, bullying may have deleterious effects on brain function. Indeed, chronic stress leads to changes in grey matter volume, smaller hippocampal regions, and memory and learning impairments (Issa, Rowe, Gauththier, & Meaney, 1990; Lupien, McEwen, Gunnar, & Heim, 2009; Sapolsky, Romero, & Munck, 2000). McEwen and Sapolsky (1995) reported that prolonged exposure to stress can result in neuron loss, particularly in the hippocampus, which is crucial for declarative memory. Moreover, Eisenberger, Lieberman, and Williams (2003) found that being socially excluded from an online ball tossing game (i.e., cyberball) differentially activated the anterior cingulate cortex (ACC), compared to being socially included in the game; this increased activity in the ACC was correlated with higher levels of self-reported distress (see also Dickerson, 2011; Eisenberger, 2011). Similar patterns of activation were also found in adolescents who were socially excluded from an online ball tossing game (Masten et al., 2009) These findings are important given that that the ACC is considered part of the "neural alarm system" that sounds at the detection that something has gone wrong. Additionally, Chen and Williams (2011) noted that, although the brain may process social pain experiences (e.g., being bullied) in a similar fashion as physical pain experiences (also see Eisenberger & Lieberman, 2004; MacDonald & Leary, 2005), social pain experiences are more likely than physical pain experiences to be relived rather than simply remembered.

These findings support other research claims that high stress levels are associated with poorer memory and altered cognitive functioning across the life span (Lupien, Maheu, Tu, Fiocco, & Schramek, 2007). In a longitudinal study, Vaillancourt et al. (2011) found evidence of a link between peer victimization and poor memory in children. There has been little direct research on the effects of being bullied and memory function in any other age group. However, given the link between chronic stress and cortisol levels negatively impacting the structure and function of neurons in the hippocampus (a brain region involved in memory), it is feasible that people who are bullied would experience cognitive problems. Future research in bullied personnel and cognitive decision-making processes may well find detriments in bullied individuals' abilities to make best practice decisions for both themselves and the organization.

Factors Influencing the Association Between Victimization and Health Outcomes

Dispositional Factors

Personality characteristics. Personality has been associated with both interpersonal relations and health (e.g., Coyne, Seigne, & Randall, 2000; Coyne, Smith-Lee Chong, Seigne, & Randall, 2003). According to Jensen-Campbell and Malcolm (2007), lack of conscientiousness is a major predictor of being bullied in adolescence. Neuroticism is negatively associated with stress tolerance (Dornick & Ekehammar, 1990) and positively associated with anxiety, depression, and medically unexplained physical symptoms (e.g., De Gucht, Fischler, & Heiser, 2004). Einarsen and Skogstad (1996) suggest that personality (e.g., conscientiousness) is a major contributing risk factor to workplace bullying rather than an outcome. Other researchers note that, although personality characteristics are associated with both interpersonal relations and health, personality does not fully account for the relationship between being bullied and poor health. For example, Knack, Iyer, et al. (2012) found that, even after controlling for personality variables among college-age students, peer victimization uniquely predicted health outcomes both concurrently and over a school year. Moreover, neuroticism appears to have an indirect influence on health via negative affect (e.g., Djurkovic, McCormack, & Casimir, 2006). These studies suggest that workplace bullying is detrimental to victims' health and well-being above and beyond individual differences in disposition or personality.

Negative affect and emotional functioning. The psychosomatic model of bullying suggests that being bullied leads to negative affect which, in turn, leads to physical symptoms (e.g., Costa & McCrae, 1980). Researchers have examined this model by testing the associations between dispositions such as negative affect (NA), self-efficacy, and bullying outcomes (Mikkelsen & Einarsen, 2002). Djurkovic et al. (2006) examined the influence of neuroticism and negative affect on poor interpersonal relations and health outcomes for Australian college students concurrently in the workplace. They found that negative affect, rather than neuroticism, mediated the link between workplace bullying and university students' physical health. Hansen et al. (2006) also examined the relationship between negative affect and victimization in the workplace. They found that participants who experienced workplace bullying reported more negative affect, as well as more symptoms of depression and anxiety and lower levels of social support, than those who were not bullied. De Gucht et al. (2004) found that negative affect was a better predictor of medically unexplained symptoms than other factors such as neuroticism.

Social Support

Social support, especially from friends, seems to shield people of all ages from the negative influences of peer abuse (e.g., Bollmer, Harris, & Milich, 2006; Hodges, Boivin, Vitaro, & Bukowski, 1999; Hoel & Cooper, 2000; Malcolm, Jensen-Campbell, Rex-Lear, & Waldrip, 2006; Nezlek, Richardson, Green, & Schatten-Jones, 2002). Social integration plays an important role in the lives of many adults (Rohr & Lang, 2009). According to the "stress-buffering hypothesis," social support is most important during stressful situations, and it helps individuals cope with stressors and diminish cortisol responses (DeLongis & Holtzman, 2005; Eisenberger et al., 2007; Knack, Waldrip, & Jensen-Campbell, 2007; Taylor, 2007; Uchino, Cacioppo, & Kiecolt-Glaser, 1996). As such, one would expect that high quality support (not quantity) from friends would protect individuals from the negative consequences of victimization (Brendgen et al., 2001; Malcolm et al., 2006; Nezlek et al., 2002). However, even the most well intentioned social support can be perceived as intrusive and unneeded. Furthermore, attempts at social support are not always positive and may instead include criticism, neglect, demand, and other insensitive or negative behaviors that detract from overall health and well-being (Pressman, Cohen, Barkin, Miller, & Rabin, 2005; Rook, 2000).

This mis-directed support can have detrimental effects on an individual's overall well-being and ability to cope with particular stressors (DeLongis & Holtzman, 2005). For example, although co-rumination is linked with feelings of closeness in relationships between girls, it has also been implicated in increased internalizing symptoms (e.g., depression, anxiety) and increased cortisol levels (Byrd-Craven, Geary, Rose, & Ponzi, 2008; Ciesla & Roberts, 2007; Nolen-Hoeksema & Morrow, 1991; Rose, Carlson, & Waller, 2007). Recent work by Haggard, Robert, and Rose (2011) has shown that co-rumination also occurs in the workplace, and has both positive and negative adjustment outcomes, especially among women. Both men and women who engaged in co-rumination reported higher quality and higher relationship satisfaction with their colleagues (regardless of level of supervisor abuse). However, women experiencing high abusive supervision and who engaged in co-rumination with colleagues reported more conflict at home than women experiencing less abusive supervision. This negative outcome of co-rumination was not seen for men who experienced high abusive supervision; rather, men who co-ruminated reported lower depression levels and higher job satisfaction. These mixed findings suggest that over-discussing personal life stressors may amplify problems in some situations rather than mitigate them.

Research conducted with adolescents suggests the importance of examining the social norms of the group in addition to examining social support. Knack, Tsar, Vaillancourt, Hymel, and McDougall (2012) found that perceptions of having high levels of characteristics valued by the peer group (i.e., physical attractiveness, wealth, academic competence, and athletic competence) buffered adolescents who were rejected from being victimized. Vaillancourt and Hymel (2006) found a similar buffering effect of characteristics; in their study aggressive adolescents high on characteristics important to the larger peer group were perceived as more popular, less disliked, and having more power than aggressive adolescents who were low on these characteristics. Although these peer-valued characteristics may be challenging to change, it may be beneficial for research on workplace bullying to examine whether nonbehavioral characteristics may reduce the likelihood of being targeted by workplace bullies and/or the negative effects associated with workplace bullying.

Cyber Bullying and the Workplace

An extension of traditional bullying tactics includes *cyber bullying* which involves using information and communication technology and devices such as cell phones and computers to knowingly harass, intimidate, and threaten to harm targeted individuals. The reasons for such behavior are as diverse as they are for traditional bullying tactics, and youth and adults are now facing the same bullying challenges in electronic interactions that occur when face-to-face. Cyber bullying tends to be associated with schools and adolescents or young adults, but employers should be aware that staff who receive offensive e-mails, phone calls, and texts from colleagues or customers could be the victims of cyber bullying in the workplace.

Along with all its benefits technology has provided a conduit to convey abusive messages via e-mails and phone calls, post images and comments on social networking Web sites such as Facebook and Twitter, as well as post videos and graphics much quicker, at any time, and to a wider audience than ever before. There is some perception that cyber bullying adds a new dimension to bullying as it is perceived to have a certain level of anonymity. According to Christopherson (2007), even though people can experience far greater contact with others than ever before the internet affords a level of social anonymity whereby one cannot identify others and they cannot identify the individual. The general tenet of cyber bullying is that the bully is not directly confronting the target (victim) but is hiding behind his/her computer or cell phone and sometimes can be difficult to trace (Christopherson, 2007).

As the nature of peer-to-peer aggression evolves the practice of online bullying among youth and young adults seems to be an integral part of the digital culture of the twenty-first century that is relatively unmonitored and unregulated. This type of bullying has been linked to psychological health problems in youth including suicidal ideation and depression (Hinduja & Patchin, 2010) with extreme cases leading to suicide. For example, in 2010 15 year old Phoebe Prince hung herself allegedly due to bullying that included threatening text messages and character-attacking comments posted on-line as well as physical and verbal harassment in and out of school. In their work with adolescents Hinduja and Patchin (2010) found that victims of cyber bullying were nearly twice as likely to have attempted suicide compared to those who had not experienced cyber bullying at all. These types of cases have brought cyber bullying under closer scrutiny of various social network companies, legislators, and communities in general but is still relatively understudied within the workplace.

Although the prevalence of cyber bullying in the workplace is still unknown there are growing concerns about the physical and psychological health of employees in multiple organizational climates exposed to cyber bullying (e.g., Baruch, 2005). In 2008, Slonje and Smith identified that adolescents experiencing some form of cyber bullying would often choose not to tell anyone of the offenses, so parents and adults might not be aware of the incidences (unless pictures or video clips were posted of the bullying acts). These findings were comparable to findings for traditional bullying. The same problems may be occurring in the workplace and may hinder any bystander intervention and development of anti-bullying programs that include cyber bullying tactics.

The most prevalent forms of cyber bullying researched so far include access via electronic mail (e-mail), Web sites, and cellular (mobile) phones. Privitera and Campbell (2009) found that recent employee complaints of bullying consisted of allegations made against them, the withholding of information, and the spreading of gossip via telephone and e-mail, alongside traditional bullying phenomena and tactics. As a result of workplace bullying including persistent harassing phone messages some employees have reported psychiatric distress including Post Traumatic Stress Disorder (PTSD) symptoms (Matthiesen & Einarsen, 2004).

Many British workers believe cyber bullying is a problem at work; a survey of 1,072 British workers found that one in five claim they experience persistent cyber bullying at work via e-mail (Dignity at Work Partnership, 2007). Some estimates project that workplace bullying (including cyber bullying) is estimated to cost United Kingdom employers more than £2bn (~$4bn) a year in sick pay, staff turnover, and lost production. The costs to American organizations where cyber bullying and face-to-face bullying concurrently occur are not yet known but they are likely to experience reduced commitment, lower productivity and morale, higher absenteeism due to ill health, higher turnover rates, and greater risk of employee retaliation and violence (Privitera & Campbell, 2009; Yamada, 2012). In turn these issues may translate into higher costs for health care, employee benefits, and workers' compensation insurance.

Conclusions and Implications

When considering peer victimization as a powerful social stressor, it is reasonable to suggest that this form of persistent, pervasive stress can have serious long-term detrimental health effects. If different processes in the stress response can ultimately result in overexposure or underexposure to stress hormones (McEwen, 1998) and fail to adequately prepare the individual to meet situational demands, individuals may subsequently experience increased susceptibility to poor health outcomes (McEwen & Wingfield, 2003). This pathway is a complex process because health outcomes may not be directly visible until years after particular stressors are presented. For example, emerging evidence suggests that bullying during school years can have long lasting effects on emotional functioning (e.g.,

Gladstone, Parker, & Malhi, 2006; Lund et al., 2009; Sourander et al., 2007). Recently, Allison, Roeger, and Reinfeld-Kirkman (2009) found in a large adult sample ($N=2,833$) that 18.7 % reported recalling being bullied at school. This study demonstrated that adults who experienced bullying as children also reported poorer physical health as adults. It is reasonable to suggest then that we have yet to identify the full health effects of workplace bullying. Longitudinal studies are needed to garner a more thorough understanding of the long-term health implications of workplace bullying.

Studies looking at the link between bullying (both in schools and the workplace) and physical health problems point to a need to continue conducting research designed to understand *why* workplace bullying is associated with more physical health problems. Research is needed to determine whether this relationship is primarily a function of factors such as negative affect or whether the stress of workplace bullying is altering physiological functioning. Much like the pattern of results that emerges throughout the child and adolescent studies, research indicates that there is indeed a relationship between being bullied and health for adults in the workplace. To date, workplace studies vary dramatically in nature, methodology, and health criteria. However, even with these differences, it is feasible to suggest that bullying does appear to have a causal link to both physical and psychological health outcomes for employees in many different and distinctive work situations. Since the empirical research presents such strong evidence for health problems, the next steps in research will be to ascertain what strategies for prevention and intervention are needed.

Employee Protections Against Being Bullied

Although the United States has had various harassment and discrimination laws in place for several years, there is no single specific statute that governs workplace bullying in particular (Mack, 2005). Scandinavians have had specific anti-bullying laws since 1993, and Great Britain has had such laws since 1997. Canada and Australia have had various laws in place providing more employees protections and prohibiting workplace bullying since the 1990s. Ireland has a health and safety code (2005) to address bullying, and many European Union nations have instigated many legal employee protections which compel employers to prevent or rectify bullying actions (e.g., Belgium in 2002). Targets of workplace bullying in the U.S. find few avenues of legal redress available to them.

Only recently has attention been paid to those *being bullied* in the workplace. Currently in the U.S. a campaign for the protection of employees against bullying and harassment is ongoing. The first anti-bullying legislation, the Healthy Workplace Bill (HWB), was introduced in California in 2003. Since then, 21 other states have proposed 60 versions of the bill based on the HWB though to date no state has passed an anti-bullying law in the workplace (Collins, 2011; Workplace Bullying Institute, 2012). The bill is designed to help both employers and employees recognize clear boundaries for what are and are not acceptable behaviors in the work environment (see Table 11.1).

As previously discussed, evidence is mounting that bullying effects are indeed real and can produce multiple traumatic effects for those bullied. Leymann and Gustafsson (1996) also reported that the longer the duration of bullying the more negative the health outcomes for the target could be expected. In other words, the research findings are pointing toward the necessity of some sort of action to reduce and eliminate workplace bullying.

Even though other nations have recognized workplace bullying and many have instituted anti-bullying policies there is little empirical research assessing the effectiveness of these anti-bullying laws. Instigating more regulations into the workplace may not be the most effective approach to protect employees or employers against workplace bullying; Title VII of the Civil Rights Act enacted in 1964 was designed to make the workplace a safer more welcoming place to be. However, the law does not appear to have been particularly effective in stemming the tide of harassment as the number of claims has continued to rise in the last decade (Sespico, Farley, & Knapp, 2007). No single strategy

Table 11.1 Healthy workplace bill guidelines

Employer benefits of the healthy workplace bill
Provides a precise definition of an *abusive work environment*
Requires proof of damaged health by licensed health and/or mental health professionals
Provides protection for conscientious employers from vicarious liability risk when internal correction and prevention mechanisms are in effect
Preserves employers rights to terminate or sanction unethical employees
Requires plaintiffs to use private attorneys
Employee benefits of the healthy workplace bill
Provides an avenue for legal redress for health harming behaviors at work
Allows the targeted individual to sue the bully as an individual
Holds employers accountable for a safe work environment
Affected individuals may pursue restoration of lost wages and benefits
Compels employers to prevent and correct future instances of bullying

Namie and Namie (2009)

or method will resolve workplace bullying and, of course, organizational culture is not going to change immediately; however, there are some key elements that can be taken into consideration to improve the workplace environment. One of the core components in dealing with workplace bullying is the engagement of the employer in recognizing and correcting bullying behaviors. Raising awareness of the bullying phenomenon and encouraging accountability on the part of all employees, both horizontally and vertically, within organizations is a key process. There are many strategies that can be implemented on an individual level as well as at the group and organizational level.

When Kevin Morissey, managing editor for the *Virginia Quarterly Review*, committed suicide in 2010, other employees had repeatedly warned university officials about his despair over alleged workplace bullying—they did nothing. There is a tendency for bystander apathy when people are unsure of what they can or cannot do in any given situation (van Heugten, 2011). It is in the best interest of individuals to be educated as to the negative impacts of workplace bullying and to be proactive in preventing it. Individual targeted employees should seek out social support within the organization to bolster any formal complaints of bullying such as, increasing others' awareness that bullying is occurring, and to include other supportive employees in activities where the target anticipates bullying (see Macintosh, 2006 for review). Early action by both the victim and the organization may prevent behaviors from escalating to out-of-control proportions where not only the victim is affected but bystander coworkers as well. Promoting conflict management and empowering other employees as bystander witnesses to aid in breaking the bullying cycle can assist in resolution processes (Namie & Namie, 2000); also, rewarding desirable social behaviors publicly can encourage more *positive* work environments (Tehrani, 2001).

Namie and Namie (2009, 2011) have published guidelines for both employers and employees on how to deal with bullying in the workplace. To protect the bullied target's health and well-being they suggest it is important to legitimize the issue by naming it (e.g., bullying, psychological harassment), as being told bullying behavior is not illegal often gives others excuses to ignore claims. Second, checking and maintaining one's mental and physical health is necessary in order to reach emotional stability; as previously mentioned stress related diseases do not manifest overnight and instead often have gradual negative effects on people's mental and physical health. Third, Namie and Namie suggest people targeted by workplace bullying gather legal advice and potential data that might be obtainable on the economic cost of the bully to the organization, for example expenses associated with employee absenteeism, sickness, lost productivity, and turnover due to bullying interference. Fourth, expose the bully and give employers a chance to work with you to correct the situation. Finally, be prepared to find alternative employment. Namie and Namie suggest that a bullied individual has a 66 % chance of losing his/her job once targeted, so do not wait to be let go, be proactive, and seek other employment.

Other advice includes finding out whether the specific employer has a bullying policy and any prevention and management plan/complaint procedures for dealing with workplace bullying. Targets of bullying should also seek advice from human resource officers, union officials, or health and safety representatives and services such as Employee Assistance Program (EAP) providers. These services are gradually becoming more sensitive to bullying issues and may be able to provide advice or potential counseling. However, one of the current drawbacks of using such programs is the lack of training that these individuals have in counseling or mentoring people who are targets of workplace bullying (Sespico et al., 2007).

Recognizing that victimization is not an individual issue but an organizational problem will be a crucial element in understanding *how* to reduce or eliminate this phenomenon. Bullying tends to be less common in organizations that promote healthy working environments and have clear identifiable policies and rules on acceptable behaviors in the workplace. Those organizations that publicly demonstrate zero-tolerance policies for disrespectful behaviors and clearly enforce those policies with consequences are the most successful at limiting bullying occurrences in the workplace.

It is important to recognize that bullying effects do not necessarily *wash out* with age. This chapter highlights that rather than disappearing during adolescence peer bullying is associated with a plethora of physical health problems throughout adolescence and through adulthood. Bullying tactics seem to become more sophisticated as individuals become adept at manipulating their surroundings, peers, and coworkers to gain a power imbalance over those they deem weaker than themselves. Bullying affects millions of American workers and as a multi- faceted problem deserves multidisciplinary solutions from researchers, practitioners, employers, employees, and policy makers.

"The world is a dangerous place to live;
Not because of the people who are evil,
But because of the people
who don't do anything about it."
Albert Einstein

References

Allison, S., Roeger, L., & Reinfeld-Kirkman, N. (2009). Does school bullying affect adult health? Population survey of health-related quality of life and past victimization. *Australian and New Zealand Journal of Psychiatry, 43*, 1163–1170. doi:10.3109/00048670903270399.

Anderson, B. L., Kiecolt-Glaser, J. K., & Glaser, R. (1994). A biobehavioral model of cancer stress and disease course. *American Psychologist, 49*, 389–404. Retrieved from http://www.ncbi.nlm.nih.gov/pmc/articles/PMC2719972/pdf/nihms90352.pdf.

Andersson, L. M., & Pearson, C. M. (1999). Tit for tat? The spiraling effect of incivility in the workplace. *Academy of Management Review, 24*, 452–471. Retrieved from http://www.jstor.org/stable/259136.

Archer, J., & Coyne, S. M. (2005). An integrated review of indirect, relational, and social aggression. *Personality and Social Psychology Review, 9*, 312–230. doi:10.1207/s15327957pspr0903_2.

Barnet, P. A., Spence, J. D., Manuck, S. B., & Jennings, J. R. (1997). Psychological stress and the progression of carotid artery disease. *Journal of Hypertension, 15*, 49–55.

Baruch, Y. (2005). Bullying on the net: Adverse behavior on e-mail and its impact. *Journal of Information Management, 42*(2), 361–371. doi:10.1016/j.im.2004.02.001.

Ben-Eliyahu, S., Page, G. G., Yirmiya, R., & Shakhar, G. (1999). Evidence that stress and surgical interventions promote tumor development by suppressing natural killer cell activity. *International Journal of Cancer, 80*, 880–888. doi:10.1002/(sici)1097-0215(19990315)80:6<880::aid-ijc14>3.0.co;2-y.

Bennett, R. J., & Robinson, S. L. (2003). The past, present, and future of workplace deviance research. In J. Greenberg (Ed.), *Organizational behavior: The state of the science* (2nd ed., pp. 247–281). Mahwah, NJ: Erlbaum.

Björkqvist, K., Lagerspetz, K. M., & Kaukiainen, A. (1992). Do girls manipulate and boys fight? Developmental trends in regard to direct and indirect aggression. *Aggressive Behavior, 18*, 117–127. doi:10.1002/1098-2337(1992) 18:2<117::AID-AB2480180205>3.0.CO;2-3.

Björkqvist, K., Österman, K., & Hjelt-Back, M. (1994). Aggression among university employees. *Aggressive Behavior, 20*, 173–184. doi:10.1002/1098-2337(1994) 20:3<173::AID-AB2480200304>3.0.CO;2-D.

Bollmer, J. M., Harris, M. J., & Milich, R. (2006). Reactions to bullying and peer victimization: Narratives, physiological arousal, and personality. *Journal of Research in Personality, 40*, 803–828. doi:10.1016/j.jrp. 2005.09.003.

Brendgen, M., Vitaro, F., Bukowski, W. M., Doyle, A. B., & Markiewicz, D. (2001). Developmental profiles of peer social influence over the course of elementary school: Associations with trajectories of externalizing and internalizing behavior. *Developmental Psychology, 37*, 308–320. doi:10.1037/0012-1649.37.3.308.

Brodsky, C. M. (1976). *The harassed worker*. Lexington, MA: Lexington Books.

Byrd-Craven, J., Geary, D. C., Rose, A. J., & Ponzi, D. (2008). Co-ruminating increases stress hormone levels in women. *Hormones and Behavior, 53*, 489–492. doi:10.1016/j.yhbeh.2007.12.002.

Chapell, M., Casey, D., De La Cruz, C., Ferrell, J., Forman, J., Lipkin, R., et al. (2004). Bullying in college by students and teachers. *Adolescence, 39*, 53–64.

Chen, Z., & Williams, K. D. (2011). Social pain is easily relived and prelived, but physical pain is not. In G. MacDonald & L. A. Jensen-Campbell (Eds.), *Social pain: Neuropsychological and health implications of loss and exclusion* (pp. 161–177). Washington, DC: American Psychological Association.

Christopherson, K. M. (2007). The positive and negative implications on anonymity in Internet social interactions: "On the internet, nobody knows you're a dog". *Computers in Human Behavior, 23*, 3038–3056. doi:10.1016/j.chb.2006.09.001.

Cicchetti, D., & Tucker, D. (1994). Development and self-regulatory structures of the mind. *Development and Psychopathology, 6*, 533–549. doi:10.1017/S0954579400004673.

Ciesla, J. A., & Roberts, J. E. (2007). Rumination, negative cognition, and their interactive effects on depressed mood. *Emotion, 7*, 555–565. doi:10.1037/1528-3542.7.3.555.

Collins, E. (2011). Healthy workplace bill. *New York Law Journal*. Retrieved from http://healthyworkplacebill.org/blog/nylj/

Cortina, L. M., Magley, V. J., Williams, J. H., & Langhout, R. D. (2001). Incivility in the workplace: Incidence and impact. *Journal of Occupational Health Psychology, 6*, 64–80. doi:10.1037//1076-8998.6.1.64.

Costa, P. T., & McCrae, R. R. (1980). Influence of extraversion and neuroticism on subjective well-being. *Journal of Personality and Social Psychology, 38*, 668–678. doi:10.1037/0022-3514.38.4.668.

Coyne, I., Seigne, E., & Randall, P. (2000). Predicting workplace victim status from personality. *European Journal of Work and Organizational Psychology, 9*, 335–49. doi:10.1080/135943200417957.

Coyne, I., Smith-Lee Chong, P., Seigne, E., & Randall, P. (2003). Self and peer nominations of bullying: An analysis of incident rates, individual differences, and perceptions of the working environment. *European Journal of Work and Organizational Psychology, 12*, 209–228. doi:10.1080/13594320344000101.

Crick, N. R., & Bigbee, M. A. (1998). Relational and overt forms of peer victimization: A multi-informant approach. *Journal of Consulting and Clinical Psychology, 66*, 337–347. doi:10.1037/0022-006X.66.2.337.

Crick, N. R., & Grotpeter, J. K. (1995). Relational aggression, gender, and social-psychological adjustment. *Child Development, 66*, 710–722. Retrieved from https://webspace.utexas.edu/lab3346/School%20Bullying/CrickGrotpeter1995/Crick%20Grotpeter%201995.pdf.

Crick, N. R., & Nelson, D. A. (2002). Relational and physical victimization within friendship: Nobody told me there'd be friends like these. *Journal of Abnormal Child Psychology, 30*, 599–607. doi:10.1023/A:1020811714064.

De Gucht, V., Fischler, B., & Heiser, W. (2004). Neuroticism, alexithymia, negative affect, and positive affect as determinants of medically unexplained symptoms. *Personality and Individual Differences, 36*, 1655–1667. doi:10.1016/j.paid.2003.06.012.

DeLongis, A., Coyne, J. C., Dakof, G., Folkman, S., & Lazarus, R. S. (1982). Relationship of daily hassles, uplifts, and major life events to health status. *Health Psychology, 1*, 119–136. doi:10.1037/0278-6133.1.2.119.

DeLongis, A., Folkman, S., & Lazarus, R. S. (1988). The impact of daily stress on health and mood: Psychological and social resources as mediators. *Journal of Personality and Social Psychology, 54*, 486–495. doi:10.1037/0022-3514.54.3.486.

DeLongis, A., & Holtzman, S. (2005). Coping in context: The role of stress, social support, and personality in coping. *Journal of Personality, 73*, 1–24. doi:10.1111/j.1467-6494.2005.00361.x.

Dersh, J., Polatin, P. B., & Gatchel, R. J. (2002). Chronic pain and psychopathology: Research findings and theoretical considerations. *Psychosomatic Medicine, 64*, 773–786.

Dickerson, S. S. (2011). Physiological responses to experiences of social pain. In G. MacDonald & L. A. Jensen-Campbell (Eds.), *Social pain: Neuropsychological and health implications of loss and exclusion* (pp. 79–94). Washington, DC: American Psychological Association.

Dickerson, S. S., & Kemeny, M. E. (2004). Acute stressors and cortisol responses: A theoretical integration and synthesis of laboratory research. *Psychological Bulletin, 130*, 355–391. doi:10.1037/0033-2909.130.3.355.

Dignity at Work Partnership. (2007). Downloaded from http://www.dignityatwork.org/the-project/default.htm

Djurkovic, N., McCormack, D., & Casimir, G. (2006). Neuroticism and the psychosomatic model of workplace bullying. *Journal of Managerial Psychology, 21*, 73–88. doi:10.1108/02683940610643224.

Dodge, K. A. (1989). Problems in social relationships. In E. J. Mash & R. A. Barkley (Eds.), *Treatment of childhood disorders* (pp. 222–244). New York, NY: Guilford.

Dougall, A. L., & Baum, A. (2001). Stress, health, and illness. In A. Baum, T. A. Revenson, & J. E. Singer (Eds.), *Handbook of health psychology* (pp. 321–337). Manwah, NJ: Lawrence Erlbaum.

Dougherty, D. S., & Smythe, M. J. (2004). Sensemaking, organizational culture, and sexual harassment. *Journal of Applied Communication Research, 32*, 293–317. doi:10.1080/0090988042000275998.

Dornick, S., & Ekehammar, B. (1990). Extraversion, neuroticism, and noise sensitivity. *Personality and Individual Differences, 11*, 989–992. doi:10.1016/0191-8869(90)90283-W.

Duffy, M. K., Ganster, D. C., & Pagon, M. (2002). Social undermining in the workplace. *The Academy of Management Journal, 45*, 331–351. Retrieved from http://www.jstor.org/stable/3069350.

Egan, S. K., & Perry, D. G. (1998). Does low self-regard invite victimization? *Developmental Psychology, 34*, 299–309. doi:10.1037/0012-1649.34.2.299.

Einarsen, S. (1996). *Bullying and harassment at work: Epidemiological and psychosocial aspects*. University of Bergen: Department of Psychosocial Science, Faculty of Psychology.

Einarsen, S. (1999). The nature and causes of bullying at work. *International Journal of Manpower, 20*, 16–27. doi:10.1108/01437729910268588.

Einarsen, S., Hoel, H., Zapf, D., & Cooper, C. L. (2003). The concept of bullying at work. In S. Einarsen, H. Hoel, D. Zapf, & C. L. Cooper (Eds.), *Bullying and emotional abuse in the workplace: International perspectives in research and practice* (pp. 3–30). London: Taylor & Francis.

Einarsen, S., Raknes, B. I., & Matthiesen, S. B. (1994). Bullying and harassment at work and their relationships to work environment quality: An exploratory study. *European Work and Organizational Psychologist, 4*, 381–401. doi:10.1080/13594329408410497.

Einarsen, S., Aasland, M. S., & Skogstad, A. (2007). Destructive leadership behaviour: A definition and conceptual model. *The Leadership Quarterly, 18*(3), 207–216. doi:10.1016/j.leaqua.2007.03.002.

Einarsen, S., & Skogstad, A. (1996). Bullying at work: Epidemiological findings in public and private organization. *European Journal of Work and Organizational Psychology, 5*, 185–201. doi:10.1080/13594329608414854.

Eisenberger, N. I. (2011). The neural basis of social pain: Findings and implications. In G. MacDonald & L. A. Jensen-Campbell (Eds.), *Social pain: Neuropsychological and health implications of loss and exclusion* (pp. 53–78). Washington, DC: American Psychological Association.

Eisenberger, N. I., & Lieberman, M. D. (2004). Why rejection hurts: A common neural alarm system for physical and social pain. *Trends in Cognitive Sciences, 8*, 294–300. doi:10.1016/j.tics.2004.05.010.

Eisenberger, N. I., Lieberman, M. D., & Williams, K. D. (2003). Does rejection hurt? An fMRI study of social exclusion. *Science, 302*, 290–292. doi:10.1126/science.1089134.

Eisenberger, N. I., Taylor, S. E., Gable, S. L., Hilmert, C. J., & Lieberman, M. D. (2007). Neural pathways link social support to attenuated neuroendocrine stress responses. *Neuro Image, 35*, 1601–1612. doi:10.1016/j.neuroimage.2007.01.038.

Escartín, J., Zapf, D., Arrieta, C., & Rodríguez-Carballeira, A. (2010). Workers' perception of workplace bullying: A cross-cultural study. *European Journal of Work and Organizational Psychology, 0*, 1–28. doi:10.1080/13594320903395652.

Forero, R., McLellan, L., Rissel, C., & Bauman, A. (1999). Bullying behaviour and psychosocial health among school students in New South Wales, Australia: Cross sectional survey. *British Medical Journal, 319*, 344–348. doi:10.1136/bmj.319.7206.344.

Gatchel, R. J. (2004). Comorbidity of chronic pain and mental health disorders: The biopsychosocial perspective. *American Psychologist, 59*(8), 795–805. doi:10.1037/0003-066X.59.8.795.

Gladstone, G. L., Parker, G. B., & Malhi, G. S. (2006). Do bullied children become anxious and depressed adults? A cross-sectional investigation of the correlates of bullying and anxious depression. *Journal of Nervous Mental Disorders, 194*, 201–208. doi:10.1097/01.nmd.0000202491.99719.c3.

Gump, B. B., & Matthews, K. A. (1999). Do background stressors influence reactivity to and recovery from acute stressors? *Journal of Applied Social Psychology, 29*, 469–494. doi:10.1111/j.1559-1816.1999.tb01397.x.

Haggard, D. L., Robert, C., & Rose, A. J. (2011). Co-Rumination in the workplace: Adjustment trade-offs for men and women who engage in excessive discussions of workplace problems. *Journal of Business and Psychology, 26*, 27–40. doi:10.1007/s10869-010-9169-2.

Hallberg, L. R., & Strandmark, K. M. (2006). Health consequences of workplace bullying: Experiences from the perspective of employees in the public service sector. *International Journal of Qualitative Studies on Health and Well-Being, 1*, 109–119. doi:10.1080/17482620600555664.

Hamilton, L. D., Newman, M. L., Delville, C. L., & Delville, Y. (2008). Physiological stress response of young adults exposed to bullying during adolescence. *Physiology & Behavior, 95*, 617–624. doi:10.1016/j.physbeh.2008.09.001.

Hansen, Å. M., Hogh, A., Persson, R., Karlson, B., Garde, A. H., & Ørbæk, P. (2006). Bullying at work, health outcomes, and physiological stress response. *Journal of Psychosomatic Research, 60*, 63–72. doi:10.1016/j.jpsychores.2005.06.078.

Hansen, Å. M., Hogh, A., & Persson, R. (2011). Frequency of bullying at work, physiological response, and mental health. *Journal of Psychosomatic Research, 70*, 19–27. doi:10.1016/j.jpsychores.2010.05.010.

Hinduja, S., & Patchin, J. W. (2010). Bullying, cyberbullying, and suicide. *Archives of Suicide Research, 14*(3), 206–221. doi:10.1080/13811118.2010.494133.

Hoel, H., & Cooper, C. L. (2000). *Destructive conflict at work*. Manchester: Manchester School of Management.

Hoel, H., Faragher, E. B., & Cooper, C. (2004). Bullying is detrimental to health, but all bullying behaviors are not necessarily equally damaging. *British Journal of Guidance and Counseling, 32*, 367–387. doi:10.1080/03069880410001723594.

Hodges, E. V. E., Boivin, M., Vitaro, F., & Bukowski, W. M. (1999). The power of friendship: Protection against an escalating cycle of peer victimization. *Developmental Psychology, 75*, 94–101. doi:10.1037/0012-1649.35.1.94.

Issa, A. M., Rowe, W., Gauthier, S., & Meaney, M. J. (1990). Hypothalamic–pituitary–adrenal activity in aged, cognitively impaired and cognitively unimpaired rats. *Journal of Neuroscience, 10*, 3247–3254. Retrieved from http://www.jneurosci.org/content/10/10/3247.full.pdf+html.

Jensen-Campbell, L. A., & Malcolm, K. T. (2007). The importance of conscientiousness in adolescent interpersonal relationships. *Personality and Social Psychology Bulletin, 33*, 368–383. doi:10.1177/0146167206296104.

Juvonen, J., Graham S., & Schuster, M. A. (2003). Bullying among young adolescents: The strong, the weak, and the troubled. Pediatrics, 112, 1231–1237. doi:10.1542/peds.112.6.1231.

Kaukiainen, A., Salmivalli, C., Björkqvist, K., Österman, K., Lahtinen, A., Kostamo, A., et al. (2001). Overt and covert aggression in work settings in relation to the subjective well-being of employees. *Aggressive Behavior, 27*, 360–371. doi:10.1002/ab.1021.

Keashly, L. (1998). Emotional abuse in the workplace: Conceptual and empirical issues. *Journal of Emotional Abuse, 1*, 85–117. doi:10.1300/J135v01n01_05.

Keashly, L., & Harvey, S. (2005). Emotional abuse at work. In P. Spector & S. Fox (Eds.), *Counterproductive workplace behaviour: An integration of both actor and recipient perspectives on causes and consequences* (pp. 201–236). Washington, DC: American Psychological Association.

Kendall-Tackett, K. (2009). Psychological trauma and physical health: A psychoneuroimmunology approach to etiology of negative health effects and possible interventions. *Psychological Trauma: Theory, Research, Practice, and Policy, 1*, 35–48. doi:10.1037/a0015128.

Kivimäki, M., Elovainio, M., & Vahtera, J. (2000). Workplace bullying and sickness absence in hospital staff. *Occupational & Environmental Medicine, 57*, 656–660. doi:10.1136/oem.57.10.656.

Kivimäki, M., Leino-Arjas, P., Luukkonen, R., Riihimäki, H., Vahtera, J., & Kirjonen, J. (2002). Work stress and risk of cardiovascular mortality: Prospective cohort study of industrial employees. *British Medical Journal, 325*, 857–860. doi:10.1136/bmj.325.7377.1386.

Kivimäki, M., Leino-Arjas, P., Virtanen, M., Elovainio, M., Keltikangas-Jarvinen, L., Puttonen, S., et al. (2004). Work stress and incidence of newly diagnosed fibromyalgia prospective cohort study. *Journal of Psychosomatic Research, 57*, 417–422. doi:10.1016/j.jpsychores.2003.10.013.

Kliewer, W. (2006). Violence exposure and cortisol response in urban youth. *International Journal of Behavioral Medicine, 13*, 109–120. doi:10.1207/s15327558ijbm1302_2.

Knack, J. M., Gomez, H., & Jensen-Campbell, L. A. (2011a). Bullying and its long-term health implications. In G. MacDonald & L. A. Jensen-Campbell (Eds.), *Social pain: Neuropsychological and health implications of loss and exclusion* (pp. 215–236). Washington, DC: American Psychological Association.

Knack, J. M., Jensen-Campbell, L. A., & Baum, A. (2011b). Worse than sticks and stones? Bullying is linked with altered HPA axis functioning and poorer health. *Brain and Cognition, 77*, 183–190. doi:10.1016/j.bandc.2011.06.011.

Knack, J.M., Iyer, P.A., & Jensen-Campbell, L.A. (2012). Not simply "in their heads:" Being bullied predicts health problems above and beyond known individual differences associated with victimization and health. *Journal of Applied Social Psychology, 42*(7), 1625–1650. doi: 10.1111/j.1559-1816.2012.00898.x.

Knack, J.M., Tsar, V., Vaillancourt, T., Hymel, S., & McDougall, P. (2012). What protects rejected adolescents from also being bullied by their peers? The moderating role of peer-valued characteristics. *Journal of Research on Adolescence, 22*(3), 467–479. doi: 10.1111/j.1532-7795.2012.00792.x.

Knack, J.M. & Vaillancourt, T. (2012). Evidence of altered cortisol levels across child maltreatment, intimate partner abuse, and peer victimization. In A.N. Hutcherson (Ed), Psychology of Victimization (pp. 205–218). Hauppauge, NY: NOVA.

Knack, J. M., Waldrip, A. M., & Jensen-Campbell, L. A. (2007). Social support. In R. Baumeister & K. D. Vohs (Eds.), *Encyclopedia of social psychology* (pp. 920–924). Thousand Oaks, CA: SAGE Publications.

Kunz-Ebrecht, S. R., Kirschbaum, C., Marmot, M., & Steptoe, A. (2004). Differences in cortisol awakening response on work days and weekends in woman and men from the Whitehall II cohort. *Psychoneuroendocrinology, 29*, 516–528. doi:10.1016/S0306-4530(03)00072-6 DOI:10.1016%2FS0306-4530%2803%2900072-6.

Kupersmidt, J. B., Coie, J. D., & Dodge, K. A. (1990). Predicting disorder from peer social problems. In S. R. Asher & J. D. Coie (Eds.), *Peer rejection in childhood* (pp. 274–305). New York, NY: Cambridge University Press.

Lazarus, R. S., & Folkman, S. (1984). *Stress, appraisal, and coping*. New York, NY: Springer.

Leymann, H. (1990a). Mobbing and psychological terror at workplaces. *Violence and Victims, 5*, 119–126. Retrieved from http://www.mobbingportal.com/leymannmain.html.

Lewis, J., Coursol, D., & Wahl, K. H. (2002). Addressing issues of workplace harassment: Counseling the targets. *Journal of Employment Counseling, 39*(3), 109–117. Downloaded from http://www.aepp.net/documents/AEPPproceedings2005final.pdf#page=82.

Leymann, H. (1990b). Mobbing and psychological terror at workplaces. *Violence and Victims, 5*(2), 119–126. Downloaded from http://www.mobbingportal.com/LeymannV%26V1990(3).pdf.

Leymann, H., & Gustafsson, A. (1996). Mobbing at work and the development of posttraumatic stress disorders. *European Journal of Work and Organizational Psychology, 5*(2), 251–275. doi:10.1080/13594329608414858.

Lund, R., Nielsen, K. K., Hansen, D. H., Kriegbaum, M., Molbo, D., Due, P., et al. (2009). Exposure to bullying at school and depression in adulthood: A study of Danish men born in 1953. *European Journal of Public Health, 19*, 111–116. doi:10.1093/eurpub/ckn101.

Lupien, McEwen, B. S. (1998). Stress, adaptation, and disease: Allostasis and allostatic load. *Annals of the New York Academy of Sciences, 840*, 33–44. doi:10.1111/j.1749-6632.1998.tb09546.x.

Lupien, S. J., Maheu, F., Tu, M., Fiocco, A., & Schramek, T. T. (2007). The effects of stress and stress hormones on human cognition: Implications for the field of brain and cognition. *Brain and Cognition, 65*, 209–237. doi:10.1016/j.bandc.2007.02.007.

Lupien, S. J., McEwen, B. S., Gunnar, M. R., & Heim, C. (2009). Effects of stress throughout the lifespan on the brain, behaviour and cognition. *Nature Reviews: Neuroscience, 10*, 434–445. doi:10.1038/nrn2639.

MacDonald, G., & Leary, M. R. (2005). Why does social exclusion hurt? The relationship between social and physical pain. *Psychological Bulletin, 131*, 202–223. doi:10.1037/0033-2909.131.2.202.

Macintosh, J. (2006). Tackling work place bullying. *Issues in Mental Health Nursing, 27*, 665–679. doi:10.1080/01612840600642984.

Mack, J. A. (2005). The law of bullying: Off the playground and into the workplace. *Bench & Bar of Minnesota, 62*(8), 20–24.

Malcolm, K. T., Jensen-Campbell, L. A., Rex-Lear, M., & Waldrip, A. M. (2006). Divided we fall: Children's friendships and peer victimization. *Journal of Social Personality Relations, 23*, 721–740. doi:10.1177/0265407506068260.

Marmot, M. G., Rose, G., Shipley, M., & Hamilton, P. J. (1978). Employment grade and coronary heart disease in British civil servants. *Journal of Epidemiology and Community Health, 32*(4), 244–249. doi:10.1136/jech.32.4.244 DOI:10.1136%2Fjech.32.4.244.

Marmot, M. G., Stansfeld, S., Patel, C., North, F., Head, J., White, I., et al. (1991). Health inequalities among British civil servants: The Whitehall II study. *The Lancet, 337*, 1387–1393. doi:10.1016/0140-6736(91)93068-K.

Matthiesen, S. B., & Einarsen, S. (2004). Psychiatric distress and symptoms of PTSD after bullying at work. *British Journal of Guidance and Counseling, 32*(3), 335–356. doi:10.1080/03069880410001723558.

Masten, C. L., Eisenberger, N. I, Borofsky, L. A., Pfeifer, J. H., McNealy, K., Mazziotta, J. C., & , Dapretto, M. (2009). Neural correlates of social exclusion during adolescence: understanding the distress of peer rejection. *Social Cognitive & Affective Neuroscience, 4*(2), 143–157. doi: 10.1093/scan/nsp007.

McDougall, P., Hymel, S., Vaillancourt, T., & Mercer, L. (2001). The consequences of childhood peer rejection. In M. R. Leary (Ed.), *Interpersonal rejection* (pp. 213–247). New York, NY: Oxford University Press.

McEwen, B. S., & Wingfield, J. C. (2003). The concept of allostasis in biology and biomedicine. *Hormones & Behavior, 43*, 2–15. doi:10.1016/S0018-506X(02)00024-7.

McEwen, B., & Sapolsky, R. (1995). Stress and cognitive function. *Current Opinion in Neurobiology, 5*, 205–216. doi:10.1016/0959-4388(95)80028-X.

McKay, R., Arnold, D. H., Fratzl, J., & Thomas, R. (2008). Workplace bullying in academia: A Canadian study. *Employee Responsibilities and Rights Journal, 20*, 77 100. doi:10.1007/s10672-008-9073-3.

Mikkelsen, E. G., & Einarsen, S. (2001). Bullying in Danish work-life: Prevalence and health correlates. *European Journal of Work and Organizational Psychology, 10*, 393–413. doi:10.1080/13594320143000816.

Mikkelsen, E. G., & Einarsen, S. (2002). Relationships between exposure to bullying at work and psychological and psychosomatic health complaints: The role of state negative affectivity and self efficacy. *Scandinavian Journal of Psychology, 43*, 397–405. doi:10.1111/1467-9450.00307.

Monteleone, P., Giovanni, N., Serritella, C., Milano, V., Di Cerbo, A., Blasi, F., et al. (2009). Hypoactivity of the hypothalamo–pituitary–adrenal axis in victims of mobbing: Role of the subjects' temperament and chronicity of the work-related psychological distress. *Psychotherapy and Psychosomatics, 78*, 381–382. doi:10.1159/000235980.

Moreno-Jiménez, B., Rodríguez-Muñoz, A., Pastor, J. C., Sanz-Vergel, A. S., & Garrosa, E. (2009). The moderating effects of psychological detachment and thoughts of revenge in workplace bullying. *Personality and Individual Differences, 46*, 359–364. doi:10.1016/j.paid.2008.10.031.

Namie, G., & Namie, R. (2006). *Workplace bullying: Introduction to the 'Silent' Epidemic*. Workplace Bullying Institute. Available at: http://www.bullyinginstitute.org

Namie, G., & Namie, R. (2009). *The bully at work: What you can do to stop the hurt and reclaim your dignity on the job*. (2nd Ed). Naperville, IL: Sourcebooks.

Namie, G., & Namie, R. (2011). *The bully-free workplace: Stop jerks, weasels, and snakes from killing your organization*. Hoboken, NJ: Wiley.

Nansel, T. R., Overpeck, M., Pilla, R. S., Ruan, J., Simons-Morton, B., & Scheidt, P. (2001). Bullying behaviors among U.S. youth: Prevalence and association with psychosocial adjustment. *Journal of the American Medical Association, 285*, 2094–2100. doi:10.1001/jama.285.16.2094.

Nansel, T. R., Haynie, D. L., & Simons-Morton, B. G. (2003). The association of bullying and victimization with middle school adjustment. *Journal of Applied School Psychology, 19*, 45–62. doi:10.1300/J008v19n02_04.

Nezlek, J., Richardson, D., Green, L., & Schatten-Jones, E. (2002). Psychological well-being and day-to-day social interaction among older adults. *Personal Relationships, 9*, 57–71. doi:10.1111/1475-6811.00004.

Nolen-Hoeksema, S., & Morrow, J. (1991). A prospective study of depression and distress following a natural disaster: The 1989 Loma Prieta earthquake. *Journal of Personality and Social Psychology, 61*, 105–121. doi:10.1037/0022-3514.61.1.115.

Olweus, D. (1993). *Bullying at school: What we know and what we can do*. Cambridge, MA: Blackwell. Retrieved from ERIC database (ED 384437).

Olweus, D. (2003). Bully/victim problems in school: Basic facts and an effective intervention programme. In S. Einarsen, H. Hoel, D. Zapf, & C. L. Cooper (Eds.), *Bullying and emotional abuse in the workplace: International perspectives in research and practice* (pp. 62–78). London: Taylor and Francis.

Ouellet-Morin, I., Danese, A., Bowes, L., Shakoor, S., Ambler, A., Pariante, C. M., et al. (2011). A discordant monozygotic twin design shows blunted cortisol reactivity among bullied children. *Journal of the American Academy of Child & Adolescent Psychiatry, 50*, 574–582. doi:10.1016/j.jaac.2011.02.015.

Padgett, D. A., Sheridan, J. F., Dorne, J., Berntson, G. G., Candelora, J., & Glaser, R. (2002). Social stress and the reactivation of latent herpes simplex virus type I. In J. T. Cacioppo, G. G. Berntson, R. Adolphs, C. S. Carter, R. J. Davidson, M. K. McClintock, B. S. McEwen, M. J. Meaney, D. L. Schacter, E. M. Sternberg, S. S. Suomi, & S. E. Taylor (Eds.), *Foundations in social neuroscience* (pp. 1185–1193). Cambridge, MA: MIT Press.

Perren, S., & Alsaker, F. D. (2006). Social behavior and peer relationships of victims, bully-victims, and bullies in kindergarten. *Journal of Child Psychology and Psychiatry, 47*, 45–57. doi:10.1111/j.1469-7610.2005.01445.x.

Perry, D. G., Kusel, S. J., & Perry, L. C. (1988). Victims of peer aggression. *Developmental Psychology, 24*, 807–814. doi:10.1037/0012-1649.24.6.807.

Pressman, S. D., Cohen, S., Barkin, A., Miller, G. E., & Rabin, B. (2005). Loneliness, social network size, and immune response to influenza vaccination in college freshmen. *Health Psychology, 24*, 297–306. doi:10.1037/0278-6133.24.3.297.

Privitera, C., & Campbell, M. A. (2009). Cyberbullying: The new face of workplace bullying? *CyberPsychology and Behavior, 12*, 395–400. doi:10.1089/cpb.2009.0025.

Puhl, R., & Brownell, K. D. (2001). Bias, discrimination, and obesity. *Obesity Research, 9*, 788–805. doi:10.1038/oby.2001.108.

Purvis, K. B., & Cross, D. R. (2006). Improvements in salivary cortisol, depression, and representations of family relationships in at-risk adopted children utilizing a short-term therapeutic intervention. *Adoption Quarterly, 10*, 25–43. doi:10.1300/J145v10n01_02.

Rayner, C. (1997). The incidence of workplace bullying. *Journal of Community and Applied Social Psychology, 7*, 199–208. doi:10.1002/(SICI)1099-1298(199706)7:3<199::AID-CASP418>3.3.CO;2-8.

Rayner, C., & Hoel, H. (1997). A summary review of literature relating to workplace bullying. *Journal of Community and Applied Social Psychology, 7*, 181–191. doi:10.1002/(SICI)1099-1298(199706)7:3<181::AID-CASP416>3.0.CO;2-Y.

Rex-Lear, M. (2011). *Not just a playground issue: Bullying among older adults and the effects on their physical health*. Dissertation manuscript, Department of Psychology, University of Texas at Arlington, Arlington, TX.

Rex-Lear, M. (2010). *Bullying and associations with physical health outcomes across the lifespan*. Unpublished manuscript, Department of Psychology, University of Texas at Arlington, Arlington, TX.

Rigby, K. (1998). The relationship between reported health and involvement in bully/victim problems among male and female secondary schoolchildren. *Journal of Health Psychology, 3*, 465–476. doi:10.1177/135910539800300402.

Rigby, K. (2000). Effects of peer victimization in schools and perceived social support on adolescent well-being. *Journal of Adolescence, 23*, 57–68. doi:10.1006/jado.1999.0289.

Rigby, K., & Slee, P. (1999). Suicidal ideation among adolescent school children, involvement in bully-victim problems, and perceived social support. *Suicide and Life-Threatening Behavior, 29*, 119–130. doi:10.1111/j.1943-278X.1999.tb01050.x.

Rodríguez-Muñoz, A., Moreno-Jiménez, B., Vergel, A. I. S., & Hernández, E. G. (2010). Post-traumatic symptoms among victims of workplace bullying: Exploring gender differences and shattered assumptions. *Journal of Applied Social Psychology, 40*, 2616–2635. doi:10.1111/j.1559-1816.2010.00673.x.

Rohr, M. K., & Lang, F. R. (2009). Aging well together—A mini-review. *Gerontology, 55*, 333–343. doi:10.1159/000212161.

Rook, K. S. (2000). The evolution of social relationships in later adulthood. In S. H. Qualls & N. Abeles (Eds.), *Psychology and the aging revolution: How we adapt to longer life* (pp. 173–191). Washington, DC: American Psychological Association.

Rose, A. J., Carlson, W., & Waller, E. M. (2007). Prospective associations of co-rumination with friendship and emotional adjustment: Considering the socioemotional trade-offs of co-rumination. *Developmental Psychology, 43*, 1019–1031. doi:10.1037/0012-1649.43.4.1019.

Rosen, T., Pillemer, K., & Lachs, M. (2008). Resident-to-resident aggression in long-term care facilities: An understudied problem. *Aggression & Violent Behavior, 13*(2), 77–87. doi:10.1016/j.avb.2007.12.001.

Sapolsky, R. M., Romero, L. M., & Munck, A. U. (2000). How do glucocorticoids influence stress responses? Integrating permissive, suppressive, stimulatory, and preparative actions. *Endocrine Reviews, 21*, 55–89. doi:10.1210/er.21.1.55.

Schneider, K. T., Hitlan, R. T., & Radhakrishnan, P. (2000). An examination of the nature and correlates of ethnic harassment experiences in multiple contexts. *Journal of Applied Psychology, 85*, 3–12. doi:10.1037//0021-9010.85.1.3.

Scott, M. J., & Stradling, S. G. (1994). Post-traumatic stress disorder without the trauma. *British Journal of Clinical Psychology, 33*(1), 71–74. doi:10.1111/j.2044-8260.1994.tb01095.x.

Sespico, P., Farley, R., & Knapp, D. (2007). Relief and redress for targets of workplace bullying. *Employee Responsibilities and Rights Journal, 19*, 31–43.

Straight, E. S., Harper, F. W., & Arias, I. (2003). The impact of partner psychological abuse on health behaviors and health status in college women. *Journal of Interpersonal Violence, 18*, 1035–1054. doi:10.1177/0886260503254512.

Striegel-Moore, R. H., Dohm, F.-A., Pike, K. M., Wilfley, D. E., & Fairburn, G. (2002). Abuse, bullying, and discrimination as risk factors for binge eating disorder. *American Journal of Psychiatry, 159*, 1902–1907. doi:10.1176/appi.ajp.159.11.1902.

Smith, P. K. (1997). Commentary III. Bullying in life-span perspective: What can studies of school bullying and workplace bullying learn from each other? *Journal of Community and Applied Social Psychology, 7*, 249–255. doi:10.1002/(SICI)1099-1298(199706)7:3<249::AID-CASP425>3.0.CO;2-2.

Smith, P. K., Singer, M., Hoel, H., & Cooper, C. L. (2003). Victimization in the school and the workplace: Are there any links? *British Journal of Psychology, 94*, 175–188. doi:10.1348/000712603321661868.

Sourander, A., Jensen, P., Rönning, J. A., Helenius, N. H., Sillanmäki, L., Kumpulainen, K., et al. (2007). What is the early adulthood outcome of boys who bully or are bullied in childhood? The Finnish 'from a boy to a man' study. *Pediatrics, 120*, 397–404. doi:10.1542/peds.2006-2704.

Taylor, S. E. (2007). Social support. In H. S. Friendman & R. C. Silver (Eds.), *Foundations of health psychology* (pp. 145–171). New York, NY: Oxford University Press.

Tehrani, N. (2001). A total quality approach to building a culture of respect. In N. Tehrani (Ed.), *Building a culture of respect: Managing bullying at work* (pp. 135–154). London: Taylor & Francis.

Thomas, M. (2005). Bullying among support staff in a higher education institution. *Health Education, 105*, 273–288. doi:10.1108/09654280510602499.

Thylefors, I. (1987). *Syndabockar. Om utstödning och mobbning i arbetslivet (Scapegoats. About social exclusion and bullying at work)*. Stockholm: Natur och Kultur.

Uchino, B., Cacioppo, J. T., & Kiecolt-Glaser, J. K. (1996). The relationship between social support and physiological processes: A review with emphasis on underlying mechanisms and implications for health. *Psychological Bulletin, 119*, 488–531. doi:10.1037/0033-2909.119.3.488.

Vaillancourt, T., Duku, E., Decatanzaro, D., Macmillan, H., Muir, C., & Schmidt, L. A. (2008). Variation in hypothalamic–pituitary–adrenal axis activity among bullied and non-bullied children. *Aggressive Behavior, 34*, 294–305. doi:10.1002/ab.20240.

Vaillancourt, T., Duku, E., Becker, S., Schmidt, L., Nicol, J., Muir, C., et al. (2011). Peer victimization, depressive symptoms, and high salivary cortisol predict poor memory in children. *Brain and Cognition, 77*, 191 199. doi:10.1016/j.bandc.2011.06.012.

Vaillancourt, T., & Hymel, S. (2006). Aggression and social status: The moderating roles of sex and peer-valued characteristics. *Aggressive Behavior, 32*, 396–408. doi:10.1002/ab.20138.

van der Wal, M. F., de Wit, C. A., & Hirasing, R. A. (2003). Psychosocial health among young victims and offenders of direct and indirect bullying. *Pediatrics, 111*, 1312–1317. Retrieved from http://pediatrics.aappublications.org/content/111/6/1312.full.html.

van Heugten, K. (2011). Theorizing active bystanders as change agents in workplace bullying of social workers. *Families in Society: The Journal of Contemporary Social Services, 92*(2), 219–224. doi:10.1606/1044-3894.4090.

Vartia, M., & Hyyti, J. (2002). Gender differences in workplace bullying among prison officers. *European Journal of Work and Organizational Psychology, 11*(1), 113–126. doi:10.1080/13594320143000870.

Verbrugge, L. M. (1985). Gender and health: An update on hypotheses and evidence. *Journal of Health and Social Behavior, 26*, 156–182. Retrieved from http://www.jstor.org/stable/2136750.

Voss, M., Floderus, B., & Diderichsen, F. (2004). How do job characteristics, family situation, domestic work, and lifestyle factors relate to sickness absence? A study based on Sweden post. *Journal of Occupational & Environmental Medicine, 46*(11), 1134–114. Retrieved from http://journals.lww.com/joem/.

Walker, S., & Richardson, D. R. (1998). Aggression strategies among older adults: Delivered but not seen. *Aggression and Violent Behavior, 3*, 287–294. doi:10.1016/S1359-1789(96)00029-8.

Wilfley, D., Pike, K., Dohm, F., Striegel-Moore, R., & Fairburn, C. (2001). Bias in binge eating disorder: How representative are recruited samples? *Journal of Consulting and Clinical Psychology, 69*, 383–388.

Williams, K. R., & Guerra, N. G. (2007). Prevalence and predictors of internet bullying. *Journal of Adolescents Health, 41*, S14–S21. doi:10.1016/j.jadohealth.2007.08.018.

Williams, K., Chambers, M., Logan, S., & Robinson, D. (1996). Association of common health symptoms with bullying in primary school children. *British Medical Journal, 3*, 17–19. doi:10.1136/bmj.313.7048.17.

Wolke, D., Woods, S., Bloomfield, L., & Karstadt, L. (2001). Bullying involvement in primary school and common health problems. *Archives of Disease in Childhood, 85*, 197–201. doi:10.1136/adc.85.3.197.

Yamada, D. (2012). *Workplace bullying is bad for business.* Downloaded from Workplace Bullying Institute at http://www.workplacebullying.org/2012/01/09/yamada-2/

Yildirim, A., & Yildirim, D. (2007). Mobbing in the workplace by peers and managers: Mobbing experienced by nurses working in healthcare facilities in Turkey and its effect on nurses. *Journal of Clinical Nursing, 16*, 1444–1453. doi:10.1111/j.1365-2702.2006.01814.x.

Zapf, D. (1999). Organisational, work group related and personal causes of mobbing/bullying at work. *International Journal of Manpower, 20*, 70–85. doi:10.1108/01437729910268669.

Zapf, D., Dormann, C., & Frese, M. (1996). Longitudinal studies in organisational stress research: A review of the literature with reference to methodological issues. *Journal of Occupational Health Psychology, 1*, 145–169. doi:10.1037/1076-8998.1.2.145.

Zapf, D., & Gross, C. (2001). Conflict escalation and coping with workplace bullying: A replication and extension. *European Journal of Work and Organizational Psychology, 10*(4), 497–522. doi:10.1080/13594320143000834.

Zogby International. (2010). *U.S. Workplace Bullying Survey.* Retrieved from http://www.workplacebullyinginstitute

Part III

Evaluation of Occupational Causes and Risks to Workers' Health

Promoting Mental Health Within Workplaces

12

Bonnie Kirsh and Rebecca Gewurtz

Introduction

Work affects the mental health and psychosocial well-being of employees through the many practices and cultures it entails. Increasingly, employers, employees, unions, insurance companies and other stakeholders are seeking guidance on ways of establishing workplaces that promote mental health and minimize risks for psychosocial distress. In some countries, this interest is being fuelled by the emergence of national standards that help employers assess and abate risks to mental health in the workplace. Such standards view protection of mental health at work as both a corporate and a social responsibility. Accordingly, risks to employee mental health arising from the organization and design of work, from the organization's leadership and corporate culture, and from the future of work for employees are in need of discussion. Only then can corporate and social policy be developed to mitigate these risks.

This chapter discusses work-related factors that influence the health of employees and, in particular, their mental health. It draws on the work of researchers in the fields of organizational development, health and safety and mental health to delineate key areas of focus and their relevance to creating mentally healthy workplaces. The factors are presented within a framework that views mental health in the workplace as the outcome of several domains that most certainly intersect, but are presented here as distinct entities. The framework is depicted in Fig. 12.1 and entails Job Design, Leadership, Organizational Culture and Job Future. Similar frameworks have been presented in the workplace health literature (see for example, CMHA & Dalla Lana School of Public Health; Wilson, Dejoy, Vandenberg, Richardson, & Mcgrath, 2004). In most of these models, including the one presented here, job design refers to work tasks and perceptions of them, leadership focuses on the qualities and practices implemented by those who lead, organizational culture refers to social and interpersonal aspects of work and job future refers to security and career development.

B. Kirsh, Ph.D. (✉)
Department of Occupational Science and Occupational Therapy, University of Toronto,
160-500 University Ave., Toronto, ON M5G 1V7, Canada
e-mail: bonnie.kirsh@utoronto.ca

R. Gewurtz, Ph.D.
Department School of Rehabilitation, McMaster University,
1280 Main Street West, Rm.447, IAHS, Hamilton, ON L8S4L8, Canada
e-mail: gewurtz@mcmaster.ca

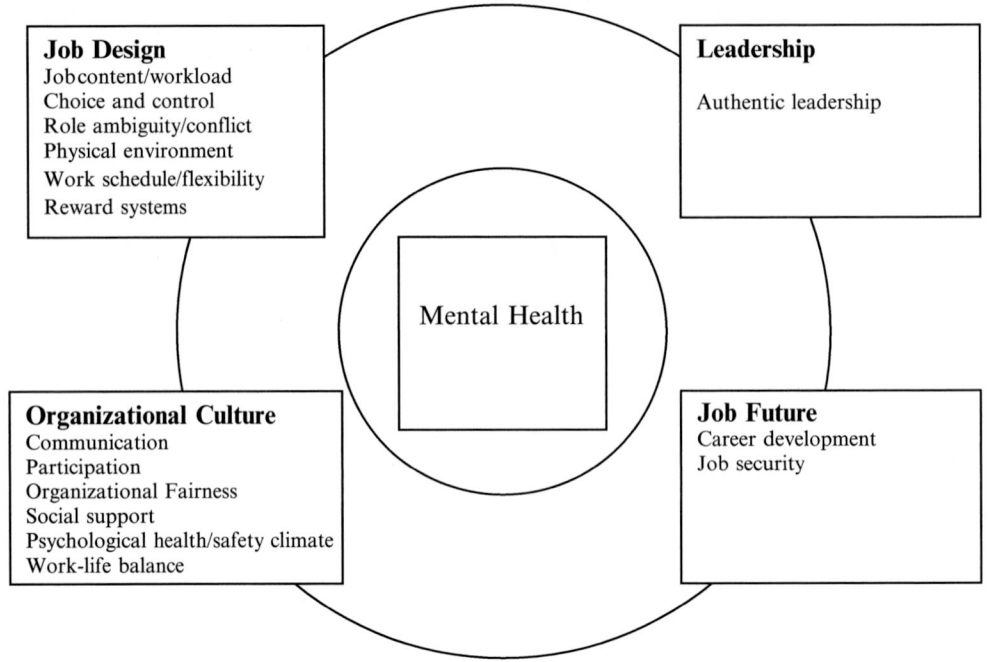

Fig. 12.1 A framework for workplace mental health

Job Design

Job design refers to aspects of the immediate work tasks, the conditions under which they are performed, and how they are perceived and experienced by individual workers. Job design consists of the rules (both explicit and implicit) that exist within all organizations and govern expectations around what employees do on a daily basis at work, when, where, and how employees complete their work, and how much discretion or choice they have within their jobs. Components of job design that have been identified as important in considering the psychosocial health of the workplace and workers within the organization include: job content and workload; choice and control; role clarity; environmental conditions; work schedules including flexible work; and reward systems (many of these issues are discussed in other chapters of this handbook). In this section we review evidence about the relationship between various components of job design and the mental health and well-being of workers.

Job Content and Workload

Job content and workload are important and related concepts within workplace health literature. Job content is a broad concept that refers to the composition of the individual's work roles, tasks, and demands. Workload refers more specifically to the amount of work or task demands assigned to a worker or group of workers in a given period of time. Both concepts have been examined in terms of their impact on the mental health and well-being of workers. The content and demands of a job should be well matched to the skills and competencies of the worker, and should provide sufficient challenge without over-taxing the worker. Work associated with excessive repetition, monotony, and the experience of boredom, or conversely, excessive demands, stress and insufficient resources have been associated with mental and physical health problems, and behaviors such as drinking and smoking (Leka & Jain, 2010).

Among health-care workers in particular, job content and workload have been identified as key determinants of the quality of the workplace environment and critical issues in the health and well-being of healthcare workers. For example, Ramirez, Graham, Richards, Cull, and Gregory (1996) found that among medical specialists, feeling overloaded, poorly managed, and dealing with patient suffering were associated with burnout and psychiatric morbidity. However, job satisfaction provided protection against work overload, as did feeling proficient in communication and management skills. This latter finding suggests that the broader concept of job content has an important role to play in the experience of work overload. Cole et al. (2009) examined the relationship between workload and health outcomes among health-care workers, and found that those with the heaviest workloads had greater odds of receiving treatment for both mental health and musculoskeletal disorders. Similarly, Hannigan, Edwards, and Burnard (2004) found that 40 % of UK clinical psychologists were experiencing high levels of personal distress. Sources of stress were found to be related to client characteristics, excessive workloads, professional self-doubt, and poor management.

In response to new insights into issues related to job content, workload and their impact on employee health, there have been increased efforts within workplaces to monitor and report on possible imbalances (Strelioff, Lavoie-Tremblay, & Barton, 2007). Such efforts have increased attention to situations of potential work overload or underload (boredom), and provided opportunities for professional development in order to maintain the health and well-being of workers, improving job performance and employee retention. These issues are especially pertinent during times of organizational restructuring when workloads and job content might undergo significant change.

Existing theoretical models highlight that job content and workload do not operate in isolation. Rather, social support in the workplace (Karasek & Theorell, 1990), systems of rewards and compensation (Siegrist, 1996), and the amount of decision-making latitude or control workers have in the workplace (Karasek, 1979) can moderate the impact that job content and workload have on the health and well-being of workers. That is, workers might tolerate or even thrive under conditions of high workload when they have adequate support, are sufficiently rewarded, compensated or recognized, when there is high job satisfaction, and if they have sufficient autonomy over their work.

Choice and Control

Choice and control have already been highlighted as key features of job design. Both theory and research within the workplace health literature suggest that choice and control (i.e., being able to actively participate in decision making at work) can counteract some of the negative effects of workplace demands and strain, and can contribute to a positive workplace climate. Drawing on national survey data from Sweden and the United States, Karasek (1979) developed a well known model suggesting that the combination of low decision latitude and heavy job demand is associated with mental strain and job dissatisfaction. Job demand within this model refers to the previously discussed concept of workload and is comprised the quantity of work assigned to an individual, the time pressure experienced at work, and mental requirements for job completion. Individuals who experience high job demand might report feeling pressured to work fast and having difficulty taking time off work. Decision latitude, on the other hand, refers to the ability to make decisions or participate in decision-making at work, exercise discretion and autonomy, and be creative (Vezina, Bourbonnais, Brisson, & Trudel, 2004). Mental strain has been linked to health conditions such as depression, anxiety, apathy, distress, burnout, exhaustion, low self-esteem, drug use, and coronary disease (Leka & Jain, 2010; Vezina et al.). Van Yperen and Snijders (2000) reported on findings that begin to clarify the relationships and interactions involved in the Karasek model. Specifically, in their study of 260 employees in 31 working groups of a national bank in the Netherlands, these researchers found that it was the specific combination of an individual's perception of his or her job demands being high compared to others, along with the group's shared evaluation of job control being low that was associated with poorer health outcomes and greater number of sick days. These findings highlight that organizations should attend to worker perceptions of their job design including workload and the degree of control and choice they experience. Providing opportunities for workers to participate in decision-making affecting their work, and exercise control over their work conditions including their work schedule and how their work should be completed, will have a positive effect on health and well-being, and contribute to the creation of a positive work environment.

Role Ambiguity and Role Conflict

The impact of role ambiguity and role conflict on well-being has been the topic of some research to date, and warrants further attention. Generally, role ambiguity refers to a lack of clarity about expected behavior from a job, whereas role conflict suggests a lack of compatibility between different expectations from a job. These variables have been shown to have negative impacts on a variety of outcomes. In a meta-analysis of research conducted on role ambiguity and role conflict in work settings, Jackson and Schuler (1985) found that role ambiguity and role conflict were strongly correlated with affective reactions such as job satisfaction, tension/anxiety, commitment, involvement, and propensity to leave. Several studies have examined health outcomes in particular. For example, Jamal (1990) found that role ambiguity was a variable that was significantly related to psychosomatic health problems in a sample of nurses, and Kelloway and Barling (1991) found emotional exhaustion to occur under conditions of role ambiguity and role conflict. International studies have supported these findings. For example, in their study of job stressors and long-term sick leave due to depressive disorders among Japanese male employees, Inoue and colleagues (2010) concluded that role ambiguity was one of two variables (the other being job control) that predicted long-term sick leave due to depressive disorders among male employees, independent of depressive symptoms and neuroticism.

In light of these findings it is incumbent upon workplaces to find ways to avoid role ambiguity and conflict as a means of promoting psychosocial health amongst their employees. Having clear and reasonable expectations and sending clear and straightforward messages are important ways of doing so. To the greatest degree possible, jobs need to be described in explicit terms with regard to scope, responsibility, authority, standards of performance, and relationships with other jobs. This process involves communication among individuals, work teams and supervisors to avoid job misunderstanding and conflict. These discussions and interactions are important, as often job descriptions list formal job duties but say little about the more subtle and informal expectations of the roles (Handy, 1999). To minimize role conflict, expectations should be consistent and account for employees' multiple roles as well as personal value systems (Danna & Griffin, 1999).

The Physical Environment

The physical work environment has received significant attention in the literature in terms of its contribution to the health and well-being of workers, worker turnover, absenteeism, and workplace productivity. In particular, there has been a focus on the physical design of work spaces and its relationship to repetitive strain and musculoskeletal injuries (Crawford, Gutierrez, & Harber, 2005; Faucett, 2005). However, the physical work environment has broader implications for the health and productivity of workers. In a qualitative study by Arwedson, Roos, and Bjorklund (2007) investigating the factors that contribute to the experience of good health at work, the participants emphasized how a good work environment, which includes natural lighting, cleanliness, and an aesthetically pleasing premise, contributes to well-being at work. These authors emphasized the importance of more psychosocial components such as a comfortable and pleasant atmosphere in the workplace in order to promote good mental health and well-being at work.

Many work organizations are implementing open-plan office designs where employees work together in large rooms, as opposed to private offices or enclosed rooms. Such physical work environments provide improved access to natural lighting for employees. Furthermore, open-plan office designs can be more conducive to team work, and support cooperation and communication among workers while reducing costs (de Croon, Sluiter, Kuijer, & Frings-Dresen, 2005; Kaarlela-Tuomaala, Helenius, Keskinen, & Hongisto, 2009). However, such office designs provide less privacy, increased noise, and have been associated with difficulty concentrating on challenging tasks (de Croon et al.; Kaarlela-Tuomaala et al.). There is some evidence that open-plan office designs can be potential workplace stressors, compromising health, motivation, and performance (Vischer, 2007), and limited evidence that such workplace designs intensify cognitive workload and compromise interpersonal relationships (de Croon et al.). Meijer, Frings-Dresen, and Sluiter (2009) evaluated the effects of an innovative open-plan office design on the health and productivity of 138 office workers at a Dutch regional governmental institute. Participants were individuals who worked at a desktop computer at least four hours per day. While there were no short-term significant differences in most outcomes, in the long-term, perceived productivity increased significantly, and there was a significant increase in general health. Conversely, Kaarlela-Tuomaala et al. (2009) evaluated the effects of moving from a private office design to an open-plan office space among professional workers. The move was associated with increased noise and distractions, reduced privacy, and increased concentration difficulties. Satisfaction with the work environment decreased after the relocation to the open-plan office. The benefits often associated with open-plan office designs did not transpire as cooperation became less pleasant and there was no change in communication or information flow.

One of the purported benefits of open-plan office designs is improved access to natural lighting, windows and green space. Most of the evidence about the health benefits associated with access to natural lighting and green space comes from research beyond the workplace. However, a review on the effects of natural lighting in the workplace conducted by the National Renewable Energy Laboratory in the United States has examined this issue in the workplace, and the findings suggest that workplace productivity increases and absenteeism decreases when a company moves into an office building with improved lighting and access to windows (Edwards & Torcellini, 2002).

The mixed findings reported in the literature on open-plan office designs suggests that the type of worker and the work tasks involved are important, and both contribute the outcomes associated with different physical work environments. Although open-plan designs might facilitate communication, teamwork, and cooperation among workers, it can cause strain and stress among those whose primary tasks involve individual effort, high concentration, and require privacy. These findings are consistent with the framework for the study of work-space stress put forth by Vischer (2007) which highlights the importance of fit between the work environment, the workers, and the work tasks. A work environment can either support workers and the work tasks being performed (good fit), or hinder them (bad fit).

Work Schedule

The work schedule is an important component of job design that contributes to the health and well-being of workers. Much of the literature to date has focused on the health consequences of shift work and working long hours. Specifically, research has highlighted that stress is common following extensive shift work, long hours of work, and interrupted sleep patterns (Leka & Jain, 2010). There is a growing body of literature that highlights the deleterious effects of shift work and long working hours on health and well-being. In their review of the literature (this literature is also reviewed in another chapter in this handbook), Leka and Jain (2010) highlight that the negative health consequences of shift work can be more pronounced among older workers and those with competing family responsibilities, while younger workers and those just beginning their careers seem to be most vulnerable to the effects of long working hours. Furthermore, Grosch, Caruso, Rosa, and Sauter (2006) found that working long hours are also associated with greater job demands, greater control through participation in decision-making, and greater opportunity for workers to develop their own special abilities. Although job satisfaction was found to be greater among workers with long work hours, working more than 70 h per week was associated with adverse health and well-being outcomes. Shields (1999) found that women who worked long hours had increased odds of subsequently experiencing depression, and increasing work hours was associated with increased weight gain among men, an increase in drinking among women, and an increase in smoking among both men and women. These findings suggest that individuals who enjoy their jobs might be more inclined to work long hours; however, too much overtime can have adverse effects on health and well-being.

Flexible Work

In some workplaces, there are provisions within the job design for workers to choose their own hours and workspaces including the option of working from home. Such flexibility can be accommodating for workers who are balancing competing responsibilities or have unique scheduling needs, and provide workers with a degree of choice and control over their job. However, flexibility associated with contract work and other temporary work arrangements often leads to job insecurity and precariousness, factors that have been associated with negative health outcomes among workers (Clarke, Lewchuk, de Wolff, & King, 2007; Lewchuk, Clarke, & de Wolff, 2008). Furthermore, such job arrangements are often associated with fluctuating periods of intense work demands to meet pressing deadlines (MacEachen, Polzer, & Clarke, 2008), and a lack of investment in the health promoting aspects of the work environment (Crawford et al., 2005). These findings suggest that flexible work schedules can have both positive and negative implications for the health and well-being of workers. It is most often associated with positive implications that allow for increased work–life balance, autonomy and control, and choice which can foster creativity and productivity. However, choice and control, which are most often considered a positive aspect of flexible work, can be circumvented by workplace demands and needs, competition, and the expectation that employees will work whenever they are needed in order to accomplish the organizational goals (Harlan & Robert, 1998; MacEachen et al.). The reality of flexible work is that it is also associated with long work hours, increased work intensity, lack of predictability in work demands, and blurred boundaries between home and worklife. MacEachen et al. argue that the practice of flexible work environments often caters to the needs of the organization rather than the worker: "Flexibility in practice relies on and requires pliant workers who 'willingly' mould their lives according to the demands of work, and who are readily available at all times including evenings and weekend" (p. 1026). Thus, flexible work can promote health and accommodate individual needs in the workplace, as well as threaten workplace health and wellness.

Furthermore, the distancing of the individual worker from the workplace through the allowance of remote and flexible workspaces and hours make it easier for organizations to disassociate themselves from the resulting health consequences. MacEachen et al. (2008) found that the managers in their study interpreted the occupational health consequences of flexible work (such as stress, strain, and challenges balancing home and work responsibilities) as individual problems rather than a problem associated with job design. Although flexible work can help workers balance competing demands in their work and personal lives, it can also be a way of meeting the needs of the organization by ensuring that workers are available to work long hours and carry heavy workloads. The resulting stress, strain, and health consequences are seen as the individual's personal concern, beyond the scope of the workplace.

Reward Systems

Workers want to feel appreciated by their employers and their colleagues. There are many ways to reward employees including acknowledgement, recognition and pay incentives. In the late 1980s, Siegrist (1996) proposed the "effort–reward imbalance" model based on findings that a work situation characterized by high effort and low reward is associated with poor health outcomes. Within the model, Siegrist further distinguished between extrinsic and intrinsic effort: extrinsic effort is associated with time pressures, interruptions, competing demands and responsibilities, and increased workload that arises from external sources; intrinsic effort or overcommitment is an internal attitude or innate drive to push forward and gain esteem or approval. According to this model, reward is primarily measured in terms of salary, esteem/respect, and job security/opportunity for advancement (Siegrist, 2002). The central process or mechanism of action is social reciprocity, the possibility of gaining or earning advantage as a result of effort expended in the workplace.

The effort/reward imbalance model has been applied to the study of precarious employment where individuals exert effort but continue to experience job insecurity and unpredictability (Clarke et al., 2007; Crawford et al., 2005; Lewchuk et al., 2008; MacEachen et al., 2008; Vezina et al., 2004), or are seen as disposable and thus tolerate unreasonable working conditions or expectations in an effort to maintain their job or get a promotion (MacEachen et al.; Vezina et al.). Such work situations have been associated with poor health outcomes, including increased anxiety, depression, substance use, and high blood pressure (Siegrist, 2002; Stansfeld, Fuhrer, Shipley, & Marmot, 1999; Vezina et al.). According to a review of the evidence supporting the model, Siegrist (2002) argued that 10–40 % of the workforce suffers from some degree of effort/reward imbalance. Based on longitudinal measures from a cohort of civil servants in the UK, Kruper, Singh-Manoux, Siegrist, and Marmot (2002) showed that effort–reward imbalance is associated with an increased risk of functional disability from mental health problems and a moderately elevated risk of newly reported mild psychiatric disorders.

These findings suggest that organizations should consider how to best reward, recognize and compensate employees for their efforts and achievements. For example, salaries, wages, benefits, and bonus structures should be kept in line with efforts and contributions made by employees. Furthermore, organizations should invest in nonmonetary rewards such as ensuring there are adequate job promotion opportunities and job security. Unfortunately, some sectors of the labor market or organizational structures rely on short-term contractual work arrangements and are unable to offer such rewards to their workers. Such workers are often particularly vulnerable and at risk for poor health outcomes.

A summary and review of the scientific evidence for the aforementioned components of *JOB DESIGN* as factors that affect mental health, is provided in Table 12.1 which lists the various studies documenting their significance.

Leadership

The importance of leadership in contributing to healthy work environments has been demonstrated across cultures, sectors and geographic boundaries. Leadership in the context of the workplace describes the overall supervisory or management style, and characterizes the culture of the organization by setting standards, norms, and expectations. It encompasses organizational justice in terms of

Table 12.1 Evidence for components of framework for workplace mental health

Job design	Leadership	Organizational culture	Job future
Job content and workload	*Effective leadership*	*Communication*	*Job security*
Leka and Jain (2010)	Kuoppala et al. (2008)	Walters (2005)	Borg et al. (2000)
Ramirez et al. (1996)		Robbins (2001)	Ferrie et al. (2002)
Cole et al. (2009)		Young and Post (1993)	McDonough (2000), Rugulies et al. (2006)
Hannigan et al. (2004)		Reina and Reina (1999)	Clarke et al. (2007)
		Cameron and Webster (2004)	
		Schabracq and Cooper (2000)	
Choice and control	*Authentic leadership*	*Meaningful participation/involvement*	*Career development*
Karasek (1979)	Shirey (2006)	Lawler (1991)	Browne (2000)
Leka and Jain (2010), Vezina et al. (2004)	Lohela et al. (2009)	Vandenberg et al. (1999)	Kaye (2010)
Van Yperen and Snijders (2000)		Freeman and Rogers (1999)	
		Simmering et al. (2003)	
		Grawitch et al. (2007)	
		Roebuck (1996)	
		McConnell (1998)	
Role ambiguity and role conflict	*Leadership development*	*Organizational justice and fairness*	
Jackson and Schuler (1985)	Woltring et al. (2003)	Kivimaki et al. (2004)	
Jamal (1990)		Kivimaki et al. (2003)	
Kelloway and Barling (1991)		Shain (2001)	
Inoue et al. (2010)		Vaananen et al. (2004)	
The physical environment		*Social support*	
Arwedson et al. (2007)		Cooper and Cartwright (1994)	
Vischer (2007)		Vecchio (1995)	
Meijer et al. (2009)		Dejonge et al. (1996), Johnson and Hall (1988), Karasek et al. (1982)	
Kaarlela-Tuomaala et al. (2009)		Karasek and Theorell (1990)	
Edwards and Torcellini (2002)		Viswesvaran et al. (1999)	
		Plaisier et al. (2007)	
		Marchand et al. (2005)	
		Stansfeld et al. (1997)	
		Ducharme and Martin (2000)	
		Beehr et al. (2000)	

Work schedule
Leka and Jain (2010)
Grosch et al. (2006)
Shields (1999)

Flexible work
Clarke et al. (2007), Lewchuk et al. (2008)
MacEachen et al. (2008)
Crawford et al. (2005)

Reward systems
Siegrist (1996)
Clarke et al. (2007), Crawford et al. (2005), Lewchuk et al. (2008), MacEachen et al. (2008), Vezina et al. (2004)
Stansfeld et al. (1999)
Kruper et al. (2002)

A psychological health/safety climate
Gilbert and Bilsker (2011)
Aldana (2001), Golaszewski (2001)
Grawitch et al. (2006)
McFarlin and Fals-Stewart (2002)
Selviket et al. (2004))
Erdogan and Enders (2007), Witt and Carlson (2006), Piercy et al. (2006)
Loi et al. (2006)
Krupa et al. (2009)

Work–life balance
Burton (2002)
Higgins and Duxbury (2009)
Scandura and Lankau (1997)
Crooker and Grover (1993)

the treatment of employees, social support through demonstrated concern for subordinates, and workplace transformation through mechanism of stimulation and motivation. Studies have examined the relationship between leadership and health and well-being at work. Kuoppala, Lamminpaa, Liira, and Vainio (2008) conducted a systematic literature review of 27 studies and found moderate evidence that good leadership is associated with improved job well-being, a decreased risk of sick absence, and a decreased risk of disability pension. Furthermore, there was weak evidence that good leadership is associated with job satisfaction but not job performance. Thus, the authors concluded that the available evidence suggests that good leadership contributes to job satisfaction and job well-being, and decreases the risk of sick leaves and early retirement. According to these authors, strong leaders, especially during times of rapid organizational change, can energize and satisfy needs for achievement and recognition.

What are the qualities of a leader that can promote health in the workplace? There is a vast literature on styles of leadership and qualities of an effective leader but far less that examines traits as they relate to workplace health. Some research in the health care domain discusses "authentic leadership" as a key ingredient for establishing and sustaining healthy work environments and the "glue" needed to hold together a healthy work environment. Avolio, Gardner, Walumbwa, Luthans, and May (2004) define authentic leaders as "those individuals who are deeply aware of how they think and behave and are perceived by others as being aware of their own and others' values/moral perspective, knowledge, and strengths, aware of the context in which they operate, and who are confident, hopeful, optimistic, resilient, and high on moral character" (2004, p. 804). Authentic leaders have the attributes of genuineness, trustworthiness, reliability, compassion, and believability, and create healthy work environments by engaging employees in promoting positive behavior (Shirey, 2006). Additional qualities of authentic leaders have been identified by Lohela, Bjorklund, Vingard, Hagberg, and Jensen (2009). In their study of 1,212 employees from four medium and large companies in Sweden, they found that changes in leadership in terms of fairness, empowerment, and the provision of social support, impact the health of subordinate workers. These findings suggest that good leadership can support workplace mental health and should be promoted in all workplaces. Indeed, leadership training programs are now common in workplaces and research across various sectors shows that they have a positive effect. For example, an 8-year evaluation of leadership development programs in the field of public health shows positive results on the personal, organizational and community levels (Woltring, Constantine, & Schwarte, 2003). Effective leaders can energize employees, provide a vision and support employees in their efforts at work.

Organizational Culture

Organizational culture is an important construct in understanding the experiences of individuals in the workplace. Defined as the shared values, beliefs, and expectations among members of an organization (Moran & Volkwein, 1992; Spataro, 2005), the culture of an organization shapes much of what occurs within it and acts as an informal system of control. Specifically, organizational culture dictates norms, rules of behavior, expectations of members, how problems and challenges are addressed, and the integration of new members and members who are different (Spataro, 2005). The culture of an organization emerges through the complex and continuous communication and interaction among members both within and across organizational structures (Keyton, 2005). Schein (1992) refers to culture as "a basic set of assumptions that defines for us what we pay attention to, what things mean, how to react emotionally to what is going on, and what actions to take in various kinds of situations" (p. 22). In short, organizational culture has been identified as the central factor that holds the modern organization together (Goffee & Jones, 1996). Within this broad concept, the safety culture of an organization has been recognized as being an important determinant of the safety and health of employees. This has held true primarily for physical health and safety, but it is becoming clear that organizational culture has a major impact on psychological or mental health as well. Components of the organizational culture that are influential in this regard are communication, meaningful participation or employee involvement, organizational fairness, social support, a psychological health and safety climate, and an emphasis on work–life balance.

Communication

Communication in the workplace is a critical factor influencing the mental health of its workers. Poor communication engenders confusion, anxiety, potential conflict with peers and in some cases, feelings of disconnection and exclusion. Surveys show that poor communication causes increases in workplace stress, absenteeism and turnover (Walters, 2005). In contrast, effective communication enables trust and cooperation to develop in the workplace, thereby fostering support and harmonious work relations. Through clear and effective communication, information is shared, workers feel included and morale improves. Identifying elements of effective communication in the workplace has been the topic of much discussion, and there appears to be agreement on a core set of principles and practices. Research by Robbins (2001) and Young and Post (1993) identifies a set of five principal communication practices common to companies with high trust cultures: (1) managers explain why decisions are made; (2) communication occurs in a timely manner; (3) important information flows continuously; (4) direct supervisors and other leaders explain the specific implications of environmental and organizational changes to each level of workers; and (5) employee responses to leader communications are validated. Honest, timely, current and consistent information-sharing is central to building trust and feelings of security within the workplace, and empowers employees by giving them the information they need to be productive in their work. In their book, *Trust and Betrayal in the Workplace*, Reina and Reina (1999) discuss information-sharing as a principal component of their Communication Trust Model.

Active listening, skillful inquiry and receptiveness are components of effective communication that have also been deemed to be essential to workplaces and to leaders in particular. Active listening includes such behaviors as empathetic body language that is consistent with verbal messages, validating others' statements, enabling others to express their thoughts without unnecessary interruption, and paraphrasing to ensure mutual understanding (Robbins & Hunsaker, 1996). Skillful inquiry, or asking good, helpful questions is a facet of active listening and conveys an interest in learning more about the issue at hand as well as the valuing of others' ideas. The creation of an open and receptive environment is created through such communication strategies, with benefits to workers' sense of well-being.

While the impact of information sharing on worker well-being has been highlighted time and time again, the pace at which information is currently being transmitted within workplaces is increasing rapidly and the impact of this change has yet to play out. Today's organizations use a variety of communication media including email, teleconferencing, videoconferencing, and more recently, Instant Messaging (IM). Using a case study approach, Cameron and Webster (2004) investigated Instant Messaging and its use in organizations and found that IM was perceived to be much less rich than face-to-face communication and carried with it some potential dangers. Employees using IM engaged in multiple forms of multitasking, leading the authors to question the impact of completing multiple communication tasks at the same time on performance and working relationships. Further, results demonstrate that IM interrupts employee work patterns and employees see its interruptive nature as unfair. Schabracq and Cooper (2000) insist that when events interfere with work routines and goals, the result is a sense of loss of control. As such, these events can be serious sources of stress with cumulative effects on individual well-being and health. The impact of rapidly developing information and communication technologies in the workplace is yet to be determined, and its effects on workers' mental health is a particularly important line of inquiry.

Meaningful Participation/Involvement

Employee involvement is a commonly cited healthy workplace practice that enables workers to bring a diverse set of ideas and perspectives to bear on solving organizational problems and increasing organizational effectiveness (Grawitch, Gottschalk, & Munz, 2006). Employee-involvement programs involve employees in decision making, and focus on such aspects as job autonomy, self-managed work teams, and empowerment (e.g., Cohen, Ledford, & Spreitzer, 1996; Karasek & Theorell, 1990; Lawler, 1991). Such strategies have been shown to produce positive consequences for both employee well-being and organizational effectiveness alike (e.g., Lawler; Vandenberg, Richardson, & Eastman, 1999). Research demonstrates a relationship between employee involvement in decision making and employee variables, such as job satisfaction and employee morale. A study by Freeman and Rogers (1999) demonstrated a significant difference between employee involvement program participants and nonparticipants, with the former reporting higher levels of loyalty and commitment to their organization, increased job satisfaction, and a more positive view of management than the latter group. Simmering, Colquitt, Noe, and Porter (2003) found evidence that employee involvement in specific development activities leads to greater perceptions of "fit" than lower levels of involvement. Furthermore, Grawitch, Trares, and Kohler (2007) found that satisfaction with employee involvement mediated the relationship between several healthy workplace practices (such as employee development, recognition, work–life balance, and health and safety programs) and the employee outcomes of organizational commitment and emotional exhaustion.

High involvement organizations create a culture of involvement and support by providing sufficient information, training, rewards, and power for employees to demonstrate the desired level of autonomy (Lawler, 1991). Opportunities for workers to provide feedback on work processes and goals offer them a voice in the workplace and empower them. Roebuck (1996) refers to such feedback as "soft feedback", defined as "information obtained from individuals that relates to ideas, opinions or perceptions and therefore requires them to make a choice as to whether or not to give it" (p. 328). Such soft feedback enables employees to identify problems hindering them in their work and may allow employees to perform better and to feel better. Workplace-based research by Roebuck (1990) indicates that requests for feedback along with a positive response and action by management have the effect of "reciprocation of concern" (p. 329), whereby employees feel that management has made positive efforts towards them and they respond positively in return. The consequences, according to Roebuck and others, include increased motivation, commitment and an improved organizational culture that contributes to the well-being of employees and organizations alike. While reciprocation of concern is the goal, oftentimes employee involvement efforts leave employees feeling more manipulated than motivated (McConnell, 1998). McConnell explains that this occurs because employee input, even when solicited, is often discounted, ignored, or altered to fit the manager's preconceptions. He suggests that managers learn to provide involvement opportunities, accompanied by clear outcome expectations, and allow employees the freedom to pursue those outcomes in their own way.

Organizational Justice and Fairness

Organizational justice is an important component of organizational culture. It has emerged in recent organizational literature on psychosocial risk factors in the workplace, and is composed of both relational and procedural components. The relational component refers to the extent to which supervisors consider the points of view of their employee and treat subordinates fairly; procedural components refer specifically to fairness within formal decision-making processes (Elovainio, Kivimaki, & Vahtera, 2002; Kivimaki, Elovainio, Vahtera, & Ferrie, 2003; Kivimaki et al., 2004). Although related to previously discussed job design components, such as work demands, control and social support, organizational justice is focused on the social structure of the organization as opposed to the individual worker. Research on organizational justice has generally reported a linear relationship, where lower levels of justice were associated with lower measures of well-being. For example, drawing on data collected as part of the prospective Whitehall II study of 10,308 mostly white collar British civil servants between 1985 and 1988, Kivimaki et al. (2004) found that low and declining relational justice is predictive of decreasing health, and favorable changes in the treatment of employees was associated with reduced health risk. Similar findings were reported by Kivimaki et al. (2003) who described findings from a longitudinal study among Finnish hospital personnel. Although Kivimaki et al. noted that low procedural and relational justice equally increased the likelihood of illness, for procedural justice there was an interaction with socioeconomic status. Furthermore, mental health problems and self-rated health status were more strongly predicted by procedural as opposed to relational components of organizational justice.

Fairness, another component of organizational justice, has also been studied in terms of its effect on health and well-being of workers. Shain (2001) has proposed that a key factor linking complex factors that are known to influence health and well-being at work is the perception of fairness. That is, the feeling among workers that workplace conditions are constructed, not by chance, but by intentional choices made by managers in light of the needs of workers. By reviewing the research exploring the health effects of power relationships, Shain argues that workers respond differently to the stress that might result from the sense of being treated unfairly. For some, it might lead to experiences of depression, anxiety, or anger (with associated implications for overall health and well-being). According to Shain, poor health outcomes such as depression and anxiety, can impair performance and lead to increased aggression, substance abuse, and physical illnesses. Such outcomes can increase absenteeism and lead to increased workplace health costs. According to Shain:

> If power is meant to garner control, then it appears to do so to a degree that can render some employees almost useless in terms of their ability to cope with or adapt to change, learn new skills, and be creative. Given outcomes like these, even in purely calculative terms, power is inefficient as a means of governing the workplace. (p. 365)

Vaananen et al. (2004) explored fairness specifically in terms of the division of labor at work among employees of a forest industry corporation in Finland, and found that perceptions of unfairness increased long sickness-related absences for blue-collar male workers, and somewhat increased short absences among blue-collar women. These authors hypothesized that the perception of fairness might be a particularly salient contributor to health among blue-collar workers whose job may offer fewer resources for their well-being compared to white-collar workers.

Social Support

Relationships with coworkers have the potential to be stressful with many negative consequences, or supportive, with numerous benefits to psychological health and well-being. Studies have found that mistrust of coworkers is related to high role ambiguity, poor communication, low job satisfaction, and poor psychosocial well-being (summarized by Cooper & Cartwright, 1994). Strong emotions, such as workplace jealousy and envy amongst employees, have been associated with such detrimental outcomes as workplace violence and harrassment (Vecchio, 1995).

On the flip side, much research has demonstrated the benefits of social support with regard to enhanced coping and well-being. Social support is broadly defined as helping relationships in the workplace and it is often thought to moderate the experience of stress and strain in the workplace (Dejonge, Jansen, & Vanbreukelen, 1996; Johnson & Hall, 1988; Karasek, Triantis, & Chaudhry, 1982). The Karasek model, discussed earlier in this chapter, as well as in another chapter of this handbook, was expanded to include social support after its initial development, in order to highlight that emotional integration, trust among coworkers and supervisors, the social cohesion of organization, and the availability of help and assistance at work, can "buffer" the poor health outcomes associated with high demand and low control among workers (Karasek & Theorell, 1990). However, some researchers have argued that social support at work has a more direct effect on workplace health than can be explained by the "buffer hypothesis." They argue that social support can either reduce the level of strain experienced, regardless of the intensity of the stressors encountered, or that the experience of strain or stress can elicit social support. For example, Viswesvaran, Sanchez, and Fisher (1999) reported in a meta-analysis of 68 studies that social support affects the work stressor–strain relationship in three ways: (1) social support reduces the experience of strain; (2) social support reduces the strength of the stressors; and (3) social support moderates the stressor–strain relationship.

Regardless of the mechanism by which social support operates—as a buffer or directly—accumulating evidence highlights its important effects on workplace health and well-being. For example, in a 2-year longitudinal study conducted by Plaisier et al. (2007), the risks for incidence of depressive and anxiety disorders tended to decrease under the conditions of high daily emotional support in combination with high levels of decision latitude, but tended to increase when both decision latitude and daily emotional support were low. Marchand, Demers, and Durand (2005) found that social support at work had an effect on preventing relapses of psychosocial distress, but had no effect on the risk of a first episode. Among British civil servants, Stansfeld, Rael, Head, Shipley, and Marmot (1997) found that support from colleagues and supervisors at work were related to lower risk of short spells of psychiatric sickness absence. These findings highlight the important role that social support at work plays in creating healthy workplaces that support worker health and well-being.

The nature of support and its impact has also been examined, albeit to a lesser extent. Ducharme and Martin (2000) isolated coworkers' relationships from supervisor-subordinate relationships, and tested the effects of two forms of coworker support—instrumental and affective—on levels of job satisfaction. They found that both affective and instrumental support contributed significantly to explanations of workers' affective reactions to their job demands, and concluded that both forms of support enhance job satisfaction and well-being regardless of the amount of job stress encountered. These authors suggest that "systematic efforts to promote both affiliative and practical ties among coworkers will enhance worker affect" (p. 240). Similarly, Beehr, Jex, Stacy, and Murray (2000) conceptualized social support in terms of emotional and instrumental types, but also included a third dimension—content of communication—as an expression of support. They found that social support predicted levels of psychosocial strain, and that the specific social support measure that had the strongest effect on strain reduction was the use of positive, job-related communications.

These workplace-based studies are consistent with findings in the broader literature on the benefits of social support. They speak to the importance of incorporating opportunities for several forms of coworker support (affective support, instrumental support, and positive work-related communication) into the workplace. To this end, it is not only important for workplaces to arrange social activities, such as gatherings that enable emotional and affective engagement, but also to implement efforts aimed at building effective work teams that enhance coworkers' abilities and opportunities to provide on-the-job assistance, advice, and information (instrumental support). In addition, a culture of respectful communication that is positive and encouraging adds to the powerful benefits of social support as it relates to mental health and well-being.

The influence of social relations and social support on the health and well-being of workers is particularly relevant given current conditions of precarious employment and short-term, insecure employment prevalent in many sectors of the labor market (Clarke et al., 2007; Crawford et al., 2005; Lewchuk et al., 2008; MacEachen et al., 2008). The findings reported by Clarke et al. (2007) in a qualitative study on the health effects of different types of precarious employment at different life/career stages suggest that the most vulnerable workers, those in precarious work situations that were described as "unsustainable," were in the greatest need of social support but had the least access to it. These findings suggest that many current work arrangements could threaten worker health by restricting opportunities to establish positive social relationships at work.

A Psychological Health/Safety Climate

An explicit organizational focus on psychological health and safety (PH&S) is an important ingredient in organizations that promote psychosocial well-being. While the need to protect *physical* health and safety in the workplace is well established and enshrined in Occupational Health and Safety (OH&S) regulations, there is a growing awareness that a holistic approach to OH&S involves the need to protect workers' *psychological* or mental health, and safety as well. In a psychological health and safety climate, there is a shared commitment to the importance of promoting and protecting the psychological well-being and safety of employees by taking actions to identify and address risks. In their guide for employers, Gilbert and Bilsker (2011) recommend a six-stage process for creating a climate focused on psychological health and safety: Policy, Planning, Promotion, Prevention, Process, and Persistence.

- The Policy stage involves commitment by organizational leadership to enhance psychological health and safety and may take the form of a statement expressing its importance or a comprehensive strategy of organizational change.
- The Planning stage involves identification of key psychological health indicators across the organization, selection of actions, and determination of desired objectives. It enables greater familiarity with the needs and issues that require attention, by collecting organizational information relevant to PH&S.
- Promotion refers to actions taken to promote the general psychological health of the workforce. The aim of psychological health promotion is to increase the capacity of employees to manage stress or emotional challenges in a way that reduces the likelihood of onset of mental disorders.
- Prevention refers to actions taken to prevent the occurrence of significant psychological problems or mental disorders, and may occur at the primary, secondary or tertiary level. *Primary prevention* changes individual or organizational conditions that contribute to psychological health problems. *Secondary prevention* identifies psychological health problems when they are in a relatively mild state, so that a timely response will prevent more serious problems. *Tertiary prevention* reduces the distress associated with a mental disorder and may involve enabling prompt access to treatment and rehabilitation, or instituting well planned return-to-work programs so that mental health problems do not cause sustained work disability.
- The Process stage involves the evaluation of implementation and monitoring results of actions taken to enhance psychological health and safety.
- Finally, Persistence refers to the sustainment of effective actions in a process of continuous improvement.

Currently, many workplaces are moving towards creating cultures that emphasize psychological health in ways that could be classified, using Gilbert and Bilsker's (2011) framework, as promotion or prevention. While implementation of these stages alone is insufficient for a sustainable culture of psychological health and safety, there have been many benefits that have resulted from such efforts. Two reviews of studies on the impact of health promotion programs (Aldana, 2001; Golaszewski, 2001) found that, across studies, health promotion programs were related to lower absenteeism and health care expenditures.

Programs such as stress management training encourage employees to engage in extra-role behaviors and also improve employee emotional well-being, defined as affect, depression, and perceived stress (Grawitch et al., 2006). The establishment of Employee Assistance Programs (EAP; comprehensively reviewed in another chapter of this handbook), such as alcohol or drug abuse counseling, has also been shown to yield positive organizational results, including a reduction in employee absences and accidents (McFarlin & Fals-Stewart, 2002). A study examining EAP outcomes on 60,000 clients at US Federal Occupational Health revealed statistically significant improvement from pre- to post-EAP intervention on a number of measures, including work productivity as affected by emotional problems, the interference of emotional issues on work and social relationships, perceived health status, job attendance and global assessment of functioning (Selviket, Stephenson, Plaza, & Sugden, 2004). Furthermore, as pointed out by Grawitch et al. (2006), implementation of programs that promote health and safety are a form of organizational support, and perceived organizational support has been linked to fulfillment of employees socio-emotional needs, higher job performance (Erdogan & Enders, 2007; Witt & Carlson, 2006), organizational citizenship behaviors (Piercy, Cravens, Lane, & Vorhies, 2006), commitment and reduced turnover (Loi, Hang-yue, & Foley, 2006).

An important component of a psychologically safe and healthy workplace is the implementation of a pro active approach to eliminating the stigma towards mental health problems that may exist in the workplace. In the workplace, stigma can produce social conditions that undermine individual efforts to meet work requirements while maintaining personal health and integrity. Many employees are reluctant to come forward and disclose a mental health problem, choosing to go untreated rather than risk being labelled as "unreliable, unproductive or untrustworthy." Krupa, Kirsh, Cockburn, and Gewurtz (2009) developed a conceptual model identifying assumptions that underlie stigma in the workplace. These assumptions revolve around notions of competence, dangerousness, legitimacy of the illness, and work as charity. Their model suggests that concerns related to task and social performance on the job influence the disposition to act in a discriminatory manner in workplaces, and that assumptions are more or less relevant to people holding different positions in the work place. Reducing or even eradicating stigma in the workplace requires a fundamental culture change to create an environment where people feel free to discuss issues openly, and to seek support and help when needed. Workplaces must review their human resource policies, practices, and behaviors to ensure that they are aligned to support the organizational changes needed for stigma reduction. Attention to reducing stigma in all phases of the employment process is warranted in order to ensure that stigma and discrimination are not at play in: hiring; achieving promotions; accessing full employment benefits; and engagement in day-to-day social interactions on the job. Workplace education about mental illness and mental health is also important in order to dismantle stereotypes and promote attitudes of acceptance and inclusion.

Work–Life Balance

Over the past two decades, work–life balance has become increasingly challenging to achieve. Work–life conflict occurs when the time and energy demands imposed by our many roles become incompatible with one another. Studies show that employees who experience work–life conflict are significantly less committed to the organization, less satisfied with their jobs, and report higher levels of job stress, absenteeism, EAP use, prescription drug use and intent to turnover (Burton, 2002). Higgins and Duxbury (2009) found that conflict between work and family roles diminish employees' perceptions of quality of both work and family life. To prevent such negative consequences, organizations can implement work–life balance programs that help individuals balance the multiple demands of their lives.

Research by Scandura and Lankau (1997) demonstrated that the existence of work–life programs was positively related to organizational commitment and job satisfaction. Crooker and Grover (1993) maintain that providing family benefits to employees is a symbolic action on the part of the employer that demonstrates sensitivity and responsiveness to employees' needs, and that employees may reciprocate with greater loyalty and better morale. While most work–life balance programs are constructed with families in mind by emphasizing elder or child care, Grawitch et al. (2006) point out that a narrow focus on the family excludes those employees who do not have such demands, but may have other responsibilities in their personal lives that require flexibility. They recommend that the exclusive category of family support programs be redefined into a more inclusive category of work–life balance programs that can provide all employees with the flexibility required to meet the demands of their work and personal lives. Gilbert and Bilsker (2011) do this by categorizing a number of effective actions that can help maintain work–life balance into two broad areas:

1. Inclusive and flexible employee supports may involve providing extended benefits to employee's partners and family members, allowing employees to choose benefits that fit their needs (e.g., support for eldercare versus childcare), flexible work schedules, work from home on certain days, or replacement of "sick days" with flexible "personal days."
2. Building employee skills to manage work-home conflict can be accomplished by using staff meetings, company newsletters and/or "lunch and learns" to provide information and training. Specific skills may focus on the job (e.g., time management, organizational skills, coping with stress) or upon personal life (e.g., financial planning, child or eldercare issues). This broad and inclusive approach to work life balance communicates universal concern and addresses the competing demands of life for all employees.

Job Future

Job Future represents a multidimensional domain that has been identified in models of healthy work organization (see for example, Wilson et al., 2004). It is about worker expectations for the future within their jobs and their organizations. Two dimensions that comprise this domain are job security and career development.

Job Security

The level of certainty associated with future employment opportunities, job security and the capacity to find and keep a job can have significant effects on the health and well-being of workers. Short-term, casual contracts are common work arrangements in Western labor markets. Although sometimes desired and sought out by employees, short-term work arrangements can restrict the development of supportive social relationships at work, and can put workers in precarious and stressful work situations where they do not have a reliable or predictable source of income. Job insecurity is often associated with lower self-reported health (Borg, Kristensen, & Burr, 2000; Ferrie, Shipley, Stansfeld, & Marmot, 2002; McDonough, 2000; Rugulies, Bültmann, Aust, & Burr, 2006). Furthermore, such work arrangements can interrupt and disrupt social and familial pursuits because of uncertainty related to employment and income.

Lewchuk et al. (2008) and Clarke et al. (2007) explored the health implications associated with precarious/insecure employment arrangements. While Lewchuk and colleagues found that the health profiles of workers in precarious/insecure employment arrangements were not consistently different or poorer than workers in permanent/secure employment arrangement, Clarke et al. found that the health effects of insecure employment varied by the reasons for the employment situation. The poorest health outcomes were reported among individuals who were in precarious/insecure employment arrangements, wanted more secure employment but were unable to find any, did not see how they could change their employment situation and had low expectations that it would change in the near future. Individuals in such "unsustainable" precarious employment arrangements have a hard time planning and organizing their finances and are often restricted in their capacity to socialize, move out on their own, take planned time off work, and make childcare arrangements. These individuals were distinguished from two other groups of workers in precarious employment situations: those "on-a-path" who saw their current precarious employment arrangement as temporary or a stepping stone to their career; and those who were in "sustainable" precarious employment situations that either offered desired flexibility or rewards. Clarke and colleagues found that precarious workers in the "unsustainable" and "on-a-path" groups were more likely to report that work was stressful, being tense at work more frequently in the last month, and that they experienced a range of health problems related to work. The workers in the "unsustainable" group in particular were more likely to report deteriorating health and a range of both physical and mental health problems. Thus, the perception of job security and the level of choice and control the worker has over their job security and work arrangement has an important influence on the mental health and well-being of workers.

Career Development

Work is a major source of identity and self-esteem, so it is understandable that opportunities for growth and development translate into higher job satisfaction and an increased sense of wellness. Employee growth and development programs provide employees with the opportunity to expand their knowledge, skills, and abilities, and to apply the competencies they have gained to new situations (e.g., Jamison & O'Mara, 1991; Pfeffer, 1998). Examples of employee growth and development programs include the following: continuing education courses; tuition reimbursement; career development or counseling services; skills training provided in-house or through outside training centers; opportunities for promotion and internal career advancement; and leadership development.

Kaye (2010) insists that "high engagement starts with career development" (p. 4), and advises companies wishing to boost satisfaction, productivity and engagement to ensure that people are in the right jobs, doing the right work, enjoying it, following a career development plan and having access to relevant tools and training. She maintains that, in order for this to happen, organizations should teach employees how to assess their skills, interests, and values and help them understand how they are viewed. Organizations should inform employees of what is happening in the company that may change how they work so as to encourage new possibilities and multiple options. In addition, companies must offer tools to create an action plan so that employees can achieve their goals. Effective career development involves assessing gaps, seeking feedback to improve capabilities, mining for career opportunities, and developing by growing in place, self-marketing, and action planning (Kaye, 2010). Opportunities for career development and learning can act as a motivator for employees and enhance job satisfaction. In an analysis of five human resource practices, Browne (2000) found training and internal career opportunities to be significant predictors of job satisfaction and job stress. Positive benefits associated with employee growth and development programs are realized by organizations as they provide employees a chance to apply the knowledge and skills acquired during development (Pfeffer, 1994).

Conclusion and Future Directions

This chapter has presented work-related factors known to affect the mental health of workers. These factors emerge from empirical research on workplace health, and have been organized into a framework consisting of four domains: Job Design, Organizational Culture, Leadership and Job Future. Within each of these domains are a number of variables that interact with one another to affect mental health. These key variables have implications for workers, employers and policymakers. Armed with information about how to contribute to the development of a psychologically healthy workplace, workers can consider how they may create a satisfying balance between job demands and control, between effort and reward, and between the many demands of work and life. Additionally, they may attend more closely to the creation of supportive environments and ensure that roles and communication within teams are clear and explicit. Employers and human resources professionals can then use this knowledge to develop and implement workplace policies and procedures that consider effective reward systems, clarify roles and expectations, promote career development and embed organizational fairness and support into the culture of the organization. Governments and policymakers can also draw on this information for the creation of national or provincial standards that encourage workplaces to assess and minimize psychological risks for employees.

While much is now known about constructing mentally healthy workplaces, the field is young and has many more issues to address. For example, as the nature of work changes, with virtual and global work increasing in prevalence, new questions about work–life balance, job security, and the impact of "place" on psychological well-being must be addressed. Additionally, while some research exists in specific work sectors, there are others that call for increased attention, particularly those that are emerging and those that are gradually disappearing from the landscape of the labor market. Finally, much research is yet to be done on workplace factors that promote successful return-to-work for those who have had to leave the workplace due to mental health issues. Research and action in these areas can contribute to a reduction in the growing rates of mental distress in the workplace and can lead to a healthier and more productive workforce.

References

Aiken, L. H., Clarke, S. P., Sloane, D. M., Sochalski, J., & Silber, J. H. (2002). Hospital nurse staffing and patient mortality, nurse burnout, and job dissatisfaction. *Journal of the American Medical Association, 288*(16), 1987–1993.

Aldana, S. G. (2001). Financial impact of health promotion programs: A comprehensive review of the literature. *American Journal of Health Promotion, 15*, 296–320.

Arwedson, I. L., Roos, S., & Bjorklund, A. (2007). Constituents of healthy workplaces. *Work: A journal of Prevention, Assessment & Rehabilitation, 28*, 3–11.

Avolio, B. J., Gardner, W. L., Walumbwa, F. O., Luthans, F., & May, D. R. (2004). Unlocking the mask: A look at the process by which authentic leaders impact follower attitudes and behaviors. *The Leadership Quarterly, 15*, 801–823.

Beehr, T. A., Jex, S. M., Stacy, B. A., & Murray, M. A. (2000). Work stressors and coworker support as predictors of individual strain and job performance. *Journal of Organizational Behavior, 21*, 391–405.

Borg, V., Kristensen, T. S., & Burr, H. (2000). Work environment and changes in self-rated health: A five year follow-up study. *Stress Medicine, 6*, 37–47.

Browne, J. H. (2000). Benchmarking HRM practices in healthy work organizations. *American Business Review, 18*, 54–61.

Burton, J. (2002). The leadership factor: Management practices can make employees sick. NQI Excellence Articles; THU. Retrieved from: http://www.nqi.ca/articles/article_details.aspx?ID=89

Cameron, A. F., & Webster, J. (2004). Unintended consequences of emerging communication technologies: Instant messaging in the workplace. *Computers in Human Behaviour, 21*(1), 85–103.

Clarke, M., Lewchuk, W., de Wolff, A., & King, A. (2007). 'This isn't sustainable': Precarious employment, stress and workers' health. *International Journal of Law and Psychiatry, 30*, 311–326. doi:10.1016/j.ijlp.2007.06.005.

CMHA and The Dalla Lana School of Public Health. *Workplace mental health promotion*. http://wmhp.cmhaontario.ca/

Cohen, S. G., Ledford, G. E., Jr., & Spreitzer, G. M. (1996). A predictive model of self managing work team effectiveness. *Human Relations, 49*, 643–676.

Cole, D. C., Koehoorn, M., Ibrahim, S., Hertzman, C., Ostry, A., Xu, F., et al. (2009). Regions, hospitals and health outcomes over time; A multi-level analysis of repeat prevalence among a cohort of health-care workers. *Health & Place, 15*(4), 1046–1057. doi:10.1016/j.healthplace.2009.05.004.

Cooper, C. L., & Cartwright, S. (1994). Healthy mind; healthy organizations—A proactive approach to occupational stress. *Human Relations, 47*, 455–471.

Crawford, L., Gutierrez, G., & Harber, P. (2005). Work environment and occupational health of dental hygienists: A qualitative assessment. *Journal of Occupational and Environmental Medicine, 47*, 623–632. doi:10.1097/01.jom.0000165744.47044.2b.

Cummins, R. (1989). Locus of control and social support: Clarifiers of the relationship between job stress and job satisfaction. *Journal of Applied Social Psychology, 19*, 772–778.

Danna, K., & Griffin, R. W. (1999). Health and well-being in the workplace: A review and synthesis of the literature. *Journal of Management, 25*(3), 357.

Dawley, D. D., Andrews, M. C., & Bucklew, N. S. (1980). Mentoring, supervisor support and perceived organizational support: What matters most? *Leadership and Organization Development Journal, 29*(3), 235–247.

de Croon, E. M., Sluiter, J. K., Kuijer, P. P. F. M., & Frings-Dresen, M. H. W. (2005). The effect of office concepts on worker health and performance: A systematic review of the literature. *Ergonomics, 48*(2), 119–134. doi:10.1080/00140130512331319409.

Dejonge, J., Jansen, P., & Vanbreukelen, G. (1996). Testing the demand-control-support model among health care professionals: A structural equation model. *Work and Stress, 10*, 209–224.

Ducharme, L. J., & Martin, J. K. (2000). Unrewarding work, coworker support, and job satisfaction: A test of the buffering hypothesis. *Work and Occupations, 27*, 223.

Edwards, L., & Torcellini, P. (2002). *A literature review of the effects of natural light on building occupants*. Golden, CA: National Renewable Energy Laboratory. Downloaded from http://www.osti.gov/bridge.

Elovainio, M., Kivimaki, M., & Vahtera, J. (2002). Organizational justice: Evidence of a new psychosocial predictor of health. *American Journal of Public Health, 92*, 105–108.

Erdogan, B., & Enders, J. (2007). Support from the top: Supervisors' perceived organizational support as a moderator of leader-member exchange to satisfaction and performance relationships. *Journal of Applied Psychology, 92*(2), 321–330.

Faucett, J. (2005). Integrating 'psychosocial' factors into a theoretical model for work-related musculoskeletal disorders. *Theoretical Issues in Ergonomics Science, 6*(6), 531–550. doi:10.1080/14639220512331335142.

Ferrie, J. E., Shipley, M. J., Stansfeld, S. A., & Marmot, M. G. (2002). Effects of chronic job insecurity and change in job security on self reported health, minor psychiatric morbidity, physiological measures, and health related behaviours in British civil servants: The Whitehall II study. *Journal of Epidemiology and Community Health, 56*, 450–454.

Freeman, R. B., & Rogers, J. (1999). *What workers want*. Ithaca, NY: Russell Sage.

Ganster, D. C., Fusilier, M., & Mayes, B. (1986). Role of social support in the experience of stress at work. *Journal of Applied Psychology, 71*, 102–110.

Gilbert, M., & Bilsker, D. (2011). *Psychological health and safety: An action guide for employers*. Calgary, AB: Mental Health Commission of Canada.

Goffee, R., & Jones, G. (1996). What holds the modern company together? *Harvard Business Review, 74*(6), 133–149.

Golaszewski, T. (2001). Shining lights: Studies that have most influenced the understanding of health promotion's financial impact. *American Journal of Health Promotion, 15*, 332–340.

Grawitch, M. J., Gottschalk, M., & Munz, D. C. (2006). The path to a healthy workplace: A critical review linking healthy workplace practices, employee well-being, and organizational improvement. *Consulting Psychology Journal: Practice and Research, 58*(3), 129–147.

Grawitch, M. J., Trares, S., & Kohler, J. M. (2007). Healthy workplace practices. *International Journal of Stress Management, 14*(3), 275–293.

Grosch, J. W., Caruso, C. C., Rosa, R. R., & Sauter, S. L. (2006). Long hours of work in the U.S.: Associations with demographic and organizational characteristics, psychosocial working conditions and health. *American Journal of Industrial Medicine, 49*(11), 943–952.

Handy, Charles (1999). Understanding organizations.Oxford University Press.

Hannigan, B., Edwards, B., & Burnard, P. (2004). Stress and stress management in clinical psychology: Findings from a systematic review. *Journal of Mental Health, 13*(3), 235–245.

Harlan, S., & Robert, P. (1998). The social construction of disability in organizations: Why employers resist reasonable accommodation. *Work and Occupations, 25*, 397-435. doi: 10.1177/0730888498025004002

Hedge, A. (2000). Where are we in understanding the effects of where we are? *Ergonomics, 43*(7), 1019–1029.

Higgins, C., & Duxbury, L. (2009). Key Findings and Recommendations From The 2001 National Work-Life Conflict Study. Health Canada. http://www.hc-sc.gc.ca/ewh-semt/pubs/occup-travail/balancing_six-equilibre_six/index-eng.php.

Hurlbert, J. S. (1991). Social networks, social circles and job satisfaction. *Work and Occupations, 18*, 415–430.

Inoue A, Kawakami N, Haratani T, Kobayashi F, Ishizaki M, Hayashi T, Fujita O, Aizawa Y, Miyazaki S, Hiro H, Masumoto T, Hashimoto S, Araki S. (2010) Job stressors and long-term sick leave due to depressive disorders among Japanese male employees: findings from the Japan Work Stress and Health Cohort study. J Epidemiol Community Health. 64(3):229–35.

Jackson, S. E., & Schuler, R. S. (1985). A meta-analysis and conceptual critique of research on role ambiguity and role conflict in work settings. *Organizational Behavior and Human Decision Processes, 36*, 16–78.

Jamal, M. (1990). Relationship of job stress and type—A behavior to employees' job satisfaction, organizational commitment, psychosomatic health problems, and turnover motivation. *Human Relations, 43*, 727–738.

Jamison, D., & O'Mara, J. (1991). *Managing workforce 2000*. San Francisco: Jossey-Bass.

Johnson, J., & Hall, E. (1988). Job strain, workplace social support and cardiovascular disease: A cross-sectional study of a random sample of the Swedish male working population. *American Journal of Public Health, 78*, 1336–1342.

Kaarlela-Tuomaala, A., Helenius, R., Keskinen, E., & Hongisto, V. (2009). Effects of acoustic environment on work in private office rooms and open-plan offices—Longitudinal study during relocation. *Ergonomics, 52*(11), 1423–1444. doi:10.1080/00140130903154579.

Karasek, R. (1979). Job demands, job decision latitude, and mental strain: Implications for job redesign. *Administrative Science Quarterly, 24*(2), 285–308.

Karasek, R., & Theorell, T. (1990). *Healthy work: Stress, productivity, and the reconstruction of working life*. New York: Basic Books.

Karasek, R., Triantis, K., & Chaudhry, S. (1982). Coworker and supervisor support as moderators of associations between task characteristics and mental strain. *Journal of Occupational Behavior, 3*, 181–200.

Kaye, B. (2010). Career development: It's a business imperative. *Leadership Excellence, 27*(1), 4.

Kelloway, E. K., & Barling, J. (1991). Job characteristics, role stress and mental health. *Journal of Occupational Psychology, 64*, 291–304.

Keyton, J. (2005). *Communication and organizational culture*. Thousand Oaks, CA: Sage Publications Inc.

Kivimaki, M., Elovainio, M., Vahtera, J., & Ferrie, J. E. (2003). Organizational justice and health of employees: Prospective cohort study. *Occupational and Environmental Medicine, 60*, 27–34.

Kivimaki, M., Ferrie, J. E., Head, J., Shipley, M. J., Vahtera, J., & Marmot, M. G. (2004). Organizational justice and change in justice as predictors of employee health: The Whitehall II study. *Journal of Epidemiology and Community Health, 58*, 931–937. doi:10.1136/jech.2003.019026.

Krupa, T., Kirsh, B., Cockburn, L., & Gewurtz, R. (2009). Understanding the stigma of mental illness in employment. *Work: A Journal of Prevention, Assessment, and Rehabilitation, 33*(4), 413–425.

Kruper, H., Singh-Manoux, A., Siegrist, J., & Marmot, M. (2002). When reciprocity fails: Effort-reward imbalance in relation to coronary heart disease and health functioning within the Whitehall II study. *Occupational and Environmental Medicine, 59*, 777–784.

Kuoppala, J., Lamminpaa, A., Liira, J., & Vainio, H. (2008). Leadership, job well-being, and health effects—A systematic review and a meta-synthesis. *Journal of Occupational and Environmental Medicine, 50*, 904–915. doi:10.1097/JOM.0b013e31817e918d.

Labriola, M., Christensen, K. B., Lund, T., Nielsen, M. L., & Diderichsen, F. (2006). Multilevel analysis of workplace and individual risk factors for long term sickness absence. *Journal of Occupational and Environmental Medicine, 48*(9), 923–929. doi:10.1097/01.jom.0000229783.04721.d2.

LaRocco, J., & Jones, A. (1978). Coworker and leader support as moderators of stress/strain relationships in work situations. *Journal of Applied Psychology, 63*, 629–634.

Lawler, E. E., III. (1991). Participative management strategies. In J. W. Jones, B. D. Steffy, & D. W. Bray (Eds.), *Applying psychology in business: The handbook for managers and human resource professionals*. Lexington, KY: Lexington Books.

Leka, S., & Jain, A. (2010). Health impact of psychosocial hazards at work: An overview. World Health Organization. Retrieved from http://whqlibdoc.who.int/publications/2010/9789241500272_eng.pdf

Lewchuk, W., Clarke, M., & de Wolff, A. (2008). Working without commitments: Precarious employment and health. *Work, Employment and Society, 22*(3), 387–406. doi:10.1177/0950017008093477.

Lohela, M., Bjorklund, C., Vingard, E., Hagberg, J., & Jensen, I. (2009). Does a change in psychosocial work factors lead to a change in employee health? *Journal of Occupational and Environmental Medicine, 51*, 195–203. doi:10.1097/JOM.0b013e318192bd2c.

Loi, R., Hang-yue, N., & Foley, S. (2006). Linking employees' justice perceptions to organizational commitment and intention to leave: The mediating role of perceived organizational support. *Journal of Occupational Psychology, 1*(79), 101–120.

MacEachen, E., Clarke, J., Franche, R.-L., Irvin, E., & The Workplace-based Return to Work Literature Review Group. (2006). Systematic review of the qualitative literature on return to work after injury. *Scandinavian Journal of Work, Environment and Health, 32*(4), 257–269.

MacEachen, E., Polzer, J., & Clarke, J. (2008). "You are free to set your own hours": Governing worker productivity and health through flexibility and resilience. *Social Science & Medicine, 66*, 1019–1033. doi:10.1016/j.socscimed.2007.11.013.

Marchand, A., Demers, A., & Durand, P. (2005). Do occupation and work conditions really matter? A longitudinal analysis of psychological distress experiences among Canadian workers. *Sociology of Health & Illness, 27*(5), 602–627.

Mayfield, J., & Mayfield, M. (2002). Leader communication strategies critical paths to improving employee commitment. *American Business Review, 20*(2), 89.

McConnell CR. (1998) Employee involvement: motivation or manipulation? Health Care Superv. 1998 Mar;16(3):69–85.

McDonough, P. (2000). Job insecurity and health. *International Journal of Health Services, 30*, 453–476.

McFarlin, S. K., & Fals-Stewart, W. (2002). Workplace absenteeism and alcohol use: A sequential analysis. *Psychology of Addictive Behaviors, 16*, 17–21.

Meijer, E. M., Frings-Dresen, M. H. W., & Sluiter, J. K. (2009). Effects of office innovation on office workers' health and performance. *Ergonomics, 52*(9), 1027–1038. doi:10.080/00140130902842752.

Moran, T. E., & Volkwein, F. J. (1992). The cultural approach to the formation of organizational climate. *Human Relations, 45*(1), 19–47.

Pfeffer, J. (1994). *Competitive advantage through people: Unleashing the power of the workforce*. Boston: Harvard Business School Press.

Pfeffer, J. (1998). *The human equation*. Boston: Harvard Business School Press.

Piercy, N. F., Cravens, D. W., Lane, N., & Vorhies, D. W. (2006). Driving organizational citizenship behaviors and salesperson in-role behavior performance: The role of management control and perceived organizational support. *Journal of the Academy of Marketing Science, 34*(2), 242–262.

Plaisier, I., de Bruijn, J. G. M., de Graff, R., ten Have, M., Beekman, A. T. F., & Penninx, B. W. J. H. (2007). The contribution of working conditions and social support to the onset of depressive and anxiety disorders among male and female employees. *Social Science & Medicine, 64*, 401–410. doi:10.1016/j.socscimed.2006.09.008.

Ramirez, A. J., Graham, J., Richards, M. A., Cull, A., & Gregory, W. M. (1996). Mental health of hospital consultants: The effects of stress and satisfaction at work. *The Lancet, 347*, 724–728.

Reina, D. S., & Reina, M. L. (1999). *Trust & betrayal in the workplace*. San Francisco: Berrett-Koehler.

Rhoades, L., & Eisenberger, R. (2002). Perceived organizational support: A review of the literature. *Journal of Applied Psychology, 87*(4), 698–714.

Robbins, S. P. (2001). *Organizational behavior: Concepts, controversies, applications* (9th ed.). Upper Saddle River, NJ: Prentice Hall.

Robbins, S. P., & Hunsaker, P. L. (1996). *Training in interpersonal skills: TIPS for managing people at work* (2nd ed.). Upper Saddle River, NJ.: Prentice-Hall.

Roebuck, C. (1996). Constructive feedback: Key to higher performance and commitment. *Long Range Planning, 29*(3), 328–336.

Rugulies, R., Bültmann, U., Aust, B., & Burr, H. (2006). Psychosocial work environment and incidence of severe depressive symptoms: Prospective findings from a 5-year follow-up of the Danish work environment cohort study. *American Journal of Epidemiology, 163*(10), 877–887.

Scandura, T. A., & Lankau, M. J. (1997). Relationships of gender, family responsibility, and flexible work hours to organizational commitment and job satisfaction. *Journal of Organizational Behavior, 18*, 377–391.

Schabracq, M. J., & Cooper, C. L. (2000). The changing nature of work and stress. *Journal of Managerial Psychology, 15*(3), 227–241.

Schein, E. (1992). *Organizational culture and leadership* (2nd ed.). San Francisco: Jossey-Bass.

Selviket, S., Stephenson, D., Plaza, C., & Sugden, B. (2004). EAP impact on work, relationship, and health outcomes. *Journal of Employee Assistance, 34*(2), 18–22.

Shain, M. (2001). Returning to work after illness or injury: The role of fairness. *Bulletin of Science Technology Society, 21*(5), 361–368.

Shields, M. (1999). Long working hours and health. *Health Reports, 11*(2), 33–48.

Shirey, M. (2006). Authentic leaders creating healthy work environments for nursing practice. *American Journal of Critical Care, 15*(3), 256.

Siegrist, J. (1996). Adverse health effects of high-effort/low-reward conditions. *Journal of Occupational Health Psychology, 1*(1), 27–41.

Siegrist, J. (2002). Reducing social inequalities in health: Work-related strategies. *Scandinavian Journal of Public Health, 30*, 49–53.

Simmering, M. J., Colquitt, J. A., Noe, R. A., & Porter, C. O. L. H. (2003). Conscientiousness, autonomy fit, and development: A longitudinal study. *Journal of Applied Psychology, 88*, 954–963.

Spataro, S. E. (2005). Diversity in context: How organizational culture shapes reactions to workers with disabilities and others who are demographically different. *Behavioral Sciences & the Law, 23*(1), 21–38.

Stansfeld, S. A., Fuhrer, R., Shipley, M. J., & Marmot, M. G. (1999). Work characteristics predict psychiatric disorder: Prospective results from the Whitehall II study. *Occupational and Environmental Medicine, 56*, 302–307.

Stansfeld, S. A., Rael, E. G., Head, J., Shipley, M., & Marmot, M. (1997). Social support and psychiatric sickness absence: A prospective study of British civil servants. *Psychological Medicine, 27*(1), 35–48.

Strelioff, W., Lavoie-Tremblay, M., & Barton, M. (2007). Collaborating to embrace evidence-informed management practices within Canada's health system. *Nursing Leadership, 20*(1), 33–39.

Vaananen, A., Kalimo, R., Toppinen-Tanner, S., Mutanen, P., Perio, J. M., Kivimaki, M., et al. (2004). Role clarity, fairness, and organizational climate as predictors of sickness absence: A prospective study in the private sector. *Scandinavian Journal of Public Health, 32*, 426–434. doi:10.1080/14034940410028136.

van Yperen, N. W., & Snijders, T. A. B. (2000). A multilevel analysis of the demands—control model: Is stress at work determined by factors at the group level or at the individual level. *Journal of Occupational Health Psychology, 5*(1), 182–190.

Vandenberg, R. J., Richardson, H. A., & Eastman, L. J. (1999). The impact of high involvement work processes on organizational effectiveness: A second-order latent variable approach. *Group and Organization Management, 24*, 300–339.

Vecchio, R. P. (1995). It's not easy being green: Jealousy and envy in the workplace. *Research in Personnel and Human Resources Management, 13*, 201–244.

Vezina, M., Bourbonnais, R., Brisson, C., & Trudel, L. (2004). Workplace prevention and promotion strategies. *Healthcare Papers, 5*(2), 32–44.

Vischer, J. C. (2007). The effects of the physical environment on job performance: Towards a theoretica model of workplace stress. *Stress and Health, 23*, 175–184. doi:10.1002/smi.1134.

Viswesvaran, C., Sanchez, J. I., & Fisher, J. (1999). The role of social support in the process of work stress: A meta-analysis. *Journal of Vocational Behaviour, 54*(2), 314–334.

Walters, J. (2005). Workplace communication essentials. *The Officer, 81*(8), 42.

Wilson, M. G., Dejoy, D. M., Vandenberg, R. J., Richardson, H. A., & Mcgrath, A. L. (2004). Work characteristics and employee health and well-being: Test of a model of healthy work organization. *Journal of Occupational and Organizational Psychology, 77*, 565–588.

Witt, L. A., & Carlson, D. S. (2006). The work-family interface and job performance: Moderating effects of conscientiousness and perceived organizational support. *Journal of Occupational Health Psychology, 11*(4), 343–357.

Woltring, C., Constantine, W., & Schwarte, L. (2003). Does leadership training make a difference? The CDC/UC Public Health Leadership Institute: 1991-1999. *Journal of Public Health Management and Practice, 9*(2), 111–130.

Young, M., & Post, J. E. (1993). Managing to communicate, communicating to manage: How leading companies communicate with employees. *Organizational Dynamics, 22*(1), 31–43.

Workplace Injury and Illness, Safety Engineering, Economics and Social Capital

13

Henry P. Cole

Overview

Throughout this past century, numerous high-profile workplace disasters occurred, some of which are listed in Table 13.1. These do not include some of the large energy industry disasters that caused long-term environmental damages, such as: the sinking of the Amoco Cadiz oil tanker off the coast of France in 1978, which was the largest oil spill of its kind in history; the partial-meltdown of the Three Mile Island nuclear energy plant in 1979; the Chernobyl nuclear power plant disaster in 1986; the Exxon Valdez oil tanker spill of 1989 in Alaska; and the recent Fukushima I nuclear plant disaster in 2011. Thus, many workplace accidents take a great human toll, as well as an environmental toll. In terms of the human toll part of the equation, as noted by Smith and Carayon (2011), even though the rates of workplace injuries and deaths in the United States have been declining ever since the Bureau of Labor Statistics first began to collect such data in 1972, the sheer numbers remain quite high, and they highlight the fact that improvements in workplace safety and illness are still needed. For example, the 2010 Bureau of Labor Statistics revealed an incidence rate of 3.5 cases per 100 workers per year for nonfatal occupational injury and illness, as well as a total of 4,547 fatal workplace injuries. Moreover, in 2007, 5,488 US workers died from workplace injuries. In that same year, an estimated 49,000 deaths were attributed to work-related diseases. In addition, it was estimated that four million workers had nonfatal work-related injury or illnesses, and about half of those required a job transfer, restricted work, or time away from their jobs. In 2004, approximately 3.4 million workers received treatment at hospital emergency departments because of a work-related injury, and about 80,000 were hospitalized (CDC/NIOSII, 2004).

Numerous empirical studies have also documented that worker occupational injuries and illness reported in government sources are grossly undercounted. Many workers, employers, and physicians fail to recognize occupational illnesses as being related to work activities. During 1988–1994, Michigan's 30,000 physicians were required by law to report occupational injuries. Only 0.7% did

H.P. Cole (✉)
Department of Preventive Medicine and Environmental Health, University of Kentucky, University of Kentucky College of Public Health, 111 Washington Avenue, Lexington, KY 40536-0003, USA
e-mail: hcole@uky.edu

Table 13.1 Examples of high-profile workplace disasters

Disaster	Date	Deaths
Monongah, WV. Nos. 6 and 8, explosion	1907	362
Chery IL, Cherry Mine, Fire	1909	259
Dawson, NM, Stag Canon No. 2, explosion	1913	263
Centrialia, IL, Centrailia No. 5, explosion	1947	111
West Frankfort, IL, Orient No. 2, explosion	1951	119
Farmington, WV, Consol No. 9, explosion	1968	78
New York City Triangle Shirtwaist Factory fire	1911	146
Port Chicago, CA, Ammunition loading explosion	1944	320
American Oil Rig North Sea, explosion	1998	167

Source for mine disasters: US Department of Labor, Mine Safety, and Health Administration, http://www.msha.gov/mshainfo/factsheets/mshafct2.htm

so. Most had never seen the occupational disease form. Most of the 115 US medical schools provide little or no training in occupational illness. The 68% that do so report a total of only 6 hours of instruction devoted to the topic over the 4-year program. It should also be noted that companies often conceal worker injury and illnesses to prevent increases in Workers' Compensation insurance premiums, as well as to avoid Occupational Safety and Health Act (OSHA) investigations. A Bureau of Labor 1987 study of 200 randomly selected manufacturing companies, with 10 or more employees, found that total worker illnesses and injuries were underreported by 10%, and lost workdays related to these events by 25%. The large majority of work-related injuries and illnesses by low-wage temporary or contingent workers are grossly undercounted for multiple reasons, including the fact that these workers needed of a daily wage to survive, fear of being fired and unable to find another job. The absence of a comprehensive occupational health data collection system in the United States has resulted in a patchwork array of systems not designed for injury surveillance (Azaroff, Levenstein, & Wegman, 2002).

This Chapter examines causes of workplace nonfatal and fatal injuries, as well as concomitant efforts toward their prevention. Moreover, the increase in "outsourcing" of work by many companies has created a new class of temporary or contingent workers, who now have unique issues and much higher rates of occupational injuries, relative to full-time long-term traditional workers.

At the outset, it should be noted that, because of the aforementioned statistics on workplace injuries and deaths, the US Congress in 1891 passed the first federal statue for regulating mine safety, including ventilation requirements to remove *methane* and prevent explosions, and prohibiting operators from employing workers less than 12 years of age. In 1910, after a decade in which coal mine fatalities exceeded 2,000 annually, Congress established the Bureau of Mines to conduct mine production and safety research, but with no authority to conduct mine safety inspections until 1941. The first code of federal regulations for mining was authorized by congress in 1947. Congress enacted The Federal Coal Mine Safety Act in 1952, and updated versions of the Act in 1966, 1969, and 1977. Major coal mine disasters were the impetus for each round of congressional legislative action that resulted in increased access for mine safety inspectors, fines and penalties for mine operators' noncompliance, and withdrawal orders that inspectors could use to close down unsafe mines. Table 13.2 lists the disasters and death tolls that prompted present day mine safety regulations and their enforcement (Kowalski-Trakofler, Alexander, Brnich, McWilliams, & Reissman, 2009; Kowalski-Trakofler, Alexander, Brnich, & Williams, 2009).

Four points need to be understood about the 11,606 mine deaths listed in Table 13.2. First, many of the miner deaths in the early 1900s were immigrants or second-generation descendants of immi-

Table 13.2 Number of Worker Deaths in US Underground Coal Mining Disasters by Cause, 1900–2006

Causal classification	Number of disasters	Worker deaths
Explosion	420	10,390
Fire	35	727
Hauling materials, workers	21	145
Roof or rib fall & outbursts	13	83
Inundation toxic gas or water	7	62
Other	17	199
Total	513	11,606

Source: MMWR January 2, 2009, 57, (51&52), 1379–1382

grants. Second, these deaths are only those that resulted in five or more miners dying as the result of a single event, like a mine fire or explosion (events that are classified as disasters). Third, most miners during this historical period, as well as at the present time, do not die in disaster events. Rather, they die individually as the results of a wide array of injury events that are historically referred to as mining accidents. Fourth, the total number of coal mine disaster deaths reported in Table 13.2 is a small fraction of total coal miner deaths during this period. This same principle applies to other workers. Construction workers and fire fighters occasionally die in groups of five or more individuals. However, these isolated disaster events account for only a small fraction of all these deaths. For example, in the United States, an average of five individual construction workers die each day in different isolated events as the result of a wide range of workplace hazards. Farmers and ranchers have occupational death rates of 32.4 per 100,000 workers per year, a rate that is 8.8 times higher than the US all industry average of 3.7 deaths per 100.000 workers per year (Bureau of Labor Census Fatal Occupational Injuries, 2008). However, farmers and ranchers nearly always die individually rather than in disaster events. Slowly accumulating deaths are less newsworthy, less noticed, and also less likely to promote congressional action for their prevention.

The US Congress passed the Occupational Safety and Health Act (OSHA) in 1970, with the goal of developing and enforcing workplace safety standards, as well as offering compliance assistance. This legislation also resulted from a history of workplace disasters and unfair work practices that spanned two centuries. In the interest of brevity, only two landmark cases that had major impacts on occupational safety and health are described. Both involve multiple deaths of immigrant workers. The first was the New York City *Triangle Shirtwaist Factory* disaster event, in which hundreds of workers died in a single fire. The second involves the much greater number of wool mill textile workers who died in Lawrence, Massachusetts, where individuals died on a nearly daily basis over a period of many years.

The Triangle Shirtwaist Fire

The Triangle Fire book by Leon Stein (2001) provides a detailed account of this 1911 workplace disaster. Among many other sources, the Wikipedia account (with its 53 reference citations) is one of the most concise descriptions. One of several Triangle Shirtwaist factories in New York City was located in the Asch building adjacent to New York University at Washington Park Square. Approximately 500 young immigrant women, then referred to as the "Shirtwaist girls," worked on the top three floors of the 10 story building. Each floor, referred to as a loft, was an open room, 100 ft long and wide. The floors and long work tables were of wood construction. The girls cut and sewed fabric to produce the popular female bodice called a shirtwaist. Large stocks of fabric were stored on the three upper floors, as were large bins of scrap fabric. Even though New York City fire codes required three stairwells for buildings this size, only two circular enclosed stairwells were present. Each had narrow steps 2 ft, 9 in. long, with the narrow ends of each step attached to a single steel pole that ran from the tenth to the bottom floor.

Although building and fire codes called for doors that opened outward, the two doors to each floor opened inward. The doors were kept locked during work hours to prevent the girls from sneaking out with fabric or completed shirtwaists. Both doors at each floor were very narrow, allowing only one person to pass through at a time. At the end of the day, the girls lined up at one door. A company foreman first unlocked the door at the front of the building, and then allowed the girls to exit one-at-a time as he inspected their open purses for stolen items. The door at the rear of the building remained locked, and the two freight elevators that were operated by men located on the ground floor were unavailable. The only way out was via the one unlocked door on each floor that was attended by a foreman or via the one external fire escape at the rear of the building (Stein, 2001). Immediately outside each door was the first narrow step on the circular stairway. There was no landing. That is why the doors had to open inward; a code violation that had been cited by a city inspector but that had been overridden by elected Borough officials who also overrode the building code violation that required three stairways. Descending the narrow stairwells required individuals to form a single line. The one fire escape in poor condition had stairs that led to the roof, as well as to the bottom of the sixth floor where, thereafter, it was damaged and unstable (Stein, 2001).

On Saturday, March 25 at approximately 4:40 PM (5 min before quitting time), people on the street below heard an explosion and observed a puff of smoke from an eighth floor window. It was later determined that the fire started in a large scrap bin on the eighth floor, likely from a discarded cigarette even though smoking was prohibited. The sound of the explosion and the puff of smoke was probably the result of a "flash-over," a condition when smoke and materials ignite instantly and fully engage the a room in fire. Almost immediately, people on the street below and in adjacent office buildings observed what they at first thought were bundles of fabric being thrown from the windows of the eighth floor by workers in an attempt to save fabric. Moments later the "bundles" were recognized as the bodies of girls, some of them with their hair and clothing in flames as they fell. Within minutes, the fire engulfed all three upper floors. There were no building fire alarms. A warning call from a book keeper on the eighth floor was received on the ninth floor at the same time that floor became engulfed in fire. The same bookkeeper received no response when she called the ninth floor. Within the next few minutes, many of the 500 workers escaped via one of three ways.

During the first few minutes, many workers exited via the Green Street spiral stairway until it became engulfed in smoke and flame. Many more left by the freight elevators when two alert male elevator operators on the ground floor made three round trips to the top floors. After the third trip, the elevators became inoperable because the heat from the fire had warped their guide rails. At that point, dozens of workers and the two company owners exited via the exterior fire escape and climbed to the roof; all survived. Others workers crowded onto the exterior fire escape and climbed downward. The portion of the fire escape below the sixth floor collapsed under the weight of the crowd of girls, dropping them to their deaths 100 ft below. At that point, a large number of girls remaining on the exterior fire escape broke the windows to the sixth floor and entered that room that was free from fire and smoke. The girls attempted to leave via the Green Street circular stairway, but the door was locked. The foreman with the key to that door had already left for the outside. Many of these girls were saved by a police officer. He sensed the problem from the girls' distressed calls from the sixth floor windows. He struggled up the stairs to the sixth floor against the line of descending girls. When he arrived at the sixth floor, he heard the girls screaming and banging on the door. After multiple lunges he broke open the door allowing many of these girls to escape. Shortly thereafter, even that only remaining escape route became impassable. At that point, the only way to escape the fire from the upper four floors was to climb onto the window ledges and jump seven to ten stories to the ground, a choice made by 62 workers only a few who were men. Others had unintentionally fallen and died when the lower portion of the external fire escape collapsed.

The last girl jumped at 4:57 PM. By that time, the bodies on the street covered the hoses that fire fighters had laid and were using to drench the upper floors. The one hand-cranked aerial fire truck ladder rescued no one because it reached only to the sixth floor. Likewise, the firefighter life nets were ineffective because the force of the falling bodies drove the nets to the pavement and injured the firefighters whose hands were looped to the nets. The fire was under control in 18 min. One hundred forty six workers died, 129 women and 17 men (Stein, 2001; Wikipedia, 2012).

The two owners of the company (Max Blanck and Isaacs Harris) were among those who climbed to the roof and survived. Later, they were indicted on first and second degree manslaughter charges, but both were acquitted by a jury. In a later civil trial in 1913, the plaintiffs won $75 for each deceased worker. The owners' insurance paid them $60,000 in excess of their losses (Stein, 2001; Wikipedia, 2012). About a year later, Blanck was cited and fined $20 when building inspectors found that, during the work day, he had locked the doors on another factory he owned (Stein, 2001). Subsequently, on November 25, 1910, 4 months before the Triangle fire, 25 workers died in a fire in a 4-story building in Newark, New Jersey. Six burned to death in the structure, and 19 jumped to their deaths. They too were locked into the building. The Triangle Company also had six previous fires at its factories in New York during the 1902 to the 1909 period. Two were in the Asch building, and the others at other locations. None resulted in injuries (Stein, 2001).

As a result of the Triangle factory disaster, *The New York State Legislature* established the *Factory Investigating Commission* to identify, report, and remediate similar hazardous conditions in other workplaces Statewide. New laws mandated improved building entrances and egress, fire proofing, fire extinguishers, sprinkler systems, fire alarms, and fire drills, and also limited the hours that children and women could work. The fire also resulted in the founding of the *American Society of Safety Engineers* (Stein, 2001; Wikipedia, 2012). The fire and its aftermath also stimulated the *Progressive Era* factory reform movement. It helped to promote the understanding and adoption of occupational injury causal theories that had not previously influenced or been included in workplace safety regulatory laws (McEvoy, 1995).

The Lawrence Woolen Textile Mill Strike

In 1789, industrial spinning machines were introduced in many New England factories Girls and young women immigrants were hired to work as spinsters (*a woman whose livelihood is spinning yarn*). Immigrants generally aroused suspicion and were disliked by established US citizens (Zinn, 2005). Later, the term spinster became a slur used to denigrate *a woman who remained unmarried beyond the usual age* (Encarta Dictionary English North America, 2012). Power looms were introduced into Waltham, Massachusetts in 1814. The new machines could be operated by unskilled workers. The looms spread rapidly throughout New England, and employed tens of thousands of workers, 28,000 in the Lawrence, MA woolen mills alone. Lawrence had 86,000 residents from 51 nations who spoke 25 different languages. All lived and worked within a seven square mile area. Most of the immigrant mill workers were unskilled laborers. They ranged in age from 12 to 50 years. The majority were less than 30 years old, and many much younger. They and their families lived in crowded, low-quality company tenements, typically with two families or more living in the same two rooms that were cold in the winter and stiflingly hot in the summer. Their typical daily diet was bread and molasses. Fresh, clean tap water was in limited supply. Poor sanitation existed within the tenements, the streets, and the factories. Many workers and their children were malnourished (Wartson, 2005).

The factories where these people worked were huge three or four story brick buildings, up to four city blocks long and 100 yards deep. When the workers entered the factories, the entrance and exit gates were chained and locked. Women and children worked on the lower floors or lofts where they sorted and cleaned cotton or wool and then spun and wound the material on spindles. The weaving rooms were on the upper floors, where rows of huge metal power looms were spaced along the length of the factory. Large metal arms on each loom hurled a steel shuttle and its thread back and forth two times a second through wooden frames that held the vertical strands. Loom operators often had to watch as many as 12 machines at once, a task that required high levels of sustained vigilance throughout the work day. The huge noise levels made conversation impossible. The average weekly wage was $8.76 for a 6-day, 9-hour work-day week (Wartson, 2005).

Averaged across all workers, death typically occurred at age 39. Fifty percent of the children who lived in the tenements died before age 6 (Wartson, 2005). A study by Dr. Elizabeth Shapleigh[1] found that *a considerable numbers of workers boys and girls died within the first 2 or 3 years after beginning work … 36 out of every 100 of all the men and women who work in the mill die before they are 25 years of age* (Zinn, 2005, p. 335; quoted from Shapleigh, 1912). Both child workers and adults died from pneumonia, tuberculosis, and brown lung pneumoconiosis from the constant inhalation of the fiber-filled factory air. Others died from anthrax, which was commonly referred to as wool sorter's disease. Anthrax spores in sheep wool typically entered workers' bodies through cutaneous lesions. In addition, traumatic occupational injuries from being entangled in machinery or crushed by falling materials often resulted in severe injury or death. During one 5-year period, 1,000 workers at the Pacific Mill sustained serious injuries at the average of one injured worker every 2 days (Wartson, 2005, p. 9). During the many years the textile mills operated, thousands of workers were fatally injured. In any 1 year, many more died than the fatality counts from the more dramatic and visible Triangle fire and major mine explosions and fire disasters.

The primary impact of the huge numbers of fatal illness and injuries to Lawrence textile mill workers began with what is called the *Bread and Roses* strike in which women workers were the key activists. The strike began when a new Massachusetts labor law reduced the work week from 56 to 54 h. The American Woolen Mill owned the four largest textile mills in Lawrence. Its president, William Wood, decided that, if work hours were to be cut, then so would workers' pay by 32 cents per week. That does not sound like much but at a weekly wage of $8.76 for 6 days work, daily take home pay was $1.46. The 32¢ cut reduced daily pay to $1.14, a sum of money needed to purchase several loaves of bread (Wartson, 2005, pp. 12–13; Zinn, 2005, pp. 336–337). Organized largely by women, the strike continued for 2 months and was the largest in US history at that time. The mill workers walked out of the factories, some damaging equipment as they left. A week after the strike started, eight companies of armed militia encamped near the mills a week after the strike started. With the help of International Workers of the World (IWW) leaders and activists throughout surrounding States, the women placed their children, from age 4 to 14, on trains from Lawrence to New York City and Philadelphia. In both cities, the children were met and cared for by immigrant relatives and friends who led the children in protest parades down main streets. Sympathizers from multiple New England States became involved and sent food and soup kitchens to the Lawrence strikers (Wartson, 2005;

---

[1] Dr. Shapleigh is the author's great aunt, the older sister of his maternal grandfather. She was one of the few women physicians at the time and one of the very first to practice occupational medicine. She died of typhus in the early 1930s in China where she worked as a missionary physician and teacher.

Zinn, 2005). The strike ended shortly after textile worker women took additional children to the Lawrence railway station to be transported to other cities. As the women and children stood in line to enter the station, they were clubbed by police. Many were injured, some seriously. The public outcry and newspaper accounts of the story resulted in State and Federal legislators pressuring the American Woolen Company to relent and negotiate with the strikers. The strike ended on March 14, 1912. Workers' wages were slightly increased, and time and a quarter pay granted for overtime time (Zinn, 2005, p. 337).

The *Bread and Roses* name for the strike is based on a song written by James Oppeheim It was printed and widely circulated (quoted in Wartson, 2005. p. 119). Two verses of the song follow.

> As we come marching, marching, in the beauty of the day,
> A million darkened kitchens, a thousand mill-lofts gray
> Are touched with all the radiance that a sudden sun discloses,
> For the people hear us singing, "Bread and Roses. Bread and Roses.
> As we come marching, marching, unnumbered women dead
> Go crying through our singing their ancient song of Bread;
> Small art and love and beauty their drudging sprits knew–
> Yes, is bread we fight for—but we fight for Roses too.

The working conditions and the worker illness and injuries that occurred in the early 1900s coal fields, the Triangle Shirtwaist factory, and the Lawrence textile mills were duplicated at thousands of transportation, construction, and manufacturing, farming, timbering, and fishing worksites throughout the United States as chronicled by Zinn (2005). The coal miner, Triangle fire and the Lawrence textile mill worker deaths were sentinel events that, over a period of years, increased public awareness of the evils and costs of occupational injuries and illnesses and, as a result, led to present day safety practices.

The Present

Finally, at the outset, it should also be pointed out that occupational safety and health issues and enforcement remain a continuously evolving process, as the nature of work in the United States has, over the past decades, changed from predominantly manufacturing to more service-based workplaces. This creates different safety and health issues. Moreover, the best methods to increase the "safety climate" of workplace environments are still greatly needed, especially in light of the fact that injuries and illnesses account for a 4–5% loss of the gross domestic product (Zohar, 2011). These "safety climate" issues range from problematic ergonomic/task activities, workplace hazards (such as chemical exposure, noise, dangerous equipment, etc.), to employer–employee cooperation in addressing and controlling such risk factors. Many of these workplace safety issues have been extensively addressed in previous publications over the years (e.g., Cohen & Colligan, 1998; DeJoy, Schaffer, Wilson, Vandenberg, & Butts, 2004; Neal & Griffin, 2006; Zohar, 2011). A recent summary of the status of current efforts to reduce occupational injuries and illnesses states that it "… requires a multifaceted approach that can define hazards, evaluate risks, establish means to control risks, and incorporate management, supervision, and employees actively in the process" (Smith & Carayon, 2011, p. 91). Many of these issues are briefly addressed in this Chapter. However, unlike previous publications, the present Chapter focuses on the changing trends in the present workplace, and new associated issues—particularly those related to contingent part-time and temporary workers. Such workers are becoming more prevalent in recent years because of the "downsizing" of the workforce by many companies, as well as the "outsourcing" of jobs to laborers who frequently are paid at or below minimum wage for difficult and dangerous work.

General Principles of Occupational Injury Prevention

General workplace injury prevention principles can be clustered into three approaches. These include: the *Haddon Injury Prevention Counter-measures* and his I*njury Phase by Factor Matrix*, the *Injury Pyramid*, and the workplace social environment and safety climate. The first two involve engineering and physical environmental interventions. The third involves the development of manager and worker social-organizational norms that promote adherence to safety policies and safe work practices.

Haddon's Injury Prevention Countermeasures

William Haddon Jr. is recognized as the person who applied the epidemiology of infectious disease science to the epidemiology of injury prevention. He conceptualized the ten injury prevention countermeasures (described in Table 13.3) that are widely used in the design of safe workplaces (Christoffel & Gallagher, 1999). He also developed the *Haddon's Injury Phase X Factor Matrix*, proposing that safety programs are effective to the extent that they intervene at the pre-event injury stage of the Matrix, and to the extent that they gather information about the human, injury agent, physical and social relationship factors that contribute to "close calls" and injury events (Haddon, 1999). Table 13.4 applies the Haddon Matrix to describe a fatal roadway crash between a heating and air conditioning contractor and a farm tractor operator. The National Safety Council reports that 40% of all workplace fatalities, and 30% of all disabling injuries, are the result of motor vehicle crashes, the majority of which occur when workers are traveling to and from their workplaces (National Safety Council, 2009).

Table 13.3 Haddon's ten basic categories of injury prevention

Counter measure		Example
1.	Prevent the initial creation of a hazard	Store flammable liquids in small closed fireproof structures away from the work area
2.	Reduce the amount of energy in the hazard	Store only the minimum amount of gasoline needed
3.	Prevent the release of a hazard	Chain and lock heavy logs securely to truck beds
4.	Modify the rate or spatial distribution of hazard forces/energy	Create energy absorbing crumple zones at the front and rear of automobiles, install seatbelts and airbags, pad dashboards and doors
5.	Separate in time or space the hazard from those to be protected	Construct enclosed overhead walkways over busy highways. Avoid operating slow-moving farm equipment on public roads during peak motor vehicle traffic periods
6.	Separate the hazard from workers by a physical barrier	Install large concrete barriers between highway construction crews and motor vehicle traffic
7.	Modify basic qualities of the hazard	Install handrails on stairways and nonslip surfaces on stair treads
8.	Make what is to be protected more resistant to damage from hazards	Balance and strength conditioning for older adults, e.g. *Silver Sneakers* programs
9.	Early intervention to begin countering the injury from a hazard	Integrated systems of on-site emergency medical care, rapid transport and hospital emergency department trauma care
10.	Stabilize, repair, and rehabilitate	Physical therapy and occupational injury rehabilitation

Table 13.4 An illustration of the Haddon injury phase by factor matrix for a roadway collision involving a HVAC contractor and a farm worker

Injury factors for a fatal roadway crash between a contractor's truck and a farm tractor

Injury Phase	Human individual	Injury agent	Physical environment	Social environment
Pre-event	Farmer and contractor are tired and rushing to get home for the weekend	Slow moving large tractor with no roll bar (ROPS) with trailing equipment and speeding truck	Hilly, narrow, heavily traveled road shared by commuters, service vehicles and farm equipment. Hay wagon and tractor engine noise prevent the farmer from hearing approaching car. High velocity of the speeding truck	Contractor's lack of knowledge, awareness, and risk perception. Farmer's lack of a trailing vehicle or turn signals, choice of driving on a public roadway during peak commuter travel time
Event	Reaction time limitations that prevent the contractor or the tractor operator from avoiding or lessening the force of the crash	Huge kinetic energy and impact forces of the crash distributed over a period of milliseconds exceed the limits of human tissue and organs	Narrow, hilly winding road limits visibility to a few hundred yards. Trees and fences block escape route to avoid a collision	Contractor and farmer cultural biases (e.g., farmers and tractors should stay off highways; city drivers are rude, aggressive, and stupid)
Post-event	Contractor and tractor operator death. Family members' anger, emotional trauma, suffering, grief, financial loss	On-scene emergency extraction of victims, investigation, and site clean-up place many others at risk	Distant EMS, long travel time to a trauma hospital and delayed care contribute to odds of the contractor's and farmer's deaths	Criminal and civil litigation, insurance claims, loss of productivity and income related to the deaths

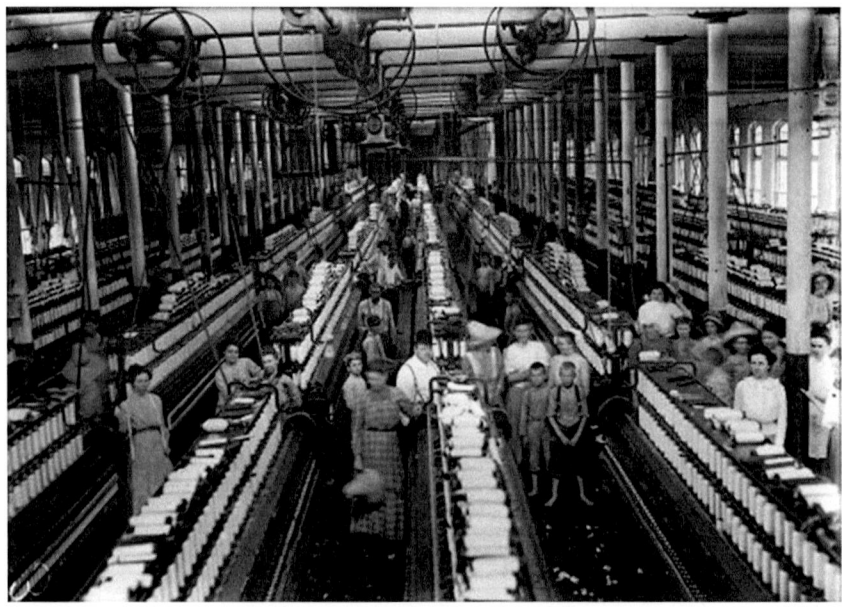

Fig. 13.1 Young Women and child workers at a Lawrence, MA textile mill circa 1912

The roadway collision scenario described below occurred on a summer Friday evening. Both the subcontractor and the farmer were working overtime, and were rushing to begin their weekends. Sam was on route to service an inoperable cooling system for a grocery store located in a rural farming county 50 miles from the city where he was employed by a HVAC service company. He drove at 65 mph (95.5 ft/s), exceeding the posted limit of 45 mph (66.0 ft/s). As he rounded a curve in the road, he saw a slow-moving loaded hay wagon 400 ft. ahead of him (see Figs. 13.1 and 13.2). He failed to notice cues of a likely left turn by the tractor, hay baler, and large hay wagon into a farm yard, even though a large barn and signs of haying were clearly visible on the left just ahead of the hay wagon. To avoid being stuck behind the farm equipment Sam accelerated to 70 mph (102.7 ft/s) to pass. Because of the loaded hay wagon and the tractor's loud diesel engine, Jake, the tractor operator, could not see or hear the Sam's truck approaching from the rear. Just as Jake turned his tractor left into the farmyard, Sam's truck crashed into the tractor at full speed. Both he and the tractor operator died at the scene. Less than four seconds elapsed from the time Sam first saw the tractor until the crash. Had he braked immediately when he first saw the slow moving hay wagon he might possibly have avoided the crash. Even then, his speed reaction time and his truck's stopping distance may have resulted in a crash, but at a lower velocity. Once he started to pass and pulled out 100 ft behind the tractor at 70 mph, there was insufficient time for him to do anything but hit the tractor and hay baler at full speed. This just described case is a collage constructed from many similar cases. It is available online from the *National Agricultural Safety Database* (Cole, Lehtola, Thomas, & Hadley, 2005). Based on 4 years (1989–1992) of Ohio public road crash data, vehicle crashes with farm equipment are most frequent during peak traffic commute times. Left-turn collisions between farm equipment and other motor vehicles like the one described above are among the most frequent (29.8%), and the most deadly (Glascock, Bean, Wood, Carpenter, & Holmes, 1995).

Collecting data only for serious injury events provides little information about frequent day-to-day departures from safe work practices, and the environmental and organizational factors that promote these unsafe actions. The conceptual tools of the *Haddon Engineering Counter-Measures* and the

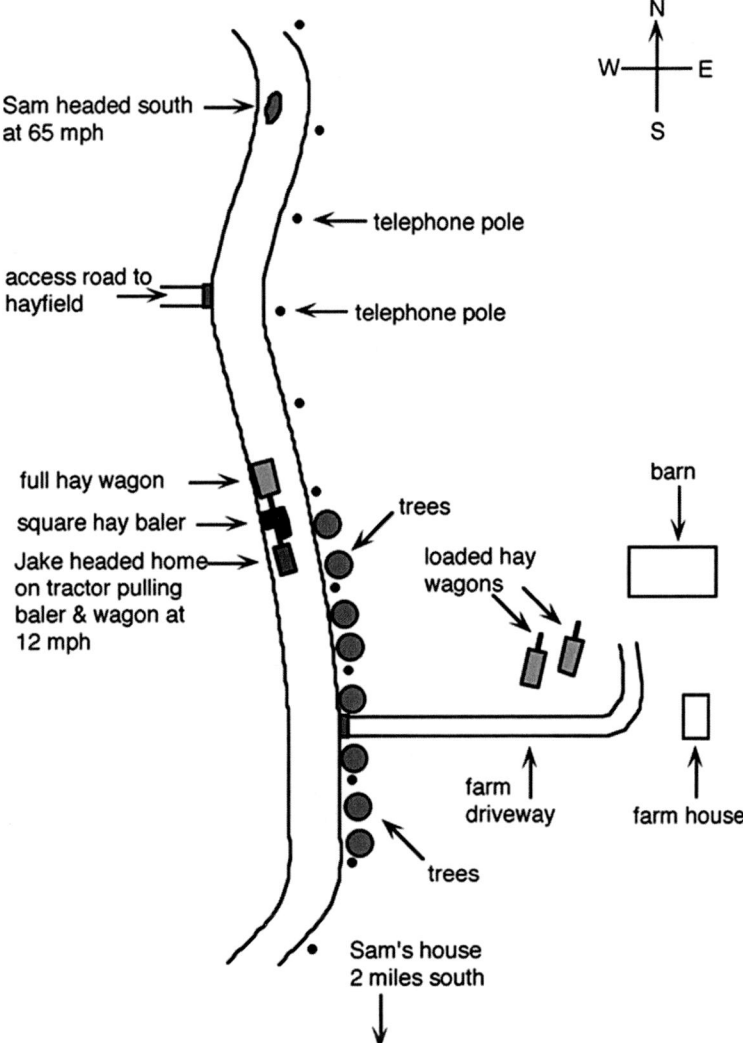

Fig. 13.2 Schematic of pre-event circumstances leading to a fatal roadway collision. (Note: The black dots at the right of the figure represent telephone poles spaced 100 ft apart. The larger gray circles represent trees.)

Injury Phase X Factors Matrix, when applied, promote regular monitoring of compliance with safe work practices. They also draw attention to workplace physical and social environment contingencies that cause workers who understand the hazards of their jobs, and the injuries that can result, to nevertheless engage in unsafe actions. Once identified, barriers to complying with safe work practices often can be removed by changes in work station design (ergonomics and engineering) and work organization (policy) procedures (Wiehagen, Lineberry, & Rethi, 1996; Vaught, Brnich, Mallett, Cole, Wiehagen, & Conti et al., 2000). Behavioral and conceptual analyses of common contingencies that cause experienced and skilled workers to engage in unsafe work practices are described in a number of papers, including the following: *Factors that Contribute to Miners Committing Unsafe Acts: A Behavioral Analysis* (Cole, 1995), *Toward a Typology of Dynamic and Hazardous Work Environments* (Scharf et al., 2001), *Cognitive-Behavioral Approaches to Farm Community Safety Education: A Conceptual Analysis* (Cole, 2002), and *Behavioral and Organizational Dimensions of Underground Mine Fires* (Vaught et al., 2000).

Impact of Haddon's Work on Safety Training

Prior to the work of Haddon and his colleagues, formal safety instruction was naively assumed to be accomplished by presenting workers with safety rules and posters. Because of Haddon's work, safety began to be understood and practiced as an ongoing process of modifying work environments to prevent injuries, developing new technologies and engineering controls to protect workers, in combination with changes in organizational structure and policy. Educational and behavioral interventions began to be understood *not* as the primary approach to injury prevention but as important means by which to promote manager and worker buy-in, as well as active participation and compliance with injury prevention technologies and work practices (Christoffel & Gallagher, 1999, pp. 32–33). Another result of Haddon and his colleagues' injury epidemiology work was the *Hierarchy of Controls Model* (The National Committee for Injury Prevention and Control, 1989). This paradigm orders the injury prevention effectiveness of three approaches. The first and most effective level of control is engineering controls that modify work stations, processes, or machinery in order to prevent workers from coming into contact with moving machinery, harmful atmospheres, chemicals, vapors, mists, dusts, or other injury agents and energy sources. Examples include constructing a work area or entire factory so that harmful dusts or vapors are completely captured or expelled to outside air, with no residual contamination remaining in the work area or factory. A second example is ground fault interrupter (GFI) electrical safety devices. If any part of a worker's body comes into contact with a "hot" or live electrical wire or machine, resulting from an improperly grounded circuit, within milliseconds, the GFI shuts off the electrical current and the worker is unharmed. Without the GFI the worker will either sustain an electrical burn or be electrocuted.

The second level of control diminishes, but does not completely remove, workers' exposure to a hazard. Examples include fresh outside intake air ventilation systems in underground coal mines. The fresh intake air sweeps through the mine entries and removes most of the coal dust generated from machines that cut and transport the coal out of the mine. It also removes and dilutes the methane gas that is released from the coal to concentrations below the explosive level. Yet, both respiratory coal dust and methane remain in the workplace, and both are higher at the face where the coal is being cut. As a result, workers still inhale small amounts of coal dust that, over time, can result in cumulative damage to the lungs called black lung or coal worker pneumoconiosis. Released *methane* also may collect in poorly ventilated sections of the mine, and may result in a deadly explosion. Another example is worker dependence on the thick and strong insulation on electrical power cables in underground mines. The cables are mounted on reels at the rear of large mining machines. As the machines advance, the cables drag on the mine floor. The cable insulation prevents worker contact with high voltage electrical energy. Over time, the large 440 V DC electrical cables that power large mining equipment can become damaged by being run over. The cable electrical insulation can become stretched, cut, cracked and frayed. When this happens, the GFI system shuts the power down because the damage allows small amounts of electrical energy to fault (escape) to the wet mine floor and/or directly through the metal body of an energized or "hot" mining machine to which the power cable is attached. At that point, the mining machines on that circuit stop. Finding and repairing such ground faults in power cables up to 900 ft long is time consuming and difficult. As a result, miners often disable the GFI apparatus in order to continue mining coal and maintain production schedules. Eight percent of coal miner deaths results from electrocutions and nonfunctional GFI systems (Reynolds, undated).

The third level of control involves workers' use of personal protective equipment (PPE) in the absence of level one and level two protective systems. Some coal mines and many surface mine sites have high levels of respirable coal and/or silica rock dust. Construction workers often cut rocks and bricks with electrical powered saws that produce thick clouds of dust. Often, the only available method of protection from long-term pneumoconiosis lung disease is the worker's use of a NIOSH approved respirator. The loud noise generated by the cutting also requires hearing protection to prevent noise-induced hearing loss. Other exposures to toxic and caustic liquids require workers' to wear fluid and chemical barrier gloves, aprons, eyewear, and sometimes full garments and self-contained breathing apparatus. PPE approaches are required when engineering controls are absent or impractical. Yet, they remain the least effective for protecting workers' health for multiple reasons, including worker discomfort, failure to properly fit, wear, clean and maintain equipment. The author once conducted an evaluation study of the NIOSH occupational respiratory training program. As part of that program, 21 used quarter-face twin-cartridge respirators were collected from factory work areas. The majority had damaged or missing straps and distorted or damaged face masks. Some had small holes punched in the face mask near the mouth area. This allowed workers to insert a soda straw or a cigarette in order to drink or smoke while wearing their respirators.

The Heinrich Injury Pyramid

For many years, the primary measure of occupational safety was the number of fatalities that occurred at a company. Few fatal events were seen as evidence of a safe workplace. Workplace fatalities are an unreliable and problematic metric by which to measure, report, and improve workplace safety and health because they tend to fluctuate widely and sometimes wildly from year to year. Even today fatality rates sometimes are the *only* metric used to report workplace safety status. This was, in part, because fatalities are more notable and are reported both within a company and also by public media.

As the Heinrich (1959) injury pyramid and its adaption by Bird and Germain and others became known and understood it focused attention on reporting and collecting data for "close calls," minor injury events and injuries and illnesses, serious and fatal injuries. This comprehensive collection of data proved to be much more informative and effective for identifying workplace hazards and then implementing preventive interventions. It is important to note that the *Injury Pyramid* in Fig. 13.3 does not include all noncompliance and "close call" events. A 2003 study by ConocoPhillips Marine reported that, for every fatality, there were at least 300,000 at-risk behaviors that were not in compliance with company safety programs, training, and work practices. Common examples included "short cuts," such as bypassing safety systems on machinery or eliminating a step in a safety procedure, because following a safety protocol was perceived as slowing production (Freibott, 2012). The pre-event contingencies that produce close calls are often identical to those that result in serious injury and death. Collecting and tabulating data for close call events leads to the proactive identification and removal or control of injury risk factors. For example, ongoing monitoring of regular workers, contractors and contingent workers' compliance with lock-out/tag-out safety protocols prevents both close calls and injury events.

With these above general principles of occupational injury prevention in mind, we now turn to the important socioeconomic issues involved in the workplace. As seen below, such issues can play a significant role in various aspects of the occupational workplace, including safety issues.

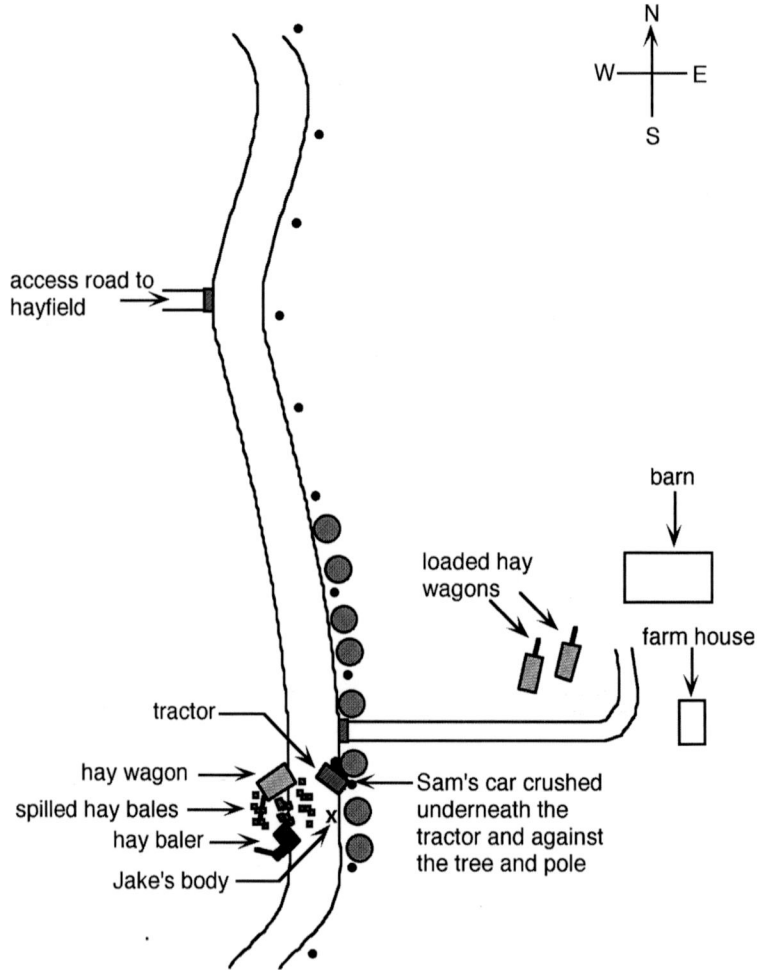

Fig. 13.3 Post-event schematic of a fatal collision between a contract worker and a farmer

Traditional Forms of Capital and Social Relations

There are basically three forms of *capital* (i.e., accumulated worth) that influence social relations among individuals across a wide range of social communities including workplace communities (Bourdieu, 1986; Putnam, 2000). The first is *economic capital*, sometimes referred to as *physical capital*. It involves owning or having control over money and other tangible assets. Economic capital can be, and often is, inherited or transferred to others. The second form is *social capital*. It refers to durable informal and formal social networks of individuals who trust, respect, and help each other. Members of social networks differ in terms of talents, wealth, and status, but are valued for their varied roles and contributions. Individuals within communities (including workplace communities) with high social capital are happier, healthier, and safer than groups with low social capital (Putnam, 2000). *Social capital*, in turn, has two forms—bonding and bridging. *Bonding social capital* occurs within groups that are tightly connected for a variety of ethnic, cultural, or economic reasons. It is common within guilds, trades, and professional organizations, with certification and licensing requirements that both protect markets and ensure that members meet professional standards. *Bonding social capital* can lead to group self-interest, exclusion, and dysfunctional social relations within larger communities, including workplace communities. *Bridging social capital* is sometimes referred to as *linking social capital*. It is present or absent in varying degrees in any community including workplace communities. In workplaces, *bridging social capital* links together individuals with varied levels of skills, social and economic status, power, and responsibility. It promotes bonds of mutual respect, trust, reciprocity, and collaboration across the worker, supervisor, and manager hierarchy. Workplaces with such structure are happier, safer, and more productive (Putnam, 2000). Social capital is sometimes thought of as social climate. Finally, the third form is *cultural capital*, sometimes referred to as *human capital*. It arises from individuals' accumulated experiences, knowledge, skills, expectations, and wisdom (Cole & Donovan, 2008; Putnam, 2000). Unlike *economic capital*, *cultural capital* cannot be inherited, but can be fostered and nurtured by coworker, supervisor, and manager mentors.

The relationship among the three forms of capital can be summarized as follows. Economic assets (*physical capital*) and individual experience and education (*human capital*), when embedded in social networks with norms of reciprocity and trustworthiness, result in individual and collective well-being, known as *social capital* (Putnam, 2000). This, in turn, can result in safe workplaces. Indeed, a multi-year Department of Interior-funded study in the early 1980s suggested that workplaces with these aforementioned social capital characteristics experienced few occupational injuries. A team of psychologists, sociologists, business administrators, rehabilitation counselors, as well as civil, mining, and human factors engineers, identified and reviewed studies reported in professional journals and government documents that identified factories and manufacturing plants with exceptionally low occupational injury rates over an extended period of years (Cole et al., 1986). These companies addressed hazard identification, risk perception, risk communication, risk reduction, and injury prevention as an ongoing process integrated into daily work practice. Safety was *not* assigned exclusively to a company safety officer or safety department, but rather to each worker, first-line supervisor and managers as well. Daily workplace safety inspections were conducted pre- and post-shift. If at any time, a safety hazard or unsafe work activity was observed, it was immediately addressed. For example, a liquid spill in a walkway observed by a worker, supervisor, or manager was immediately cleaned up and reported, as were incidents involving unsafe work practices such as failure to wear a hard hat or eye protection, backing a forklift without looking to the rear, or climbing on a chair to replace a light bulb instead of using a step ladder. The seven common characteristics of these safe workplaces are listed in Table 13.5 (Cole et al., 1986).

The very low occupational injury rates among the companies identified in the Cole et al. (1986) study can be understood within the *Haddon Injury Prevention Counter-Measures*, the *Injury Phase X Factor Matrix*, and the of the 1959 *Heinrich Injury Pyramid*, and its 1996 adaptation by Bird and Germain, as earlier depicted in Fig. 13.4. At the individual company level, fatal occupational injuries are rare events that, when investigated, can lead to safer work environments and practices. However, fatality investigations alone provide limited utility for robust surveillance and epidemiological analyses. "Close call" events (near misses) occur much more frequently than do even minor injuries. One of the reasons that safety programs like those described in the previous section are successful is that they monitor ongoing compliance and noncompliance with safe work practices. "Close calls" are understood to have the same array of contingencies that result in minor, serious and fatal injuries. Safety programs that involve workers, supervisors and managers in ongoing monitoring and abating or mitigating workplace hazards prevent "close calls," as well as minor, serious and fatal injuries. Safety programs that focus primarily on collection and review of injury events promote *hindsight* at the expense of *foresight*. Foresight is necessary to anticipate, recognize, control, and prevent emergent hazards that occur in all workplaces (Fischoff, 1975; Cole, 1997; Cole, Vaught, Wiehagen, Haley, & Brnich, 1998). Companies using prevention methods, like those described earlier in Table 13.3 and 13.4,

Table 13.5 Characteristics of safe factories and mines

1.	Strong management commitment to safety • Safety matters regularly included on meeting agenda • Safety of workers viewed as a management responsibility • All levels of management committed to and involved in safety
2.	Positive and proactive organizational climate • Supportive and open relationship between management and workers • Frequent, easy two-way communication among workers, supervisors, and managers
3.	Management efficiency in planning and operations • Good housekeeping materials handling/storage • Shared knowledge and well-coordinated activities among departments, workers, supervisors, and managers • Good record keeping in production, job performance, safety, etc., and widespread sharing of this information • Frequent use of data in planning and decision making
4.	Decentralized wide involvement of persons in safety matters • First line supervisors and workers involved in daily inspections, hazard detection/correction • Top managers encourage preventive/corrective safety activity and are themselves frequently involved • Little reliance upon a centralized safety officer/staff for being solely responsible for maintaining a safe work environment

5.	Behavioral specificity in safety and job procedures
	• Rules for proper performance are clearly and operationally specified
	• Regular and redundant communication of safety and proper job performance by multiple means including
	   – Informal meetings/dialog at the work section
	   – Formal safety meetings
	   – Posters, fliers including safety rules, procedures, reminders, etc.
	   – Formal investigations of accidents and near accidents (close calls)
	   – Consistent and fair enforcement of safety procedures

6.	A stable workforce • Good worker morale and attendance • Little employee turnover • An experienced and older workforce
7.	Strong financial solvency of the company • Company/division is earning profits • Good backlog of orders for products ensures future

Although it is informative to know the characteristics of safe work places, it is not an easy matter to change those which are not safe. Some of the characteristics are not subject to change by the company itself, the industry, or by regulatory agencies (e.g., characteristics of the workforce, financial solvency of the company, changes in technology. Changes to improve both safety and production may require long-term comprehensive approaches (Cohen & Swift, 1999)

proactively avoid injuries and their associated costs by ongoing monitoring of workplace hazards and compliance with safe work practices.

Work as a Social Activity

The above section documented the importance of *social capital* in the workplace. Indeed, work is a social activity, with the same types of social needs and interactions common to other social groups. Prior to the 1980s and early 1990s, many manufacturing companies and a wide variety of other

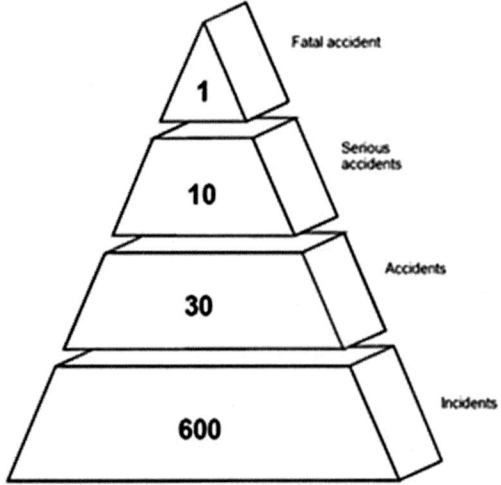

Fig. 13.4 Bird and Germain's adaptation of the Heinrich Injury Pyramid

businesses hired workers on a long term-basis. What often resulted was a social community with reciprocal relationships of trust, mutual respect, and cooperation among workers and managers that benefited the company, the workers and the larger society. Workplaces with these characteristics and long-term worker employment typically are safe and productive (Cohen & Prusak, 2001, Gochfeld & Mohr, 2007, Putnam, 2000). Indeed, prior to the 1980s, a widely practiced and central assumption of employee-management relations was an unwritten but tacit understanding by both parties that workers hired who performed well would become career employees. In many cases, this expectation occurred. Full-time employment of workers in steel mills, automobile and manufacturing plants, as well as in many service industries, was commonplace from the 1940s up to the 1980s (Putnam, 2000)

The Changing Face of the Workplace

With rapid changes in technology, production and globalization, tacit long-term employment contracts became increasingly rare during the downsizing, restructuring, re-engineering and outsourcing that occurred in the 1980s and 1990s. During 1993–1994, nearly 50% of all US firms downsized their employees by an average of 10%. This trend continues for both blue and white color workers who are increasingly employed in temporary or part-time positions across nearly all private and public sectors (Putnam, 2000; Hipple, 2001). The Department of Labor refers to members of this population as *alternative* or *contingent workers*, that is, individuals who report that their jobs are temporary without an implicit or explicit contract or expectation for continued employment (Department of Labor, 2005). Contingent workers range across socioeconomic and educational levels, from unskilled and unschooled to highly educated and skilled. They work as day laborers, freelancers, on-call workers, independent contractors, and leased hires from contract labor firms. They are employed in agriculture, construction, manufacturing, transportation, hazardous waste work, health care, public service, law enforcement, the military, and nearly all other sectors. Across many sectors contingent workers tend to be young, inexperienced and at increased risk for both nonfatal and fatal injury (Department of Labor, 2005; Guerrina, Burns, & Conlon, 2011; Gochfeld & Mohr, 2007; Hipple, 2001; Oh & Shin, 2003). Contingent workers often are without workers' compensation insurance and health insurance. A recent study identified 1,023 patients who visited an emergency department at a university medical center during 2005 because of a work-related injury that was confirmed by the medical staff. Twenty percent (209/1,023) were not covered by workers' compensation insurance. Of the 209 without workers' compensation insurance, 92% also lacked health insurance (Nicholson, Bunn, & Costich, 2008).

Reasons for Outsourcing and Subcontracting

Outsourcing work to subcontractors is widely practiced to lower costs, to employ workers with special skills, and to diversify risk (Gochfeld & Mohr, 2007). Individuals or contracting companies that win contracts often do so by operating at the lowest possible cost. This economic constraint often means there is little time for safety training, as well as too little time and money to properly maintain and upgrade equipment. Examples include general contracting companies that operate equipment with damaged or missing machine guards, and whose workers are without personal protective equipment. For example, rock drill rigs and crews are familiar sights at highway, building construction, and surface mine sites. In the author's experience, rarely does one observe drill rig contract workers wearing respiratory protection, and frequently no hearing protection even when exposed to very high concentrations of rock dust and high decibel noise levels. Small business general contractors and small farm operators and their contract laborers also often work with older equipment that, while functional, is compromised by a range of safety problems that place workers at increased injury risk. For example, mobile powered equipment with missing shields on PTO drivelines, inoperable backup alarm warning systems, broken or faulty lighting and marking, absence of fully charged and functional fire extinguishers, as well as bent, broken, or missing access steps and hand-holds for mounting and dismounting equipment, are widely prevalent (Cole et al., 2009). These conditions and unfamiliarity with hazards peculiar to a series of different work sites during short-term job placements increase contract risk for injury (Gochfeld & Mohr, 2007).

Contract Workers and Injury Risk

Park and Butler (2001) identified contract workers' injury risk by comparing workers' compensation costs for full-time workers with two types of contingent workers—"regular part-time workers" and "leased workers." Both the full-time and regular part-time workers were paid by the companies where they performed work, and both received worker's compensation insurance. The leased workers were paid by a contractor and received no wages or worker's compensation coverage from the host companies where they worked. Regular full-time workers were more likely to be male, older, and better paid than regular part-time workers. Yet, they did not differ in terms of their workers' compensation claim frequency, injury severity, or claim denial rates, even though they differed demographically. However, the "leased" workers' compensation injuries were *three times* greater than for regular workers, and *ten times* greater than for regular part-time workers, even when controlling for age, gender, industry, type and date of injury. The leased employees had a much higher number of claims, and also significantly higher injury severity claims. This strongly suggests that contracted or self-employed transient workers, who come onto a company property only occasionally for short periods, have limited contact with other workers and little opportunity for integration into the company work organization social structure and its safety practices. Errors in hazards communication between the company's full-time workforce and the contract workers often result (Gochfeld & Mohr, 2007; Park & Butler, 2001). Because of the transient nature of their jobs, contingent workers often are excluded from the safety instruction, safety policies and safety supervision at the sites where they work (Kalleberg, 2000).

Small independent contracting companies and their workers generally do not participate in host company safety training or in local or regional safety training sessions, even when such sessions are available at no cost. Taking time to attend a safety session is perceived as too costly. While away from their jobs sites, small contractors risk unsafe or improperly completed work by unsupervised workers, missed deadlines, earning a "bad reputation," and losing customers (Kidd, Parshall, Wojcik, & Struttmann, 2004). Small labor contractors also work in a constantly changing environment that includes not only weather changes, but also the availability and costs of materials and a changing workforce. For example, a small roofing contractor company owner with two long-term experienced workers can complete most jobs safely, efficiently, and well. However, when one worker leaves to start his own roofing company, and/or when a bigger job is contracted, the owner may have to hire unskilled labor from a general labor contract organization or unemployment office. Having two or three inexperienced roofers slows the rate at which work can be completed, risks compromising work quality and safety. It not only also increases the risk of injury to the transient inexperienced workers, but to the contractor and his skilled workers as well. Many contract workers are not covered by workers' compensation insurance, and a majority lack health insurance (Kidd et al., 2004; Lineberry, Scharf, & Wiehagen, 2003).

Economics and Injury Consequences of Subcontracting

A case study examined the Department of Energy and its prime subcontractors' practices of outsourcing work to subcontractors at hazardous chemical and nuclear waste sites, as well as similar practices in the US petrochemical industry (Gochfeld & Mohr, 2007). In each case, the short-term benefits for hiring subcontractor contingent workers as opposed to "regular hires" were the same. Hiring temporary workers reduces payroll and worker benefit costs. It facilitates hiring workers with technical expertise or unskilled laborers on an "as needed" basis for short periods of time. It also transfers parent company and prime contractor responsibility for the safety training and supervision of contingent workers, as well as compliance with the OSHA Rules of Construction (29 CFR 1926.16), even though the rules state that companies and their subcontractors, each individually and jointly, assume responsibility for worker safety and health. OSHA increasingly relies on voluntary compliance rather than enforcement. Subcontractors often do not report their workers' injuries. Thus, total the number of contingent workers and their annual hours of exposure are unknown. As a result, injury epidemiological studies by OSHA or by the National Institute of Occupational Safety and Health (NIOSH) Fatality Assessment and Control Evaluation (FACE) program are compromised because denominator data are missing. Deaths are more likely to be reported than nonfatal injuries or illnesses, but not even all deaths are reported.

One study with incomplete data found that 59% of workers who died in trench collapse on Department of Energy (DOE) job sites were subcontractor employees (Gochfeld & Mohr, 2007). Alfonso Alverez's death in a trench in 2002 is a typical case. While working for a Texas construction company the 17-yearo old was laying a water line in an un-shored trench. A trench cave-in buried the lad to his waist. During the 30 min required to free him he Alfonso remained alive but died later that day from asphyxia and other injuries. Asphyxia deaths of this type result when heavy earth pushes the internal organs in the abdomen upward against the diaphragm. The individual then is unable to inhale and fill his or her lungs with air. OSHA cited the company for nine health and safety violations, three of which were willful (Hopkins, 2003). Trenching and excavating are recognized as one of the most hazardous construction operations. OSHA revised Subpart P, Excavations, 29 CFR 1926.650, 29 CFR 1926.651, and 29 CFR 1926.652 require that all trenches through soil and unstable material must be shored or widely angled at the top to prevent cave ins and worker entrapment.

In hazardous waste work and in the petrochemical industry, contingent workers hired by subcontractors tend to be younger and less experienced than regular workers. In addition, some companies that employ subcontracted temporary workers advise managers to avoid assuming responsibility for safety training and supervision of the workers in order to avoid liability issues (Gochfeld & Mohr, 2007).

Underground coal mining companies also outsource complex, difficult and dangerous jobs to subcontractors. For example, after a large mining company's workers have completed "room and pillar" mining, they sometimes contract with small mining companies whose workers extract the coal pillars. The pillars are rectangular blocks of coal with dimensions of 80×100 ft. The pillars are left in place between parallel sets of entries (longitudinal tunnels) and cross cuts (perpendicular tunnels) from which the coal is cut. The pillars are left in place during mining to prevent the mine roof from collapsing. The small contractor companies hired to remove the pillars proceed in a carefully planned sequence. When performed correctly, the mine roof collapses in a controlled manner as the contract miners and their equipment cut the coal from the pillars and retreat toward the outside. Although inherently dangerous, removing the pillars is highly profitable because it yields a high coal tonnage with a minimum of equipment, time and effort. By outsourcing removal of pillars, the larger mining company shifts the risk of injury and the associated costs and liability from its regular workers to the contractors. During his years of coal mine safety research, the author met with such a small retreat mining contracting company. The entire workforce consisted of two brothers and their six sons who worked with old and used equipment.

Small roofing companies, building framers, and general construction companies also often work as contractors for other host companies. These workers seldom have time to attend safety meetings or to participate in other types of safety training, except for the training they receive on the job from the owner-operator and their coworkers. As part of a NIOSH-funded project, Dr. Pamela Kidd at the University of Kentucky, Dr. Ted Scharf at the NIOSH Taft Laboratory, the author, and others worked with the Kentucky Employees Mutual Insurance Company (KEMI) on a project to lower injury rates among construction companies with ≤10 employees. The incentive was KEMI's lowering workers' compensation premiums for construction companies whose owners and workers participated in the program. Six tabletop interactive narrative simulation exercises that depicted construction-related fall and back injury cases were developed. The simulations were designed to teach and simultaneously assess workers' decision making with respect to selecting safe work practices versus quicker but high-risk actions (Cole, 1994). Random samples of owner-operators, supervisors, and workers completed the simulations and judged them to be relevant and useful for identifying and preventing errors that lead to injuries (Wojcik, Kidd, Parshall, & Struttmann, 2003). However, it proved difficult to deliver the interventions because most small contractors and their workers were so busy working at their trade that they had little time for any form of formal safety training. In addition, many believed that they already knew how to work safely. Group administrations of the simulations at local meetings proved ineffective because of poor attendance. Completing the simulations individually at home was more popular, but the overall participation rate was only 26.7% (Kidd et al., 2004). In addition, completing the simulations at home deprived the workers of the valuable and vigorous dialog and interaction that occur when small groups of workers collaborate in completing the tabletop simulation exercises. While at work, individuals frequently talk about, and evaluate approaches to problems that arise. To the extent possible, workplace technical and safety training should do the same (Cole, 1994; 1997; Cole et al., 1998). In addition, farmers who regularly hire part-time and seasonal workers, face similar problems in finding workers who can competently operate farm machinery. Like small contractors, many farmers are too busy to attend local safety training sessions (Cole, Kidd, Isaacs, Parshall, & Scharf, 1997).

Immigrant Workers at Highest Risk of Injury

Immigrants comprise 12.5% of the US Population and 15.6% of the labor force. Many are employed as contingent workers with no health or retirement benefits. They tend to work in low-wage, low-skill and what is referred to as 3 D jobs (dirty, dangerous, and difficult). (Schenker, 2010). Hispanics are among the most rapidly growing members of the US workforce. During the 2003–2006 period, 67% of the Hispanic workers who died in workplace injury events were foreign born. Approximately 70% of these deaths were persons born in Mexico (MMWR, 2008). During 2000 Hispanics comprised 15% of US construction workers, but 23.5% of the fatalities (Schenker, 2010). From 1992 to 2001 during the US economic boom period, workplace fatality rates for Hispanic workers rose 15.1% while, during that same period, the rate for all other workers fell by 15.4% (Bureau of Labor, Census of Fatal Occupational Injuries, 2008). Deaths of Hispanic workers were distributed as follows: construction 34%; administrative and waste services 11%; agriculture forestry and fishing 10%; and transportation warehousing 10% (MMWR, 2006).

Injury Risk Is Greater in Dynamic Work Environments

Many of the models for identifying, communicating, and managing injury risks were developed for manufacturing plants and similar workplaces. In such places, much of the equipment and many of the workers are in relatively fixed locations, and are engaged in relatively ordered and routine sets of tasks. Other workplaces are more dynamic and less static (Scharf et al., 2001). Examples include underground mines where the workers daily carve out and enlarge their work space on a daily basis, and constantly advance their equipment, supply lines, and their product output and transport system. This is accomplished while working in dark, restricted spaces in close proximity to noisy and very large equipment. As the mine advances, even the best geological maps and technology cannot predict all the potential hazards that may emerge. These include, among others, cutting into old works and rapid inundations of "black damp" (oxygen deficient atmospheres) or water, and encountering sections with small geologic faults and/or nonconformities that can result in roof falls. Working in an underground mine is much more dynamic and unpredictable than working on the assembly line of a typical manufacturing plant.

Other highly dynamic work environments include logging, commercial fishing, and many types of agricultural production. The large majority of US electrical power company linemen are contractors. Electrical linemen contractors conduct emergency repair work during and following major ice and wind storms. During major outages they typically travel long distances from other States to areas with damage. They conduct repair work while working at heights with combinations of "live" and "dead" power lines that can become energized by local farmers' and businesses' emergency electrical generators feeding back into the system. As linemen work, they also are at risk from strong wind, falling trees and debris from damaged structures. Additional risks are associated with working in unfamiliar territory, in combination with local emergency response crews whose individuals and collective work practices may differ from theirs. For example, on January 29, 2009, a 35-year old guest utility worker from a small Minnesota contracting company died when he and a local lineman fell 40 ft from a utility pole while repairing a power line damaged in a major Kentucky ice storm. Visibility was limited because of darkness and sleet. A utility truck that slid into a ditch was being towed out of the ditch by a second truck. In the darkness and bad weather, no one noticed that the truck being towed had become entangled in a steel support cable attached to the utility pole. As the towed truck advanced the support cable snapped the utility pole in half. Both linemen fell. A 300 pound transformer fell on the worker who died. The local lineman sustained non-life-threatening injuries (The Crittenden Press Online, 2009).

Subcontracted iron workers and construction crews also work in highly dynamic, emerging structures and unstable environments that include changes in wind and weather conditions, working at heights on temporary structures, and in close proximity to heavy loads of materials being moved and lifted by large machinery. In addition, construction sites usually include many contract laborers who are needed for short periods of time. Construction of large multistory buildings in restricted spaces adjacent to busy city streets and adjacent buildings confine a wide range of workers, equipment, and materials in close proximity. Removal of soil and rock, delivery, unloading, storage, movement, and hoisting of equipment and construction materials is an ongoing process that exposes large numbers and varieties of contract workers to potential injury. Contract and part-time workers at such sites, which span a wide range of trades and experience, are the rule rather than the exception. Traffic and construction noise tend to drown out backup alarms that occur so frequently from multiple machines that workers on foot have difficulty discriminating a source. Workers also can habituate to such frequent warning signals. It is unlikely that a single hazard identification, risk perception, and risk communication model will fit all combinations of the various populations of contract workers, and the wide array of static and dynamic environments in which they work (Scharf et al., 2001).

Robert Peters and his colleagues at the NIOSH Pittsburgh Research Laboratory studied the contingencies that cause experienced underground coal miners to intentionally move under unsupported mine roof and risk severe injury or death from a roof fall, even when they are aware of the potential fatal injury (Peters & Randolph, 1991). The contingencies that motivate this behavior are primarily economic. Going under an unsupported roof, while dangerous, is a safety shortcut. A miner working at the face (where coal is cut) can move quickly to a parallel entry (tunnel) by dashing 80 ft through a cross cut (tunnel) where the roof is not yet supported. The safe alternative route is for the miner to circle three sides of an 80 × 100 foot coal pillar in passage ways where the mine roof has been bolted to the upper rock strata. Coal seams in Eastern Kentucky mines average around 52 in. in height. Taking the safe route requires the miner to stoop walk 280 ft, while perhaps carrying 30–40 pounds of equipment. The safe route results in high physical energy costs for the miner, and lost production time for the mine section crew. Both conspire to encourage managers to "look the other way" and provide miners with tacit approval to engage in this dangerous and MSHA-prohibited practice. Because of these workplace contingencies, 90% of miners have engaged in this behavior on a few occasions, but fewer than 5% do so on a regular basis (Peters & Randolph, 1991).

Promoting Safety Practices by Examining the Cost

For multiple years, teams of researchers at the University of Kentucky have used occupational injury simulation exercises and case materials, in combination with economic analyses of occupational injuries related to farming. These intervention materials demonstrate the huge cost of low probability but serious work-related injuries, and the low cost of safety equipment and safety practices that prevent costly injury events (Cole et al., 1997; Isaacs, Cole, & Gross, 1997; Myers, Cole, & Mazur, 2005; Myers, Cole, Mazur, & Isaacs, 2006, 2008). Decision analysis and cost tools developed by Melvin Myers are used to calculate the probabilities of the injuries, their direct and indirect costs, and the cost effectiveness of their prevention through readily available protective interventions. The tools demonstrate graphically the huge costs of low probability events, such as operator disability or death from overturning a tractor without a roll bar, and the effect of the injury costs on revenue. If a farm or other business with a profit margin of 10% experiences even a relatively minor injury that results in $10,000 of direct costs, the operation must produce an additional $100,000 of revenue to offset the direct cost associated with the injury event. In addition, indirect costs associated with the injury event, such as lost work time, also negatively impact cash flow and revenue (Myers et al., 2008). It is not possible for most small farm operators and many larger operations to increase either their production or markets to overcome the revenue lost related to even relatively minor injury events. Serious occupational injuries, especially those that result in full or partial disability, can result in direct costs of hundreds of thousands or millions of dollars. Criminal and civil law suits can impose additional staggering losses. When potential injury events and their costs are examined in this way, the revenue protection value of investing in safety equipment and safe work practices becomes more apparent. Larger and well-managed companies generally are aware of these facts. Smaller farm operations and small business contractors, though, are often less aware and less capable of surviving such injury events. Unfortunately, changing farmers' ingrained attitudes against taking actions to improve safety often requires a severe injury event or death, and its associated huge personal and economic costs. A key aspect of using stories based on real farming injury cases, in combination with economic analysis cost tools, is that attitudes and behavior changes that support safe work practices can emerge before a catastrophic injury event occurs (Cole, 2002). Perhaps similar methods can be developed and used with small business contractors whose workers are not well integrated into larger companies' work organization and safety practices.

Narrative Guides and Directs Behavior, Including Safety Behavior

A large body of research suggests that a primary method by which humans understand what they should value and believe, and how they should act in their personal, social, and work roles, is based on internalized stories or narratives (Bandura, 1989; Bruner, 1990; Cole, 1997; Sarbin, 1986). Sometimes these narratives are referred to as *culture tales* (Cole, 1997; Howard, 1991). The *culture tales* of workers and managers in mines, factories, agricultural, and other businesses are pervasive and powerful influences on workers' attitudes, what they believe are effective safety practices, and what they are willing to do or not do with respect to working safely. People who are otherwise intelligent, self-efficacious, and safety-conscious may believe that seat belts do not protect them, but instead place them at increased risk of being trapped in a burning vehicle during a crash. Consequently, they will not wear seat belts. Workers exposed to silica dust as they saw concrete or operate rock drilling rigs, and suffer no apparent ill effects from unprotected dust exposures, often will not wear respirators because they believe that doing so does not protect them from lung disease. Witte's (1992) extended *Parallel Process Model* of human behavior refers to this type of reasoning as *response efficacy*. If workers believe that a prescribed safety behavior is effective for preventing injury or illness, they are likely to comply. If they believe a safety procedure is ineffective for preventing injury or illness, they will not comply. Such beliefs often are based on internalized stories or *culture tales* that are not easily changed, even by scientifically sound evidence. This is especially true when the ill effects of a harmful behavior do not appear until well into the future, and at that point become punishing. At that point in time, the immediate reinforcement for the harmful behavior "short cut" pales in comparison as the severe illness or injury consequences emerge. Common health examples include smokers who derive immediate and powerful reinforcement from smoking and, in most cases, for which the profoundly and painful adverse punishers do not become apparent until years later. Chronic overeating, obesity, and drug and alcohol dependency are difficult to overcome for similar reasons. The same principles apply to many workers' reluctance or refusal to wear respiratory, hearing, eye protection, and seat belts.

How Attitudes are Learned

Knowledge of how to work productively and safely within a factory or mine is shared safety information (often called *declarative knowledge*). It can be taught by providing workers with oral, visual or printed language explanations. Safe work practice procedures (often called *procedural knowledge*) can be taught by demonstrating the proper completion of a series of actions, and having the worker practice and perfect the performance. Both of these methods are referred to as *direct instruction*. However, the teaching of beliefs and attitudes related to the injury prevention value of wearing a respirator, wearing hearing protection, and always wearing a seat belt when operating motor vehicles is a different matter. In these and similar cases, direct instruction is typically ineffective or counterproductive (Bandura, 1989; Gagne, 1984; Cole, 2002). The noncompliant individual may not be influenced by the instruction, or may resent being told what he or she should believe and value. Two indirect methods of instruction that are effective for teaching safety attitudes and beliefs are the behaviors of human models with whom workers identify, and the *culture tales* (stories) that permeate the work environment. These stories describe whom workers should trust and what they should believe and do to work safely and effectively (Cole, 1997, 2002; Cole et al., 1998; Vaught, Mallett, Brnich, Reinke, & Kowalski-Trakofler et al., 2006).

Conclusions and Future Directions

One of the most insightful papers regarding workers' self-protective behaviors and the theoretical models that attempt to explain such behavior was published 16 years ago (DeJoy, 1996). That paper classified previous workplace safety studies into three broad categories. The first are studies of employee personal and demographic characteristics as they relate to workers' safety performance. The second are behavioral intervention studies that use operant conditioning learning theory and contingent reinforcement to shape specific desired safety behaviors and to extinguish unsafe behaviors. The third are studies that focus on the correlates of safe work practices by identifying and studying common characteristics of factories and other workplaces that have very low injury rates over multiple year periods. DeJoy also summarized three major theoretical models that attempted to predict health behaviors. The first are cost-benefit models that describe individual worker choices based on value-expectancy theory (e.g., *Why should I put up with the discomfort a respirator and being unable to talk or drink? I know that only a small percentage of coal miners die from black lung disease!*). The second are environmental-contextual models that focus not only on individual worker personal characteristics as predictors of behavior, but also on workers' decisions that arise from interactions with each other, mangers and changing physical environment variables (e.g., *The overhead conveyor chain is jammed for the third time tonight. The foreman is screaming at me to fix it immediately or we will not meet our production schedule. I don't have time to get the ladder and the plywood tank cover. I'll climb up on the dip tank frame, reach up and clear the jam.*[2]). The third are stages-of-change models developed by Prochaska and DiClemente and their colleagues (1982) in relation to eliminating addictive behaviors such as smoking. The process of behavior change was conceptualized in five sequential stages: Pre-contemplation, contemplation, preparation, action, and maintenance. The stages-of-change approach was also applied to many occupational injury prevention programs including studies conducted by the author and his colleagues. DeJoy also noted that all of the models when applied tended to focus on the person, and excluded the influence of the larger system variables. Most studies also were conducted in factories or other workplaces with static as opposed to dynamic work environments, and with long-term as opposed to short-term contingent workers.

A major contribution is DeJoy's (1996) matrix of self-protective behavior constructs and stages of worker self- protective behavior (p. 69). He suggested that workers often can recognize a hazard and

---

[2] This scenario describes a permanently disabling injury event that resulted when the author's younger brother fell into a large tank filled with a 140 °F solution of water and phosphoric acid that was used to degrease metal components for large commercial electrical meters. He spent 6 months in the Massachusetts General Hospital burn unit and an additional 4 years in physical therapy and rehabilitation. He never was able to return to work. The event was investigated by OSHA.

respond with behavior that mitigates the threat. However, a worker's self-efficacy does not necessarily lead to a safe decision. In the interest of maintaining production, a supervisor may issue an order to a worker to engage in and unsafe action. On other occasions, a contingency may require an immediate action. In such circumstances, the worker may not be able to follow a prescribed safety policy for dealing with a problem. DeJoy's final factor is the safety climate in which the worker is embedded. Safety climate also can be described by the presence or absence of social capital. When managers do not value and respect workers' decisions, and when workers are reluctant to disagree with supervisor for fear of being punished, little social capital is present and the supervisors make the decision. This is illustrated in what happened in the Triangle fire and the Lawrence textile mills. DeJoy also notes that even well trained and highly motivated workers often will not respond appropriately to workplace injury threats if their actions are not valued, recognized and reinforced by managers. He states that safe workplaces depend on collective control, a set of group norms or beliefs shared by workers, managers, and supervisors. He also notes that these group norms are similar to Zohar's safety climate construct (DeJoy, 1996, p. 67). On page 67 DeJoy et al. have this to say about safety climate.

> Long-term adherence ultimately requires constructing task and work environments that support safe behavior, even under the most adverse workload conditions.
> …high levels of both individual and collective controls may be critical to long-term adherence.

On the same page he continues with the following statement.

> …safety climate serves as a frame of reference for guiding relevant behavior in the workplace and that employees develop reasonable expectations regarding behavior-outcome contingencies in their environment…. It follows that collective control or safety climate should be an important consideration in fostering long-term and broad based adherence to safe work practices.

A 2009 meta-analysis study examined workplace safety with respect to the roles of person and situation factors (Christin, Bradley, Wallace, & Burke, 2009). The work was based in part on an earlier study by Clarke (2006) that found safety climate predicts worker safety performance behavior, but is only weakly related to workplace injury events. Christin and his colleagues conducted a literature review of journal articles dealing with prediction of worker safety performance and injuries. They identified 90 studies and 1,744 effect sizes. Of those, 477 were used in a predictor-criterion path analysis model. Safety climate was significantly related to worker safety motivation which, in turn, was significantly related to worker safety knowledge that, in turn, was significantly related to safety performance and this entire path to lower injury rates.

Contingent workers are typically not included in the larger workplace shared safety community norms and practice of the companies for which they work. This is especially true for workers involved in dirty, dangerous, and difficult work that frequently involves temporary, unskilled, under educated, and often non-English speaking workers. The OSHA General Duty Clause and contract worker laws require employers to be responsible for contract workers' safety training and supervision across the hierarch from employer, to prime contractor, to subcontractor, and sub-subcontractors. The reality is that these workers frequently are excluded from safety training, safety supervision, access to safety equipment, and worker's compensation insurance. The plights of the miners, shirtwaist factory and textile workers in the early 1900s were ignored for many years. Those "invisible" workers were the ones at greatest risk for occupational illness and injury.

Unfortunately, this past history is being repeated in this twenty-first century. A new and also largely invisible population suffers the same plights and an excessive burden of occupational illness and injury. Not all such at-risk workers are within the United States. Many more are found in the sweatshops and dangerous workplaces in other countries, to which much tedious and dangerous work is outsourced. Yet, there is hope and the potential for lowering the very high injury rates among contingent workers. Table 13.2 reveals a huge drop in workplace disasters in coal mines and loss of life over

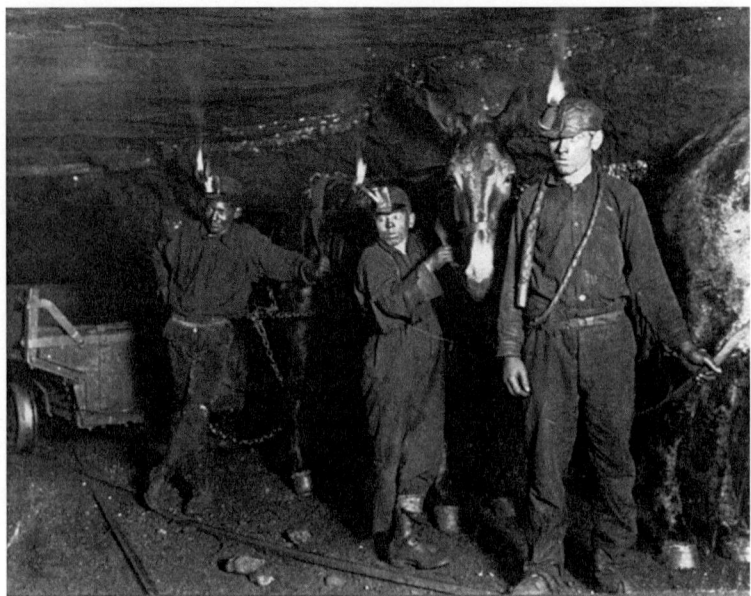

Fig. 13.5 Child Coal Miners 1900. Source http://en.wikipedia.org/wiki/History_of_coal_mining

the period from 1900 to 2006. The reduction in fatalities may be attributed to three factors. First, early coal mine immigrants became integrated into American society and, along with that, became more informed and empowered. Second, technology not only made coal mining easier and more profitable, but also safer. Third, as the dangerous conditions under which miners worked became widely known, coal mine health and safety laws were passed and enforced. All three played a major role in the reduction of workplace injuries. Similar patterns occurred not only in textile mills, but at foundries, railways, smelters, construction sites and scores of other workplaces. The images in Figs. 13.4 and 13.5 reveal much about working conditions in the early 1900s. Nevertheless, at the present time, much remains to be done and many partners need to be involved, including poets, film makers, reporters, artists, unions, professional organizations, business, newspapers, researchers, teachers, health-service providers, attorneys, local officials, trade organizations, state and federal legislators, and regulatory agencies, among others (Fig. 13.5).

Acknowledgments Preparation of this paper was supported by the efforts of hundreds of researchers over many years. The author's education and research was supported by a series of research grants from the National Science Foundation, US Department of Interior, the United Nations International Labor Organization, and the National Institute for Occupational Safety and Health, Centers for Disease Control and Prevention.

References

Azaroff, L. S., Levenstein, C., & Wegman, D. H. (2002). *American Journal of Public Health, 92*, 1421–1429.
Bandura, A. (1989). Human agency in social cognitive theory. *American Psychologist, 44*, 1175–1184.
Bird, F. E., & Germain, G. L. (1996). Loss control management: Practical loss control leadership, Revised Edition. *Det Norske Veritas*, U.S.A. Retrieved from Roughton, J. The accident pyramid. *Safety Culture Plus* http://emeetingplace.com/safetyblog/2008/07/22/the-accident-pyramid/. 21 February 2012.
Bourdieu, P. (1986). Forms of capital. In J. G. Richardson (Ed.), *Handbook of theory and research for the sociology of education* (pp. 241–258). New York: Greenwood Press.

Bruner, J. S. (1990). *Acts of meaning*. Cambridge, MA: Harvard University Press.
Bureau of Labor Statistics. *Census of fatal occupational injuries 2008 chart book*. Retrieved from http://www.bls.gov/iif/oshwc/osh/os/oshs2008_18.pdf
CDC/NIOSH. (2004). Worker Health Chartbook. *Chapter 2—Fatal and nonfatal injuries and illnesses*. Retrieved from http://www.cdc.gov/niosh/docs/2004-146/pdfs/2004-146.pdf
Christin, M. S., Bradley, J. C., Wallace, J. C., & Burke, M. J. (2009). Workplace safety: A meta-analysis of the roles of person and situation factors. *Journal of Applied Psychology, 94*, 1103–1127.
Christoffel, J. D., & Gallagher, S. S. (1999). *Injury prevention and public health*. Gaithersburgh, MD: Aspen Publishers, Inc.
Cohen, A., & Colligan, M. J. (1998). *Assessing occupational safety and health training: A literature review*. Cincinnati, OH: U.S. Department of Health and Human Services, National Institute for Occupational Safety and Health.
Cohen, L., & Swift, S. (1999). The spectrum of prevention: Developing a comperehensive approach to injury prevention. *Injury Prevention, 5*, 203–207.
Cohen, D., & Prusak, L. (2001). *In good company: How social capital make organizations work*. Boston, MA: Harvard Business School Press.
Cole, H. P. (1994). Embedded performance measures as teaching and assessment devices. *Occupational Medicine: State of the Art Reviews, 9*, 261–281.
Cole, H. P. (1995, 13 June). Factors that contribute to miners committing unsafe acts: A behavioral analysis. *Invited keynote paper presented to the 85th Annual Convention of the Mine Inspectors' Institute of America*. Canaan Valley Resort, WV.
Cole, H. P. (1997). Stories to live by: A narrative approach to health-behavior research and injury prevention. In D. S. Gochman (Ed.), *Handbook of health behavior research methods* (Vol. 4, pp. 325–349). New York: Plenum.
Cole, H. P. (2002). Cognitive-behavioral approaches to farm community safety education: A conceptual analysis. *Journal of Agricultural Safety and Health, 8*, 145–159.
Cole, H. P., Berger, P. K., Garrity, T. F., Auvenshine, C. D., Szwilski, A. B., Hernandez, M. S., Blythe, D. K., & Lacefield, W. E. (1986). Medical compliance behavior and miner health and safety. *Annals of the American Conference of Governmental Industrial Hygienists, 14*, 425–433.
Cole, H. P., & Donovan, T. A. (2008). Oder farmers' prevalence, capital, age-related limitations and adaptations. *Journal of Agromedicine, 13*, 81–94.
Cole, H. P., Kidd, P., Isaacs, S., Parshall, M., & Scharf, T. (1997). Difficult decisions: A simulation that illustrates cost effectiveness of farm safety behaviors. *Journal of Agromedicine, 4*(1/2), 117–124.
Cole, H. P., Lehtola, C. J., Thomas, S. R., & Hadley, M. (2005). *No way to meet a neighbour*. National Agricultural Safety Database. Retrieved from http://nasdonline.org/document/1014/9/d000997/the-kentucky-community-partners-for-healthy-farming-rops-project.html#sims1. 25 February 2012.
Cole, H. P., Piercy, L. R., Heinz, K. L., Westneat, S. C., Arrowsmith, H. E., & Raymond, K. M. (2009). Safety status of farm tractors that operate on public highways in four rural Kentucky counties. *Journal of Agricultural Safety and Health, 15*, 207–223.
Cole, H. P., Vaught, C., Wiehagen, W. J., Haley, J. V., & Brnich, M. J., Jr. (1998). Decision making during a simulated mine fire escape. *IEEE Transactions of Engineering Management, 45*, 153–162.
DeJoy, D. M., Schaffer, B. S., Wilson, M. G., Vandenberg, R. J., & Butts, M. M. (2004). Creating safer workplaces: assessing the determinants and role of safety climate. *Journal of Safety Research, 35*(1), 81–90. doi:10.1016/j.jsr.2003.09.018.
DeJoy, D. M. (1996). Theorectical models of health behaviour and workplace self-protective behaviour. *Journal of Safety Research, 27*, 2, 61–72.
Department of Labor. (2005, February). *Contingent and alternative employment arrangements*. Retrieved from http://www.bls.gov/cps/lfcharacteristics.htm#contingent. 19 February 2012.
Encarta Dictionary English North America. (2012). Retrieved from http://www.google.com/#hl=en&sugexp=frgbld&gs_nf=1&cp=40&gs_id=4&xhr=t&q=Encarta+Dictionary+English+North+America&pf=p&output=search&sclient=psy-ab&oq=Encarta+Diction
Fischoff, B. (1975). Hindsight ≠ foresight: The effect of outcome knowledge on judgment under uncertainty. *Journal of Experimental Psychology: Human Perception and Performance., 1*, 288–299.
Freibott, B. (2012). Sustainable safety management: Incident management as a cornerstone of a successful safety culture. *Paper presented at the American Society of Safety Engineers—Middle East Chapter, 10th Professional Development Conference & Exhibition*, February, 18–22. Retrieved from http://scholar.googleusercontent.com/scholar?q=cache:YX2KdTgLBmAJ:scholar.google.com/+ConocoPhillips+Marine+Safety+Injury+Pyramid+April+2003&hl=en&as sdt=0,18
Gagne, R. M. (1984). Learning outcomes and their effects: Useful categories of human performance. *American Psychologist, 39*, 377–385.
Glascock, L. A., Bean, T. L., Wood, R. K., Carpenter, T. G., & Holmes, R. G. (1995). A summary of roadway accidents involving agricultural machinery. *Journal of Agricultural Safety and Health, 1*, 93–104.
Gochfeld, M., & Mohr, S. (2007). Protecting contractor workers: Case study of the US Department of Energy's nuclear and chemical waste management. *American Journal of Public Health, 97*, 1607–1613.

Guerrina, R. T., Burns, C. M., & Conlon, H. (2011). Contingent workers. *American Association of Occupational Health Nurses Journal., 59*, 107–109.

Haddon, W., Jr. (1999). The changing approach to the epidemiology, prevention, and amelioration of trauma: the transition to approaches etiologically rather than descriptively based. *Injury Prevention, 5*, 231–235.

Occupational Safety and Health Administration (1926.16(c)). *Code of Federal Regulations General Interpretations 1926.16 Rules of construction.* Retrieved from http://www.osha.gov/pls/oshaweb/owadisp.show_document?p_id=10605&p_table=STANDARDS

Heinrich, H. W. (1959). *Industrial accident prevention* (4th ed.). New York: McGraw Hill Book Company.

Hipple, S. (2001, March). Contingent work in the late—1990s. *Monthly Labor Review.* U.S. Department of Labor.

Hopkins, J. (2003, 13 March). *Fatality rates increase for Hispanic workers.* USA Today Final Edition. Money Section, Thursday, p. 1B.

Howard, G. S. (1991). Culture tales: A narrative approach to cross-cultural psychology and psychotherapy. *American Psychologist, 46*, 197–197.

Isaacs, S., Cole, H. P., & Gross, B. (1997). *Spread sheet-based farm planning tools for site-specific applications in developing a safer and more productive work environment.* Morgantown, WV: Paper presented at the NIOSH Agricultural Health and Safety Conference.

Kalleberg, A. L. (2000). Nonstandard employment relations: Part-time, temporary, and contract work. *Annual Review of Sociology, 26*, 341–365.

Kidd, P., Parshall, M., Wojcik, S., & Struttmann, T. (2004). Overcoming recruitment challenges in construction safety intervention research. *American Journal of Industrial Medicine, 45*, 297–304.

Kowalski-Trakofler, K. M., Alexander, D. W., Brnich, M. J., McWilliams, L. J., & Reissman, D. B. (2009). Underground coal mining disasters and fatalities—United States, 1900–2006. *Morbidity and Mortality Weekly Report, 57*(51 & 52), 1379-1382. Retrieved from http://www.cdc.gov/mmWR/preview/mmwrhtml/mm5751a3.htm

Kowalski-Trakofler, K. M., Alexander, D. W., Brnich, M. J., & Williams, M. S. (2009). *Underground coal mining disasters and fatalities—United States 1900–2006.* Retrieved from www.cdc.gov/niosh/mining/pubs/pdfs/ucmdn.pdf

Lineberry, G. T., Scharf, T., & Wiehagen, W. J. (2003). A multi-use educational intervention for reducing injury risk in the set-up and use of extension ladders. *Maine Occupational Research Agenda, 2nd Regional Conference.* Portland, ME: Department of Labor.

McEvoy, A. F. (1995). The Triangle Shirtwaist Factory Fire of 1911: Social change and industrial accidents. *Law & Social Inquiry, 20*, 621–651.

Mine Safety and Health Administration. (Undated). *History of mine safety and health legislation.* Retrieved from http://www.msha.gov/mshainfo/mshainf2.htm

MMWR. (2008). *Work-related Injury deaths among Hispanics—United States, 1992—2006.* Retrieved from http://www.cdc.gov/mmwr/preview/mmwrhtml/mm5722a1.htm

Myers, M. L., Cole, H. P., & Mazur, J. M. (2005). *Cost analysis tool for promoting safety awareness.* Wintergreen, VA, June: Paper presented at the annual conference of the National Institute for Farm Safety. 28.

Myers, M. L., Cole, H. P., Mazur, J. M., & Isaacs, S. (2006). Promoting safety through economics education. Paper No. 065009. *Presented at the American Society of Agricultural and Biological Engineers*, Portland Convention Center, Portland, OR, July 9–12.

Myers, M. L., Cole, H. P., Mazur, J., & Isaacs, S. (2008). *April)* (pp. 37–45). Economics and safety: Understanding the cost of injuries and their prevention. Professional Safety.

National Committee for Injury Prevention and Control. (1989). *Injury Prevention: Meeting the Challenge.* New York: Oxford University Press.

National Safety Council. (2009). *The most dangerous part of a job is getting to work.* National Safety Council. Retrieved from http://www.nsc.org/news/nr111803.aspx

Neal, A., & Griffin, M. A. (2006). A study of the lagged relationships among safety climate, safety motivation, safety behavior, and accidents at the individual and group levels. *Journal of Applied Psychology, 91*(4), 946–953. doi:10.1037/0021-9010.91.4.946.

Nicholson, V. J., Bunn, T. L., & Costich, J. F. (2008). Disparities in work-related injuries associated with work compensation coverage status. *American Journal of Industrial Medicine, 51*, 393–398.

Occupational Safety and Health Administration. Trenching and Excavation, 29 CFR 1926.650, 29 CFR 1926.651, and 29 CFR 1926.652. *Code of Federal Regulations.* Retrieved from http://www.osha.gov/SLTC/trenchingexcavation/index.html

Oh, J. H., & Shin, E. H. (2003). Inequalities in nonfatal work injury: The significance of race, human capital, and occupations. *Social Science Medicine, 57*, 2173–21782.

Park, Y. S., & Butler, R. J. (2001). The safety costs of contingent work: Evidence from Minnesota. *Journal of Labor Research, 22*, 831–849.

Peters, R. H., & Randolph, R. F. (1991). *Miners' views about why people go under unsupported roof and how to stop them. Bureau of Mines IC 9300.* Washington, DC. Superintendent of Documents No. I 28:27:9300.

Putnam, R. D. (2000). *Bowling alone—The collapse and revival of American community*. New York: Simon & Schuster. Chapter 5: Connections in the workplace.

Reynolds, R. L. (Undated). *History of coal mine electrical fatalities since 1970*. Pittsburgh, PA: Mine Safety and Health Administration. Retrieved from http://www.msha.gov/S&HINFO/TECHRPT/ELECTRICAL/HISTORY.pdf

Sarbin, T. R. (1986). *Narrative psychology: The storied nature of human conduct*. New York: Praeger.

Scharf, T., Vaught, P., Steiner, L., Kowalski, K., Wiehagen, B., Rethi, L., & Cole, H. (2001). Toward a typology of dynamic and hazardous work environments. *Human and Ecological Risk Assessment, 7*, 1827–1841.

Schenker, M. B. (2010). A global perspective of migration and occupational health. *American Journal of Industrial Medicine, 53*, 329–337.

Shapleigh, E. (1912, December 29). Occupational disease in the textile industry. *New York Call,* 13.

Smith, M. J., & Carayon, P. (2011). Controlling occupational safety and health hazards. In J. C. Quick & L. E. Tetrick (Eds.), *Handbook of occupational health psychology* (2nd ed.). Washington, D.C.: American Psychological Association.

Stein, L. (2001). *The triangle fire*. Ithaca, NY: Cornell University Press.

The Crittenden Press Online (2009, 13 February). *Crittenden County Kentucky*. Retrieved from http://crittendenpress.blogspot.com/

Vaught, C., Brnich, M. J. Jr., Mallett, L. G., Cole, H. P., Wiehagen, W. J., Conti, R. S., Kowalski, K., & Litton, C. D. (2000). *Behavioral and organizational dimensions of underground mine fires*. Pittsburgh, PA: IC 9450, DHHS (NIOSH) Publication No. 2000-2126.

Vaught, C., Mallett, L., Brnich, M. J., Reinke, D., Kowalski-Trakofler, K., & Cole, H. P. (2006). Knowledge management and transfer for mine emergency response. *International Journal of Emergency Management, 3*(2/3), 178–190.

Wartson, B. (2005). *Mills, Migrants and the Struggle for the American Dream*. New York: Viking Penguin.

Wiehagen, W. J., Lineberry, G. T., & Rethi, L. L. (1996). The work crew performance model: A method for defining and building upon the expertise within an experienced work force. *SME Transactions, 298*, 1925–1931.

Wikipedia, the Free Encyclopaedia. (2012). *Triangle shirtwaist factory fire*. Retrieved from http://en.wikipedia.org/wiki/Triangle_Shirtwaist_Fire

Witte, K. (1992). Putting the fear back into fear appeals: The extended parallel process model. *Communication Monographs, 59*, 329–349.

Wojcik, A. M., Kidd, P. S., Parshall, M. B., & Struttmann, T. W. (2003). Performance and evaluation of small construction safety training simulations. *Occupational Medicine, 53*, 279–286.

Zinn, H. (2005). *A Peoples History of the United States, 1492—Present*. New York: Harper Perennial Modern Classics.

Zohar, D. (2011). Safety climate: Conceptual and measurement issues. In J. C. Quick & L. E. Tetrick (Eds.), *Handbook of occupational health psychology* (2nd ed.). Washington, D.C.: American Psychological Association.

The Role of Work Schedules in Occupational Health and Safety

14

Jeanne M. Geiger-Brown, Clark J. Lee, and Alison M. Trinkoff

Adverse work schedules increase the risk of accidents, injuries, acute illness and chronically impaired health for workers. As society moves toward providing many services 24 h per day and 7 day per week, the need is increasing for work schedules characterized by shift work, rotating shifts, and early start times. According to the 2004 Current Population Survey, 18% of full-time workers in the USA spend some portion of their work schedule outside of a 6 a.m. to 6 p.m. time frame (McMenamin, 2007). Extended work hours (more than 8 h per day, or more than 40 h per week) also are increasing steadily (Caruso, Hitchcock, Dick, Russo, & Schmidt, 2004) for a variety of reasons. Some workers elect to take secondary employment to boost their earnings, particularly those with low wages or whose household income has decreased because of a partner's unemployment. Others choose, or are required to, work extended hours because of shift design (for example, 12-h shifts as a norm). Since the economic downturn that began in late 2008, there has been a trend for employers to use overtime to manage excess demand, which allows them to maintain productivity without hiring new workers (Maher & Aeppel, 2009). In the USA and Canada, employees work 200–300 h more per year than in France, Germany, or Sweden because of an absence of legal minimums for paid vacation days or holidays (Yelin, 2009).

There is little awareness of, or substantial disregard for, social determinants of health, with work schedules being one of the most salient of these social factors. This chapter is written at a time of economic downturn in the USA, and across Europe. Anecdotal comments from workers suggest that they fear loss of employment and are unwilling to advocate for improved working conditions, including work schedules, because there are scores of unemployed workers eager to replace them. Furthermore, organized labor sometimes advocates for workers' rights to work overtime rather than limiting work hours (as they have in the past). Given this climate, the incentive for employers to improve work schedules, and for employees to respond to their own need for reasonable schedules, may be challenged.

J.M. Geiger-Brown, Ph.D., R.N. (✉) • A. M. Trinkoff, Sc.D., R.N., F.A.A.N.
Department of Family and Community Health, University of Maryland School of Nursing, 655 W. Lombard Street, Baltimore, MD 21201, USA
e-mail: jgeiger@son.umaryland.edu

C.J. Lee, J.D.
Center for Health and Homeland Security, University of Maryland, Baltimore, 500 W. Baltimore Street, Baltimore, MD 21201, USA

This chapter begins with a description of adverse work schedule patterns. Next, the research literature about health and safety risks of adverse schedules is summarized. Then, the components of an ideal fatigue risk management system are explained, with documentation of the effectiveness of this approach to reduce occupational risk among workers. We then explain how governments and public policies regulate work schedules. Finally, we conclude with suggested future directions for research and policy in order to improve the health and safety of workers by improving work schedules.

Adverse Work Schedules

Shift Work

Shift work (any shift where most of the hours fall outside the typical 8 a.m. to 5 p.m. period) is common in the service industry (e.g., food service, medical and emergency workers, safety, transportation, utilities, hospitality), as well as in production industries where processes are continuous (e.g., refining, chemicals), and in capital-intensive industries that demand high production (e.g., oil drilling, maritime, construction, mining). Shift work falls disproportionately on males, racial minorities, and workers with less education (McMenamin, 2007). The most common reason given by workers for working shifts is that the job required it, with other common reasons being higher wages, less supervision, time for schoolwork, and better arrangement for family and childcare (Camarino et al., 2008; McMenamin, 2007). About 15% of US and 18–24% European full-time workers have some night work (BLS, 2005; Parent-Thirion, Fernandez-Macias, Hurley, & Vermeylen, 2007).

Night shift workers have a high risk of occupational accidents, injuries, and illnesses (Caruso et al., 2004). The mechanism for this effect is physiologically complex. Working at night against the normal endogenous circadian rhythm (misalignment), and then switching back to a nighttime sleep schedule on off-days, disrupts the body's homeostatic mechanisms. Furthermore, shift workers get about 10 h less sleep per week (Akerstedt, 2003) and poorer quality sleep than those who work daytime or evening schedules. Extensive research over the past several decades has shown that the effects of shift work can be cumulative and may be an under-recognized contributor to later ill health (Oishi et al., 2005; Suwazono et al., 2006; Suwazono et al., 2008).

Shift Rotation

Rotating shifts between day and night (or day, evening, and night) is challenging from a circadian biological perspective. The most hazardous aspect of rotating shifts is the "quick return," a pattern where the worker has fewer than 10 h off between shifts. Shifts can rotate forward (day to evening to night), or backward, and rotation can be quick (several different shifts within 1 week, or slow (blocks of shift work lasting several weeks). Both the speed and direction of rotation affect sleep duration and quality. Few full-time night shift workers (<3%) ever really make a complete circadian adjustment to their shift (Folkard, 2008), and rotating shift workers are even less likely to make this adaptation. Permanent night workers achieve slightly more sleep than workers who rotate to night shift (Pilcher, Lambert, & Huffcutt, 2000), perhaps because they learn to make accommodations over time. Night shift workers benefit from higher incomes due to shift differentials (Camarino et al., 2008), and they often prefer the autonomous nature of the work itself (fewer "bosses").

Because in 24/7 operations, evening and night shifts will always need to be covered, most employers look at the issue of worker fatigue from shifts as inevitable and are unaware of the science that supports using fatigue risk tools to examine current scheduling practices to improve outcomes. Many employers also believe that workers want to compress work schedules to "get it over with" so that they can have larger blocks of time off. This belief was contradicted recently in a study of police officers that examined the implementation of a non-compressed pattern of rotating shifts. Even though the officers had fewer days off per month with this pattern, they now had at least 16 h off between shifts, and were more satisfied with their work schedules (Kecklund, Eriksen, & Åkerstedt, 2008). In general, evening shift workers have the longest and best quality sleep of 8 h shift workers (Akerstedt, 2003).

Early Start Times

Work start times are usually dictated by the employer. Start times before 9 a.m. are common in the transportation, mining, construction, and health care industries (BLS, 2010a, 2010b). Early start times can interfere with sleep. Because most adults are unable to sleep at all between 7 and 9 p.m. due to a circadian waking pressure in the early evening, their bedtimes often occur at 10 p.m. or later. Ingre, Kecklund, Akerstedt, Soderstrom and Kecklund (2008) showed that, for shift start times between 4:30 a.m. and 9:00 a.m., there was a linear increase in sleep time of 0.7 h for every hour that the shift start time was delayed. An experimental study where start times were manipulated showed that workers whose start time was delayed had an increased duration of sleep prior to work, and improved alertness during the shift (Rosa, Harma, Pulli, Mulder, & Nasman, 1996). Sleep deprivation is well known to increase the risk for occupational accidents (Philip & Akerstedt, 2006). The problem of curtailed sleep with early start times is often compounded by long commute times. In dense urban areas and in sparse rural areas, commutes can be an hour or more (National Academies, 2006). Teenagers with developmentally delayed sleep phase (i.e., cannot fall asleep until after midnight) are particularly vulnerable to accidents or injuries since they will have insufficient sleep with early start times (Crowley, Acebo, & Carskadon, 2007). In contrast, older workers who fall asleep early because their circadian phase has advanced may be able to accommodate early start times more easily than others (Dijk, Duffy, & Czeisler, 2000).

Other Factors Related to Work Schedules

The actual work schedule of any employee is dependent on the overall policies, procedures, and economics of the organization. In order for workers to have reasonable schedules, there must be adequate staffing to satisfy the work demands at hand. Without adequate staffing, there is no possibility of achieving adequate scheduling for workers even when management is aware of how to implement healthful schedule patterns. Some personal responsibility also falls on the individual worker. If the schedule provides adequate sleep opportunity, does the worker take advantage of time off to obtain needed rest and recovery? Is the worker free of impediments to sleep (e.g., sleep disorder or home responsibilities such as child care or elder care)? It is useful to think of the work schedule as the foundation upon which other aspects of health risk are built.

Health and Safety Consequences of Adverse Work Schedules

Adverse work schedules have been shown to increase the risk for several health conditions, and to make workers less safe on the job and on the drive home. Overtime hours have been associated with increased mortality in several population-based studies (Nylen, Voss, & Floderus, 2001; Johansson, 2004). We review several health and safety conditions in this section.

Accidents and Injuries

Shift work and extended work hours are both associated with increased accidents and injuries across a number of occupations (Dembe, Delbos, & Erickson, 2008; de Castro et al., 2010). Moore-Ede (1993) estimated the annual economic impact (in 1993 US dollars) of sleep problems due to late shifts were as follows: 50 billion in reduced manufacturing productivity; 5.7 billion in increased motor vehicle accidents; four billion in industrial accidents; 2.5 billion in accidents, injuries and deaths at work; two billion in increased medical and psychiatric illness; and one billion to account for personnel turnover and training. During the night shift, most workers are sleepier, have reduced reaction times, poorer neuromuscular coordination, and poorer cognitive executive functioning, which can contribute to injury risk. The increased risk for night shift accidents is 30% higher than for day shift workers, and this risk increases over consecutive night shifts and with longer work shifts (Folkard, Lombardi, & Tucker, 2005; Folkard & Akerstedt, 2004). Within an extended shift, the risk for injury increases after the eighth hour of work, regardless of time of day (Haneke, Tiedemann, Nachreiner, & Grzech-Sukalo, 1998). Researchers have shown industry-specific data (e.g., healthcare, aviation, maritime, etc.) that support the relationship between work schedules and injuries; detailed in a NIOSH/CDC report (Caruso et al., 2004).

Motor Vehicle Crashes

Driving accidents are a common source of injury and death for workers and the driving public. In the USA, the National Transportation Safety Board estimates that 71,000 injuries and 1,550 deaths per year are due to drowsy driving, although they admit this is probably an underestimate because of reporting problems (Moore, Kaprielian, & Auerbach, 2009). In European nations and Australia, where crash reporting is more consistent, the estimate of drowsy driving as a cause of motor vehicle crashes is 10–30% (National Sleep Foundation, 2008). In a study of 100 video-instrumented cars driven over 42,000 miles where drivers were continuously observed during naturalistic driving, 22% of all motor vehicle crashes and 16% of near-crashes could be attributed to drowsy driving (Dingus et al., 2006). Drowsy driving accidents tend to be more severe than others because the sleepy driver fails to brake before a collision.

Drowsy driving is increased in workers with extended shifts (Robb, Sultana, Ameratunga, & Jackson, 2008), after night shifts (Rogers, Holmes, & Spencer, 2001; Stutts, Wilkins, Scott Osberg, & Vaughn, 2003; Barger, Cade, Ayas et al., 2005), and with inadequate sleep prior to working (Valent, Di Bartolomeo, Marchetti, Sbrojavacca, & Barbone, 2010; Philip & Akerstedt, 2006; Gander, Marshall, Harris, & Reid, 2005). However, because of significant interindividual differences in tolerance to sleep deprivation that can be traced to genetic polymorphisms (Czeisler, 2009), there is a subpopulation of workers who may be less tolerant of sleep deprivation and thus have an even greater risk for drowsy driving. Drivers with sleep disorders, such as sleep apnea, narcolepsy, insomnia, and restless leg syndrome, also have a higher risk for drowsy driving independent of their work schedule (Volna & Sonka, 2006).

Musculoskeletal Disorders

Recent reports of nonfatal occupational injuries show nursing and health care facilities as leading the incidence rates, followed by fire protection, sports and general aviation (BLS, 2010a, 2010b). According to the US Bureau of Labor Statistics, musculoskeletal injuries (MSD) accounted for 28% of all nonfatal worker injuries (BLS, 2009). The occupations with the highest MSD incidence rates were nursing aides and orderlies, emergency medical technicians and psychiatric aides (ranging from 226 to 256 per 100 full-time employees). The next highest groups included laborers, truck drivers and fire fighters (ranging from 134 to 146 per 100 full-time employees) (BLS, 2009). As many occupations have experienced staff cuts, job restructuring and redesign, increasingly heavy demands have been placed on the remaining workers. This is especially true in occupations with strong physical demands as part of their jobs. Such demands have been associated with increased risk of MSD (Ariens, Bongers, Hoogendoorn, van der Wal, & van Mechelen, 2002; Davis, Marras, Heaney, Waters, & Gupta, 2002; Smedley et al., 2003), leading to sick days, disability, and turnover.

Adverse work schedules can also affect the sleep–wake cycle, and working 12+ hour shifts can lead to MSD due to extended exposure to physical demands combined with insufficient recovery time between work shifts (Waersted & Westgaard, 1991; Larese & Fiorito, 1994). In workers with employment-related myalgia, symptoms increased with each successive workday and only remitted by the second day off (Lundberg et al., 1999). These workers had shorter periods of muscle rest, suggesting that continuous muscle tension was associated with musculoskeletal symptoms. Without adequate time in between shifts or enough time off to rest and sleep prior to resuming a long shift, employees are required to come to work while still injured or in pain. This situation compounds the difficulty of recovery from the injury.

Workers on schedules requiring long hours and frequent overtime are at higher risk for MSD and pain (Gordon, Cleary, Parker, & Czeisler, 1986; Parkes, 1999; Folkard, Spelen, & Toterdell, 1995). Hoogendoorn et al. (2000), using video observations and questionnaires in a 3-year study of workers, found that extreme flexion and frequent heavy lifting had a strong impact on worker low back pain. Movements that require flexion and rotation, such as in health care with patient transfers from a bed to stretcher, increase the injury risk due to a combination of compression, rotation, and shear forces and, if unavoidable, can lead to further injury (Forde, Punnett, & Wegman, 2002; Hoogendoorn et al., 2000, 2002; Hoozemans et al., 2004). Heavy lifting has also been associated with shoulder pain or injury in many occupational groups (Allen, 1990; Nahit, Macfarlane, Pritchard, Cherry, & Silman, 2001; Punnett, Fine, Keyserling, Herrin, & Chaffin, 2000). In a survey of 1428 registered nurses (RNs), over one-third had extended work schedules, and such schedules were associated with an increased likelihood of MSD (Trinkoff, Le, Geiger-Brown, Lipscomb, & Lang, 2006). The relationship was diminished when physical demands were controlled, suggesting that work schedule served to increase exposure to hazardous tasks.

Cardiovascular Disease (CVD)

Cardiovascular disease is the leading cause of death globally, with 7.3 million deaths due to coronary heart disease and 6.2 million due to stroke in 2008 (WHO, 2011). Public media campaigns focus on preventing this disease by encouraging individuals to engage in healthy behaviors, with little recognition of the role of work organization in the genesis of these serious health conditions (Landsbergis, Schnall, & Dobson, 2009). Adverse work schedules have a direct effect on CVD risk, and also an indirect effect through their detrimental influence on health risk behaviors among workers (Thomas & Power, 2010).

Health Risk Behaviors

A number of studies have examined the impact of shift work or long-work hours on healthy behaviors. Usually these ask questions about diet, weight, and smoking or alcohol use, and compare those with adverse schedules to daytime workers. A recent study of workers in a manufacturing company compared workers on 8 vs.10 and 12 h shifts, as well as daytime, night, and rotating shift workers, using 8 h daytime workers as the reference group (Bushnell, Colombi, Caruso, & Taki, 2010). Those on 12-h shifts were significantly more likely to smoke regardless of shift; rotating workers were the least likely to exercise, and night workers were significantly more likely to be obese.

A Spanish study also showed an increased likelihood of smoking among those working 51–60 hours per week (Artazcoz, Cortès, Escribà-Agüir, Cascant, & Villegas, 2009). Reeves, Newling-Ward and Gissane (2004) found the same patterns among nursing home workers, as night workers were more likely to smoke than daytime workers. Kivimäki, Kuisma, Virtanen and Elovainio, (2001) and Trinkoff and Storr (1998) also found a higher rate of smokers among night shift nurses. However, Kivimäki et al. (2001) found almost no difference in smoking by shift among workers under age 45, and almost three times the rate of smoking among night-shift workers greater than age 45. Zhao and Turner (2007) reviewed these and other studies from Europe, North America, and Asia that assessed shift work and accompanying behaviors; most noted an increase in smoking among shift workers compared to those working days only. . Nakamura et al. (1997) noted no smoking differences in Japanese workers, but the smoking prevalence was over 70% in their sample; those who rotated among all three shifts reported the highest prevalence of alcohol use. One study reported that a greater proportion of evening and night shift workers were found to be smokers prior to their entry into the workforce, suggesting that selection issues may be an additional factor to consider (Nabe-Nielsen, Garde, Tuchsen, Hogh, & Diderichsen, 2008).

Alcohol use is typically examined as part of studies conducting prevalence surveys for lifestyle behaviors in relation to adverse work schedules, including some mentioned above. Findings have been conflicting. Hermansson et al. (2003) found no differences in alcohol consumption by shift using a variety of alcohol screening tools, although workers who rotated among two-shifts (as opposed to three-shifts or not at all) had the lowest alcohol prevalence. Zhao and Turner (2007) note a study of Brazilian workers who reported higher alcohol consumption among those on the night shift, and another in which shift workers did not differ compared to day time employees. Kivimäki et al. (2001) reported some differences in alcohol use, though not significant, with more heavy drinkers and nondrinkers among nurses working night shifts. They postulate that the relationship between alcohol use and work schedule is likely nonlinear, with lower health risk among moderate drinkers; thus, studies examining a linear trend for alcohol and shift work may be mischaracterizing the relationship. Little data are available for those with long work hours in relation to alcohol and drug use. Trinkoff and Storr (1998) found that rates for drug use and alcohol, as well as smoking, were all increased among nurses working greater than 8 h shifts compared to shorter length shifts.

Reasons for disparities in risk among shift workers or those with long work hours are manifold, and include that health behaviors are altered as consequences of the work environment, sleep deprivation, and circadian rhythm disturbance (Bushnell et al., 2010). The opportunity to exercise is reduced in persons with adverse work schedules. Although exercise has been found to be an important component of weight control and CVD prevention, shift work and other nonstandard work schedules have been shown to impede participation in exercise programs, largely due to decreased opportunity to engage in sports or participate at a consistent time of day (Atkinson, Fullick, Grindey, Maclaren, & Waterhouse, 2008). A study of workers in Catalonia, Spain found that men who worked long hours were significantly more likely to report that they engaged in no physical exercise during their leisure time, although this was not true among women (Artazcoz et al., 2009). Kivimaki's (2001) study of nurses also showed no overall effect of schedule on sedentary lifestyle, although older shift workers were more likely to get little to no exercise compared to younger workers. Sleep deprivation incurred from rotating shifts or extended work schedules may further limit the desire to exert oneself. Most of the studies done on the benefits of exercise have not included shift workers (e.g., Li et al., 2004). In addition, there may be altered benefits of exercise to those who work shifts or nontraditional hours, possibly due to hormonal alterations when exercise occurs during hours that circadian rhythms support for sleep (Atkinson et al., 2008). More work is needed to explain these relationships.

CVD and Metabolic Disease Risk

Cardiovascular disease (high blood pressure, heart attack, stroke) is often a late effect of metabolic disease (glucose and insulin dysregulation, obesity). In order to understand the relationship between work schedules, metabolic and cardiovascular disease risk, one needs to appreciate the role of the circadian system in the pathogenesis of these disorders. Extensive genetic, cell, and tissue biology research clearly demonstrates that human metabolic activities are regulated by circadian pacemakers that oscillate based on the light–dark cycle of the 24-h clock (Huang, Ramsey, Marcheva, & Bass, 2011). Nearly all body cells are responsive to this pacemaker. Functionally, behaviors such as food intake and physical activity, as well as metabolic processes (e.g., glucose regulation, thermogenesis, adipose deposition, lipid regulation, bile synthesis), are regulated by circadian cycles (Cajochen et al., 2005). Shift work and long shifts increase autonomic arousal, alter neurohormones, such as cortisol, causing deranged glucose and lipid metabolism, and increase inflammatory cytokine production (Miller & Cappuccio, 2007). These processes can lead to obesity, Type-II diabetes, and atherosclerosis (Puttonen, Harma, & Hublin, 2010).

Studies linking work schedules to incident cardiovascular diseases have shown conflicting results. In two review papers summarizing 20 years of population-based studies, an increased CVD risk of 40% was evident for shift workers (Kristensen, 1989; Bøggild & Knutsson, 1999). However, this association was absent in a more recent review (Frost, Kolstad, & Bonde, 2009). Boggild (2009) suggested that methodological issues are the source of this inconsistency in association. Epidemiologic studies have shown that cardiovascular changes may begin during the earliest years of shift work, with one study showing a near doubling of the risk for metabolic syndrome in rotating shift workers in only 6 years of observation (De Bacquer et al., 2009). Another study showed increased atherosclerotic changes in the carotid artery before age 40 in shift workers, after adjusting for other health and lifestyle factors (Puttonen et al., 2009).

Researchers have moved beyond incidence studies to begin to understand the mechanisms by which adverse work schedules cause cardiovascular changes. Recent studies have shown desynchronization of cellular clock genes to the circadian day as a primary mechanism for increases in CVD in shift work (Suessenbacher et al., 2011; Manfredini, Pala, Fabbian, & Manfredini, 2011). Studies of subclinical precursors to heart disease have shown increased plasma resistin (an inflammatory cytokine) (Burgueño, Gemma, Fernández, Sookoian, & Pirola, 2010), carotid intimal thickening (Puttonen et al., 2009), increased blood pressure (Fialho, Cavichio, Povoa, & Pimenta, 2006), and increased cardiac rhythm disturbances in shift workers (van Amelsvoort, Schouten, Maan, Swenne, & Kok, 2001). Extended work hours have also been implicated in CVD risk (Landsbergis, Schnall, & Dobson, 2009).

Gastrointestinal Disorders

Night shift workers often experience gastrointestinal symptoms and disorders (gastric reflux, gastritis, peptic ulcers, irritable bowel conditions, abdominal discomfort), and use more antacids and proton-pump inhibitors than those working day shift (Bilski, 2006: Nojkov, Rubenstein, Chey, & Hoogerwerf, 2010; Sveinsdottir, 2006; Zhen Lu, Ann Gwee, & Yu Ho, 2006). Infection with *Helicobacter pylori* increases the risk of gastritis and ulcer disease, and shift work increases the risk that colonization with this bacterium will progress to disease (Pietroiusti et al., 2006). Relatedly, workers on off-shifts often lack healthful food resources when the company cafeteria and local restaurants are closed, and vending machines are the only available choice. These workers often eat to remain awake despite lower hunger at night (Lowden et al., 2001), and drink caffeinated beverages to sustain alertness, which can cause gastrointestinal distress. Many report that food is harder to digest at night (Bilski, 2006), which may be due to misalignment of food intake with circadian-controlled gastric secretion and intestinal motility.

Infectious Disease

Exposure to infectious agents is a feature of many work settings (Trajman & Menzies, 2010), most prominently in health care settings such as hospitals, dental offices, and long-term care facilities (Hosoglu et al., 2009; Leggat, Kedjarune, & Smith, 2007). Other settings with infectious exposures include social assistance (day care, funeral service, prisons, taxi and bus drivers) (Eriksen, Bruusgaard, & Knardahl, 2004; Slack-Smith, Read, Darby, & Stanley, 2006; Davidson & Benjamin, 2006; Valway et al., 1994; Hannerz & Tuchsen, 2001), as well as animal slaughtering and processing (Johnson & Ndetan, 2011). There has been little investigation into the role of work schedules in either risk exposure or host resistance. However, sleep researchers have described a reduction in immune response to infection among those who are sleep deprived, which is a common situation among shift workers (Bryant, Trinder, & Curtis, 2004). As highly infectious disease strains exist and are becoming resistant to antibiotic therapy (Brouqui, 2009), additional research is needed to understand the role of work schedules in immune response for high risk workers.

Cancer

Recent epidemiologic evidence has shown an increased risk of breast cancer among shift workers, with the International Agency on Research on Cancer (World Health Organization) classifying shift work as a "probable carcinogen" (Costa, Haus, & Stevens, 2010; IARC, 2007). Other cancers with weaker evidence for association with shift work include prostate, colorectal, endometrial, and non-Hodgkin's lymphoma (Costa et al., 2010). Light exposure during night time working hours suppresses melatonin production. Melatonin acts as a powerful antioxidant to reduce reactive oxygen species in cells, and provides an antiestrogen effect to modify cellular responses to estrogen. Sleep deprivation (which is common in night workers) also suppresses immune function that can allow cells to proliferate in abnormal ways. Moreover, shifting back and forth to sleeping at night on, days off, can cause phase disruption of circadian clock genes that regulate cell growth. There are thus multiple mechanisms by which shift work can increase the risk for cancer formation (Costa et al., 2010). Of course, shift work will always be necessary in some industries, but the increased risk for cancer in shift workers points to the need for employers and occupational sleep medicine specialists to work together to create shift schedules that are the least disruptive to circadian cycles, and to provide adequate screening, diagnosis and treatment for adverse sequelae of shift work, such as cancer. It also points to the need for workers to limit their lifetime "dose" of shift work.

Reproduction

Compared to other occupational disorders, there is less literature describing the association between shift work and reproductive outcomes, and the studies that exist are inconsistent. Studies of fertility and pregnancy outcomes must take into account many confounding factors, such as the mothers' general and reproductive health and health risk behaviors, as well as many aspects of the job and work environment (e.g., schedule, standing and other physical demands). Becoming pregnant and carrying a baby to term is physiologically complex; many occupational factors can influence the reproductive outcome. In a small sample of nurses under age 40, 53% reported changes in menstrual function when working a night shift. However, the characteristics of the change were inconsistent across workers (e.g., longer and shorter periods, heavier and lighter flow, etc.) (Labyak, Lava, Turek, & Zee, 2002). The nurses who did report changes also averaged less sleep and had other somatic complaints (gastrointestinal symptoms, malaise, reduced concentration), and the author concluded that menstrual changes during shift work could be a marker for shift work intolerance. Fecundity (time to pregnancy for planned pregnancies) was reduced in evening and night shift workers in a large Danish study of pregnant women although, once adjusted for confounders, was not significantly different from day shift (Zhu, Hjollund, Boggild, & Olsen, 2003). However, unplanned pregnancies were higher among night shift workers (Zhu et al., 2003, Zhu, Hjollund, & Olsen, 2004). Several large cohort studies have shown that fixed (but not rotating) night shifts increase the risk of pregnancy loss, with risk ranging from 60 to 85% (Zhu, Hjollund, Andersen, & Olsen, 2004; Whelan et al., 2007). The biological mechanism for this effect is still unclear, but may be related to hormonal changes associated with circadian misalignment. Preterm deliveries were elevated by 50% in night shift workers and in those with prolonged work hours (Pompeii, Savitz, Evenson, Rogers, & McMahon, 2005; Bonzini, Coggon, & Palmer, 2007), and small-for-gestational-age births were increased in shift workers (Pompeii et al., 2005). Given these findings, it is prudent for maternal health professionals to take a careful occupational history and counsel pregnant women to limit night shift work during their pregnancy.

Managing Fatigue Risk in Occupational Settings

The risks of occupational fatigue can be partially mitigated by health-preserving actions taken by individual workers and their employers. Fatigue risk management programs are one component of workplace safety management systems, and are a shared responsibility of workers, occupational health and safety officers, and management (Geiger-Brown & McPhaul, 2011).

Employer Occupational Health Programs

The primary elements of a comprehensive occupational safety and health program include management commitment and employee involvement, hazard analysis and accident investigation, prevention activities, training, and recordkeeping and evaluation. A further component of an overall safety and health program is a health and safety committee. However, the state of occupational fitness-for-duty testing to detect sleep deprivation in workers is in its infancy. There are instruments of high quality that are used in research settings to detect fatigue and microsleep (uncontrollable and unintended episodes of sleep lasting up to 30 s) in ambulatory research conditions, but these are not used for "real time" testing of employees in actual work situations. Because real time detection of fatigue is not feasible at the present time, a better approach is to reduce the work-related inhibitors of sleep by making sure that work schedules allow sufficient sleep opportunity. Software is commercially available and in common use in some settings to "flag" fatigue-inducing schedules in workers (Moore-Ede et al., 2004). In the next section, we review organizational measures to reduce the impact of work on sleep duration and quality.

Organizational Interventions to Improve Schedule-Related Health and Safety

Worksite health promotion programs often target employee health risk behaviors (such as diet and exercise) to reduce cardiovascular risk, sickness absence, and disability (Parks & Steelman, 2008). Work schedules are often not examined as a source of morbidity. A robust worksite health program should conduct an exposure assessment of working hours as part of the health history and ongoing surveillance activities (Geiger-Brown & McPhaul, 2011). But addressing the work schedule in isolation will not reduce worker fatigue unless all aspects of fatigue risk are examined.

Occupational Screening for Sleep Disorders

The transportation industry is a leader in screening workers for sleep disorders in order to reduce accident risk (Hartenbaum et al., 2006). A large scale occupational sleep disorder screening program was successful in reducing injury rates among those with excessive sleepiness, with rates dropping by 30% after screening and a sleep hygiene educational intervention (Melamed & Oksenberg, 2002). In this study of 532 industrial workers (power plants, medical fabrication plants, heavy machinery repair), the odds of an occupational injury with excessive daytime sleepiness was twice that of those without sleepiness after controlling for age, sex, BMI, job tenure, type of factory, physical demands, and noise. Workers often have unrecognized sleep disorders, and generally do not seek medical attention. Lavie (2002) proposed that aggressive screening programs should be used to identify individuals with sleep-disordered breathing at the youngest age possible (similar to hypertension and diabetes screening) in order to prevent cardiovascular morbidity and mortality. In addition, shift workers with high levels of fatigue, who discount this as an unavoidable reaction to shift work, may actually have a sleep disorder (Hossain, Reinish, Kayumov, Bhuiya, & Shapiro, 2003). This is particularly true where the worker population is older or obese.

Shift Work Sleep Disorder

Nearly all shift workers have some sleepiness during the circadian low point of the night shift, and most cannot achieve adequate sleep during the day. Workers experiencing extreme shift work symptoms (sleepiness during the shift and daytime insomnia) have *Shift Work Sleep Disorder* (SWSD) (Box 14.1) (Barion & Zee, 2007), SWSD is estimated to affect 32% of night shift workers, and 26% of rotating shift workers based on one population-based sample (Drake, Roehrs, Richardson, Walsh, & Roth, 2004). Many workers accept difficulty sleeping during daytime hours and high levels of sleepiness during the night shift, thinking that this is a normal part of shift work. Most are not aware that there are treatments available for this physiologically based disorder. Risk for SWSD may be higher in older worker and females with social obligations (Sack et al., 2007). Also, workers who are exposed to bright light in the early morning may develop maladaptive phase shifting that reduces their ability to sleep in the daytime. Employers should provide accommodations under the Americans with Disabilities Act (ADA, Pub. L. No. 101-336, 104 Stat. 327 (1990) (codified as amended at 42 U.S.C. § 12101–12213)) to workers with SWSD by reducing night shift participation, allowing planned naps during the night shift and stimulant medication, and restructuring the work environment to increase ambient light. Occupational health departments should be instrumental in screening and detecting workers with this disorder, and working with the employer to tailor the job to improve the workers' health and safety as well as on-the-job performance.

Box 14.1. ICD-9 Criteria for Circadian Rhythm Sleep Disorder: Shift-Work Type (327.36)

1. Complaint of insomnia or excessive sleepiness that is temporarily associated with a recurring work schedule that overlaps the usual time for sleep.
2. Symptoms are associated with the shift work schedule over the course of at least 1 month.
3. Sleep log or actigraphy monitoring (with sleep diaries) for at least 7 days demonstrates disturbed circadian and sleep time misalignment.
4. Sleep disturbance is not better explained by another current sleep disorder, medical or neurological disorder, mental disorder, medication use, or substance use disorder.

Source: Center for Medicare and Medicaid Services, ICD-9 Manual

Shift Work and Long Work Hours Education for Workers

Guidance for coping with shift work and extended work hours often receives little attention during worker orientation programs, yet this has reduced fatigue in workers with adverse schedules. In a worksite intervention to prevent "occupational jet lag" for shift workers, sleep quality and quantity improved in the treatment group when sleep health education was provided in combination with exercise (Atlantis, Chow, Kirby, & Singh, 2006). Major industries, such as the Saturn automobile manufacturing company (Round-the-Clock-Systems, 2011) and Canadian Transport affiliated companies (Transport Canada, 2003), have instituted fatigue education programs for their workers The US National Transportation Safety Board (NTSB) cites fatigue as one of the major modifiable causes of accidents, and recommends worker education and safe scheduling as two important interventions to reduce accident risk (Rosekind, 2011). In fact, the NTSB has included fatigue-related factors on its list of "Most Wanted Safety Improvements" since 1990 (NTSB, 2011).

Creating Healthful Work Schedules

In 24/7 operations, there will always be a need for some workers to do shift work and to work with some level of cognitive impairment during the circadian low point. Most managers have not been trained in the principles of scheduling to avoid fatigue risk. However, fatigue risk management software can be used to model performance impairment based on specific work and rest schedules (Caldwell, Caldwell, & Schmidt, 2008). Managers can use this software to preplan work schedules, as well as to modify them "on the fly" to cover peak demands or worker absences. This software has been used since the mid 1990s in safety-sensitive industries such as rail, bus, chemical, nuclear, and offshore operations in the UK (Folkard, Lombardi, & Spencer, 2006), and for military, rail, and airline applications in the USA (Hursh et al., 2004) . The variables for fatigue prediction are as follows: (1) a cumulative component where patterns of work on previous shifts influence the current shift, (2) timing of work including start time, shift length, and time of day throughout the shift, and (3) the nature of the work (job intensity), as well as patterns of breaks taken during the shift (Folkard & Lombardi, 2006). In a US study where managers and dispatchers were trained in scheduling methods and fatigue risk software to reduce truck driver fatigue while still maintaining 24/7 h of service, fatigue risk scores (range 0–100, with higher score = more risk) fell significantly from 46.8 1 month prior to the intervention to 28.9 nine months after the intervention (Moore-Ede et al., 2004). A substantial change in overall patterns of work resulted from this intervention, with fewer accidents, lower cost of accidents, and lower insurance premiums for the company. The company maintained this program for several years after the intervention, supporting the contention that, once successful changes are made in organizations, they are generally sustained over time (Swerissen & Crisp, 2004). Managers sometimes fear workers' reactions to schedule modifications to reduce fatigue risk. However, in a study of 2,000 police officers where shift systems were experimentally altered to avoid compressed work schedules, officers preferred the healthier shift system to the compressed schedules that were thought to be favored, despite having two fewer days off per month (Kecklund et al., 2008).

Modifying Light Conditions During Night Shift

Dim lighting conditions are present in some workplaces during the night shift, and can increase workers' sleepiness during the circadian low period (usually between 3 and 5 a.m.) (Caldwell et al., 2008). Employers can provide brighter light during this time to improve workers' alertness (Santhi, Aeschbach, Horowitz, & Czeisler, 2008). This light provides a direct alerting effect, and also suppresses melatonin which can phase-shift the circadian rhythm (Cajochen et al., 2005). Night workers have used blue light in 10–15 min bursts every 3 h to sustain alertness during their workshift, and amber glasses to block blue light and promote sleep upon returning home (Boivin, Tremblay, & James, 2007; Boivin & James, 2005; Shechter, James, & Boivin, 2008). Light has also been used to reduce decrements in alertness during the post-prandial dip in dayshift workers after lunch (Hayashi, Masuda, & Hori, 2003).

Planned Napping During Work Breaks

In the USA, napping during working hours is prohibited by most employers as it is thought of as "sleeping on the job"; however, many night-shift workers do nap covertly during breaks. Planned, but unsanctioned naps interfere with safe operations, with a recent example being air traffic controllers falling asleep on the job (Czeisler, C.A. (26 April, 2011). Unplanned napping also occurs when the biological drive to sleep overcomes the worker's ability to remain alert while on duty. It is unfortunate that napping is held in such low regard, as naps have been shown to be an effective way to increase alertness during shift work or extended work shifts (Ficca, Axelsson, Mollicone, Muto, & Vitiello, 2010). Both laboratory and workplace studies have confirmed (by EEG) that a brief 15–20 min nap during a workshift confers additional alertness, especially for workers with partial sleep deprivation or those working in monotonous tasks (Driskell & Mullen, 2005). A study of 12-h night shift workers' response times on a vigilance task revealed that, at the end of the first night shift, reaction times were quicker after a 20 min nap was taken between 1 and 3 a.m. (Purnell, Feyer, & Herbison, 2002). Because sleep inertia (i.e., grogginess upon awakening) can impair performance if the duration of napping is too long, naps ideally should last about 20 min. Excessive noise inhibits sleep initiation during planned napping; if employers create appropriate conditions for napping, it improves the outcome (Lenne, Dwyer, Triggs, Rajaratnam, & Redman, 2004). Most workers will decline to nap if work demands cannot be adequately covered during their absence.

Individual Worker Strategies to Improve Schedule-Related Health and Safety

Workers themselves can be proactive to manage their health and safety when working shifts, extended hours and early start times. These personal behaviors can reduce drowsiness and improve alertness.

Planned Caffeine and Stimulant Use

Caffeine is a universally used substance that helps workers to maintain alertness during shift work (Ker, Edwards, Felix, Blackhall, & Roberts, 2010). Night shift workers often drink caffeinated beverages throughout their shift in order to be alert enough to drive home. But, because the half-life of caffeine is about 4–5 h, this can cause premature awakening in the early afternoon before a full sleep period is achieved. The most commonly recommended strategy to avoid this is to drink 200–300 mg of a caffeinated beverage at 11 p.m. (e.g., 16 ounces of strong coffee), and then avoid caffeine for the rest of the night. More recently, Wyatt, Cajochen, Ritz-De-Cecco and Czeisler (2004) demonstrated a dosing regime that uses small intermittent doses of caffeine throughout the night to provide adequate and sustained stimulation without residual caffeine interfering with daytime sleep.

Sleep Timing

Because night shift workers usually revert to sleeping at night on their days off, their circadian systems can become dysregulated, creating poor sleep throughout the work schedule cycle. Eastman's extensive laboratory research on timing sleep to produce alertness during the night demonstrates that it is possible to improve nighttime performance in carefully controlled conditions. Her most recent study recommends that night shift workers adopt a compromise sleep position by remaining awake into the early morning hours (go to bed at 3 a.m.) on nights off, and then sleep during part of the day (arise at 12 noon) to avoid fully shifting their circadian system to increase night shift alertness (Smith, Fogg, & Eastman, 2009). Night shift workers should use blue-light blocking glasses in the morning to avoid triggering the normal upswing in circadian waking pressure from bright morning light (Sasseville, Benhaberou-Brun, Fontaine, Charon, & Hebert, 2009).

Pharmacotherapy

There are several drugs that can be prescribed to promote either sleep or alertness for workers with SWSD. Hypnotics and melatonin can be used to induce and sustain sleep when the worker is unable to achieve adequate sleep independently. Stimulants are used to sustain alertness. Drugs are often prescribed as a first-line therapy by primary care providers without a full diagnostic assessment for sleep disorders; patients seen by sleep specialists are often patients who were unresponsive to medication from primary care settings. Drug treatment should not be a replacement for spending adequate time in bed.

Regulation of Work Hours: Governmental Regulation and Public Policy

Governments around the World have attempted to address some of the societal problems associated with work schedules and drowsiness as a matter of law and public policy, particularly where public and occupational health and safety are threatened (Jones, Lee, & Rajaratnam, 2010). One of the most common governmental actions has been the development, adoption, and implementation of hours of service (HOS) regulations to limit the number of work hours and to prescribe minimum rest periods for workers in particular occupational groups (Table 14.1). Many governments also have used their legal authority to regulate public health and safety by adopting broad regulatory schemes relating to occupational health and safety (OH&S) that place a general legal duty on employers to address drowsiness as a workplace safety hazard.

The USA

The principle legal authority protecting worker health and safety rights in the USA is the federal Occupational Safety and Health Act of 1970 (OSH Act; Pub. L. No. 91-596, 84 Stat. 1590), and the regulations promulgated under it that establish federal occupational safety and health standards (*see* 29 C.F.R. pts. 1900–2400). The OSH Act covers most employers and employees in the USA, including all of those in the private sector (*see* OSH Act § 3(5) (definition of "employer"), *codified at* 29 U.S.C. § 652(5); OSHA Workers website), and requires employers to "furnish to each of his employees employment and a place of employment which are free from recognized hazards that are causing or are likely to cause death or serious physical harm to his employees" (OSH Act § 5 ("General Duty Clause"), *codified at* 29 U.S.C. § 654). In effect, the OSH Act provides workers with a right to working conditions that do not pose a risk of serious harm to their person and health. Enforcement of workplace safety and health regulations is administered by the federal Occupational Safety and Health Administration (OSHA, which is now part of the US Department of Labor). Under the regulatory scheme created by the OSH Act, States are free to address occupational safety or health issues for which OSHA has not promulgated federal standards; States also may work with OSHA to develop and enforce their own standards where OSHA has issued standards (OSH Act § 18, *codified at* 29 U.S.C. § 667).

To date, there are no formal OSHA federal standards relating to hours of service or to unusual or extended work shifts in any occupational group, despite requests from advocates to do so. For example, a group of health and safety advocates has petitioned OSHA to regulate work hours for resident physicians in US hospitals on two occasions over the past decade (Public Citizen et al.,

Table 14.1 Sample of Federal Hours of Service (HOS) Regulations in the USA

HOS regulation	Industry or profession regulated	Examples of types of workers covered	Promulgation year (oldest regulatory provision)
49 U.S.C. § 21103 and 49 C.F.R. pt. 228	Rail	Locomotive engineers Railroad signalmen	1907 (49 U.S.C. § 21103)
14 CFR §§ 121.465 to 121.525 and 135.261 to 135.273	Aviation	Airplane pilots Air crews	1964 (Various Provisions)
49 CFR pt. 395	Commercial Motor Carriers	Long-haul truck drivers Intercity bus drivers	1979 (§ 395.13–Drivers declared out of service)
46 U.S.C. § 8104 and 46 CFR §§ 15.705, 15.710, and 15.1111	Maritime Crews	Seamen Merchant marine officers	1983 (46 U.S.C. § 8104)
10 C.F.R. §§ 26.201 to 26.211	Nuclear Power Personnel	Nuclear power reactor operators	2008

2001, 2010). However, OSHA recently has provided guidance materials to educate workers in certain occupational groups about the health and safety hazards associated with unusual or extended work shifts (OSHA Safety and Health Guide; OSHA, Workers we can help.), and has signified that it is taking the issue of work schedules and occupational health and safety seriously. In his formal statement acknowledging receipt of the 2010 petition from Public Citizen and its allies, the US Assistant Secretary of Labor for Occupational Safety and Health acknowledged that:

> [t]he relationship of long hours, worker fatigue and safety is a concern beyond medical residents, since there is extensive evidence linking fatigue with operator error.... It is clear that long work hours can lead to tragic mistakes, endangering workers, patients and the public." (OSHA, Dr. David Michaels, 2010)

Other federal agencies in the USA appear to have already adopted this position (for quite some time in some cases), and have promulgated HOS regulations for workers in a number of industries and professions (Table 14.1) Furthermore, New York and Puerto Rico have promulgated HOS regulations for physicians in training at the State and Territory level, given the lack of federal HOS regulations for this occupational group (N.Y. COMP. CODES R. & REGS. tit. 10, § 405.4 and P.R. LAWS ANN., tit. 24, §§ 10005–10009).

European Working Time Directive

Europeans have paid more attention to work schedules as a quality of life issue than US employers. For example, the European Union (EU) has adopted a society-wide approach to addressing drowsiness in the work place as a matter of public policy by issuing the European Working Time Directive [EWTD; Directive 2003/88/EC of the European Parliament and of the Council (November 4, 2003), *repealing* Council Directive 93/104/EC (November 23, 1993)]. Instituted as a health and safety measure, the EWTD has changed working hours for citizens of EU Member States substantially by generally requiring all EU Member States to enact provisions limiting working time throughout all sectors of their respective economies (European Commission, 2010).

These provisions are to entitle all workers to work schedules that provide appropriate rest periods, including:

- A limit of 48 h of working time per week, including overtime (where "working time" is defined as "any period during which the worker is working, at the employer's disposal and carrying out his activity or duties, in accordance with national laws and/or practice")
- A minimum rest period of 11 continuous hours for every 24-h period (where "rest period" is defined as any period which is not "working time")
- A minimum rest period of 24 continuous hours for every 7-day period (in addition to the 11 h daily rest)
- Rest breaks during working time for shifts of 6 h or longer
- A minimum of 4 weeks of paid annual leave per year
- Restrictions on night work to an average of 8 h per 24-h periods and on heavy or dangerous work at night to 8 h in any 24-h period

The EWTD also provides night workers with a right to free regular health assessments and to transfer off of night duty when medically indicated. It also sets out special rules for working time in certain sectors (e.g., doctors in training, offshore workers, seagoing fishing workers, workers in urban passenger transport (Articles 17–21). Article 22 of the EWTD, however, allows EU Member States to "opt-out" of certain EWTD provisions restricting weekly working time under certain specified circumstances.

Organized Labor

Organized labor plays a significant role in decisions relating to work schedules and engages in a number of initiatives and activities to address the safety and health issues relating to long hours of work. For example, certain unions affiliated with the American Federation of Labor and Congress of Industrial Organizations (AFL-CIO) formed the Overtime Work Group (now the Work Organization Work Group) in 2001 for the purposes of "gather[ing] and disseminat[ing] information on health and safety hazards associated with long work hours, develop[ing] materials for unions and their members to educate and assist them in addressing problems with excessive hours at work, draft[ing] model legislation, encourag[ing] research," and initiating other efforts to protect workers (Kojola, 2004). Many labor organizations have negotiated contract language in their collective bargaining agreements that place some limitations and restrictions on employers' ability to make working overtime hours mandatory, and to protect workers who refuse such hours (Kojola, 2004; AFL-CIO, 2002). In some cases, unionized workers have gone on strike over the issue of work schedules containing excessive hours and mandatory overtime. Such strikes in the past among certain health care workers (e.g., nurses, resident physicians) have resulted in some notable concessions from their hospital employers (Kojola, 2004; Lee, 2006).

Labor unions and other organizations also have been involved in a variety of governmental and legal activities relating to work schedules and excessive hours. For example, labor unions have been active in legislative efforts in the USA at the Federal and State levels relating to restrictions on mandatory overtime (Kojola, 2004). The Committee of Interns and Residents, a union affiliated with the Service Employees International Union (SEIU), has been one of the organizations to petition OSHA to regulate resident physician work hours in the USA (Public Citizen et al., 2001, 2010). In Canada, organized labor recently took legal action to bring about reforms in the work hours of resident physicians in Québec (FMRQ, 2011). The Québec Charter of Human Rights and Freedoms and the Canadian Charter of Rights and Freedoms were invoked to challenge certain extended work hour requirements for medical residents at a Montréal hospital under an existing collective agreement (McGill University Health Centre, 2011); FMRQ, 2011.

Finally, labor unions in the USA actively encourage and engage with government (viz., NIOSH) and academic researchers to "conduct scientific studies that deepen our understanding of the relationships between long work hours and worker health and safety and to identify effective intervention measures that protect workers." Of particular interest to organized labor is research on intervention and prevention efforts that are focused on "making changes in the workplace that reduce or eliminate exposure to hazards rather than at the level of the individual worker and his or her coping skills"; and do not "blame victims or discipline those who are injured or made sick" (Kojola, 2004).

It should be noted, however, that the interests of organized labor do not always align with the interests of advocates for healthy and safe work schedules. As a writer for the business travel blog on *The Economist* website noted when commenting on the recent controversy over sleeping air traffic controllers in the USA:

> [I]t's not always obvious whether labour, management or both are behind [drowsiness-inducing work schedules].... On its face, [such scheduling] seems like the result of understaffing and of management cutting corners. But unions love overtime, so it's possible that labour was okay with this practice. Either way, let's all be glad that a few naps forced some major, necessary changes, and that no one was hurt. This could have been a lot worse. (NB, 2011)

These arguments could be framed as a workers' rights issue. Czeisler (2010) believes that adverse work schedules are unethical in safety-sensitive industries. He posits that employers often justify extended work hours by comparing schedules to the extremely onerous and unsafe physician-in-training work hours. The authors think that action is necessary at several levels. The provision of fatigue counter-measures and interventions should occur at the worksite, be evident in company policies, and at the level of industry regulation in order to prevent and mitigate the adverse health and safety consequences of work-related drowsiness and to promote worker sleep health. Such activities could be characterized as a meaningful response to the call for action of one Industrial Hygienist for the AFL-CIO:

> Organized labor will continue its efforts at the bargaining table to address issues of long hours of work, mandatory overtime and work organization through contract language with its employers. And we will remain involved in legislative efforts to resolve problems such as mandatory overtime in the health care industry. But dealing with individual employers and small sectors of our economy will not likely move the ball forward enough to address these problems for all workers who are impacted. To ultimately be successful, we will need to have broader public policy discussions and decisions over these matters. At this point in time, our colleagues in Europe and Canada are far ahead of us in this regard. They are examining issues of work organization and work–family balance, including long working hours, on a policy scale that far surpasses what we are doing in the United States (Kojola, 2004).

Summary and Conclusions

Adverse work schedules increase the risk for accidents, injuries, errors, acute health conditions and the development of chronic health problems. Work schedule characteristics such as early start times, shift work, and rotating shifts cause physiologic disruption in the body's homeostatic mechanisms. Adverse work schedules will continue to be a feature of employment worldwide, as some companies will always require continuous operations. Although employers cannot totally eliminate the impact of adverse work schedules, there are organizational interventions that can be implemented to mitigate risk. Employees must also maintain healthy behaviors, especially getting adequate sleep. As this is a societal issue, regulation could be improved to equal the playing field among employers and to protect workers against the risk of fatigue-induced injury and illness. Indeed, adverse work schedules affect nearly 1 in 5 workers in the USA (substantially larger proportion in some industry sectors), with the burden falling disproportionately on low-wage employees. This chapter documents the effect of work schedules on increases in workplace accidents, drowsy driving, acute health conditions (e.g., infections, reproductive outcomes) as well as chronic diseases (e.g., cardiovascular disease, cancer). The consequences of working these adverse schedules can be serious, but are often not attributed to this risk exposure. For example, when a worker develops high blood pressure at age 35, he is unlikely to think "it must have been all that shift work I did for the past 15 years"; instead, he is more likely to think "I guess I'm not getting enough exercise and have gained a few pounds." The culture of individuality in the USA stresses personal responsibility for health, which is bolstered by public health campaigns that stress diet and exercise (but not sleep). Yet, most workers have little control over the types of schedules that are created by their employer, and thus, the more logical target for intervention is the employer.

There is a business case for preserving alertness and reducing drowsiness in workers. States can prosecute drivers who leave work drowsy and kill another driver in a motor vehicle crash under "reckless homicide" statutes (Jones et al., 2010). Moreover, the family members of victims in such cases have sued the employer on several occasions, arguing that the employer knew or should have known that their employee was too drowsy to drive based on their work schedule and failed to take preventative action (Robertson v. LeMaster, 301 S.E.2d 563 (W.Va. 1983); Faverty v. McDonald's Restaurants of Or., Inc., 892 P.2d 703 (Or. Ct. App. 1995), *appeal dismissed, petition for review dismissed*, 971 P.2d 407 (Or. 1998); Escoto v. Estate of Ambriz, 200 S.W.3d 716 (Tex. App. 2006), but *judgment reversed by* Nabors Drilling, USA, Inc. v. Escoto, 288 S.W.3d 401(Tex. 2009)) (Table 14.2). Moreover, the cost of workplace injuries is high for businesses that self-insure, and instituting fatigue-reducing schedules can reduce injuries as well as insurance costs (Moore-Ede et al., 2004).

Large employers who have active occupational health and safety departments already have adopted some elements of fatigue risk management program. Smaller employers are less aware of the need for such programs, and many are ill equipped to implement them. Small businesses account for about 45% of the non-Federal non-farm economy in the USA, and are projected to be a source of economic growth in the coming years (Popkin, 2001). There is a need to educate these employers, who are often operating on slim margins and may not have an awareness of occupational health and safety policies and practices.

Future Directions

Future research should focus on several areas. First, because adverse work schedules will continue to be a feature of work life for a substantial portion of the population, attention should be directed towards discovering strategies to help workers with these schedules to be safer. As was shown in this chapter, there are strategies known to be efficacious, but they need to be mainstreamed into the working culture. For example, it is accepted as "normal" for night shift workers to have extreme drowsiness on the drive home from work and, until workplace planned napping programs become a part of the work culture, this dangerous situation will continue. Workplace health promotion strategies should begin to emphasize sleep and safety, but must go beyond worker education and include the development and implementation of policies that ensure the opportunity for workers to achieve adequate rest. This must occur across industries where adverse work schedules are common, and must include motivated and resistant employers. Horrey et al. (2011) details other research needs, including identifying high risk populations and conditions for workplace sleepiness using stronger study designs and more objective measures of fatigue. In addition, he advocates for researchers to examine populations with chronic health conditions, and to consider interaction effects of various demographic and personality factors in fatigue research. As mathematical models of fatigue still have considerable unexplained

Table 14.2 Sample of Appellate Cases from US States Involving Lawsuits Against Employers of Drowsy Drivers

Case name	Citation	Summary of facts	Summary of decision	Subsequent judicial history
Robertson v. LeMaster	301 S.E.2d 563 (W.Va. 1983)	A 19 year-old railroad laborer fell asleep while driving home after being required to work for ~27 h without rest, resulting in a nonfatal crash with another vehicle	Ruling in which West Virginia's state supreme court declined to hold as a matter of West Virginia law that an employer's conduct in requiring its employee to work ~27 h and then "setting [the employee] loose upon the highway in an obviously exhausted condition" did not "create a foreseeable risk of harm to others which the [employer] had a duty to guard against"	The case was sent back to the trial court for further legal proceedings consistent with the state supreme court's opinion
Faverty v. McDonald's Restaurants of Or., Inc.	892 P.2d 703 (Or. Ct. App. 1995)	An 18 year-old employee of a fast-food restaurant fell asleep while driving home after working three shifts in a 24-h period and five nights during the preceding week, resulting in a crash with another vehicle that killed the employee and severely injured an occupant of the other vehicle	Ruling by an intermediate appeals court in Oregon that: • Upheld a trial court verdict for a plaintiff injured by the defendant corporation's fatigued employee driving home from work • Held that the defendant corporation knew or should have known that its employee was a hazard to himself and others when he drove home from his work place after working numerous hours	A subsequent appeal to Oregon's state supreme court ultimately was dismissed (971 P.2d 407 (Or. 1998)). [*N.B.*: This action does not necessarily mean that the Oregon state supreme court agreed with the outcome or legal reasoning behind the lower court's decision, nor does it mean that the state supreme court disagreed with the lower court's decision. Making such inferences from the state supreme court's action would be improper and invalid]
Escoto v. Estate of Ambriz	200 S.W.3d 716 (Tex. App. 2006)	A 19 year-old oil field worker driving home after a 12-hour night shift (6 p.m. to 6 a.m.) crashed into another vehicle, killing the worker and all 4 occupants of the other vehicle. During the ~4 months before the crash, the worker had been required by his employer to work 12-hour day shifts (6 a.m. to 6 p.m.) 1 week, take a week off, and then work 12-hour night shifts (6 p.m. to 6 a.m.) the following week	Case in which an intermediate appeals court in Texas ruled that: • An employer had a legal duty to an accident victim under Texas law because it was aware of the dangers of fatigue and knew that one of its employees was fatigued but "nonetheless permitted him to drive home to the foreseeable peril of himself and others" • The evidence adduced at trial "supports that [the employer] breached its duty by failing to act as a reasonably prudent employer in [the] same or similar circumstances" • The evidence adduced at trial was legally and factually sufficient to support a finding that the employer's conduct was "instrumental in causing its employee's fatigue and the subsequent accident in question"	The ruling in *Escoto* ultimately was reversed by Texas' state supreme court, which held that an employer had "no duty [under Texas law] to prevent injuries resulting from fatigue following an employee's shift-work schedule [or] to train its employees regarding the dangers of fatigue" (*Nabors Drilling, USA, Inc. v. Escoto*, 288 S.W.3d 401 (Tex. 2009))

Case name	Citation	Summary of facts	Summary of decision	Subsequent judicial history
Brewster v. Rush-Presbyterian-St. Luke's Med. Ctr.	836 N.E.2d 635 (Ill. App. 1 Dist. 2005)	A first-year resident physician at a hospital (i.e., hospital intern) fell asleep while driving home after a 36-hour work shift during which the resident worked (and thus was awake for) 34 of the 36 h scheduled, resulting in a crash with another vehicle that seriously injured the driver of the other vehicle	Ruling by an intermediate appeals court in Illinois holding in part that, under Illinois law, a hospital does not have a legal duty to a plaintiff "injured by an off-duty resident doctor allegedly suffering from sleep deprivation as a result of the hospital's policy on working hours"	The Illinois state supreme court declined to hear an appeal of this decision (844 N.E.2d 964 (Table) (Ill. 2006)). [*N.B.*: This action does not mean that the Illinois state supreme court agreed with the outcome or legal reasoning behind the lower court's decision, nor does it mean that the state supreme court disagreed with the lower court's decision. Making such inferences from the state supreme court's action would be improper and invalid]

variance, research should be directed towards identifying additional factors to account for these. Technological advances can be studied that can both predict and intervene when a fatigued worker is at risk. Finally, implementing fatigue risk management in organizations successfully is critical to reducing the burden of adverse work schedules on workers and the public at large.

In addition to studying workplaces, there needs to be a concerted effort to map out or examine systematically the current legal and policy landscape for protections against the occupational and public health and safety hazards posed by work-related sources of fatigue and drowsiness in the USA. There is a compelling public health and societal need for further work in this important area of public health law and policy. Once such a mapping effort is completed, it will be possible to investigate whether any gaps exist between governmental regulatory and enforcement activities, as well as to identify legal authorities and public policies where established fatigue and sleep knowledge is disregarded to the detriment of workers. The findings from such analyses potentially could allow legal professionals, researchers, legislators, policy-makers, workers, employers, and other stakeholders to consider thoughtful next steps to improve the health of the working population.

Acknowledgment The authors would like to thank Russell A. Sanna, PhD (Harvard Medical School, Division of Sleep Medicine) for providing the thematic inspiration for portions of this chapter.

References

Akerstedt, T. (2003). Shift work and disturbed sleep/wakefulness. *Occupational Medicine (Oxford, England), 53*, 89–94.

Allen, A. (1990). On-the-job injury: A costly problem. *Journal of Post Anesthesia Nursing, 5*(5), 367–368.

American Federation of Labor and Congress of Industrial Organizations, & Safety and Health Department. (2002). *Restrictions on mandatory overtime—Examples of contract language*. Available at: http://www.aflcio.org/issues/safety/issues/otexamples.cfm. Accessed on October 20, 2011.

Ariens, G. A., Bongers, P. M., Hoogendoorn, W. E., van der Wal, G., & van Mechelen, W. (2002). High physical and psychosocial load at work and sickness absence due to neck pain. *Scandinavian Journal of Work, Environment & Health, 28*(4), 222–231.

Artazcoz, L., Cortès, I., Escribà-Agüir, V., Cascant, L., & Villegas, R. (2009). Understanding the relationship of long working hours with health status and health related behaviours. *J Epidemiology and Community Health., 63*, 521–527.

Atkinson, G., Fullick, S., Grindey, C., Maclaren, D., & Waterhouse, J. (2008). Exercise, energy balance and the shift worker. *Sports Medicine, 38*(8), 671–685.

Atlantis, E., Chow, C. M., Kirby, A., & Singh, M. A. (2006). Worksite intervention effects on sleep quality: A randomized controlled trial. *Journal of Occupational Health Psychology, 11*(4), 291–304.

Barger, L. K., Cade, B. E., Ayas, N. T., et al. (2005). Extended work shifts and the risk of motor vehicle crashes among interns. *The New England Journal of Medicine, 352*, 125–134.

Barion, A., & Zee, P. C. (2007). A clinical approach to circadian rhythm sleep disorders. *Sleep Medicine, 8*(6), 566–577.

Bilski, B. (2006). Influence of shift work on the diet and gastrointestinal complains among nurses. A pilot study. [Wplyw pracy zmianowej na sposob odzywiania sie i patologie przewodu pokarmowego wsrod pieliegniarek--wyniki badania pilotowego]. *Medycyna Pracy, 57*(1), 15–19. English abstract only.

Boggild, H. (2009). Settling the question- the next review on shiftwork and heart disease in 2009. *Scandinavian Journal of Work, Environment & Health, 35*, 157–161.

Bøggild, H., & Knutsson, A. (1999). Shift work, risk factors and cardiovascular disease [review]. *Scandinavian Journal of Work, Environment & Health, 25*, 85–99.

Boivin, D. B., & James, F. O. (2005). Light treatment and circadian adaptation to shift work. *Industrial Health, 43*(1), 34–48.

Boivin, D. B., Tremblay, G. M., & James, F. O. (2007). Working on atypical schedules. *Sleep Medicine, 8*(6), 578–589.

Bonzini, M., Coggon, D., & Palmer, K. T. (2007). Risk of prematurity, low birthweight and pre-eclampsia in relation to working hours and physical activities: a systematic review. *Occupational and Environmental Medicine, 64*(4), 228–243.

Brouqui, P. (2009). Facing highly infectious diseases: new trends and current concepts. *Clinical Microbiology and Infection, 15*(8), 700–705.

Bryant, P. A., Trinder, J., & Curtis, N. (2004). Sick and tired: does sleep have a vital role in the immune system? *Nature Reviews Immunology, 4*, 457–467.

Bureau of Labor Statistics. (2010). *American time use survey (2003–2007)*. Available at http://www.bls.gov/tus/tables/a5_0307htm. Accessed on August 17, 2011.

Bureau of Labor Statistics. (2010). TABLE SNR06. *Highest incidence rates of total nonfatal occupational injury cases, 2010* Available at http://www.bls.gov/iif/oshwc/osh/os/ostb2806.pdf. Accessed on October 24, 2011.

Bureau of Labor Statistics. *Nonfatal occupational injuries and illnesses requiring days away from work, 2009*. Available at http://www.bls.gov/news.release/osh2.nr0.htm/ Accessed on October 24, 2011.

Burgueño, A., Gemma, C., Fernández, G., Sookoian, S., & Pirola, C. J. (2010). Increased levels of resistin in rotating shift workers: A potential mediator of cardiovascular risk associated with circadian misalignment. *Atherosclerosis, 210*(2), 625–629.

Bushnell, P. T., Colombi, A., Caruso, C. C., & Taki, S. W. (2010). Work schedules and health behavior outcomes at a large manufacturer. *Industrial Health, 48*, 395–405.

Cajochen, C., Munch, M., Kobialka, S., Krauchi, K., Steiner, R., Oelhafen, P., et al. (2005). High sensitivity of human melatonin, alertness, thermoregulation, and heart rate to short wavelength light. *The Journal of Clinical Endocrinology and Metabolism, 90*(3), 1311–1316.

Caldwell, J. A., Caldwell, J. L., & Schmidt, R. M. (2008). Alertness management strategies for operational contexts. *Sleep Medicine Reviews, 12*(4), 257–273.

Camarino, D., Conway, P. M., Sartori, S., Campanini, P., Estryn-Behar, M., van der Heijden, B. I., & Costa, G. (2008). Factors affecting work ability in day and shift-working nurses. *Chronobiology International, 25*, 425–442.

Caruso, C.C., Hitchcock, E.M., Dick, R.B., Russo, J.M., & Schmidt, J.M. (2004). Overtime and extended work shifts: Recent findings on injuries, illnesses and health behaviors. Washington, D.C., National Institute of Occupational Safety and Health., NIOSH Publication 2004:143.

Costa, G., Haus, E., & Stevens, R. (2010). Shiftwork and cancer- considerations on rationale, mechanisms, and epidemiology. *Scandinavian Journal of Work, Environment & Health, 36*, 163–179.

Crowley, S., Acebo, C., & Carskadon, M. (2007). Sleep, circadian phase, and delayed phase in adolescence. *Sleep Medicine, 8*, 602–612.

Czeisler, C. A. (2009). Medical and genetic differences in the adverse impact of sleep loss on performance: Ethical considerations for the medical profession. *Transactions of the American Clinical and Climatological Association, 120*, 249–285.

Czeisler, C. A. (2010). Ethical considerations for the scheduling of work in continuous operations: physicians in training as a case study. In F. P. Miller, M. A. Cappucio, & S. W. Lockley (Eds.), *Sleep, Health & Society. From Aetiology to Public Health* (pp. 435–456). Oxford University Press: New York.

Czeisler, C.A. (26 April 2011). FAA knew controllers nap, ignored fatigue issue. CNN Opinion, Available at: http://www.cnn.com/2011/OPINION/04/26/czeisler.sleep.air.traffic.controllers/.

Davidson, S. S., & Benjamin, W. H., Jr. (2006). Risk of infection and tracking of work-related infectious diseases in the funeral industry. *American Journal of Infection Control, 34*(10), 655–660.

Davis, K. G., Marras, W. S., Heaney, C. A., Waters, T. R., & Gupta, P. (2002). The impact of mental processing and pacing on spine loading: 2002 Volvo Award in biomechanics. *Spine, 27*(23), 2645–2653.

De Bacquer, D., Van Risseghem, M., Clays, E., Kittel, F., De Backer, G., & Braeckman, L. (2009). Rotating shift work and the metabolic syndrome: a prospective study. *International Journal of Epidemiology, 38*(3), 848–854.

de Castro, A. B., Fujishiro, K., Rue, T., Tagalog, E. A., Samaco-Paquiz, L. P., & Gee, G. C. (2010). Associations between work schedule characteristics and occupational injury and illness. *International Nursing Review, 57*(2), 188–194.

Dembe, A. E., Delbos, R., & Erickson, J. B. (2008). The effect of occupation and industry on the injury risks from demanding work schedules. *Journal of Occupational and Environmental Medicine, 50*(10), 1185–1194.

Dijk, D. J., Duffy, J. F., & Czeisler, C. A. (2000). Contribution of circadian physiology and sleep homeostasis to age-related changes in human sleep. *Chronobiology International, 17*, 285–311.

Dingus, T.A., Klauer, S.G., Neale, V.L., Petersen, A., Lee, S.E., Sudweeks, J., Perez, M.A., Hankey, J., Ramsey, D., Gupta, S., Bucher, C., Doerzaph, Z.R., Jermeland, J., & Knipling, RR. (2006). The 100-car naturalistic driving study; Phase II –Results of the 100-car field experiment. Washington, D.C., National Highway Traffic Safety Administration. DOT HS 31 810 593: 1–352.

Drake, C. L., Roehrs, T., Richardson, G., Walsh, J. K., & Roth, T. (2004). Shiftwork sleep disorder. Prevalence and consequences beyond that of symptomatic day workers. *Sleep, 27*(8), 1453–1462.

Driskell, J. E., & Mullen, B. (2005). The efficacy of naps as a fatigue countermeasure: A meta-analytic integration. *Human Factors, 47*(2), 360–377.

Eriksen, W., Bruusgaard, D., & Knardahl, S. (2004). Work factors as predictors of sickness absence attributed to airway infections; a three month prospective study of nurses' aides. *Occupational and Environmental Medicine, 61*(1), 45–51.

European Commission, Employment, Social Affairs and Inclusion. *Working conditions working time directive.* 2010. Available at: http://ec.europa.eu/social/main.jsp?catId=706&langId=en&intPageId=205. Accessed on October 19, 2011.

Fédération des médecins résidents du Québec [FMRQ]. 16-hour call duty: Arbitrator rules in FMRQ's favour. June 14, 2011. Available at: http://www.fmrq.qc.ca/formation-medicale/actualitesDetails_ang.cfm?noActualite=199. Accessed on October 20, 2011.

Fialho, G., Cavichio, L., Povoa, R., & Pimenta, J. (2006). Effects of 24-h shift work in the emergency room on ambulatory blood pressure monitoring values of medical residents. *American Journal of Hypertension, 19*(10), 1005–1009.

Ficca, G., Axelsson, J., Mollicone, D. J., Muto, V., & Vitiello, M. V. (2010). Naps, cognition and performance. *Sleep Medicine Reviews, 14*, 249–258.

Folkard, S. (2008). Do permanent night workers show circadian adjustment? A review based on the endogenous melatonin rhythm. *Chronobiology International, 25*(2), 215–224.

Folkard, S., & Akerstedt, T. (2004). Trends in the risk of accidents and injuries and their implications for models of fatigue and performance. *Aviation, Space, and Environmental Medicine, 75*(3 Suppl), A161–A167.

Folkard, S., & Lombardi, D. A. (2006). Modeling the impact of the components of long work hours on injuries and "accidents". *American Journal of Industrial Medicine, 49*, 953–963.

Folkard, S., Lombardi, D. A., & Spencer, M. B. (2006). Estimating the circadian rhythm in the risk of occupational injuries and accidents. *Chronobiology International, 23*(6), 1181–1192.

Folkard, S., Lombardi, D. A., & Tucker, P. T. (2005). Shiftwork: safety, sleepiness and sleep. *Industrial Health, 43*(1), 20–23.

Folkard, S., Spelen, E., & Toterdell, P. (1995). The use of survey measures to assess circadian variation in alertness. *Sleep, 18*, 355–361.

Forde, M. S., Punnett, L., & Wegman, D. H. (2002). Pathomechanisms of work-related musculoskeletal disorders: conceptual issues. *Ergonomics, 45*(9), 619–630.

Frost, P., Kolstad, H. A., & Bonde, J. P. (2009). Shift work and the risk of ischemic heart disease: a systematic review of the epidemiologic evidence. *Scandinavian Journal of Work, Environment & Health, 35*, 163–179.

Gander, P. H., Marshall, N. S., Harris, R. B., & Reid, P. (2005). Sleep, sleepiness and motor vehicle accidents: A national survey. *Australian and New Zealand Journal of Public Health, 29*(1), 16–21.

Geiger-Brown, J., & McPhaul, K. (2011). Sleep promotion in occupational health settings. In N. S. Redeker & G. Phillips Mc Enany (Eds.), *Sleep Disorders and Sleep Promotion in Nursing Practice* (pp. 355–370). New York: Springer Publishing Co.

Gordon, N. P., Cleary, P. D., Parker, C. E., & Czeisler, C. A. (1986). The prevalence and health impact of shiftwork. *American Journal of Public Health, 76*(10), 1225–1228.

Haneke, K., Tiedemann, S., Nachreiner, F., & Grzech-Sukalo, H. (1998). Accident risk as a function of hour at work and time of day as determined from accident data and exposure models for the German working population. *Scandinavian Journal of Work, Environment & Health, 24*(Suppl 3), 43–48.

Hannerz, H., & Tuchsen, F. (2001). Hospital admissions among male drivers in Denmark. *Occupational and Environmental Medicine, 58*(4), 253–260.

Hartenbaum, N., Collop, N., Rosen, I. M., Phillips, B., George, C. F., Rowley, J. A., et al. (2006). Sleep apnea and commercial motor vehicle operators: Statement from the Joint Task Force of the American College of Chest Physicians, American College of Occupational and Environmental Medicine, and the National Sleep Foundation. *Journal of Occupational and Environmental Medicine, 48*(9 Suppl), S4–S37.

Hayashi, M., Masuda, A., & Hori, T. (2003). The alerting effects of caffeine, bright light and face washing after a short daytime nap. *Clinical Neurophysiology, 114*(12), 2268–2278.

Hermansson, U., Knutsson, A., Brandt, L., Huss, A., Rönnberg, S., & Helander, A. (2003). Screening for high-risk and elevated alcohol consumption in day and shift workers by use of the AUDIT and CDT. *Occupational Medicine (London), 53*(8), 518–526.

Hoogendoorn, W., Bongers, P., de Vet, H., Ariens, G., van Mechelen, W., & Bouter, L. (2002). High physical work load and low job satisfaction increase the risk of sickness absence due to low back pain: results of a prospective cohort study. *Occupational and Environmental Medicine, 59*, 323–328.

Hoogendoorn, W., Bongers, P., deVet, H. C., Douwes, M., Koes, B., Miedema, M., Ariëns, G., & Bouter, L. (2000). Flexion and rotation of the trunk and lifting at work are risk factors for low back pain: results of a prospective cohort study. *Spine, 25*, 3087–3092.

Hoozemans, M. J., Kuijer, P. P., Kingma, I., van Dieën, J. H., de Vries, W. H., van der Woude, L. H., Veeger, D. J., van der Beek, A. J., & Frings-Dresen, M. H. (2004). Mechanical loading of the low back and shoulders during pushing and pulling activities. *Ergonomics, 47*(1), 1–18.

Horrey, W. J., Noy, Y. I., Folkard, S., Popkin, S. M., Howarth, H. D., & Courtney, T. K. (2011). Research needs and opportunities for reducing the adverse safety consequences of fatigue. *Accident Analysis and Prevention, 43*, 591–594.

Hosoglu, S., Akalin, S., Sunbul, M., Otkun, M., Ozturk, R., & Occupational Infections Study Group. (2009). Predictive factors for occupational bloodborne exposure in Turkish hospitals. *American Journal of Infection Control, 37*(1), 65–69.

Hossain, J. L., Reinish, L. W., Kayumov, L., Bhuiya, P., & Shapiro, C. M. (2003). Underlying sleep pathology may cause chronic high fatigue in shift-workers. *Journal of Sleep Research, 12*(3), 223–230.

Huang, W., Ramsey, K. M., Marcheva, B., & Bass, J. (2011). Circadian rhythms, sleep and metabolism. *The Journal of Clinical Investigation, 121*(6), 2133–2141.

Hursh, S. R., Redmond, D. P., Johnson, M. L., Thorne, D. R., Belenky, G., Balkin, T. J., et al. (2004). Fatigue models for applied research in warfighting. *Aviation, Space, and Environmental Medicine, 75*(3 Suppl), A44–A53.

Ingre, M., Kecklund, G., Akerstedt, T., Soderstrom, M., & Kecklund, L. (2008). Sleep length as a function of morning-shift start time in irregular shift schedules for train drivers: self-rated health and individual differences. *Chronobiology International, 25*(2&3), 349–358.

International Agency for Research on Cancer, World Health Organization. (2007). IARC monograph on the evaluation of carcinogenic risks to humans. Volume 98. Painting, firefighting and shiftwork. Lyon, France. Accessed on August 25, 2010 at http://monographs.iarc.fr/ENG/Monographs/vol98/mono98.pdf

Johansson, E. (2004). A note on the impact of hours worked on mortality in OECD countries. *The European Journal of Health Economics, 5*(4), 335–340.

Johnson, E. S., & Ndetan, H. (2011). Non-cancer mortality in poultry slaughtering/processing plant workers belonging to a union pension fund. *Environment International, 37*(2), 322–327.

Jones, C. B., Lee, C. J., & Rajaratnam, S. M. W. (2010). Sleep, law and policy. In F. P. Cappuccio, M. A. Miller, & S. W. Lockley (Eds.), *Sleep, Health and Society: From Aetiology to Public Health* (pp. 417–434). Oxford: Oxford University Press.

Kecklund, G., Eriksen, C. A., & Åkerstedt, T. (2008). Police officers attitude to different shift systems: Association with age, present shift schedule, health and sleep/wake complaints. *Applied Ergonomics, 39*(5), 565–571.

Ker, K., Edwards, P.J., Felix, L.M., Blackhall, K., & Roberts, I. (2010). Caffeine for the prevention of injuries and errors in shift workers. *Cochrane Database of Systematic Reviews* 2010, Issue 5. Art. No.: CD008508.

Kivimäki, M., Kuisma, P., Virtanen, M., & Elovainio, M. (2001). Does shift work lead to poorer health habits? A comparison between women who had always done shift work with those who had never done shift work. *Work and Stress, 15*(1), 3–13.

Kojola B. Organized Labor's Response to Long Work Hours. Extended Abstract from Conference: Long Working Hours, Safety, and Health: Toward A National Research Agenda, University of Maryland, Baltimore, Maryland. April 29-30, 2004. Available at: http://www.cdc.gov/niosh/topics/workschedules/abstracts/kojola.html. Accessed on October 19, 2011.

Kristensen, T. S. (1989). Cardiovascular diseases and the work environment: a critical review of the epidemiologic literature on nonchemical factors. *Scandinavian Journal of Work, Environment & Health, 15*, 165–179.

Labyak, S., Lava, S., Turek, F., & Zee, P. (2002). Effects of shiftwork on sleep and menstrual function in nurses. *Health Care for Women International, 23*(6–7), 703–714.

Landsbergis, P. A., Schnall, P. L., & Dobson, M. (2009). The workplace and cardiovascular disease. In P. L. Schnall, M. Dobson, & E. Rosskam (Eds.), *Unhealthy work: causes, consequences, cures* (pp. 89–112). Amityville, NY: Baywood Publishing Company, Inc.

Larese, F., & Fiorito, A. (1994). Musculoskeletal disorders in hospital nurses: A comparison between two hospitals. *Ergonomics, 37*(7), 1205–1211.

Lavie, P. (2002). Sleep apnea in the presumably healthy working population–revisited. *Sleep, 25*(4), 380–387.

Lee, C. J. (2006). Federal Regulation of Hospital Resident Work Hours: Enforcement with Real Teeth. *J Health Care Law Policy., 9*, 162–216.

Leggat, P. A., Kedjarune, U., & Smith, D. R. (2007). Occupational health problems in modern dentistry: a review. *Industrial Health, 45*(5), 611–621.

Lenne, M. G., Dwyer, F., Triggs, T. J., Rajaratnam, S., & Redman, J. R. (2004). The effects of a nap opportunity in quiet and noisy environments on driving performance. *Chronobiology International, 21*(6), 991–1001.

Li, F., Fisher, K. J., Harmer, P., Irbe, D., Tearse, R. G., & Weimer, C. (2004). Tai chi and self-rated quality of sleep and daytime sleepiness in older adults: a randomized controlled trial. *J American Geriatric Society, 52*(6), 892–900.

Lowden, A., Holmback, U., Akerstedt, T., Forslund, A., Forslund, J., & Lennernas, M. (2001). Time of day type of food--relation to mood and hunger during 24 hours of constant conditions. *Journal of Human Ergology, 30*(1-2), 381–386.

Lundberg, U., Melin, B., Ekstrom, M., Elfsberg Dohns, I., Sandsjo, L., Palmerud, G., Kadefors, R., & Parr, D. (1999). Psychophysiological stress responses, muscle tension, and neck and shoulder pain among supermarket cashiers. *Journal of Occupational Health and Safety, 4*(3), 245–255.

Maher, K., & Aeppel, T. (2009). Overtime creeps back before jobs. *Wall Street Journal—Eastern Edition, 254*(126), A3.

Manfredini, R., Pala, M., Fabbian, F., & Manfredini, F. (2011). Peripheral endothelial function, shift work, and circadian rhythm disturbances. *Am. J. Cardiology, 107*, 1870–1871.

McGill University Health Centre and Association de Résidents de McGill. Grievance No. 4-CUSM-0809-01 (Arbitration Board, Québec, Canada, June 7, 2011) (Jean-Pierre Lussier, Arb.), English translation from the original French available at http://www.fmrq.qc.ca/PDF/2011-06-07_Griefhorairesgarde_DecisiondeMeJPLussier_VA.pdf.

McMenamin, T. M. (2007). A time to work: recent trends in shiftwork and flexible schedules. *Monthly Labor Review, 130*(12), 3–15.

Melamed, S., & Oksenberg, A. (2002). Excessive daytime sleepiness and risk of occupational injuries in non-shift daytime workers. *Sleep, 25*(3), 315–322.

Miller, M. A., & Cappuccio, F. P. (2007). Inflammation, sleep, obesity and cardiovascular disease. *Current Vascular Pharmacology, 5*(2), 93–102.

Moore, R.T., Kaprielian, R., Auerbach, J. (2009). Asleep at the Wheel. *Report of the special commission on drowsy driving. massachusetts department of public health.* Available as a download from sleep.med.harvard.edu/file_download/103. Accessed on October 1, 2011.

Moore-Ede, M. C. (1993). The twenty-four hour society: Understanding human limits in a world that never stops. Reading, MA: Addison-Wesley. In H. R. Colton & B. M. Altevogt (Eds.), *Sleep disorders and sleep deprivation, an unmet public health problem.* Washington, DC: Institute of Medicine, National Academies Press.

Moore-Ede, M., Heitmann, A., Guttkuhn, R., Trutschel, U., Aguirre, A., & Croke, D. (2004). Circadian alertness simulator for fatigue risk assessment in transportation: Application to reduce frequency and severity of truck accidents. *Aviation, Space, and Environmental Medicine, 75*(3 Suppl), A107–A118.

Nabe-Nielsen, K., Garde, A. H., Tuchsen, F., Hogh, A., & Diderichsen, F. (2008). Cardiovascular risk factors and primary selection into shift work. *Scandinavian Journal of Work, Environment & Health, 34*(3), 206–212.

Nahit, E. S., Macfarlane, G. J., Pritchard, C. M., Cherry, N. M., & Silman, A. J. (2001). Short term influence of mechanical factors on regional musculoskeletal pain: a study of new workers from 12 occupational groups. *Occupational and Environmental Medicine, 58*, 374–381.

Nakamura, K., Shimai, S., Kikuchi, S., Tominaga, K., Takahashi, H., Tanaka, M., Nakano, S., Motohashi, Y., Nakadaira, H., & Yamamoto, M. (1997). Shift work and risk factors for coronary heart disease in Japanese blue-collar workers: serum lipids and anthropometric characteristics. *Occupational Medicine, 47*(3), 142–146.

National Sleep Foundation. (2008). *State of the states report on drowsy driving.* Retrieved on August 18,2011 from: http://drowsydriving.org/resources/2008-state-of-the-states-report-on-drowsy driving/

National Transportation Safety Board. (2011). *Most wanted list.* Accessed at http://www.ntsb.gov/safety/mwl.html. Retrieved on November 1, 2011.

National Academies, Transportation Research Board. (2006). Commuting in America III. *The third national report on commuting patterns and trends.* Retrieved on August 18, 2011 from http://onlinepubs.trb.org/onlinepubs/nchrp/ciaiii.pdf

NB. Sleeping air-traffic controllers: Another napper in the airport tower [Gulliver Blog]. Economist.com. April 17, 2011. Available at: www.economist.com/blogs/gulliver/2011/04/sleeping_air-traffic_controllers?fsrc=nlw|gul|04-19-11|gulliver. Accessed on October 19, 2011.

Nojkov, B., Rubenstein, J. H., Chey, W. D., & Hoogerwerf, W. A. (2010). The impact of rotating shift work on the prevalence of irritable bowel syndrome in nurses. *The American Journal of Gastroenterology, 105*(4), 842–847.

Nylen, L., Voss, M., & Floderus, B. (2001). Mortality among women and men relative to unemployment, part time work, overtime work, and extra work: a study based on data from the Swedish twin registry. *Occupational and Environmental Medicine, 58*(1), 52–57.

Oishi, M., Suwazono, Y., Sakata, K., Okubo, Y., Harada, H., Kobayashi, E., Uetani, M., & Nogawa, K. (2005). A longitudinal study on the relationship between shiftwork and the progression of hypertension in male Japanese workers. *Journal of Hypertension, 23*(12), 2173,2178.

Parent-Thirion, A., Fernandez-Macias, E., Hurley, J., & Vermeylen, G. (2007). *Fourth European Working Conditions Survey.* Dublin: European Foundation for the Improvement of Living and Working Conditions.

Parkes, K. (1999). Shiftwork, job type, and the type of work environment as joint predictors of health related outcomes. *Journal of Occupational Health Psychology, 4*(3), 256–268.

Parks, K. M., & Steelman, L. A. (2008). Organizational wellness programs: a meta-analysis. *Journal of Occupational Health Psychology, 13*(1), 58–68.

Philip, P., & Akerstedt, T. (2006). Transport and industrial safety, how are they affected by sleepiness and sleep restriction? *Sleep Medicine Reviews, 10*, 347–356.

Pietroiusti, A., Forlini, A., Magrini, A., Galante, A., Coppeta, L., Gemma, G., Romeo, E., & Bergamaschi, A. (2006). Shift work increases the frequency of duodenal ulcer in H pylori infected workers. *Occupational and Environmental Medicine, 63*(11), 773–775.

Pilcher, J. J., Lambert, B. J., & Huffcutt, A. I. (2000). Differential effects of permanent and rotating shifts on self-report sleep length: A meta-analytic review. *Sleep: Journal of Sleep Research & Sleep Medicine, 23*(2), 155–163.

Pompeii, L. A., Savitz, D. A., Evenson, K. R., Rogers, B., & McMahon, M. (2005). Physical exertion at work and the risk of preterm delivery and small-for-gestational-age birth. *Obstetrics and Gynecology, 106*(6), 1279–1288.

Popkin, J. (2001). *Small business share of economic growth*. Retrieved on October 1, 2011 and accessed at: http://archive.sba.gov/advo/research/rs211.pdf

Public Citizen et al. Petition to the U.S. *Occupational safety and health administration requesting medical residents work hour limits*. April 30, 2001. Available at: http://www.citizen.org/hrg1570. Accessed on October 19, 2011.

Public Citizen et al. Petition to the U.S. *occupational safety and health administration to reduce medical resident work hours*. September 2, 2010. Available at: www.citizen.org/hrg1917. Accessed on October 19, 2011.

Punnett, L., Fine, L. J., Keyserling, W. M., Herrin, G. D., & Chaffin, D. B. (2000). Shoulder disorders and postural stress in automobile assembly work. *Scandinavian Journal of Work, Environment & Health, 26*, 283–291.

Purnell, M. T., Feyer, A. M., & Herbison, G. P. (2002). The impact of a nap opportunity during the night shift on the performance and alertness of 12-h shift workers. *Journal of Sleep Research, 11*(3), 219–227.

Puttonen, S., Harma, M., & Hublin, C. (2010). Shift work and cardiovascular disease—pathways from circadian stress to morbidity. *Scandinavian Journal of Work, Environment & Health, 36*(2), 96–108.

Puttonen, S., Kivimaki, M., Elovainio, M., Pulkki-Raback, L., Hintsanen, M., Vahtera, J., Telama, R., Juonala, M., Viikari, J. S., Raitakari, O. T., & Keltikangas-Jarvinen, L. (2009). Shift work in young adults and carotid artery intima-media thickness: The Cardiovascular Risk in Young Finns study. *Atherosclerosis, 205*(2), 608–613.

Reeves, S. L., Newling-Ward, E., & Gissane, C. (2004). The effect of shift-work on food intake and eating habits. *Nutrition & Food Science, 34*(5), 216–221.

Robb, G., Sultana, S., Ameratunga, S., & Jackson, R. (2008). A systematic review of epidemiological studies investigating risk factors for work-related road traffic crashes and injuries. *Injury Prevention, 14*(1), 51–58.

Rogers, A., Holmes, S., & Spencer, M. (2001). The effect of shiftwork on driving to and from work. *Journal of Human Ergology, 30*(1–2), 131–136.

Rosa, R. R., Harma, M., Pulli, K., Mulder, M., & Nasman, O. (1996). Rescheduling a three shift system at a steel rolling mill: Effects of a one hour delay of shift starting times on sleep and alertness in younger and older workers. *Occupational and Environmental Medicine, 53*, 677–685.

Rosekind, M. R. (2011). *An NTSB perspective on Sleep/Fatigue Risks in Transportation: Accidents, recommendations, and future needs*. The Sleepy Brain, Stockholm, Sweden: Conference presentation.

Round-the-Clock-Systems, Shiftwork Education, The Saturn, Strategy. Accessed at http://www.roundtheclocksystems.com/library3_cs_01saturn.html on August 29. 2011.

Sack, R. L., Auckley, D., Auger, R. R., Carskadon, M. A., Wright, K. P., Vitiello, M. V., & Zhdanova, I. V. (2007). Circadian rhythm sleep disorders: Part I. Basic principles, shift work and jet lag disorders. An American Academy of Sleep Medicine Review. *Sleep, 30*(11), 1460–1483.

Santhi, N., Aeschbach, D., Horowitz, T. S., & Czeisler, C. A. (2008). The impact of sleep timing and bright light exposure on attentional impairment during night work. *Journal of Biological Rhythms, 23*(4), 341–352.

Sasseville, A., Benhaberou-Brun, D., Fontaine, C., Charon, M., & Hebert, M. (2009). Wearing blue-blockers in the morning could improve sleep of workers on a permanent night schedule: a pilot study. *Chronobiology Int., 26*(5), 913–925.

Shechter, A., James, F. O., & Boivin, D. B. (2008). Circadian rhythms and shift working women. *Sleep Med Clin., 3*, 13–24.

Slack-Smith, L. M., Read, A. W., Darby, J., & Stanley, F. J. (2006). Health of caregivers in child care. *Child: Care, Health and Development, 32*(1), 111–119.

Smedley, J., Inskip, H., Trevelyan, F., Buckle, P., Cooper, C., & Coggon, D. (2003). Risk factors for incident neck and shoulder pain in hospital nurses, *Occupational and Environmental Medicine, 60*, 864–869.

Smith, M. R., Fogg, L. F., & Eastman, C. I. (2009). A compromise circadian phase position for permanent night work improves mood, fatigue and performance. *Sleep, 32*(11), 1481–1489.

Stutts, J. C., Wilkins, J. W., Scott Osberg, J., & Vaughn, B. V. (2003). Driver risk factors for sleep-related crashes. *Accident Analysis and Prevention, 35*(3), 321–331.

Suessenbacher, A., Potocnik, M., Dorler, J., Fluckinger, G., Wanitschek, P. O., Frick, M., & Alger, H. F. (2011). Comparison of peripheral endothelial function in shift versus nonshift workers. *The American Journal of Cardiology, 107*, 945–948.

Suwazono, Y., Dochi, M., Sakata, K., Okubo, Y., Oishi, M., Tanaka, K., Kobayashi, E., Kido, T., & Nogawa, K. (2008). A longitudinal study on the effect of shift work on weight gain in male Japanese workers. *Obesity, 16*(8), 1887–1893.

Suwazono, Y., Sakata, K., Okubo, Y., Harada, H., Oishi, M., Kobayashi, E., Uetani, M., Kido, T., & Nogawa, K. (2006). Long-term longitudinal study on the relationship between alternating shift work and the onset of diabetes mellitus in male Japanese workers. *Journal of Occupational and Environmental Medicine, 48*(5), 455–461.

Sveinsdottir, H. (2006). Self-assessed quality of sleep, occupational health, working environment, illness experience and job satisfaction of female nurses working different combination of shifts. *Scandinavian Journal of Caring Sciences, 20*(2), 229–237.

Swerissen, H., & Crisp, B. R. (2004). The sustainability of health promotion interventions for different levels of social organization. *Health Promotion International, 19*(1), 123–130.

Thomas, C., & Power, C. (2010). Shift work and risk factors for cardiovascular disease: a study at age 45 years in the 1958 British birth cohort. *European Journal of Epidemiology, 25*(5), 305–314.

Trajman, A., & Menzies, D. (2010). Occupational respiratory infections. *Current Opinion in Pulmonary Medicine, 16*(3), 226–234.

Transport Canada, Civil Aviation Policy & Regulatory Services (2003). *Position paper on fatigue risk management with the aviation maintenance industry.* Accessed at http://www.tc.gc.ca/eng/civilaviation/standards/sms-frms-menu-634.htm, retrieved on October 15, 2011.

Trinkoff, A., Le, R., Geiger-Brown, J., Lipscomb, J., & Lang, G. (2006). The longitudinal relationship of long work hours and mandatory overtime to MSD in Nurses. *American Journal of Industrial Medicine, 49*, 964–971.

Trinkoff, A. M., & Storr, C. L. (1998). Work schedule characteristics and substance use in nurses. *American Journal of Industrial Medicine, 34*, 266–271.

U.S. Bureau of Labor Statistics. *Occupational outlook handbook 2005.* Accessed on August 25, 2011 at http://www.bls.gov/OCO/

U.S. Department of Labor. Occupational Safety and Health Administration [OSHA]. Emergency Preparedness and Response, Safety and Health Guides—Extended/Unusual Work Shifts. Available at: www.osha.gov/SLTC/emergencypreparedness/guides/extended.html. Accessed on October 19, 2011.

U.S. Department of Labor. Occupational Safety and Health Administration [OSHA]. Statement by US Department of Labor's OSHA Assistant Secretary Dr. David Michaels on long work hours, fatigue and worker safety (Release Number: 10-1238-NAT). September 2, 2010. Available at: www.osha.gov/pls/oshaweb/owadisp.show_document?p_table=NEWS_RELEASES&p_id=18285. Accessed on October 19, 2011.

U.S. Department of Labor. Occupational Safety and Health Administration [OSHA]. Workers, We Can Help. Available at: http://www.osha.gov/workers.html. Accessed on October 20, 2011.

Valent, F., Di Bartolomeo, S., Marchetti, R., Sbrojavacca, R., & Barbone, F. (2010). A case-crossover study of sleep and work hours and the risk of road traffic accidents. *Sleep, 33*(3), 349–354.

Valway, S. E., Richards, S. B., Kovacovich, J., Greifinger, R. B., Crawford, J. T., & Dooley, S. W. (1994). Outbreak of multi-drug resistant tuberculosis in a New York State prison. *American Journal of Epidemiology, 140*(2), 113–122.

van Amelsvoort, L. G., Schouten, E. G., Maan, A. C., Swenne, C. A., & Kok, F. J. (2001). Changes in frequency of premature complexes and heart rate variability related to shift work. *Occupational and Environmental Medicine, 58*(10), 678–681.

Volna, J., & Sonka, K. (2006). Medical factors of falling asleep behind the wheel. *Prague Medical Report, 107*(3), 290–296.

Waersted, M., & Westgaard, R. H. (1991). Working hours as a risk factor in the development of musculoskeletal complaints. *Ergonomics, 34*(3), 265–276.

Whelan, E. A., Lawson, C. C., Grajewski, B., Hibert, E. N., Spiegelman, D., & Rich-Edwards, J. W. (2007). Work schedule during pregnancy and spontaneous abortion. *Epidemiology, 18*(3), 350–355.

World Health Organization. (2011). Global atlas on cardiovascular disease prevention and control. Accessed at http://whqlibdoc.who.int/publications/2011/9789241564373_eng.pdf on October 13, 2011.

Wyatt, J. K., Cajochen, C., Ritz-De-Cecco, A., & Czeisler, C. A. (2004). Low-dose repeated caffeine administration for circadian phase-dependent performance degradation during extended wakefulness. *Sleep, 27*(3), 374–381.

Yelin, E. (2009). The changing nature of work in the United States. In P. Schnall, M. Dobson, & E. Rosskam (Eds.), *Unhealthy work: causes, consequences, cures* (pp. 79–86). Amityville, NY: Baywood Publishing Co.

Zhao, I., & Turner, C. (2007). The impact of shift work on people's daily health habits and adverse health outcomes. *The Australian Journal of Advanced Nursing, 25*, 8–22.

Zhen Lu, W., Ann Gwee, K., & Yu Ho, K. (2006). Functional bowel disorders in rotating shift nurses may be related to sleep disturbances. *European Journal of Gastroenterology & Hepatology, 18*(6), 623–627.

Zhu, J. L., Hjollund, N. H., Andersen, A. M., & Olsen, J. (2004). Shift work, job stress, and late fetal loss: The National Birth Cohort in Denmark. *Journal of Occupational and Environmental Medicine, 46*(100), 1144–1149.

Zhu, J. L., Hjollund, N. H., Boggild, H., & Olsen, J. (2003). Shift work and subfecundity: a causal link or an artefact? *Occupational and Environmental Medicine, 60*(9), E12.

Zhu, J. L., Hjollund, N. H., & Olsen, J. (2004). Shift work, duration of pregnancy, and birth weight. *American Journal of Obstetrics and Gynecology, 191*(1), 285–291.

Work–Family Balance Issues and Work–Leave Policies

15

Rosalind B. King, Georgia Karuntzos,
Lynne M. Casper, Phyllis Moen, Kelly D. Davis,
Lisa Berkman, Mary Durham, and Ellen Ernst Kossek

Work–Family Balance Issues

The contemporary US workforce differs dramatically from that of the mid-twentieth century, yet workplace structures and human resource policies and practices addressing work–family balance issues have changed relatively little. Moreover, technological, economic, and globalization forces are reducing job security, while simultaneously increasing productivity expectations and time pressures for those who retain their jobs (Kossek, Lewis, & Hammer, 2010). Employees are increasingly subjected to greater job demands and are asked to be available to work all hours of the day and all days of the week, often with neither schedule consistency (Kossek, 2006; Presser, 2003) nor schedule control (Kelly & Moen, 2007). With the majority of women in the paid workforce, relatively stable fertility levels, increases in single-parent families, and an aging population, many workers are confronted with the need to care for family members while coping with increased work demands. In the USA, few public and limited private sector policies enable workers to balance the dual needs of work and family. The resulting disconnect has increased work–family conflict (Nomaguchi, 2009), a type of

---

This chapter was supported through the Work, Family and Health Network (www.WorkFamilyHealthNetwork.org), which is funded by a cooperative agreement through the National Institutes of Health and the Centers for Disease Control and Prevention: Eunice Kennedy Shriver National Institute of Child Health and Human Development (Grant # U01HD051217, U01HD051218, U01HD051256, U01HD051276), National Institute on Aging (Grant # U01AG027669), Office of Behavioral and Science Sciences Research, and National Institute for Occupational Safety and Health (Grant # U01OH008788, U01HD059773). Grants from the William T. Grant Foundation, Alfred P Sloan Foundation, and the Administration for Children and Families have provided additional funding. The contents of this publication are solely the responsibility of the authors and do not necessarily represent the official views of these institutes and offices. Special acknowledgement goes to Extramural Staff Science Collaborator, Rosalind B. King, PhD and Lynne Casper, PhD for design of the original Work, Family, Health and Well-Being Network Initiative.

R.B. King, Ph.D. (✉)
Eunice Kennedy Shriver National Institute of Child Health and Human Development, National Institutes of Health,
9000 Rockville Pike, Bethesda, MD 20892, USA
e-mail: kingros@mail.nih.gov

G. Karuntzos, Ph.D.
RTI International, 3040 East Cornwallis Road, 12194, Research Triangle Park, NC 27709-2194, USA
e-mail: gtk@rti.org

inter-role conflict where work and family roles are incompatible (Greenhaus & Beutell, 1985), resulting in reduced employee, family, and community health and well-being (Allen, Herst, Bruck, & Sutton, 2000; Bianchi, Casper, & King, 2005; Christensen & Schneider, 2010; Eby, Casper, Lockwood, Bordeaux, & Brinley, 2005; Kossek et al., 2010). Moreover, increased job insecurity, high unemployment, and declining wages for men, along with shifts in gender roles, have generated a steady increase in the proportion of wives and mothers engaged in paid market labor outside the home (Casper & Bianchi, 2002; Sayer, Cohen, & Casper, 2004). In most households with children, all adults are in the workforce, and dual-earner families must coordinate the schedules of two jobs along with responsibilities at home, with no member solely dedicated to family needs (Chesley & Moen, 2006; Jacobs & Gerson, 2004; Moen, 2003; Moen & Hernandez, 2009). To add even more complexity, in 2010, almost seven million Americans (ages 16 and older) were working two or more jobs (Bureau of Labor Statistics, 2011b). Role incompatibility is especially experienced by parents of children who are too young for elementary school, and by families with older relatives who need care (Casper & Bianchi; Moen & Chesley, 2008; Moen & Roehling, 2005).

Increasing rates of nonmarital childbearing and high levels of divorce also result in more single-parent families that have fewer adults available to fulfill work and caregiving obligations (Casper & Bianchi, 2009). Nonmarital childbearing comprised only 10 % of all births in the 1960s, but recent estimates indicate that 40 % of births are now to unmarried mothers (Hamilton, Martin, & Ventura, 2009). Divorce probabilities remain high; about one-third of marriages last less than 10 years, and only about half of married couples are still together at their 20th anniversary (Goodwin, Mosher, & Chandra, 2010). In 1970, 6 % of family households with children were maintained by a single mother,

---

L.M. Casper, Ph.D.
Department of Sociology, University of Southern California,
KAP 352, Los Angeles, CA 90089, USA
e-mail: lcasper@usc.edu

P. Moen, Ph.D.
Department of Sociology, University of Minnesota,
909 Social Sciences, 267 19th Ave S, Minneapolis, MN 55455, USA
e-mail: phylmoen@umn.edu

K.D. Davis, Ph.D.
Department of Human Development and Family Studies, Penn State University,
118 N. Henderson etc., 005 Henderson Building, University Park, PA 16802-1294, USA
e-mail: kdavis@psu.edu

L. Berkman, Ph.D.
Department of Society, Human Development and Health, Harvard University,
9 Bow Street, Cambridge, MA 02138, USA
e-mail: lberkman@hsph.harvard.edu

M. Durham, Ph.D.
The Center for Health Research, Kaiser Permanente, Center for Health Research,
3181 S.W. Sam Jackson Park Rd., Portland, OR 97239-3098, USA
e-mail: Mary.Durham@kpchr.org

E.E. Kossek, Ph.D.
School of Human Resources and Labor Relations, Michigan State University,
South Kedzie Hall, 368 Farm Lane, Room 428, East Lansing, MI 48824, USA

Purdue University Krannert School of Management & Susan Bulkeley Butler Leadership Center, West Lafayette, Indiana West Lafayette, IN 47907, USA
e-mail: kossek@msu.edu

and 1 % by a single father. By 2007, these figures were 23 and 5 %, respectively. When cohabiting couples are excluded from the tally of single parents, current estimates suggest single parents account for about one quarter of households with children under 18 (Kreider & Elliott, 2009). Additional shifts in demographic behaviors, such as delayed or foregone marriage and postponed or reduced childbearing, also reflect the growing incompatibility between jobs and families. Young adults increasingly delay marriage—in 2009, the median age at first marriage rose to 28 years for men and 26 years for women (US Census Bureau, 2010). Greater demands of work in terms of both time and energy also result in the postponement of children, especially among the better educated segments of the population. Currently, 20 % of American women aged 40–44 have never had a child, double the percentage of 30 years ago (Dye, 2008). Research that tracked a highly educated cohort of women from 1979 until the end of their childbearing years showed that the women's stated intentions averaged about half a child more than their completed fertility, suggesting that they may have had difficulty reaching their childbearing goals (Morgan, 2010). A plausible explanation for this trend is the demanding nature of jobs highly educated women and their partners are likely to occupy.

Care demands are also heavy for "sandwich" families, who must provide care for young and old alike (Casper & Bianchi, 2002; Neal & Hammer, 2007). Increased mobility for education and employment takes many families geographically away from extended family and other childhood social support networks. Future generations of elderly are likely to have fewer of their own children on whom they can rely for care. At the same time, the number of step-children is expanding due to high levels of union disruption and repartnering. Thus, caregiving is likely to be shared among fewer adult siblings and those who may be more tenuously related. These changes in working families suggest the need for policies promoting greater workplace flexibility and leave access to provide care in circumstances where backup from other family members is becoming less likely (Bianchi et al., 2005; Christensen & Schneider, 2010; Executive Office of the President Council of Economic Advisors, 2010). In addition, the aging US population is another factor pushing workplace flexibility to the forefront of national discussions. The fraction of the population aged 65 and over is projected to increase from the current 12 to 20 % in 2030 (He, Sengupta, Velkoff, & DeBarros, 2005). Older workers may be driven from the workforce earlier than their health dictates by overly demanding jobs or work schedules that do not allow them to fulfill the care needs of aging companions (Dentinger & Clarkberg, 2002; Moen, 2007; Moen & Altobelli, 2007; Sweet, Moen, & Meiksins, 2007). Older workers in full-time jobs with little schedule flexibility risk experiencing both health and safety difficulties (National Research Council and the Institute of Medicine, 2004). New ways of work that incorporate flexibility and part-time possibilities may enable older workers to remain actively engaged. Thus, employees face a variety of stressful situations that lead to work–family balance issues: time deadlines and speedups, increased workloads and overloads, dual-earner and single-parent conflicts and strains, and even routine obligations at work and home are often at odds with one another. Individuals and families may have exhausted their ability to rearrange their lives to fit the existing social organization of work, and so examining workplace policies and practices that can address the dual demands of work and family becomes a priority.

Work–Leave Policies

In the USA, the primary responsibility for providing release time from work responsibilities rests with companies and employers (Kelly, 2005; Stebbins, 2001). The federal government oversees employer compliance with legislation such as the Fair Labor Standards Act and protections such as nondiscrimination requirements, but the enactment of work–leave policies beyond the Family and Medical Leave Act (FMLA) are left to states and municipalities. Most current work-hour and supervisory policies and practices were designed in the mid-twentieth century, with the unstated assumption that employees have few nonwork responsibilities since another family member, usually the wife, primarily handles the home responsibilities (Moen & Chesley, 2008; Moen & Roehling, 2005; Neal & Hammer, 2007; Perlow, 1997; Rapoport, Bailyn, Fletcher, & Pruitt, 2002; Williams, 2000). Standard types of employer-provided leave in contemporary US workplaces are sick and annual. Sick leave is intended to cover an employee's time needed to obtain medical care for himself/herself, and possibly for dependent family members. Annual leave is intended to cover vacations or other leisure time. Some companies simply offer "personal time off (PTO)" that the employees may use at their discretion for any purpose. These types of leave are invaluable for the households with all adults in the workforce; but there are often restrictions on these types of leave that limit their usefulness for handling work–family balance issues. Annual leave often requires advance approval, which eliminates its use in emergencies. Sick leave is often restricted to the employee themselves, or may be utilized only as entire days rather than on an hourly basis, in which case follow-up visits for a single illness may use up an entire year's allotment. Additionally, access to these types of leave options varies substantially by occupation and wage level, with lower wage and manufacturing or production industries having the least access (Crouter & Booth, 2009). Strikingly, 30 % of American workers lack access to sick and annual leave, and approximately 60 % lack access to nonspecific paid personal time off (Bureau of Labor Statistics, 2011a). Moreover, in 2008, 21 % of US employees had no access to paid vacation days, 37 % had fewer than 5 days of paid personal sick leave (including those with no leave), and 37 % of those with children had fewer than 5 days of paid time off to care for sick children (Tang & Wadsworth, 2010).

The most recently enacted national leave legislation was the FMLA, passed in 1993. It mandates that employers with 50 or more employees provide up to 12 weeks of unpaid sick leave annually for workers to use for themselves or dependent family members. The employer must allow employees to return to their same or a similar job at the same pay and benefits. The mandate provides a right to take leave to the subgroup of US workers who work for large employers and can afford to not receive wages for a period of time. In recent years, some states and municipalities (e.g., Connecticut; San Francisco, CA; Washington, D.C.) have passed paid sick leave mandates for employers within their jurisdictions. The California Family Leave Act is a unique program that uses the workman's compensation model to provide up to 6 weeks of partially paid leave to bond with a new child or care for a parent, child, or spouse/domestic partner. Workers pay into the State Disability Insurance (SDI) program through their regular paychecks. All workers who pay in are eligible, regardless of full-time or part-time status, and benefits are paid out as a percent of wages. However, workers must still rely on provisions from the FMLA or the state-level California Family Rights Act to protect their job (information from www.working-families.org/learnmore/ca_family_leave_guide.pdf.) The success of the program thus far has been difficult to evaluate because public awareness is low, which has resulted in minimal use (Schuster et al., 2008).

Currently, at the federal level, President Obama created The White House Forum on Workplace Flexibility within The White House Council on Women and Girls (www.whitehouse.gov/work-flex-kit). A kickoff event in March 2010 brought together representatives from academic and practitioner professional societies, advocacy groups, and employers. The program has since hosted multiple regional forums to encourage dialogue and action at the local level. A report from the Council on Economic Advisors details the potential economic benefits of workplace flexibility, including paid leave (www.whitehouse.gov/files/documents/100331-cea-economics-workplace-flexibility.pdf).

While public policy moves slowly forward, some employers and unions have made changes at their own initiative. Over the past few decades, organizations have adopted "family-friendly" or "work-life" policies, although these initiatives are often implemented unevenly across and within organizations (Eaton, 2003; Kelly & Kalev, 2006; Kossek et al., 2010). These policies include a range of strategies: time-based (e.g., flexible schedules and leave programs), information-based (e.g., referral programs and provider fairs), money-based (e.g., dependent care spending accounts), and direct services (e.g., on-site child care) (Thompson, Beauvais, & Allen, 2006). However, even when worker supportive policies are implemented in US companies, the existence of a policy does not necessarily translate into an employee's ability to access it in practice. Work–family policies are often treated as accommodations available to some employees—often those with a record of superior performance—rather than work process adaptations useful to a wide range of employees (Kelly & Moen, 2007; Lee, MacDermid, & Buck, 2000; Williams, 2000). As a result, employee usage of these policies and practices is low; workers fear, and often experience, career penalties such as slower wage growth as a consequence of using them (Blair-Loy & Wharton, 2002; Glass, 2004). Finally, work leave policies and "family friendly" policies may effectively substitute for each other. For example, employees may not require sick leave if flexible hours allow them to shift their schedules around a physician's appointment. Telework may also alleviate the need for annual leave to be present in the home with an older child on a school holiday. Because of the range of policy levers and practices utilized by organizations, we include work–leave policies and other work supportive policies within a larger umbrella of work–family policies for the remainder of this Chapter.

Testing a Biopsychosocial Model of Work–Family Balance and Health

Rigorous evaluations of how policies and programs affect work–family balance issues are rare (for some exceptions, see Hammer, Neal, Newsom, Brockwood, & Colton, 2005; Hammer, Kossek, Bodner, Anger, & Zimmerman 2011; Kelly, Moen, & Tranby, 2011; Thomas & Ganster, 1995). Few studies have systematically modeled the pathway from the reduction of work–family conflict to improved health, and most have not included the psychosocial mechanisms by which these factors affect health across work units and at home (see Bianchi et al., 2005; Kelly et al., 2008; Melchior, Berkman, Niedhammer, Zins, & Goldberg, 2007). Health interventions usually focus on changes at the individual level, and rarely include organizational-level changes such as work process designs (Rapoport et al., 2002). No study, to our knowledge, has tested the existence of a causal relationship between workplace-level policies and practices, work–family conflict, employee health, and organizational health in a longitudinal, experimental design. Furthermore, none has investigated how such policies and practices may have implications for the health of family members. The Work Family and Health Network (WFHN), a multisite longitudinal randomized field experiment, currently underway, was designed to address this scientific gap. The WFHN is a collaborative network of researchers, formed with grant support from several federal government agencies and foundations, to design and test an innovative psychosocial intervention aimed at reducing work–family conflict in order to improve physical and mental health (www.workfamilyhealthnetwork.org). The WFHN comprises research expertise in a wide array of disciplines: biobehavioral health; demography; developmental psychology; economics; industrial/organizational psychology; medicine; occupational health psychology; organizational behavior; social epidemiology; sociology; study design, methodology, and data collection; and the science of translation and dissemination. For its first 3 years (2005–2008), the WFHN conducted observational and intervention pilot studies with hourly workers in the long-term nursing care, hotel, and grocery industries, and in the white-collar headquarters of a multinational, retail corporation. The observational studies examined basic biopsychosocial processes through which workplace conditions affected work–family balance which impacted employee health. These researchers collected data on current usual workplace practices in these industries and examined their associations with objectively measured health, self-reported health, family relationship quality, and workplace outcomes. In the long-term care setting, employees' cardiovascular risk and sleep patterns were associated with supervisors' management of work–family balance issues (Berkman, Buxton, Ertel, & Okechukwu,

2010; Ertel, Koenen, & Berkman, 2008). The study in the hotel industry used a daily diary design to understand the daily stressors and reactivity to stress experienced by hotel managers and hourly employees. In order to extend the conceptual model to the social unit of the family in order to understand how daily work and family experiences can influence one another, the study added data collection with the hotel managers' spouses and hourly employees' children. There, a lack of workplace flexibility was associated with both greater daily stressor exposure and reactivity in the employee, as well as greater potential for stress transmission from employees to their children (Almeida & Davis, 2011; Davis, 2008). These findings also demonstrated the importance of managerial support for employee work–family integration (O'Neill et al., 2009). Other research teams tested interventions that changed policies and practices around work demands and control and workplace social support from supervisors and colleagues. These interventions aimed at all levels of prevention (primary, secondary, and tertiary), as they were designed to prevent work–family conflict among those not yet experiencing it and to ameliorate work–family conflict among those already strained by it. These studies together generated evidence to support a causal relationship between work–family policies, work–family balance issues, and employee health across different populations. The first intervention changed both structure and culture in the workplace in order to increase employees' control over the time and timing of their work. The goal of the intervention was to orient work-group culture away from emphasizing time spent on work activities and toward results achieved (Kelly et al., 2011; Kelly, Ammons, Chermack, & Moen, 2010; Moen, Kelly, & Hill, 2011). The pilot study in the retail corporate headquarters (www.rowe.iambestbuy.com) confirmed that employees in the intervention groups reported greater schedule control, lower levels of negative work-to-family spillover, better sleep, more energy, and better health management (such as seeing a doctor when sick; Kelly et al., 2011; Moen, Kelly, Tranby, & Huang, 2011). This study also showed that reduced work–family conflict improved employee health behaviors and reduced behavioral pathogens (Moen, Kelly, Tranby et al., 2011). Research has also shown that functionally impoverished environments—those lacking in socially supportive interactions—influence a range of negative health outcomes (Taylor, Repetti, & Seeman, 1997). Therefore, a second set of interventions increased supervisors' social support for work–family balance issues. In the grocery industry, managers received training in interpersonal processes, and participated in self-monitoring of their subsequent behaviors. Employees whose supervisors received the family-supportive training had improved reports of physical and mental health, self-reported sleep quality, lower turnover intentions, less actual turnover, and better performance appraisals than employees whose supervisors were in the control group (Hammer et al., 2011; Hammer, Kossek, Yragui, Bodner, & Hansen, 2009; Kossek, Hammer, Michel, Petty, & Yragui, 2009). Significantly, the first intervention study provided evidence for a mediational model in which changes in workplace policies reduce stress from work–family conflict, and this decrease in work–family conflict then leads to increased time adequacy, increased hours of sleep, and improved health behaviors (Kelly et al., 2011; Moen, Kelly, Tranby et al., 2011). The second intervention demonstrated that enriching the social environment improved self-reported physical health for workers with high levels of work–family conflict, a moderated meditational model (Hammer et al., 2011).

The Work, Family, and Health Network Theoretical Model

Based on these above pilot results, an interdisciplinary literature review (Kelly et al., 2008), and previous scholarship by network members, the WFHN created a theoretically and empirically derived biopsychosocial model (see Fig. 15.1). The model represents the critical indicators and causal pathways linking an intervention to increased employee temporal control within the context of family-supportive supervision and job redesign. Figure 15.1 presents the core components of this theoretical model.

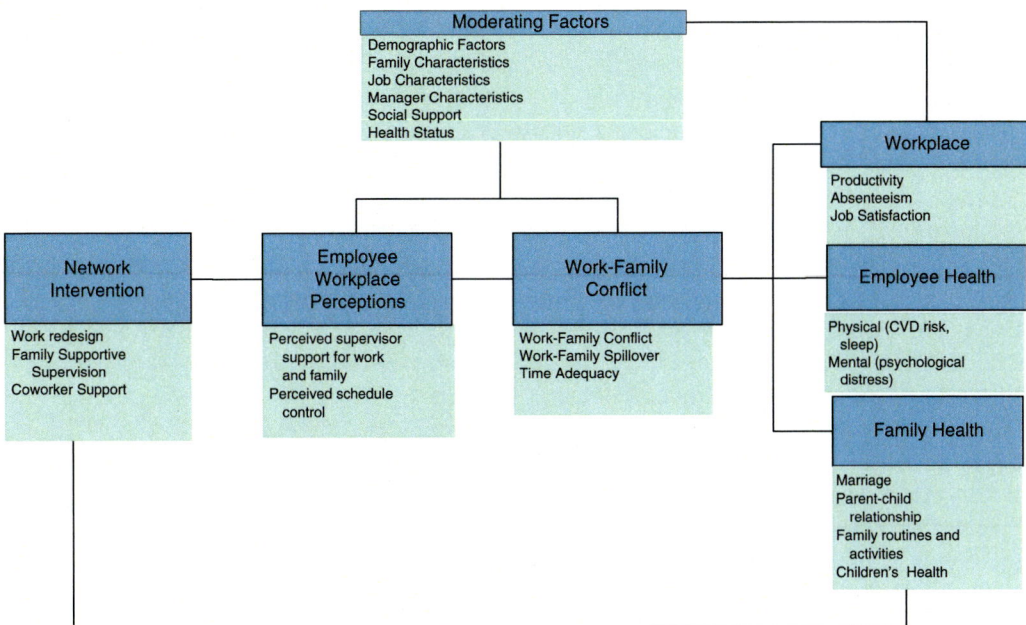

Fig. 15.1 Work, family, and health conceptual model

We theorized that a successful intervention will influence employee perceptions of control and support and reduce work–family conflict, which will improve the health and well-being of employees and their families. We linked the health of the work environment stress, health outcomes for the individual, and the health quality of the individual's work and family social environments (Taylor et al., 1997). The reduction of this stressor should also improve workplace outcomes such as productivity, absenteeism, turnover, and overall job satisfaction. We hypothesized that moderating factors affecting work–family conflict and the intervention's effectiveness include: demographic characteristics; job, family, and manager characteristics; employee health; and social support outside the workplace.

Workplace Intervention and Work–Family Conflict

The evidence discussed above suggests that supervisors' support for family and personal life, as well as employees' control over their work time, is a crucial component for interventions to reduce work–family conflict. Theory from a number of disciplines (Bronfenbrenner, 2005; Karasek & Theorell, 1990; Landsbergis, 1988) postulates an orthogonal relationship between employee schedule control and social support, and that, within the context of reasonable demands, both together produce healthy environments that encourage individual development and well-being. The Network intervention is not a one-size-fits-all or one-time treatment but, rather, a facilitated process in which supervisors and employees look carefully at current supervisory and temporal practices, and then identify concrete changes that may improve their work conditions to ameliorate work–family conflict. The intervention is designed to prompt reflection and improve workplace practices regarding two questions: (1) What concrete actions can work groups take to increase the control team members have over when, where, and how work is done (i.e., hours and/or predictability) while simultaneously meeting business goals? (2) What concrete actions can supervisors take to demonstrate their support of employees' lives and family responsibilities? Workplace change efforts should focus on improving these constructs to generate measureable change in outcome measures. Specifically, this workplace intervention consists of: (1) a *work redesign*; and (2) increasing *support* from supervisors and coworkers. Both supervisor training and work redesign promoting flexibility occur in the context of an organization's existing policies, regulations, staffing strategies, and financial constraints. Some organizational constraints may be reevaluated in light of the intervention while others, such as collective bargaining agreements, are less amenable to change in the short-term. Family-supportive supervisor training, coupled with actions to ensure transfer of training, such as behavioral self monitoring, provides supervisors with managerial tools to assist employees as they gain more control over their work time. Previous research has found wide variability in supervisors' implementation of flexible work and scheduling policies (Blair-Loy & Wharton, 2002; Hammer, Kossek, Zimmerman, & Daniels, 2007; Kelly & Kalev, 2006; Kossek, 2005). It is therefore essential to teach supervisors how to enable greater schedule control and facilitate greater social support on the part of their employees.

The proposed work redesign initiative is innovative, compared to customary flexible work arrangements (Kelly & Moen, 2009; Moen, Kelly, & Chermack, 2009). It aims to change the organizational structure by having employees and managers focus solely on the desired result of an assignment, not the time that employees spend at the workplace. Employees are instructed that they now have autonomy to decide when and where they work so long as they are meeting their objectives and contributing to their team's goals and effectiveness. Unlike typical arrangements that may accommodate individual employees, this redesign process is implemented by work groups ("teams" of employees and supervisors). Interactive training sessions guide each work group through a critical assessment of their traditional work culture; prompt group members to clarify specific work outcomes and expectations; and help group members identify new strategies for meeting job expectations while providing employees more control over their work time. Measurable changes resulting from the intervention are expected to include increases in employee schedule control, changes in organizational systems supportive of employee time control, changes in managerial self-awareness and supportive behaviors, and changes in employee behavior and organizational citizenship. We hypothesize, as depicted in our model (Fig. 15.1), that the intervention effects are mediated through employee perceptions of the support that the supervisors and coworkers provide (Hammer et al., 2007), and the perceived schedule control they have over the timing and location of work (Kelly & Moen, 2007). These perceptions about the psychosocial work environment then affect employees' experience of work–family balance (Kelly et al., 2008). Changes in workplace behaviors and work-time expectations may also directly affect more objective measures, such as the proportion of schedule changes that are initiated by employees versus managers and turnover.

Work–Family Conflict and Workplace Outcomes

Meta-analyses and reviews show that work–family conflict is significantly correlated with higher work stress, turnover intentions, absenteeism, and family stress (Allen et al., 2000). It is also correlated with lower family, marital, life, and job satisfaction, and lower organizational commitment and productivity (e.g., Allen et al.; Eby et al., 2005; Kossek & Ozeki, 1998). Recent research has demonstrated that higher levels of work–family conflict are also related to lower levels of participation in workplace safety procedures (Cullen & Hammer, 2007). Negative stress in the workplace also creates consequences for businesses, including reduced employee productivity and increased turnover (e.g., Grandey & Cropanzano, 1999; Kelly et al., 2008; Moen & Huang, 2010; Moen, Kelly, & Hill, 2011; Netemeyer, Boles, & McMurrian, 1996; O'Neill & Davis, 2011). Outcomes in our model for employers include turnover, absenteeism, productivity, higher job satisfaction of workers, better safety compliance, and return on investment (ROI). Employers will not implement new policies and practices, unless they can ensure that the benefits of the implementation outweigh the costs, or that there is a positive return on investment.

Work–Family Conflict and Employee Health

Work–family conflict is correlated with both the mental and physical health of employees (Frone, Russell, & Cooper, 1997). Over time, the effects of work–family conflict appear in objectively measured and self-reported health indicators, such as high blood pressure (e.g., Belkic, Landsbergis, Schnall, & Baker, 2004; Landsbergis et al., 2002), sleep complaints (Lallukka, Rahkonen, Lahelma, & Arber, 2010), and other mental and physical health problems (Frone, 2000; Ganster & Schaubroeck, 1991; Greenhaus, Allen, & Spector, 2006; Grzywacz & Bass, 2003). A recent national study showed that increases in work–family conflict predicted increases in the number of chronic health conditions and self-rated health problems over a 10-year period (Dmitrieva, Baytalskaya, & Almeida, 2007). Negative work-to-family spillover, when an individual's experiences at work continue to affect him or her even after leaving the worksite, is related to lower self-reported health status, more chronic disease, and higher levels of dysphoria, psychological distress, and sickness absence (Grzywacz, 2000; Vaananen et al., 2004). Limited research has also examined the implications of work–family conflict for health behaviors. However, researchers have demonstrated a link between work pressure and problem drinking (Grzywacz & Marks, 2000; Roos, Lahelma, & Rahkonen, 2006), and heavy alcohol and cigarette use (Frone, Barnes, & Farrell, 1994). In addition, Grzywacz and colleagues (2007) found promising support that workplace flexibility can contribute to healthy lifestyle behaviors, including better sleep habits and participation in stress management practices. Furthermore, higher job control has been linked to more regular physical activity (Grzywacz & Marks, 2001). We hypothesize that these effects work in much the same way as classical job strain measures based on high demand and low control. Often, low workplace support has impacted a host of outcomes, especially cardiovascular-related outcomes (Karasek et al., 1998). Health outcomes included in our model for employees include cardiovascular risk, sleep behaviors, tobacco and alcohol use, other indicators of chronic conditions and function, and mental health (e.g., psychological distress, depression).

Work–Family Conflict and Family Outcomes

Drawing from an emotional transmission paradigm (Larson & Almeida, 1999) and family systems theory (Cox & Paley, 1997), our model also considers that employees' work experiences can spill over into their home lives and cross over to their family members' health. Families are a nexus of social exchanges, and the emotional tone of family interactions varies in intensity and valence in ways that have implications for family members' individual well-being and family relationships (Repetti, Taylor, & Seeman, 2002). Extant research has demonstrated that workplace stressors can spill over to family life and strain parent–child and marital relationships evidenced by more conflict or withdrawal (Almeida, Wethington, & Chandler, 1999; Crouter, Bumpus, Head, & McHale, 2001; Repetti, 2005). Furthermore, time conflicts between work and family can interfere with families' daily routines and activities, such as family meals and effective parenting. For example, McLoyd and colleagues (2008) found that among single mothers, work demands were linked to higher work–family conflict which, in turn, was associated with fewer family routines. Family routines provide children with a sense of family cohesion, intimacy, and stability that are important for psychological well-being and for buffering the effects of daily stress (Fiese, Foley, & Spagnola, 2006; Jacob, Hill, Mead, & Ferris, 2008). Family relationship quality and satisfaction are important not only for individual family members' well-being, but also their experiences at work; there is evidence of spillover from family to work, an often neglected side of the work–family interface (Dilworth, 2004). Growing evidence suggests that the stress employees experience on the job can also cross over to family members. Crossover occurs when the stress and strain of an individual are then experienced by another person in the course of social interactions (Westman, 2001). For example, increased work–family conflict is associated with depression among spouses (Hammer, Allen, & Grigsby, 1997; Hammer, Cullen, Neal, Sinclair, & Shafiro, 2005). Most of the crossover research focuses on spouses (e.g., Hammer et al., 1997; Westman; Westman, Etzion, & Horovitz, 2004), but some research also shows crossover from parents to children (Crouter, Davis, Updegraff, Delgado, & Fortner, 2006; Davis, 2008; McLoyd, Toyokawa, & Kaplan, 2008), and even the children's caregivers (Kossek, Pichler, Meece, & Barratt, 2008). Davis' daily diary study (2008) of female hourly hotel workers and their children demonstrated that work stressors on a given day were associated with boys' lower positive affect that same day. Therefore, based on existing research and family theory, outcomes in our model for family health include marital relationship quality, parent–child relationship quality, effective parenting practices, family routines, and children's psychological and physical health.

Moderating Factors

The links between working conditions (and changes in them), work–family conflict, and health-related outcomes occur in particular social-locational contexts. Accordingly, our model includes the potential for moderating effects. Demographic factors, such as gender, marital status, race, age or life stage, and socioeconomic status, shape family status, the types of jobs people hold, and their health (Casper & Bianchi, 2002). They are also associated with the contexts in which people deal with work and family issues. For example, low wage employees and those in poor neighborhoods are less likely to have access to goods and services that would lessen work–family conflict and improve health. Other factors affecting employees' abilities to manage work–family conflict might include the degree of social support they have in their families and communities and family characteristics, such as the number of children and adults in family or the presence of a disabled family member. These factors help to define the number and types of work–family issues that arise and the availability of others who can be counted on for help should assistance become necessary. The health of employees is also likely related to their ability to perform work and family duties. Manager characteristics may affect employees' level of work–family conflict and their health, irrespective of the job characteristics and the intervention being applied. Thus, moderators in our model include demographic and contextual factors, social support, family characteristics, health status, and manager characteristics.

Summary

Mounting evidence suggests that Americans are experiencing difficulty in meeting work and family responsibilities, leading to negative consequences for the health and well being of employees, their families, and the workplace. Work–family balance issues have been defined more as a "private trouble" (cf Mills, 1959) of individual workers and their families than as a public issue. While family-friendly and leave policies in US workplaces have changed dramatically in recent years (Bond, Galinsky, Kim, & Brownfield, 2005; Glass & Estes, 1997; Kelly, 2003; Kossek, 2005), they are frequently only "on the books" or otherwise defined on the margins, not challenging the basic organization of work (Kelly & Moen, 2007; Kossek et al., 2010). These work–family balance issues cause acute and chronic stress which have negative health consequences. Work–leave and more general family-friendly policies may serve as a leverage point for psychosocial interventions to forestall or ameliorate this stress, and thus improve physical and mental health. The Work, Family, and Health Network theorizes that changing working conditions is the best prevention strategy for the dilemmas faced by working families. Few theoretically driven longitudinal studies are using experimental designs to evaluate how specific work–family interventions affect work–family conflict and health outcomes. The conceptual model described in this chapter addresses limitations in current studies, and provides a framework for an intervention study that can be applied to diverse industries and employees. We expect to see improvements in both worker's perceptions of their health through self-reported measures and objective improvements in health measured through biomarkers. Because employees' experience of stress tends to last beyond the boundaries of the workday, and because emotional stress is likely to be transmitted to other family members, we also include measures to allow us to examine potential positive effects in social units at home. These interventions should also benefit employers by improving workplace productivity.

Conclusions

Given the limitations at the micro-level (the individual) and the macro-level (the government), the meso-level, or the workplace itself, may be the best scientific focus for designing and evaluating work–leave and related interventions in order to ameliorate work–family balance issues and improve health. Interventions on this level may later inform more macro-level policies in the public and private sectors. Survey and interview evidence links policies and practices, such as flextime, schedule control, and supervisor support, for work–family balance issues to a variety of positive outcomes. These outcomes include increases in job and life satisfaction and organizational commitment, and decreases in work–family conflict, absenteeism, intentions to quit, actual turnover, and health behaviors that are pathogenic (Berkman et al., 2010; Kelly et al., 2008; Kossek et al., 2011; Moen, Kelly, & Hill, 2011; Moen, Kelly, Tranby et al., 2011; O'Neill et al., 2009). Both structure and culture count at the workplace. Work–family conflict increases with both a functionally impoverished social environment and ineffective workplace policies and programs regarding employees' control over the time and timing of work (e.g., Hammer et al., 2007, 2009; Kelly et al., 2011; Kelly & Moen, 2007; Kossek et al.; Kossek & Michel, 2011; Moen, Kelly & Huang, 2008). Therefore, successfully intervening at workplaces may lower work–family conflict; have salutary impacts on workers, their spouses, and their children; and improve the employer's bottom line.

Future Directions

A full evaluation of our theoretical model requires a number of subsequent studies. As noted in the literature, health interventions tend to be programmatically complex and context-dependent, and require: comprehensive evaluations that delineate the efficacy of the implementation of these interventions; the contextual and structural factors that influence the interventions' effectiveness; and the efficacy of the interventions themselves along a continuum of theoretically derived outcomes (Danaher & Seeley, 2009; Rychetnik, Frommer, Hawe, & Shiell, 2002). To accomplish this in future research, we will first undertake a comprehensive test of the model parameters, through a series of methodological studies assessing the reliability and validity of our measures, and testing the mediating and moderating hypothesis. Additionally, because this model relies on a workplace intervention, we have included a process evaluation to document fully the program and the context in which it is implemented. This process evaluation will describe the theoretical underpinnings of the WFHN intervention, the design strategies for customizing the intervention to meet the program's objectives while adhering to fiscal and regulatory requirements at the workplace, and the implementation strategies for fully deploying a job redesign and adaptive change processes aimed at reducing work and family conflict. These efforts are consistent with existing research which suggests that workplace interventions focusing on job stress and employee well-being require deliberate attention to the linkages among the program objectives, the context, and the intended outcomes (Kelly et al., 2008). However, this redesign will vary depending on the nature of the industry and the job to be performed.

As a means of assessing program fidelity, we will analyze data from our protocols to measure treatment receipt and treatment enactment as measures of program implementation (Bellg et al., 2009; Lichstein, Riedel, & Grieve, 1994). Treatment receipt or program exposure involves an assessment of the extent to which the program participants received critical elements of the program and demonstrate knowledge of, and ability to use, this knowledge or skills. We documented program dosage using observations and tracking logs for each intervention session. Treatment enactment assesses the degree to which the program participant applies the skills or knowledge acquired in the program. We documented program enactments or outputs through structured interviews with key stakeholders and through participant self-report measures. Our implementation study will facilitate the interpretation of the main study findings. Future research should map the terrain of variation in terms of what characteristics allow for which successful adaptations, and document whether some workplaces are simply not fixable. We will also look carefully at variation by our moderators. Particular combinations of work and family characteristics may make individuals more or less vulnerable to stress, and may influence how movable their stress is with this type of intervention. We may need to provide alternate theoretical models of pathways and mechanisms for different employee populations. We may also find that stress manifests in different aspects of health by moderators. For example, we would already expect gender differences in the likelihood of demonstrating internalizing versus externalizing negative health behaviors. If work–family balance issues are more salient for women, then we might find stronger prevention effects of our intervention on depression than alcohol use.

Our outcome analyses will assess program effectiveness using statistical methods accounting for multiple levels of measurement, including the employee, work group, manager, and family. Our study data include longitudinal self report measures, biometric measures, and a daily diary study to examine effects on family functioning and daily stress. Our model examines the intervention effects at each measurement level, and could be extended to include measures of the crossover between levels. Understanding the interactive relationship between work outcomes and health can inform future program development and research. For example, targeted interventions (including non-workplace-based programs) that improve family function might have positive crossover effects on workplace outcomes. Our model could also be extended to include a feedback loop to understand the lasting effects of the intervention and the need for ongoing health promotion interventions. The theoretical model presented here ends with improved health and positive workplace outcomes. Logically, healthier workers in healthier families will both perform more efficiently, and thus face decreased demands for health promotion efforts for themselves and at home. For example, weight loss maintenance is less demanding than the treatment period of exercise and nutritional change. Likewise, alleviation of depression and psychosocial distress should result in an improved outlook on one's work and home situations Thus, changes in our outcomes should theoretically then influence both actual work–family balance demands and the need for leave, as well as perceptions of schedule control and supervisor support in a positive direction. In this scenario, a one-time intervention has lasting effects through feedback over time.

Our theoretical model also directs our efforts toward adapting the environment rather than the individual. The opening chapter to this Handbook notes that adaptation to stress responses may occur in a maladaptive way over time if stressors are unusually persistent. Given that routine family caregiving demands are a feature of major life course stages, stressors from work–family balance issues fall into this category, calling into question efforts to "fix" the worker. Our workplace redesign includes tracking and evaluation of effects of the adaptation on the workplace to ensure that the outcomes are functional. Finally, we evaluate economic implications for the employers through a robust "return on investment" study, and assess translational potential by identifying key factors related to program adoption and diffusion. We anticipate that our findings will challenge the existing organization of work, which was designed for a workforce in the middle of the last century, without the family care responsibilities prevalent in today's workforce.

References

Allen, T. D., Herst, D. E. L., Bruck, C. S., & Sutton, M. (2000). Consequences associated with work-to-family conflict: A review and agenda for future research. *Journal of Occupational Health Psychology, 5*, 278–308.

Almeida, D. M., & Davis, K. D. (2011). Workplace flexibility and daily stress processes in hotel employees and their children. *The Annals of the American Academy of Political and Social Science, 638*(1), 123–140. Special issue on workplace flexibility.

Almeida, D. M., Wethington, E., & Chandler, A. (1999). Daily spillover between marital and parent child conflict. *Journal of Marriage and the Family, 61*, 49–61.

Belkic, K. L., Landsbergis, P. A., Schnall, P. L., & Baker, D. B. (2004). Is job strain a major source of cardiovascular disease risk? *Scandinavian Journal of Work, Environment & Health, 30*, 85–128.

Bellg, A. J., Borrelli, B., Resnick, B., Hecht, J., Minicucci, D. S., Ory, M., et al. (2009). Enhancing treatment fidelity in health behavior change studies: Best practices and recommendations from the NIH Behavior Change Consortium. *Health Psychology, 23*, 443–451.

Berkman, L. F., Buxton, O., Ertel, K., & Okechukwu, C. (2010). Managers' practices related to work-family balance predict employee cardiovascular risk and sleep duration in extended care settings. *Journal of Occupational Health Psychology, 15*, 316–329.

Bianchi, S. M., Casper, L. M., & King, R. B. (Eds.). (2005). *Work, family, health, and well-being*. Mahwah, NJ: Lawrence Erlbaum.

Blair-Loy, M., & Wharton, A. S. (2002). Employee's use of work–family policies and the workplace social context. *Social Forces, 80*, 813–845.

Bond, J., Galinsky, E., Kim, S., & Brownfield, E. (2005). *National study of employers*. New York: Families and Work Institute.

Bronfenbrenner, U. (2005). *Making human beings human: Bioecological perspectives on human development*. Thousand Oaks, CA: Sage.

Bureau of Labor Statistics. (2011a). Employee benefits in the United States—March 2011. Accessed at November 21, 2011 http://bls.gov/ncs/ebs/sp/ebnr0017.txt.

Bureau of Labor Statistics. (2011b). *Employment and Earnings On-line, 58*(1), 49. Accessed at http://www.bls.gov/cps/cpsaat36.pdf.

Casper, L. M., & Bianchi, S. M. (2002). *Continuity and change in the American family: Anchoring the future*. Thousand Oaks, CA: Sage.

Casper, L. M., & Bianchi, S. M. (2009). The stalled revolution: Gender and time allocation in the United States. In B. Mousli-Bennett & E. Roustang-Stoller (Eds.), *Women, feminism, and femininity in the 21st century: French and American perspectives*. New York: Palgrave Macmillan.

Chesley, N., & Moen, P. (2006). When workers care: Dual earner couples' caregiving strategies, benefit use, and psychological well-being. *American Behavioral Scientist, 49*(9), 1248–1269.

Christensen, K., & Schneider, B. (Eds.). (2010). *Workplace flexibility: Realigning 20th-century jobs for a 21st-century workforce*. Ithaca, NY: Cornell University Press.

Cox, M. J., & Paley, B. (1997). Families as systems. *Annual Review of Psychology, 48*, 243–267.

Crouter, A. C., & Booth, A. (2009). *Work-life policies*. Washington, DC: Urban Institute.

Crouter, A. C., Bumpus, M. F., Head, M. R., & McHale, S. M. (2001). Implications of overwork and overload for the quality of men's family relationships. *Journal of Marriage and the Family, 63*, 404–416.

Crouter, A. C., Davis, K. D., Updegraff, K., Delgado, M., & Fortner, M. (2006). Mexican American fathers' occupational conditions: Links to family members' psychological adjustment. *Journal of Marriage and the Family, 68*, 843–858.

Cullen, J. C., & Hammer, L. B. (2007). Developing and testing a theoretical model linking work-family conflict to employee safety. *Journal of Occupational Health Psychology, 12*, 266–278.

Danaher, B. G., & Seeley, J. R. (2009). Methodological issues in research on web-based behavioral interventions. *Annals of Behavioral Medicine, 38*, 28–39.

Davis, K. D. (2008). *Daily positive and negative work-family spillover and crossover between mothers and children*. Dissertation, The Pennsylvania State University.

Dentinger, E., & Clarkberg, M. (2002). Informal caregiving and retirement timing among men and women. *Journal of Family Issues, 23*, 857–879.

Dilworth, J. E. L. (2004). Predictors of negative spillover from family to work. *Journal of Family Issues, 25*, 241–261.

Dmitrieva, N., Baytalskaya, N., & Almeida, D. M. (2007). Longitudinal changes in work-family conflict predict changes in health. Poster presented at the 60th Annual Scientific Meeting of the Gerontological Society of America, San Francisco, CA.

Dye, J. L. (2008). *Fertility of American Women 2006. Current Population Reports, P20-558*. Washington, DC: U.S. Census Bureau.

Eaton, S. (2003). If you can use them: Flexibility policies, organizational commitment, and perceived performance. *Industrial Relations, 42*, 145–167.

Eby, L. T., Casper, W. J., Lockwood, A., Bordeaux, C., & Brinley, A. (2005). Work and family research in IO/OB: Content analysis and review of the literature (1980–2002). *Journal of Vocational Behavior, 66*, 124–197.

Ertel, K. A., Koenen, K. C., & Berkman, L. F. (2008). Incorporating home demands into models of job strain: Findings from the work, family, and health network. *Journal of Occupational and Environmental Medicine, 50*, 1244–1252.

Executive Office of the President Council of Economic Advisors. (2010). *Work-Life Balance and the Economics of Workplace Flexibility*. Accessed March 31, 2010 http://www.whitehouse.gov/blog/2010/03/31/economics-workplace-flexibility.

Fiese, B. H., Foley, K. P., & Spagnola, M. (2006). Routines and ritual elements in family mealtimes: Contexts for child well-being and family identity. *New Directions for Child and Adolescent Development, 111*, 67–89.

Frone, M. R. (2000). Work-family conflict and employee psychiatric disorders: The national comorbidity survey. *Journal of Applied Psychology, 85*, 888–895.

Frone, M. R., Barnes, G. M., & Farrell, M. P. (1994). Relationship of work-family conflict to substance use among employed mothers: The role of negative affect. *Journal of Marriage and the Family, 56*, 1019–1030.

Frone, M. R., Russell, M., & Cooper, M. L. (1997). Relationship of work-family conflict to health outcomes: A four-year longitudinal study of employed parents. *Journal of Occupational and Organizational Psychology, 70*, 325–335.

Ganster, D. C., & Schaubroeck, J. (1991). Work, stress and employee health. *Journal of Management, 17*, 235–271.

Gareis, K. C., Barnett, R. C., Ertel, K. A., & Berkman, L. F. (2009). Work-family enrichment and conflict: Additive effects, buffering, or balance? *Journal of Marriage and the Family, 71*, 696–707.

Glass, J. (2004). Blessing or curse? Work–family policies and mother's wage growth over time. *Work and Occupations, 31*, 367–394.

Glass, J. L., & Estes, S. B. (1997). The family responsive workplace. *Annual Review of Sociology, 23*, 289–313.

Goodwin, P. Y., Mosher, W. D., & Chandra, A. (2010). Marriage and cohabitation in the United States: A statistical portrait based on Cycle 6 (2002) of the National Survey of Family Growth. National Center for Health Statistics. *Vital Health Stat, 23*(28). http://www.cdc.gov/nchs/data/series/sr_23/sr23_028.pdf.

Grandey, A., & Cropanzano, R. (1999). The conservation of resources model and work-family conflict and strain. *Journal of Vocational Behavior, 54*, 350–370.

Greenhaus, J. H., Allen, T. D., & Spector, P. E. (2006). Health consequences of work-family conflict: The dark side of the work-family interface. In P. L. Perrewe & D. C. Ganster (Eds.), *Research in occupational stress and well-being* (Vol. 5, pp. 61–98). Amsterdam: Elsevier.

Greenhaus, J. H., & Beutell, N. J. (1985). Sources of conflict between work and family roles. *Academy of Management Review, 10*, 76–88.

Grzywacz, J. G. (2000). Work–family spillover and health during midlife: Is managing conflict everything? *American Journal of Health Promotion, 14*, 236–243.

Grzywacz, J. G., Almeida, D. M., & McDonald, D. A. (2002). Work-family spillover and daily reports of work and family stress in the adult labor force. *Family Relations, 51*, 28–36.

Grzywacz, J. G., & Bass, B. L. (2003). Work, family, and mental health: Testing different models of work-family fit. *Journal of Marriage and the Family, 65*, 248–262.

Grzywacz, J. G., Casey, P. R., & Jones, F. A. (2007). The effects of workplace flexibility on health behaviors: A cross-sectional and longitudinal analysis. *Journal of Occupational and Environmental Medicine, 49*, 1302–1309.

Grzywacz, J. G., & Marks, N. F. (2000). Family, work, work-family spillover, and problem drinking during midlife. *Journal of Marriage and the Family, 62*, 336–348.

Grzywacz, J. G., & Marks, N. F. (2001). Social inequalities and exercise during adulthood: Toward an ecological perspective. *Journal of Health and Social Behavior, 42*, 202–220.

Hamilton, B. E., Martin, J. A., & Ventura, S. J. (2009). *Births: Preliminary Data for 2007, National Vital Statistics Reports (Vol. 57, No. 12)*. Hyattsville, MD: National Center for Health Statistics.

Hammer, L., Allen, E., & Grigsby, T. (1997). Work-family conflict in dual-earner couples: Within-individual and crossover effects of work and family. *Journal of Vocational Behavior, 50*, 185–203.

Hammer, L. B., Cullen, J. C., Neal, M. B., Sinclair, R. R., & Shafiro, M. (2005). The longitudinal effects of work-family conflict and positive spillover on experiences of depressive symptoms among dual-earner couples. *Journal of Occupational Health Psychology, 10*, 138–154.

Hammer, L. B., Kossek, E. E., Bodner, T., Anger, K., & Zimmerman, K. (2011). Clarifying work-family intervention processes: The roles of work-family conflict and family supportive supervisor behaviors. *Journal of Applied Psychology, 96*, 134–150.

Hammer, L., Kossek, E., Yragui, N., Bodner, T., & Hansen, G. (2009). Development and validation of a multi-dimensional scale of family supportive supervisor behaviors (FSSB). *Journal of Management, 35*, 837–856.

Hammer, L. B., Kossek, E. E., Zimmerman, K., & Daniels, R. (2007). Clarifying the construct of family supportive supervisory behaviors (FSSB): A multilevel perspective. In P. L. Perrewe & D. C. Ganster (Eds.), *Research in occupational stress and well-being* (Vol. 6, pp. 171–211). Oxford: Elsevier.

Hammer, L. B., Neal, M. B., Newsom, J. T., Brockwood, K. J., & Colton, C. L. (2005). A longitudinal study of the effects of dual-earner couples' utilization of family-friendly workplaces supports on work and family outcomes. *Journal of Applied Psychology, 90*, 799–810.

He, W., Sengupta, M., Velkoff, V., & DeBarros, K. (2005). *65+ in the United States: 2005. Current Population Reports, P23-209*. Washington, DC: U.S. Census Bureau.

Jacob, J. I., Hill, E. J., Mead, N. L., & Ferris, M. (2008). Work interference with dinnertime as a mediator and moderator between work hours and work and family outcomes. *Family and Consumer Sciences Research Journal, 36*, 310–327.

Jacobs, J. A., & Gerson, K. (2004). *The time divide: Work, family, and gender inequality*. Cambridge, MA: Harvard University Press.

Karasek, R. A., Jr., & Theorell, T. (1990). *Healthy work: Stress, productivity, and the reconstruction of working life*. New York: Basic Books.

Karasek, R., Brisson, C., Kawakami, N., Houtman, I., Bongers, P., & Amick, B. (1998). The job content questionnaire (JCQ): An instrument for internationally comparative assessment of psycholosical job characteristics. Journal of Occupational Health Psychology, 3, 322–355.

Kelly, E. L. (2003). The strange history of employer-sponsored child care: Interested actors, uncertainty, and the transformation of law in organizational fields. *The American Journal of Sociology, 109*, 606–649.

Kelly, E. L. (2005). Discrimination against caregivers? Gendered family responsibilities, employer practices, and work rewards. In L. B. Nielsen & R. L. Nelson (Eds.), *Handbook of employment discrimination research* (pp. 353–374). Berlin/Heidelberg: Springer.

Kelly, E. L., Ammons, S. K., Chermack, K., & Moen, P. (2010). Gendered challenge, gendered response: Confronting the ideal worker norm in a white-collar organization. *Gender and Society, 24*, 281–303.

Kelly, E. L., & Kalev, A. (2006). Managing flexible work arrangements in US organizations: Formalized discretion or 'a right to ask'. *Socio-Economic Review, 4*, 379–416.

Kelly, E., Kossek, E., Hammer, L., Durham, M., Bray, J., Chermack, K., et al. (2008). Getting there from here: Research on the effects of work-family initiatives on work-family conflict and business outcomes. *The Academy of Management Annals, 2*, 305–349.

Kelly, E. L., & Moen, P. (2007). Rethinking the clockwork of work: Why schedule control may pay off at work and at home. *Advances in Developing Human Resources, 9*(4), 487–506.

Kelly, E. L., Moen, P., & Tranby, E. (2011). Changing workplaces to reduce work-family conflict: Schedule control in a white-collar organization. *American Sociological Review, 76*, 1–26.

Kennedy, S. & Bumpass, L. (2007). Cohabitation and Children's Living Arrangements: New Estimates from the United States. *Center for Demography and Ecology Working Paper, 2007-2020*, Madison, WI

Kossek, E. E. (2005). Workplace policies and practices to support work and families. In S. Bianchi, L. Casper, & R. King (Eds.), *Work, family, health, and well-being* (pp. 97–116). Mahwah, NJ: Lawrence Erlbaum.

Kossek, E. E. (2006). Work and family in America: Growing tensions between employment policy and a changing workforce. A thirty year perspective. In E. Lawler & J. O'Toole (Eds.), *America at work: Choices and challenges* (pp. 53–72). New York: Palgrave MacMillan.

Kossek, E., Hammer, L., Michel, J., Petty, R., & Yragui, N. (2009). *An embedded leadership and work group context perspective on work-family conflict*. Paper presented at Society of Industrial Organizational Psychology National Meetings, New Orleans, Louisiana.

Kossek, E. E., Lewis, S., & Hammer, L. (2010). Work-life initiatives and organizational change: Overcoming mixed messages to move from the margin to the mainstream. *Human Relations, 63*, 1–17.

Kossek, E. E., & Michel, J. (2011). Flexible work scheduling. In S. Zedeck (Ed.), *Handbook of industrial-organizational psychology* (pp. 535–557). Washington, DC: American Psychological Association.

Kossek, E. E., & Ozeki, C. (1998). Work-family conflict, policies, and the job-life satisfaction relationship: A review and directions for organizational behavior/human resources research. *Journal of Applied Psychology, 83*, 139–149.

Kossek, E., Pichler, S., Bodner, T., & Hammer, L. (2011). Workplace social support and work-family conflict: A meta-analysis clarifying the influence of general and work-family specific supervisor and organizational support. *Personnel Psychology, 64*(2), 289–313.

Kossek, E., Pichler, S., Meece, D., & Barratt, M. (2008). Family, friend and neighbor child care providers and maternal well-being in low income systems: An ecological social perspective. *Journal of Organizational and Occupational Psychology, 81*, 369–391.

Kreider, R. M., & Elliott, D. R. (2009). *America's Families and living arrangements 2007. Current population reports, P20-561*. Washington, DC: U.S. Census Bureau.

Lallukka, T., Rahkonen, O., Lahelma, E., & Arber, S. (2010). Sleep complaints in middle-aged women and men: The contribution of working conditions and work-family conflicts. *Journal of Sleep Research, 19*, 466–477.

Landsbergis, P. A. (1988). Occupational stress among health care workers: A test of the job demands-control model. *Journal of Organizational Behavior, 9*, 217–239.

Landsbergis, P. A., Schnall, P. L., Belkic, K. L., Baker, D., Schwartz, J. E., & Pickering, T. G. (2002). The workplace and cardiovascular disease: Relevance and potential role for occupational health psychology. In J. C. Quick & L. E. Tetrick (Eds.), *Handbook of occupational health psychology* (pp. 265–288). Washington, DC: American Psychological Association.

Larson, R. W., & Almeida, D. M. (1999). Emotional transmission in the daily lives of families: A new paradigm for studying family process. *Journal of Marriage and the Family, 61*, 5–20.

Lee, M. D., MacDermid, S. M., & Buck, M. L. (2000). Organizational paradigms of reduced load work: Accommodation, elaboration, and transformation. *Academy of Management Journal, 43*(6), 1211–1226.

Lichstein, K. L., Riedel, B. W., & Grieve, R. (1994). Fair tests of clinical trials: A treatment implementation model. *Advances in Behavior Research and Therapy, 16*, 1–29.

McLoyd, V. C., Toyokawa, T., & Kaplan, R. (2008). Work demands, work-family conflict, and child adjustment in African American families: The mediating role of family routines. *Journal of Family Issues, 29*, 1247–1267.

Melchior, M., Berkman, L. F., Niedhammer, I., Zins, M., & Goldberg, M. (2007). The mental health effects of multiple work and family demands: A prospective study of psychiatric sickness absence in the French GAZEL study. *Social Psychiatry and Psychiatric Epidemiology, 42*, 573–582.

Mills, C. W. (1959). *The sociological imagination*. New York: Oxford University Press.

Moen, P. (2003). *It's about time: Couples and careers*. Ithaca, NY: Cornell University Press.

Moen, P. (2007). Not so big jobs (and retirements): What older workers (and retirees) really want. *Generations, 31*(1), 31–36.

Moen, P., & Altobelli, J. (2007). Strategic selection as a retirement project: Will Americans develop hybrid arrangements? In J. James & P. Wink (Eds.), *The crown of life: Dynamics of the early postretirement period* (pp. 61–81). New York: Springer Publishing Company.

Moen, P., & Chesley, N. (2008). Toxic job ecologies, lagging time convoys, and work-family conflict: Can families (re)gain control and life course "fit"? In K. Korabik, D. S. Lero, & D. Whitehead (Eds.), *Handbook of work–family integration: Theories, perspectives, and best practices* (pp. 95–122). New York: Elsevier.

Moen, P., & Hernandez, E. (2009). Social convoys: Studying linked lives in time, context, and motion. In G. Elder Jr. & J. Giele (Eds.), *The craft of life course research* (pp. 258–279). New York: Guilford Press.

Moen, P., & Huang, Q. (2010). Customizing careers by opting out or shifting jobs: Dual-earners seeking life-course 'fit'. In K. Christensen & B. Schneider (Eds.), *Workplace flexibility: Realigning 20th century jobs to 21st century workers* (pp. 73–94). New York: Cornell University Press.

Moen, P., Kelly, E., & Chermack, K. (2009). Learning from a natural experiment: Studying a corporate work-time policy initiative. In A. C. Crouter & A. Booth (Eds.), *Work-life policies that make a real difference for individuals, families, and organizations* (pp. 97–131). Washington, DC: Urban Institute Press.

Moen, P., Kelly, E. L., & Hill, R. (2011). Does enhancing work-time control and flexibility reduce turnover? A naturally occurring experiment. *Social Problems, 58*(1), 69–98.

Moen, P., Kelly, E. L., & Huang, Q. (2008). Work, family, and life-course Fit: Does control over work time matter? *Journal of Vocational Behavior, 73*, 414–425.

Moen, P., Kelly, E., Tranby, E., & Huang, Q. (2011). Changing work, changing health: Can real work-time flexibility promote health behaviors and well-being? *Journal of Health and Social Behavior, 52*(4), 404–429.

Moen, P., & Roehling, P. (2005). *The career mystique: Cracks in the American dream*. Lanham, MD: Rowman and Littlefield.

Morgan, S. P. (2010). Thinking about demographic family differences. In M. Carlson & P. England (Eds.), *Changing families in an unequal society*. Unpublished Book Manuscript.

National Research Council and the Institute of Medicine. (2004). Health and safety needs of older workers. Committee on the health and safety needs of older workers. In D. H. Wegman & J. P. McGee (Eds.), *Division of behavioral and social sciences and education*. Washington, DC: The National Academies Press.

Neal, M. B., & Hammer, L. B. (2007). *Working couples caring for children and aging parents: Effects on work and well-being*. Mahwah, NJ: Lawrence Erlbaum Associates.

Netemeyer, R. G., Boles, J. S., & McMurrian, R. (1996). Development and validation of work-family conflict and family-work conflict scales. *Journal of Applied Psychology, 81*, 400–410.

Nomaguchi, K. M. (2009). Change in work-family conflict among employed parents between 1977 and 1997. *Journal of Marriage and the Family, 71*, 15–32.

O'Neill, J. W., & Davis, K. D. (2011). Differences in work and family stress experienced by managers and hourly employees in the hotel industry. *International Journal of Hospitality Management, 30*, 385–390.

O'Neill, J. W., Harrison, M. M., Cleveland, J., Almeida, D., Stawski, R., & Crouter, A. C. (2009). Work-family climate, organizational commitment, and turnover: Multilevel contagion effects of leaders. *Journal of Vocational Behavior, 74*, 18–29.

Perlow, L. (1997). *Finding time: How corporations, individuals, and families can benefit from new work practices.* Ithaca, NY: Cornell University Press.

Presser, H. (2003). Race-ethnic and gender differences in nonstandard work shifts. *Work and Occupations, 30*(4), 412–439.

Rapoport, R., Bailyn, L., Fletcher, J., & Pruitt, B. (2002). *Beyond work–family balance: Advancing gender equity and work performance.* London: Wiley.

Repetti, R. (2005). A psychological perspective on employment and family well-being. In S. Bianchi, L. Casper, & R. King (Eds.), *Work, family, health, and well-being.* Mahwah, NJ: Erlbaum.

Repetti, R. L., Taylor, S. E., & Seeman, T. E. (2002). Risky families: Family social environments and the mental and physical health of offspring. *Psychological Bulletin, 128*(2), 330–366.

Roos, E., Lahelma, E., & Rahkonen, O. (2006). Work-family conflicts and drinking behaviours among employed women and men. *Drug and Alcohol Dependence, 83*, 49–56.

Rychetnik, L., Frommer, M., Hawe, P., & Shiell, A. (2002). Criteria for evaluating evidence on public health interventions. *Journal of Epidemiology and Community Health, 56*, 119–127.

Sayer, L. C., Cohen, P. N., & Casper, L. M. (2004). Women, men, and work. In R. Farley & J. Haaga (Eds.), *The American people: Census 2000.* New York: Russell Sage.

Schuster, M. A., Chung, P. J., Elliott, M. N., Garfield, C. F., Vestal, K. D., & Klein, D. J. (2008). Awareness and use of California's Paid Family Leave Insurance among parents of chronically ill children. *Journal of the American Medical Association, 300*, 1047–1055.

Stebbins, L. (2001). *Work and family in America: A reference handbook* (annotatedth ed.). Santa Barbara, CA: ABC-CLIO.

Sweet, S., Moen, P., & Meiksins, P. (2007). Dual earners in double jeopardy: Preparing for job loss in the new risk economy. *Research in the Sociology of Work, 17*, 445–469.

Tang, C., & Wadsworth, S. M. (2010). *Time and workplace flexibility.* New York: Families and Work Institute.

Taylor, S. E., Repetti, R. L., & Seeman, T. (1997). Health psychology: What is an unhealthy environment and how does it get under the skin? *Annual Review of Psychology, 48*, 411–447.

Thomas, L. T., & Ganster, D. C. (1995). Impact of family-supportive work variables on work-family conflict and strain: A control perspective. *Journal of Applied Psychology, 80*, 6–15.

Thompson, C. A., Beauvais, L. L., & Allen, T. D. (2006). Work and family from an industrial/organizational psychology perspective. In M. Pitts-Catsouphes, E. E. Kossek, & S. Sweet (Eds.), *The work and family handbook: Multi-disciplinary perspectives and approaches.* Mahwah, NJ: Erlbaum.

U.S. Census Bureau. (2010). Press Release (January 15, 2010). http://www.census.gov/Press-release/www/releases/archives/families_households/014540.html

Vaananen, A., Kevin, M. V., Ala-Mursula, L., Pentti, J., Kivimaki, M., & Vahtera, J. (2004). The double burden of and negative spillover between paid and domestic work: Associations with health among men and women. *Women & Health, 40*(3), 1–18.

Westman, M. (2001). Stress and strain crossover. *Human Relations, 54*, 717–751.

Westman, M., Etzion, D., & Horovitz, S. (2004). The toll of unemployment does not stop with the unemployed. *Human Relations, 57*, 823–844.

Williams, J. (2000). *Unbending gender: Why family and work conflict and what to do about it.* New York: Oxford University Press.

Workers' Compensation and Its Potential for Perpetuation of Disability

Michael E. Schatman

Overview

Workers' compensation, in its various forms, was developed as a means of protecting employees, injured while working, from financial ruin. Over more recent years, a secondary purpose of this type of insurance has developed, which is to protect employers from lawsuits by injured workers (Davis, n.d.). In relationship to the history of workers' compensation, vocational retraining is relatively new, originating in the "human investment" literature that rose to prominence in the 1960s (Mincer, 1962). Pocius (n.d.), however, has noted that returning injured workers to vocational activity has already become "a forgotten aspect of workers' compensation," and that by providing such activity should be considered one of several "humanitarian" aspects of the system. According to Pocius, vocational reactivation helps not only the employer and the insurer, but the workers' compensation recipient as well. This is a perspective from which this chapter is written. It will examine the potential role of workers' compensation systems in inadvertently perpetuating disability in cases in which doing so is unnecessary. Taking a global view, it begins with a history of workers' compensation throughout the world, examining differences in systems not only between nations, but between different States in the United States. Some of the primary factors that cause the perpetuation of disability in certain systems are examined. Finally, this chapter examines one particularly dysfunctional workers' compensation system, with case studies illustrating the perpetuation of disability by the system as a means of highlighting the glaring problems that can occur when a system is neither adequately developed nor appropriately administered.

Brief History of Workers' Compensation

While workers' compensation represents a relatively new phenomenon in the United States, Guyton (1999) has noted that: "The history of compensation for bodily injury begins shortly after the advent of written history itself" (p. 106). Ancient Sumerian scriptures date monetary compensation for work-related

M.E. Schatman, Ph.D., CPE (✉)
Schatman-Robinson Pain Psychology Associates, Foundation for Ethics in Pain Care,
1601 114th Ave. SE, Suite 100, Bellevue, WA 98004, USA
e-mail: headdock@comcast.net

injuries back to 2050 BC (Kramer, 1958), with the *Code of Hammurabi* in Mesopotamia dating similar compensation back to 1750 BC (Smith, 1931). Additionally, Ancient Greek, Chinese, and Roman laws included sets of compensation schedules (Geerts, Kornblith, & Urmson, 1977), each of which specified circumscribed payments for losses of body parts. In the feudalistic Middle Ages, however, compensation for work-related injuries essentially disappeared, as indemnification was left to the arbitrary whims of feudal lords (Guyton, 1999). For many subsequent years, injured workers were left without appropriate protection, and needless suffering occurred due to this lack of oversight and regulation.

Modern workers' compensation was pioneered in Germany in the 1870s and 1880s through autonomous industry insurance funds referred to as *"Berufsgenossenschaften"* (Clayton, 1997). This process was actually championed by the socially conservative Prussian Chancellor, Otto von Bismarck, as a pragmatic move to neutralize the influence of the worker-friendly Marxist movement that was growing at the time (Perlin, 1985). Although Britain enacted the *Employer's Liability Act* as early as 1880, proof of employer negligence was still required in order for an injured worker to receive compensation. It was not until 1897 that Parliament passed a "no fault" doctrine (Hadler, 1995). In the United States, policies protecting injured workers came about more slowly. Although several States attempted to enact workers' compensation laws as early as 1898, it was not until Congress passed the *Employers' Liability Acts* of 1906 and 1908 that a genuine workers' compensation program became effective. Unfortunately, these Acts covered only railroad workers involved in interstate commerce (Baker, 1992). In 1911, Wisconsin became the initial State to pass a comprehensive workers' compensation law, and 36 other States followed suit by the end of the decade. Mississippi became the final state to pass workers' compensation legislation in 1948 (Fishback & Kantor, 2000).

At any given time, 10 % of the US work force is experiencing work disability due to industrial injury or illness (Weil, 2001). However, there exists considerable heterogeneity in workers' compensation systems from State to State, including rates of work-related disability within workers' compensation systems. Private insurance carriers are the largest provider of workers' compensation policies, with all but four States—North Dakota, Ohio, Washington, and Wyoming—allowing private carriers to provide workers' compensation benefits (Sengupta, Reno, & Burton, 2009). Twenty-one States allow private carriers to provide workers' compensation benefits, despite the availability of competing State-sponsored coverage. Some may consider such competition between the private sector and the government to be ideal, as it will theoretically foster efficacy and efficiency. The proportion of benefits for which competitive State funds account varies from a low of 5.4 % in South Carolina to a high of 59.5 % in Arizona. With the exception of North Dakota and Wyoming, which require all employers to obtain coverage through their State funds, all States allow employers to self-insure for workers' compensation. The rates of self-insurance in States that allow it vary from a low of 13.3 % in Rhode Island to a high of 50.8 % in Alabama. All but five States allow for policies with deductibles. Shares of workers' compensation benefits by type of insurer have also been found to vary considerably across the States (Sengupta et al., 2009). Complicating the situation in the United States is the continued federal workers' compensation covering federal employees and coal miners diagnosed with black lung disease, longshore and harbor workers, employees of overseas contractors with the US government, energy employees exposed to hazardous material, workers involved in the manufacturing of atomic bombs, and veterans injured on active duty in the Armed Forces. A 2004 report (Hunt, 2004) noted the extreme variance across States regarding the adequacy of medical and earning replacement benefits. It is clear that the United States does not have "a workers' compensation system," but rather a myriad of systems that provide benefits in very different manners. The relationships between the insurance industry and each State's regulations has been empirically determined to impact businesses' willingness to acknowledge reports of industrial injuries and to commence benefits in workers' compensation systems (Boden & Ruser, 2003).

Data indicate that the rates at which employees return to the workforce following industrial injury vary dramatically between countries. For example, a six-country cohort study of chronic low back patients indicated a sustainable return-to-work (RTW) rate, ranging from 22 % in a German cohort to 62 % in a Dutch cohort at 2 years of follow up (Anema, Schellart, & Cassidy, 2009). The authors of the study attributed this wide range to variance in applied work interventions and the eligibility criteria for long-term disability benefits. Some in the United States have lambasted the American "welfare mentality" as contributing to deficiencies in returning injured workers to work, presenting a "moral hazard" (Bolduc, Fortin, Labreqecque, & Lanoie, 2002). This conceptualization is certainly consistent with criticism that our work ethic has devolved into a "something-for-nothing" mentality.

The infeasibility of even directly comparing States' workers' compensation data has recently been noted. Stover and Seixas (2009) attributed this problem to a number of factors, including inconsistencies in "statutes of limitations" for filing, employer-selection vs. worker-selection of initial physician seen for treatment, exclusion of certain industries and occupations, exclusion by employer size, exclusion of self-insured companies, and specific illnesses or injuries covered by State systems. Moreover, a recent study assessed the heterogeneity of treatment of work-related acute pain from a geographical perspective. Webster and colleagues (2009) examined workers' compensation claims for acute low back pain, and found that the rate of opioid prescription ranged from 5.7 % of patients in Massachusetts, to 52.9 % in South Carolina. Given the prodigious body of evidence that suggests that workers' compensation patients who are prescribed opioid analgesics are less likely to return to work and experience prolonged disability (Dersh et al., 2007; Gross et al., 2009; Kidner, Mayer, & Gatchel, 2009; Mahmud et al., 2000; Volinn, Fargo, & Fine, 2009; Webster, Verma, & Gatchel, 2007), the implications of these findings are formidable. Irrespectively, more empirical investigation is necessary before concrete conclusions regarding this relationship can be comfortably drawn.

States vary in their regulations regarding compromise and release (C&R) as a means of mitigating expenses to carriers for medical services and/or lost wage indemnity, with a recent analysis determining that the vast majority of States allow such agreements (Hunt & Barth, 2010). The authors note, however, that certain States actively discourage C&R in workers' compensation. Considerable variance is seen in the average amount of these "lump-sum" payments, ranging from approximately $13,000.00 in Indiana to $49,000.00 in Pennsylvania (Telles, Eccleston, Radeva, Yang, & Tanabe, 2009). It has been speculated that the practice of C&R serves to discourage return to employment (Reville, Boden, Biddle, & Mardesich, 2001), with a study conducted by the Minnesota Office of the Legislative Auditor in 2009 (State of Minnesota Office of the Legislative Auditor, 2009) indicating a tendency for injured workers receiving settlements to accept their lump-sum payment and leave the work force. However, it should be noted that the complexity of the relationship between lost wage indemnity and disability has likely been underestimated, and that results of a single-State study, such as that performed in Minnesota, do not necessarily generalize to other geographic regions.

The Complex Relationship Between Workers' Compensation Indemnity and Disability

Common sense suggests that those who are entitled to lost wage indemnity through workers' compensation deserve such financial support because they are truly disabled. However, many theorists and empirical investigators have attempted to unravel the very complicated relationship between financial compensation and disability, with the heterogeneity of results suggesting that doing so is a challenging endeavor. Much of the research aimed at understanding how financial compensation impacts disability has examined differences in disability between compensated vs. non-compensated patients, with early research (Abram, Anderson, & Maitra-D'Cruze, 1981; Brena, Chapman, & Bradford,

1980; Sander & Meyers, 1986; Trief & Stein, 1985) suggesting, for the most part, that those receiving compensation experienced poorer treatment outcomes compared to those who were not being compensated. However, results of a more methodologically robust study by Dworkin and colleagues in 1985 (Dworkin, Handlin, & Richlin, 1985) suggest that when employment and compensation are jointly used to predict outcome, only employment status is significant. The authors utilized their results to bring question to the potentially deleterious effects of the concept of *"compensation neurosis."* A 1988 study by Jamison and colleagues (1988) found that *time-limited* compensation did not necessarily adversely affect clinical outcomes or return-to-work status, although *unlimited* compensation may do so. Accordingly, the authors concluded that those receiving time-limited financial benefits may not represent a "problem" subgroup of chronic pain patients. This is logically sound, as many in the Jamison et al. study (Jamison et al.), whose vocational outcomes were not adversely affected, were *acute* pain sufferers rather than *chronic* pain patients. The tremendous variance in psychosocial sequelae of chronic vs. acute pain sufferers, although beyond the scope of this analysis, is obvious.

Although many subsequent studies (Biondi & Greenberg, 1990; Hanley & Levy, 1989; Herron & Mangelsdorf, 1991; Kleinke & Spangler, 1988; Tollison, Satterthwaite, Kriegel, & Hinnant, 1990) have suggested that receiving compensation payments is related to inferior clinical outcomes, other investigations (Barnes, Smith, Gatchel, & Mayer, 1989; Connally & Sanders, 1991; Jamison et al., 1988) have indicated the likely presence of intervening variables in determining the relationship. Through reviews, Mendelson (1986, 1988, 1991) and, more recently, others (Bryant, 2003; Spearing & Connelly, 2010) have strongly challenged the validity of the concept of *"compensation neurosis"*— despite its continued utilization to "explain" failure to recover from work-related injuries by insurance carriers and defense attorneys. Interestingly, numerous studies and systematic reviews conducted on populations outside of the United States (Abbott, Rounsefell, Fraser, & Goss, 1990; Allaz, Vannotti, & Desmeules, 1998; Mendelson, 1995; Ownsworth, Fleming, & Hardwick, 2006; Schlesinger, Hering-Hanit, & Dagan, 2001; Scholten-Peeters, Verhagen, & Bekkering, 2003; Shin, Chang-Bong, & Min-Su, 2010; Wood & Rutterford, 2006) were even less likely to identify a relationship between receiving compensation and poor clinical outcomes when compared to American investigations. This suggests that there exists something inherent in the American system(s) of compensation that provides a greater disincentive to return to work than is the case in other nations' systems. Accordingly, one can speculate that, compared to workers in other industrialized nations in which health care is guaranteed through the government, injured American workers may be reluctant to allow their workers' compensation benefits to be terminated partially due to a fear that they will no longer have *any* access to necessary medical treatment for residuals of their injuries. Although not yet empirically investigated, this author's practice is replete with anecdotal reports from patients that this scenario indeed occurs. Campbell (2006) has suggested that *"compensation neurosis"* is related to the wide divisions between classes in society and, accordingly, represents a reaction of anger toward social injustice. Few would argue that the divisions between classes in the United States are not more glaring than in other industrialized nations, with this assertion supported by recent Organisation for Economic Co-operation and Development (OECD) data (n.d.). It is also interesting that Hungerer and colleagues (2011) recently noted that the German workers' compensation system is more heavily focused on rehabilitative efforts as opposed to compensation payments. American systems, on the other hand, vary in the extent to which they focus on rehabilitation vs. compensation, perhaps explaining the variance from State-to-State in return-to-work rates. Unfortunately, as most States do not maintain data on return-to-work rates of their workers' compensation recipients, we are forced to rely upon anecdotal reports in drawing this conclusion. Again, more accurate record maintenance will allow for research that may substantiate this position.

Irrespective of the empirical data refuting the concept of *litigation or compensation neurosis*, the roles of potential secondary and tertiary gain have to be considered in any discussion of a workers' compensation system's perpetuation of disability. "Secondary gain," a concept that originated in the psychoanalytical literature, refers to an "…interpersonal or social advantage attained by the patient as a consequence of… illness" (Freud, 1959). However, the term has, over the years, become largely a legal concept (Kwan & Friel, 2002), with Finneson (1976) suggesting 35 years ago that the term had come to refer to financial awards associated with disability. Although Freud considered secondary gain to represent unconscious behavior, the term has unfortunately become strongly equated with malingering, which is a conscious behavior (Dersh, Polatin, Leeman, & Gatchel, 2004). This inadequate distinction between unconscious secondary gain and consciously motivated malingering seems to be most prevalent in situations in which potential financial gain is an issue (King, 1994). There is no simple test for the detection of malingering, and assumptions based on limited data can be quite dangerous. According to the American Academy of Clinical Neuropsychology Consensus Conference Statement (Heilbronner et al., 2009), "…the context of the evaluation and overall presentation of the examinees, including background information, history information gathered during interview, observations, neuropsychological tests, and measures of response bias, should be considered in this process" (pp. 1097–1098). Although the concept of secondary gain is highly speculative, its relative lack of negative connotation, compared to the label of "malingering," suggests that it clearly safer to use, with a considerably less pejorative connotation.

Some empirical investigation has supported the phenomenon of secondary gain in the workers' compensation arena. For example, Loeser and colleagues (1995) determined that the higher the percentage of one's working wages that were provided as workers' compensation lost wage indemnity, the greater the frequency and duration of workers' compensation claims. However, other studies have failed to support secondary gain as relevant in workers' compensation cases (Sprehe, 1984; Tarsh & Royston, 1985), with Harris and colleagues (2005) noting that many of the studies that lend support to the concept of secondary gain are methodologically flawed. Additionally, it is important to note that the empirical literature (Fishbain, Rosomoff, Cutler, & Rosomoff, 1995; Bellamy, 1997) does not necessarily support the notion that symptoms "magically" resolve with the resolution of compensation or litigation, thereby serving to detract from the strength of the argument supporting the salience of the secondary gain concept.

Despite the lack of clarity regarding the existence and impact of secondary gain, workers' compensation systems seem to accept and even exploit the concept, at times using it to take advantage of injured workers. This process of exploitation serves as a severe stressor to many claimants (Benner, 2007), resulting in anger, demoralization, and frustration with the system. As injured workers suffer more emotionally due to carrier accusations (often further muddled by insurers' failure to distinguish accurately between "secondary gain" and "malingering," as discussed above), their exacerbated depression can potentially have a demotivating impact on their efforts toward vocational reactivation. This de-motivational effect of depression has been strongly supported empirically (Cléry-Melin et al., 2011; Elliott et al., 1996; Lane, 1980; Richards & Ruff, 1989), with depression identified as a predictor of failure to return to work following injury (Ash & Goldstein, 1995). Accordingly, the pejorative labeling of injured workers' symptoms can have a significant emotional impact on them, thereby serving to further perpetuate disability. Although it is quite likely that unconscious secondary gain motivating work-avoidance plays a role in preventing vocational reactivation in many workers' compensation cases, it is also evident that the over-attribution of its causal role can also indirectly impede the return-to-work process.

Beyond secondary gain, the concept of *tertiary gain* in workers' compensation needs to be considered in any discussion of perpetuation of disability. "Tertiary gain" is a concept introduced by Dansak in 1973 (Dansak, 1973) that refers to benefits gained from one's illness by one other than the actual patient. In discussing the role of tertiary gain in disability syndromes in 2001, Kwan and colleagues (2001) noted that little research or discussion of the topic appeared in the literature during the 28 years following Dansak's introduction of the concept. Unlike secondary gain, which was originally posed as an unconscious process, tertiary gain was conceptualized by the term's originator as the result of some self-serving intent (Dansak). Accordingly, it is a term that has always been utilized pejoratively, unlike secondary gain—whose meaning evolved over time into an almost universally negative one. Kwan & colleagues make an effort to present the concept as a "neutral phenomenon" rather than a "malignant" one by suggesting that the benefits "are attained automatically from the caregiver role, and their existence does not necessarily imply a motivation to receive gain" (p. 461). However, this effort has not necessarily been successful in the medicolegal arena. Although the authors emphasize the beneficence of the caregiver role in their analysis, they also acknowledge the potential for one to be motivated to pursue tertiary gain for non-altruistic reasons. They write, "While in that caregiver role, however, the individual may be motivated to again care not simply for 'caring's sake', but to pursue the recognized opportunity for tertiary gain, and this pursuit is then the underlying motivation for their behavior" (p. 461). Dersh and colleagues (2004) are kinder than most in assessing the motivation behind tertiary gain, stating that conscious, unconscious, and preconscious processes are all involved in its development.

Although several theoretical analyses of the impact of tertiary gain in potentially perpetuating disability in general have been written, there appears to be a paucity of literature regarding the role of tertiary gain in perpetuating disability specifically in cases involving workers' compensation. While much that has been written on the potential impact of tertiary gain on disability makes reference to family members and other caretakers, the potential for claimants' attorneys to seek tertiary gain in workers' compensation cases should not be underestimated. Schatman (2009), for example, notes that "medical bills function as a yardstick for indication of injury severity….the potential exists for personal injury victims to 'inflate' the sum of their medical bills by seeking medical treatment beyond that which is necessary to address the personal injuries that have been sustained." (p. 157). He goes on to observe that this behavior may be encouraged by injury victims' attorneys, as doing so will also potentially increase any settlement for disability, and thereby increase their contingency fees. Although family members certainly have the potential to gain from an injured workers' misfortune, the uniquely contentious medicolegal environment associated with workers' compensation provides an opportune setting in which workers' attorneys can benefit through the process of tertiary gain. This position is certainly consistent with the results of numerous studies that have associated claimants' attorneys' involvement with reduced likelihood of vocational reactivation (Ash & Goldstein, 1995; Bernacki & Tao, 2008; Blackwell, Leirerer, Haupt, & Kampotsis, 2003; Chibnall & Tait, 2010; Gardner, 1991; Hester, Decelles, & Gaddis, 1986; Tate, 1992). Yet, workers' compensation claimants' attorneys are not the only players in the system that can perpetrate tertiary gain-related disability. Defense attorneys representing insurance carriers are, of course, paid for their services, typically on an hourly basis (unlike plaintiffs' attorneys, who are typically paid on a contingency basis (Mnookin, 1998)). Reports of personal injury defense attorneys unnecessarily running up costs certainly can be found in the literature. For example, according to a RAND report, "…some defense attorneys increase their revenue by churning a case for a while, mediating the case for a while, and then settling,…" (Carroll, Dixon, Anderson, Hogan, & Sloss, n.d.) (p. 22). When this occurs, the potential for the legal process associated with the case to be prolonged exists, shifting the focus from vocational reactivation to generating maximal legal fees. Carriers need to be vigilant regarding their legal representatives' actions, as unscrupulous defense attorneys have the potential to alter the emphasis of the process from a rehabilitative one to a remunerative one. When legal battles take center stage, issues of vocational reactivation may lose their salience, and claimant disability can be inadvertently perpetuated.

What are some of the other determinants that account for the variance across workers' compensation systems' abilities to return their injured workers to gainful employment? While a number of factors seem to be involved, the *overall competence* of various systems seems to be a crucial factor. Such competence cannot be created by the workers' compensation carrier alone, as there exist myriad parties that are involved in determining vocational reactivation. Depending upon the system, these parties may include injured workers, their workers' compensation carriers, treating health care providers, attorneys (who may assist or impede vocational reactivation, depending upon their motivations), vocational counselors, labor unions, and, certainly, employers. The relative influence of each of these interested parties varies from system to system. Hunt (n.d.) provides us with an important analysis of comparative disability management between workers' compensation programs in 2009, looking at programs in Canada, as well as in the United States. The author takes a unique approach, examining disability management from an historical perspective. In describing the goal of disability management, Hunt writes, "Its purpose is to interrupt the negative progression of an injury or disease" (p. 1). The question arises whether all workers' compensation systems are genuinely invested in interruption of such negative progression, as opposed to having alternative agendas that have little to do with negative progression of injury or disease per se. Although disability avoidance through accident prevention has been considered a central component of disability management for many years (Habeck, Leahy, Hunt, Chan, & Welch, 1991), prevention is clearly beyond the scope of this present chapter. Realistically, irrespective of the rigor of accident prevention efforts, unwanted job-related injuries will occur. Given this unfortunate reality, the salient question becomes how different workers' compensation systems deal with injured workers once they are actually injured.

According to Hunt (n.d.), "Successful resolution relies primarily on the flexibility and willingness of the workplace to make accommodations and modifications, either temporary or permanent, to enable the worker to perform productive work successfully and safely" (p. 3). With so much focus on the claimant, treating health care providers, and, of course, the workers' compensation carrier, the role of the employer in determining vocational reactivation and disability management is often underestimated. Although the success of return-to-work efforts is traditionally attributed to worker characteristics such as beliefs, attitudes, and motivation, a 2003 Canadian study (Baril, Clarke, Friesen, Stock, & Cole, 2003) found that injured workers, their representatives, and health and safety managers attribute successful vocational reactivation to the workplace culture and consideration of the worker's well-being. Early international disability prevention and management studies, such as that conducted in the 1970s on Finnish municipal workers, involved workplace assessment (Järvikoski & Tuunainen, 1978), which occurs far too infrequently in most systems. While it has been claimed that there was a shift in the emphasis of workers' compensation in the United States to vocational reactivation over the last 20 years of the last century (Spieler & Burton, 1998), Hunt notes that the leadership role in disability management in the Canadian workers' compensation system has recently shifted to unions, employers, and other "interested individuals" working together in the interests of all involved. A recent Canadian qualitative study (MacEachen, Kosny, Ferrier, & Chambers, 2010) determined that, when an imbalance in power between these parties occurs, communication problems and impediment of return-to-work efforts arise, thereby potentially perpetuating disability unnecessarily. Following the Canadian example, the International Labour Organization has conceptualized disability management as optimally involving a combined union-management effort that includes the goal of maintenance of injured worker employment (International Labour Organization, 2002).

Employer goodwill toward injured employees has been empirically linked to a successful return to work (MacEachen, Clarke, Franche, Irvin, & the Workplace-Based Return to Work Literature Review Group, 2006). For example, when employers are unwilling to provide workplace accommodations to an injured employee, the likelihood of successful vocational reactivation decreases—with the literature suggesting that this phenomenon occurs in multiple nations' workers' compensation systems (Habeck, Scully, VanTol, & Hunt, 1998; Kirsh, 2001). However, it is likely that a broader approach of goodwill beyond that of the employer is necessary in order to optimize the likelihood of vocational reactivation following industrial injury. Although a spirit of *rapprochement* between all involved parties is likely ideal, goodwill on the part of the workers' compensation carrier is imperative to successful vocational reactivation and disability mitigation. While the literature (Lipscomb, Moon, Li, Pompeii, & Kennedy, 2002; Kennedy, Badger, Pompeii, & Lipscomb, 2003) suggests that managed care systems have the potential to facilitate healthy working relationships between employers, health care providers, and workers, and in doing so foster successful return-to-work, the *overly managed* care dictated by some workers' compensation systems can have just the opposite effect.

Workers' compensation system rigidity and unresponsiveness in the United Kingdom have been considered as a cause of previously fit workers becoming physically deconditioned (Disler & Pallant, 2001), with deconditioning empirically established as contributing to disability (Okawa, Nakamura, Kudo, & Ueda, 2009). Yet another disability-perpetuating behavior that may be evidenced by workers' compensation systems is claim manager misinterpretation of the scientific data necessary to accurately interpret medical conditions. This was established in a Canadian study (Lippel, 2003) as particularly problematic in regard to musculoskeletal injuries among women, resulting in a greater rate of denial of claims than among men. The author of the study writes, "Erroneous refusal of claims may thus exacerbate the gravity of the disability, and in many cases leads to permanent damage when early treatment could have prevented the onset of handicap" (p. 254). Few would argue that unjust delay or refusal of workers' compensation benefits—particularly health care—will potentially have a negative impact on one's health and contribute to the development of disability (Herbert, Janeway, & Schecter, 1999). The findings of the study on non-clinician decision-makers' misinterpretation of scientific data and its impact on the clinical decision-making process (Lippel) present a potentially frightening picture of workers' compensation systems. In an ideal system, all clinical decisions made on the administrative side would be made by well-qualified clinicians. Doing so, however, would obviously be cost-prohibitive. However, is there not a minimal level of clinical knowledge that decision-makers should possess if they are to make potentially life-altering determinations? The majority of workers' compensation case managers, who serve as liaisons between claimants and workers' compensation systems, are registered nurses (State of Vermont Department of Labor, n.d.). However, case managers are typically advisors to systems, and are not the clinical decision-makers. According to the United States Department of Labor Bureau of Labor Statistics (n.d.), "There are no formal education requirements for any of these occupations, and a high school degree is typically the minimal requirement needed to obtain employment." The absurdity of such medically uneducated individuals typically lacking any medical background whatsoever making decisions regarding the treatment that a board-certified physician can provide to injured workers is obvious. Theoretically, claims managers are under the direct supervision of medical directors, who are tasked with reviewing medical aspects of claims and correcting claim managers' errors in judgment. Unfortunately, there are often insufficient numbers of medical directors, resulting in an over-abundance of independent decision-making by unqualified parties. Given the established disregard for the insurance industry in general for principles of medical ethics in favor of the "business ethic" of cost-containment and profitability (Schatman, 2006, 2007), this failure to hire sufficient medical experts is not necessarily surprising. However, some practices by insurers are so outrageous that they defy belief. For example, in a recent case, this author determined that the "medical director" to whom a chronic musculoskeletal pain patient appealed her claim was actually a fertility specialist. When this was brought to the insurer's attention, the denial was quickly overturned. Unfortunately, in some workers' compensation systems, all appeals of claim manager decisions regarding allowance of treatment are handled *internally*. In such cases in which the workers' compensation carrier is permitted to function as "judge, jury, and executioner," obvious ethical issues arise. On a practical level, the end result is that, often, much-needed treatment is denied, thereby perpetuating a claimant's disability.

In addition to lacking adequate educational backgrounds and medical knowledge, many claims' managers are thought by claimants (as well as the physicians that treat their work-related injuries) to have an "ax to grind" against certain injured workers. In writing on the increasing immunity of claims adjusters, Stempel (2009) suggests that they should be held legally accountable for their misconduct, including for "bad faith." The author writes, "Faced with reduced incentive to discharge their duties well, the other intermediaries frequently act negligently, recklessly, or even in bad faith, needlessly creating claims imbroglios that could be avoided, minimized, or streamlined" (p. 603). While Stempel (2009) writes about insurance claims adjusters in general, his thesis is certainly applicable to workers' compensation claims managers. This creation of an adversarial relationship is not unique to the American system of workers' compensation. In a qualitative Australian study (Roberts-Yates, 2003), the author identified a theme of the perception that the workers' compensation carrier assumes that claimants are "either fraudulent or malingerers until they have proven otherwise" (p. 903). A very similar theme was identified in a Canadian qualitative study (Beardwood, Kirsh, & Clark, 2005), in which injured workers experienced responses from their insurers that they considered "demeaning and inappropriate."

Yet another feature of many workers' compensation systems that serves to perpetuate claimant disability is their lack of access to sufficient numbers of qualified health care professionals to treat injured workers. Many physicians choose not to accept workers' compensation patients into their practices, as the time spent in dealing with the bureaucratic "red tape" is typically overwhelming and not sufficiently remunerative. In a qualitative Canadian study (Beardwood et al., 2005), injured workers identified the amount of paperwork required by their physicians as a deterrent to adequate treatment. In the United States, physician refusal to participate in workers' compensation programs is rampant, particularly among certain specialties. In Texas and Hawaii, for example, neurologists' participation in workers' compensation decreased by 75 % following the adoption of a Medicare fee schedule (Illinois State Medical Society, 2011). A 2007 study (Levine, n.d.) identified a downward trend in medical specialists' willingness to accept workers' compensation for the previous 10 years. Orthopedist participation ranged from 23 to 46 % in the States that were included in the study, which is particularly alarming given the crucial role of orthopedists in workers' compensation. In a study conducted in New York State (Lax & Manetti, 2001), the investigators found that the lack of a guarantee of payment for services rendered deterred physicians from seeing injured workers. Research has already identified a shortage of pain specialists in the United States (Breuer, Pappagallo, Tai, & Portenoy, 2007). A progressive reduction of specialists such as neurologists and orthopedists, who treat so many workers' compensation injuries, will serve to exacerbate the impact of this shortage. As a result, fewer injured workers will receive the treatment that they need, thereby potentially perpetuating their disability.

While it is well beyond the scope of this chapter to compare every aspect of every nation's and every State's workers' compensation system, this analysis will turn to an examination of one State's woeful performance in returning injured workers to the work force (Washington State), and how its inadequacy serves to perpetuate disability among injured workers. Although Malloy (2003) has suggested that "If an employee who has reached maximum medical improvement fails to seek employment, the employer may discontinue disability benefits" (p. 836), this is clearly not true under all workers' compensation systems. In systems in which the carrier and the employer are essentially powerless to enforce vocational reactivation, considerable "gaming" by work-avoidant claimants may occur. The potential for disincentive for vocational reactivation is obvious in such cases, with disability needlessly perpetuating workers' abilities to remain free of the "burdens" of work, while continuing to be compensated. Whether consciously or unconsciously motivated, one would be naïve to believe that instances of secondary do not occur in these cases.

The Unfortunate Example of Washington State

A 2008 study found that the rates of Total Permanent Disability (TPD) in the Washington's workers' compensation system were four to eight times than those that could be expected given national data (Hunt, 2008). The author of this study suggests that Washington's statute prohibiting compromise and release (C&R) in workers' compensation cases "leads to longer durations of time loss and ultimately more total permanent disability pension (TPD) awards" (p. 3). Indeed, between 1998 and 2007, the number of L&I cases that were pensioned increased by over 20 %. Additionally, Hunt and colleagues (n.d.) note that Washington's system has the highest TPD rate in the United States. Hunt has noted that "…the workers' compensation system in Washington offers only two relatively extreme options, a low impairment rating with consequent small benefit, or a total permanent disability pension, with no compromise in between" (p. 3)—also contributing to subtle encouragement of disability. Compared to other States, Washington's law calls for awarding permanent partial disability payments based on relatively low impairment ratings, resulting in the payment of relatively small benefits. Accordingly, "The permanent partial disability benefit can be perceived as inadequate and all that can be done for the worker is to leave him/her on time-loss benefits or award a pension" (Barth & Hunt, 2010) (p. 2). Barth and Hunt (2010) link the likelihood of pensions in Washington to time-loss claims of long duration, which they note is an important cost driver within the State system. They also note that vocational rehabilitation services act as a "temporary way station on the way to a pension award." Washington lacks a coherent disability management program within the structure of L&I (i.e., one that would prevent acute injuries from becoming chronic) (Barth & Hunt). They observe that developing such a program would require a substantial "change in orientation, structure, and function at L&I." Given the rigidity of the system, however, significant changes seem to be at least passively discouraged. Barth and Hunt also recently reported that "the incidence of pensions under Washington's workers' compensation program appeared to be very high and out of line with the experience of most jurisdictions in the U.S." (Barth & Hunt) (p. 1). For the past 100 years, however, there has been an option for a commutation of cases, despite the lack of an option for C&R. However, due to a limit of $8,500, this option has fallen into disuse (Hunt & Barth, 2010).

So much of L&I's obsessive and fanatical efforts have been aimed at reducing opioid consumption among its enrollees (Franklin et al., 2005, 2008; Franklin, Rahman, Turner, Daniell, & Fulton-Kehoe, 2009; Franklin et al., 2012; Stover et al., 2006) that attention to vocational reactivation has been minimal. Because of the weakness of the vocational component of Washington State Workers' Compensation, two studies of multidisciplinary pain center outcomes among workers' compensation patients (Robinson, Fulton-Kehoe, Franklin, & Wu, 2004; Robinson, Fulton-Kehoe, Martin, & Franklin, 2001) actually found *no* effect for such programs on disability status, despite the myriad of American and international investigations and reviews that have been performed and that strongly support multidisciplinary treatment's efficacy in reducing work disability (Bosy, Etlin, Corey, & Lee, 2010; Bültmann et al., 2009; Gatchel & Okifuji, 2006; Gatchel et al., 2009; Greenberg & Bello, 1996; Guzmán et al., 2002; Harden & Cole, 1998; Huge et al., 2006; Mayer, Anagnostis, Gatchel, & Evans, 2002; Nordström-Björverud & Moritz, 1998; Schultz et al., 2008; Taylor, Simpson, Gow, & McNaughton, 2001; Vowles, Gross, & Sorrell, 2004; Wright, Mayer, & Gatchel, 1999). Curiously, despite the findings of the studies conducted by employees and associates of L&I, the agency continues to fund multidisciplinary treatment and, in fact, is the only insurer that does so in the State of Washington. However, this set of circumstances results in an ethical quandary, as when an interdisciplinary pain clinic depends on a single payer source, the payer is "always right" in situations of conflict between L&I and patients—which are common in disability situations. Anecdotal reports indicate that many claimants drop out of these programs in

Washington due to the perception of bias toward L&I on the part of the clinics that are treating them. These premature discontinuations of treatment, of course, result in claimants not receiving the treatment that the empirical evidence indicates is most likely to help them—thereby serving to further perpetuate their disability. Although the role of the health insurance industry in perpetuating sub-optimal pain care in the United States has recently been elucidated (Schatman, 2011), further discussion regarding the power of private insurers' attitudes toward interdisciplinary chronic pain treatment and their more subtle impact on injured workers in certain states, such as Washington, will certainly be merited.

Fortunately, the archaic Washington State L&I worker's compensation system is finally beginning to change in a positive direction. For example, in 2011, the State Legislature passed a bill that allows for Compromise and Release for recipients of benefits ages 55 and above (Washington Engrossed House Bill 2123, n.d.), which was signed into law by the Governor and took effect on June 15, 2011. As the average age of full retirement is increasing (Social Security Online, n.d.) progressively, due to economic and demographic factors as well as age of eligibility for Social Security benefits, this policy change will allow recipients to move forward with their lives by re-entering the workforce. It can be noted that this new legislation will currently impact only a small percentage of injured workers in Washington. However, the age requirement decreases to 53 in 2015 and to 50 in 2016, thereby increasing the number of workers' compensation recipients who may be positively affected by the legislation. Despite the benefits that may ultimately be associated with this new legislation, the failure of Washington L&I to return workers' compensation recipients to active employment is due primarily to the weakness of the vocational component of the program. Anecdotally, this clinician/researcher and colleagues treating workers' compensation recipients have concluded that anyone who desires to avoid vocational reactivation following a work-related injury can do so, particularly if that individual is represented by an attorney who is at least moderately competent. These tertiary gain issues among plaintiffs' attorneys have already been addressed earlier in this chapter. The system assigns injured workers, in certain cases, to contracted vocational counselors, whose obvious aims are to return the worker to employment. However, irrespective of the capabilities of the vocational counselors, injured workers can easily sabotage their efforts in a variety of ways. For example, a worker who is uninterested in returning to the workforce can endorse vocational options that he/she knows are outside of his/her physical limitations, or perhaps would require such extensive retraining that L&I is reluctant to make the type of financial investment that would make obtaining such a position realistic. Similarly, an injured worker can endorse vocational activity that is beyond his/her intellectual capacities—even if extensive vocational retraining were to be provided. In speaking to a number of vocational counselors, it has become apparent that they see themselves as impotent if an injured worker is "dead-set" against returning to active employment. After a period of time, the vocational counselor is deemed by L&I to have been unsuccessful in his or her efforts to facilitate vocational reactivation, and that counselor is removed from the case—subsequent to which any remote possibility of vocational reactivation ceases to exist. Once there is no longer a vocational counselor working on a case, perpetual disability is almost guaranteed.

Case Studies

The following are two case studies that illustrate the ways in which workers' compensation can serve to perpetuate disability. As this clinician/author practices in the State of Washington—a State in which the government-managed L&I system is so dysfunctional—these case studies will pertain to clients whose injuries (and rehabilitation) are the responsibility of Washington L&I.

Case Study #1

"Margie" is a 53-year-old white female who was employed as a house painter for over 20 years. In 2003, she fell off of a ladder while working, sustaining three fractured ribs, a collapsed lung, a ruptured spleen, and fractured thoracic vertebrae. She was immediately transported to a regional trauma center in Seattle, where she underwent several intensive surgeries. Following a period of convalescence, she initiated physical therapy. She was prescribed high-dosage opioid analgesics, which she has continued to take for 9 years. In addition to the development of physiological and psychological dependence, the claimant developed addictive behaviors associated with her opioid use. Eventually, L&I discontinued paying for her opioids, despite the fact that her attending physician (AP) continued to prescribe them. L&I cited a statute within the Washington Administrative Codes (WACs) stating that, in regard to chronic non-cancer pain, payment will be provided only for treatment that "must be of a type to cure the effects of a work-related injury or illness, or it must be rehabilitative. Curative treatment produces permanent changes, which eliminate or lessen the clinical effects of an accepted condition. Rehabilitative treatment allows an injured or ill worker to regain functional activity in the presence of an interfering accepted condition. Curative and rehabilitative care produce long-term changes" (Washington State Legislature, n.d.). Based on this WAC, L&I is *legally* justified, although not necessarily justified *ethically*, as L&I failed to provide any alternative treatment that this patient would tolerate that would ameliorate her suffering. Certainly, few would argue that opioids represent a "cure" for chronic non-cancer pain, with a number of studies (Darchuk, Townsend, Rome, Bruce, & Hooten, 2010; Dersh et al., 2008; Hooten, Townsend, Sletten, Bruce, & Rome, 2007; Kidner et al., 2009; Townsend et al., 2008) suggesting that chronic opioid therapy can actually either *interfere* or at least not contribute positively to the success of rehabilitative efforts. However, given this patient's issues of addiction, she was quickly able to find a so-called "pain specialist" operating a "cash-only" practice, and her opioid reliance has continued. Several psychiatric Independent Medical Examinations (IMEs) have attributed the maintenance of this claimant's depression to the effects of chronic high-dosage opioid usage, consistent with the empirical literature on opioid-induced mood disorder (Leventhal et al., 2011; Mowla, Kianpor, Bahtoee, Sabayan, & Chohedri, 2008; Sullivan, Von Korff, Banta-Green, Merrill, & Saunders, 2010). Unfortunately, despite its anti-opioidist stance, L&I is ultimately powerless to compel this claimant to discontinue chronic opioid therapy, or even to undergo treatment for opioid dependence and addiction.

In the period of time during which this author has worked clinically with Margie, she has repeatedly voiced a disinterest in vocational reactivation, stating that "there are no jobs that (she) wants to do." Efforts to discuss ethical issues associated with allowing L&I to financially support her when she is functionally capable of holding down some type of employment have been rejected by the claimant, due to her formidable sense of entitlement in conjunction with an ability to "play" a system whose policies toward vocational reactivation have been impotent. Margie underwent a functional capacity evaluation (FCE) per her attending physician, in which she failed the majority of the validity criteria—indicating likely submaximal effort. Despite paying for this expensive evaluation and receiving a report detailing the evaluation's findings, L&I chose not to act upon her efforts at deception. The claimant was sent to multiple interdisciplinary pain management programs, all of which at least purport to involve vocational rehabilitation components. Although figures identifying return-to-work rates of these programs are not readily available, it is evident that the efficacies of their vocational reactivation efforts are limited when compared to the return-to-work rates of the nation's top interdisciplinary programs. For example, the Productive Rehabilitation Institute of Dallas for Ergonomics (PRIDE) functional restoration program has reported return-to-work rates following program completion of over 85 % in a cohort of 1,316 consecutively treated patients (Proctor, Mayer, Gatchel, & McGeary, 2004). In addition to sending the claimant to interdisciplinary pain programs, L&I assigned a contracted vocational counselor to her case. Despite valiant efforts to return Margie to work (many of which were observed firsthand by this author), the claimant was sufficiently "savvy" to make vocational training and reactivation impractical. The concept of secondary gain, in its most negative utilization and understanding, clearly applies in this case. Currently, Margie is awaiting receipt of a pension for total disability from L&I, which has been her goal for many years. Not only has L&I not lived up to its proclaimed fiduciary obligation to the taxpayers of Washington State, but its own incompetence in the area of vocational reactivation has all but assured this claimant disability status for the rest of her potential working years.

Case Study #2

"Sally" is a 46-year-old white female who sustained a severe blow to her head at work, throwing her several feet into a brick wall in 2007. In this accident, she sustained injuries to her low back and neck, as well as a moderate to severe traumatic brain injury (TBI). She had been involved in another work-related accident 2 years earlier in which she slipped and fell, striking her head and injuring her low back and neck. However, according to the patient and her physicians, she had fully recovered from this initial injury, and had been able to return to work on a full-time basis well prior to her 2007 accident. Following her second accident, she sought treatment from a physiatrist with whom she had been successfully treated for injuries sustained in her first accident. The physiatrist noted pronounced depression (in addition to cognitive deficits), and referred her for a behavioral medicine evaluation through this author's practice. While psychosocial factors, including moderate to severe depression, pronounced somatic focus, and a behavioral pacing excess were identified, she was determined to be a poor candidate for behavioral medicine services at that time due to the severity of her cognitive deficits. Shortly following her behavioral medicine evaluation, she was referred to a neurologist specializing in TBI, who has subsequently continued to serve as her attending physician. L&I then sent her for a neuropsychological evaluation through an "independent" neuropsychologist, whose report indicated that she was experiencing no gross cognitive abnormalities. Interestingly, in a more recent "independent" neuropsychological evaluation funded by L&I, the same neuropsychologist noted significant cognitive gains since the time of his last evaluation of the claimant. The corruption and bias associated with the Independent Medical Evaluation system has been addressed elsewhere (Schatman & Sullivan, 2010), however, and is beyond the scope of this chapter. Let it suffice to note that the claimant was deeply distressed by the very biased and grossly inaccurate findings of these L&I-funded evaluations, exacerbating her depression temporarily. As a result of these exacerbations, the claimant experienced temporarily increased symptoms of depression, with associated motivational deficits exerting a negative impact on her performance in cognitive remediation. This is consistent with the reports of Benner (2007), a chronic pain sufferer and medical professional, who eloquently addressed the sense of depersonalization associated with the IME process and its contribution to despair and depression. Again, the egregious and unnecessary actions of her L&I Claim manager (CM) served to negatively affect the claimant's recovery, albeit temporarily, thereby serving to perpetuate her disability.

Since sustaining her injuries in 2007, Sally's case management by L&I has been marked by severe obstructionism by the insurer, which this author considers cruel and inhumane, as well as contributing to the perpetuation of her disability. For example, while demonstrating a willingness to provide treatment for her TBI, certain evidence-based treatments for her chronic pain have been denied by L&I. As one who has more than passively observed Sally's case, it appears that L&I is unwilling to accept the fact that a claimant can suffer from the cognitive effects of a TBI *while simultaneously suffering from debilitating chronic pain*. This seeming refusal to fully recognize and accept the comorbidity is bewildering, particularly given the substantial body of literature that addresses the frequent concomitant existence of these disorders and the need to treat both the pain and the cognitive deficits in order to restore quality of life (Branca & Lake, 2004; Gironda et al., 2009; Iezzi, Duckworth, Mercer, & Vuong, 2007; Lew et al., 2009; Martelli, Zasler, Bender, & Nicholson, 2004; Nampiaparampil, 2008; Patil et al., 2011). Various treating health care professionals have commented that they have been forced to "fit a square peg into a round hole" in their efforts to address the multiple work-related injuries and their sequelae associated with her accident. Based on the WACs, L&I-funded workers' compensation allows for one AP; if that physician is a specialist in TBI (as is true in Sally's case), what is the likelihood that sufficient focus will be placed on the amelioration of her suffering secondary to her chronic pain? This misguided policy also begs the question of whether a claimant can overcome her disability without all of the debilitating injuries associated with her work-related accident being appropriately addressed. Complicating this particular case was the AP's move to a university medical school-based practice. Upon recommendation, the claimant was referred to the Department of Anesthesiology at that medical center, where she was evaluated by one of the world's leading interventional pain specialists. After running a number of tests and providing several diagnostic injections, this physician determined that the patient's headaches would be ameliorated through a neurotomy. Unfortunately, due to political issues within her department, the anesthesiologist was "chased" out of the university, and was compelled to return to private practice in another State. When Sally was referred to a less accomplished anesthesiologist at the university, he refuted everything that the world-renowned physician had concluded through her evaluation, and L&I chose not to cover the originally recommended procedure. Once again, the claimant has been left without adequate pain management, and has been forced to rely upon medications that incapacitate her for up to 3 days each time she experiences a severe headache. According to Sally, her headaches, rather than her cognitive deficits, remain the primary factor impeding successful vocational reactivation. The claimant is aware that it will be impossible to maintain employment when she is forced to spend several days in bed at a time. This has been expressed to her CM on multiple occasions. Irrespective, nothing has been done to appropriately treat her headaches, further perpetuating her disability.

Obtaining appropriate psychiatric care for Sally has also been nightmarish. At one point, her L&I's CM questioned why she would need a psychiatrist when she is already receiving psychological counseling. Due to uncertain factors, the claimant has been extremely sensitive to psychotropic medications, demonstrating a limited capacity for tolerating their side effects as dosages are titrated toward therapeutic ranges. While she has been under the constant care of a well-qualified pain psychologist, that psychologist has been aware for several years of the absolute necessity of psychopharmacological intervention. Referrals have been made to psychiatrists, none of whom (until very recently) has had training or experience in dealing with chronic pain sufferers. Accordingly, these psychiatrists have been extremely insensitive to her needs, seeing her as a "difficult" patient, and often giving up on treating her. Compounding the problem is L&I's practice of forcing the claimant to wait for months at a time prior to providing authorizations for treatment. This practice, of course, prolongs disability, and, perhaps more egregiously, perpetuates human suffering.

It has been interesting for this author to observe L&I's response to his efforts to serve as this unfortunate claimant's advocate. Within the WACs, there is no provision for a patient advocate by L&I, irrespective of how crucial advocacy may be in a particular case. Despite citing work emphasizing the importance of serving as patients' *moral* agents as well as *therapeutic* agents (Giordano & Schatman, 2008a, 2008b), exposure of the insurer's obstructionist policies has certainly served to incur the wrath of L&I. At one point, bills for psychological services were denied, necessitating appeal. In speaking to the CM, this author questioned who would be "responsible" should the claimant commit suicide due to L&I's refusal to cover very necessary psychological services at a time at which the claimant was actively voicing suicidal ideation. To this query, the CM responded that culpability could not be determined until after the fact! In this single instance in this case, L&I actually *assisted* the patient in her efforts to escape from disability, as their behavior seemed to temporarily motivate her through increasing her anger. However, it is unlikely that the CM's motivation in this instance actually had any relationship to a desire to assist the claimant in overcoming her disability.

Summary and Conclusions

Workers' compensation, in various forms, has existed for over 4,000 years, and has the potential to ease human suffering, improve quality of lives, and, theoretically, reduce disability. However, not only do the purpose and effectiveness of different systems vary between nations but, unfortunately, vary tremendously from State to State within the United States. As a result, American workers' compensation systems are inconsistent, ranging from "the good, the bad, to the ugly." Attitudes of workers' compensation systems toward injured workers are generally negative, with claimants often considered fraudulent until proven otherwise. Beardwood and colleagues (2005) wrote of systems' attitudes toward claimants as characterized by "blame and marginalization," stating: "The difference in the case of injured workers is that this attitude is hidden beneath the rhetoric of return to work and rehabilitation" (p. 30). Because of a lack of system support, even injured workers who are motivated for vocational reactivation are often unsuccessful in their efforts. Chronic pain sufferers in workers' compensation systems are most vulnerable, with empirical data indicating that after 6 months, 50 % never return to work, and after a year, only 10–15 % ever work again (Gamborg, Elliott, & Curtis, 1992). Systems' abilities to reduce disability ultimately depend upon their overall competence. Although the Washington State L&I was highlighted in this analysis in order to illustrate a system that is totally inept at returning many injured workers to vocational activity, this is not to say that other States' systems all do a particularly good job at reducing disability either. Accordingly, future analyses need to be research-based, examining the specific elements of workers' compensation systems that are successful in efforts at vocational reactivation and disability reduction. Unfortunately, even when an optimal system is identified, individual States are likely to support the autonomy of their own systems, as failure to do so would be acknowledging many years of failure. One area of research that would potentially be valuable would involve comparison of outcomes of federal workers' compensation programs to those of the individual States. In this era of a growing likelihood of an eventual single-payer health care system, perhaps a federally administered workers' compensation system would provide data supporting the government's ability to cost-efficiently restore individuals to wellness, enhanced quality of lives, and reduced problems with perpetual disability. As it has been noted that the Social Security system in the United States is already a major (if not the primary) source for insurance for workplace disabilities (LaDou, 2011), perhaps a transition to a federally run system would be less dramatic than some may fear. Although the State-run system of workers' compensation in Washington State that was discussed above has proven that it is inept in ameliorating disability, the success of the Public Health approach taken by European systems (LaDou) may provide the answer(s) to the American workers' compensation disability dilemma.

References

Abbott, P., Rounsefell, B., Fraser, R., & Goss, A. (1990). Intractable neck pain. *The Clinical Journal of Pain, 6*, 26–31.

Abram, S. E., Anderson, R. A., & Maitra-D'Cruze, A. M. (1981). Factors predicting short-term outcome of nerve blocks in the management of chronic pain. *Pain, 10*, 323–330.

Allaz, A. F., Vannotti, M., Desmeules, J., et al. (1998). Use of the label "litigation neurosis" in patients with somatoform pain disorder. *General Hospital Psychiatry, 20*, 91–97.

Anema, J. R., Schellart, A. J. M., Cassidy, J. D., et al. (2009). Can cross country differences in return-to-work after chronic occupational back pain be explained? An exploratory analysis on disability policies in a six country cohort study. *Journal of Occupational Rehabilitation, 19*, 419–426.

Ash, P., & Goldstein, S. I. (1995). Predictors of returning to work. *The Bulletin of the American Academy of Psychiatry and the Law, 23*, 205–210.

Baker, T. E. (1992). Why Congress should repeal the Employers' Liability Act of 1908. *Harvard Journal on Legislation, 29*, 79–122.

Baril, R., Clarke, J., Friesen, M., Stock, S., Cole, D., & The Work-Ready Group. (2003). Management of return-to-work programs for workers with musculoskeletal disorders: A qualitative study in three Canadian provinces. *Social Science & Medicine, 57*, 2101–2114.

Barnes, D., Smith, D., Gatchel, R. J., & Mayer, T. G. (1989). Psychosocioeconomic predictors of treatment success/failure in chronic low-back pain patients. *Spine, 14*, 427–430.

Barth, P. S., & Hunt, H. A. (2010). *Workers' compensation reemployment programs options for modifying the pension system: final report.* Available at: http://research.upjohn.org/cgi/viewcontent.cgi?article=1182&context=reports&sei-redir=1&referer=http%3A%2F%2Fscholar.google.com%2Fscholar%3Fstart%3D80%26q%3DWashington%2BL%2526I%26hl%3Den%26as_sdt%3D0%2C48%26as_ylo%3D2005#search=%22Washington%20L%26I%22. Accessed on December 12, 2011.

Beardwood, B. A., Kirsh, B., & Clark, N. J. (2005). Victims twice over: Perceptions and experiences of injured workers. *Qualitative Health Research, 15*, 30–48.

Bellamy, R. (1997). Compensation neurosis: Financial reward for illness as nocebo. *Clinical Orthopaedics and Related Research, 336*, 94–106.

Benner, D. E. (2007). Ethical dilemmas of chronic pain from a patient's perspective. In M. E. Schatman (Ed.), *Ethical issues in chronic pain management* (pp. 15–32). New York: Informa Healthcare.

Bernacki, E. J., & Tao, X. (2008). The relationship between attorney involvement, claim duration, and workers' compensation costs. *Journal of Occupational and Environmental Medicine, 50*, 1013–1018.

Biondi, J., & Greenberg, B. J. (1990). Redecompression and fusion in failed back syndrome patients. *Journal of Spinal Disorders, 3*, 362–369.

Blackwell, T. L., Leirerer, S., Haupt, S., & Kampotsis, A. (2003). Predictors of vocational rehabilitation return to work outcomes in workers compensation. *Rehabilitation Counseling Bulletin, 46*, 108–114.

Boden, L. I., & Ruser, J. W. (2003). Workers' compensation 'reforms', choice of medical care provider, and reported workplace injuries. *The Review of Economics and Statistics, 85*, 923–929.

Bolduc, D., Fortin, B., Labreqecque, F., & Lanoie, P. (2002). Workers' compensation, moral hazard, and the composition of workplace injuries. *Journal of Human Resources, 37*, 623–652.

Bosy, D., Etlin, D., Corey, D., & Lee, J. W. (2010). An interdisciplinary pain rehabilitation programme: Description and evaluation of outcomes. *Physiotherapy Canada, 62*, 316–326.

Branca, B., & Lake, A. E. (2004). Psychological and neuropsychological integration in multidisciplinary pain management after TBI. *The Journal of Head Trauma Rehabilitation, 19*, 40–57.

Brena, S. F., Chapman, S. L., & Bradford, L. A. (1980). Conditioned responses to treatment in chronic pain patients: Effects of compensation for work-related accidents. *Bulletin of the Los Angeles Neurological Society, 44*, 48–52.

Breuer, B., Pappagallo, M., Tai, J. Y., & Portenoy, R. K. (2007). U.S. Board-certified pain physician practices: Uniformity and census data of their locations. *The Journal of Pain, 8*, 244–250.

Bryant, R. A. (2003). Assessing individuals for compensation. In D. Carsoneds & R. Bull (Eds.), *Handbook of psychology in legal contexts* (2nd ed., pp. 89–107). West Sussex, England: John Wiley & Sons.

Bültmann, U., Sherson, D., Olsen, J., Hansen, C. L., Lund, T., & Kilsgaard, J. (2009). Coordinated and tailored work rehabilitation: A randomized controlled trial with economic evaluation undertaken with workers on sick leave due to musculoskeletal disorders. *Journal of Occupational Rehabilitation, 19*, 81–93.

Campbell, F. K. (2006) Litigation neurosis: Pathological responses or rational subversion? Disability Studies Quarterly, 26(1), online version. Available at: http://www.dsq-sds.org/article/view/655/832. Accessed on August 1, 2011.

Carroll, S. J., Dixon, L., Anderson, J. M., Hogan, T., & Sloss, E. M. (n.d.). The abuse of medical diagnostic practices in mass litigation: The case of silica. Available at: http://www.rand.org/content/dam/rand/pubs/technical_reports/2009/RAND_TR774.pdf. Accessed on February 6, 2012.

Chibnall, J. T., & Tait, R. C. (2010). Legal representation and dissatisfaction with workers' compensation: Implications for claimant adjustment. *Psychological Injury and Law, 3*, 230–240.

Clayton, A. (1997). Workers compensation—The third way. *Safety Science Monitor, 1*, 1–12.

Cléry-Melin, M. L., Schmidt, L., Lafargue, G., Baup, N., Fossati, P., & Pessiglione, M. (2011). Why don't you try harder? An investigation of effort production in major depression. *PLoS One, 6*(8), e23178.

Connally, G. H., & Sanders, S. H. (1991). Predicting low back pain patients' response to lumbar sympathetic nerve blocks and interdisciplinary rehabilitation: The role of pretreatment overt pain behavior and cognitive coping strategies. *Pain, 44*, 139–146.

Dansak, D. A. (1973). On the tertiary gain of illness. *Comprehensive Psychiatry, 14*, 523–534.

Darchuk, K. M., Townsend, C. O., Rome, J. D., Bruce, B. K., & Hooten, W. M. (2010). Longitudinal treatment outcomes for geriatric patients with chronic non-cancer pain at an interdisciplinary pain rehabilitation program. *Pain Medicine, 11*, 1352–1364.

Davis, S. (n.d.). Learn the ABCs of workers compensation insurance. Business.com. Available at: http://www.business.com/insurance/workers-compensation-insurance/. Accessed January 8, 2012.

Dersh, J., Mayer, T. G., Gatchel, R. J., Polatin, P. B., Theodore, B. R., & Mayer, E. A. (2008). Prescription opioid dependence is associated with poorer outcomes in disabling spinal disorders. *Spine, 33*, 2219–2227.

Dersh, J., Mayer, T., Gatchel, R. J., Towns, B., Theodore, B., & Polatin, P. (2007). Psychiatric comorbidity in chronic disabling occupational spinal disorders has minimal impact on functional restoration socioeconomic outcomes. *Spine, 32*, 1917–1925.

Dersh, J., Polatin, P. B., Leeman, G., & Gatchel, R. J. (2004). The management of secondary gain and loss in medicolegal settings: Strengths and weaknesses. *Journal of Occupational Rehabilitation, 14*, 267–279.

Disler, P., & Pallant, J. (2001). Vocational rehabilitation. *British Medical Journal, 323*, 121–123.

Dworkin, R. H., Handlin, D. S., Richlin, D. M., et al. (1985). Unraveling the effects of compensation, litigation, and employment on treatment response in chronic pain. *Pain, 23*, 49–59.

Elliott, R., Sahakian, B. J., McKay, A. P., Herrod, J. J., Robbins, T. W., & Paykel, E. S. (1996). Neuropsychological impairments in unipolar depression: The influence of perceived failure on subsequent performance. *Psychological Medicine, 26*, 975–989.

Finneson, B. (1976). Modulating effect of secondary gain on the low back syndrome. *Advances in pain research and therapy, 1*, 949–952.

Fishback, P. V., & Kantor, S. E. (2000). *Prelude to the welfare state: The origins of workers' compensation*. Chicago: University of Chicago Press.

Fishbain, D. A., Rosomoff, H. L., Cutler, R. B., & Rosomoff, R. S. (1995). Secondary gain concept: A review of the scientific evidence. *The Clinical Journal of Pain, 11*, 6–21.

Franklin, G. M., Mai, J., Turner, J., Sullivan, M., Wickizer, T., & Fulton-Kehoe, D. (2012). Bending the prescription opioid dosing and mortality curves: Impact of the Washington state opioid dosing guidelines. *American Journal of Industrial Medicine, 55*(4), 325–331.

Franklin, G. M., Mai, J., Wickizer, T., Turner, J. A., Fulton-Kehoe, D., & Grant, L. (2005). Opioid dosing trends and mortality in Washington State workers' compensation, 1996–2002. *American Journal of Industrial Medicine, 48*, 91–99.

Franklin, G. M., Rahman, E. A., Turner, J. A., Daniell, W. E., & Fulton-Kehoe, D. (2009). Opioid use for chronic low back pain: A prospective, population-based study among injured workers in Washington state, 2002–2005. *The Clinical Journal of Pain, 25*, 743–751.

Franklin, G. M., Stover, B. D., Turner, J. A., Fulton-Kehoe, D., Wickizer, T. M., & Disability Risk Identification Study Cohort. (2008). Early opioid prescription and subsequent disability among workers with back injuries: The Disability Risk Identification Study Cohort. *Spine, 33*, 199–204.

Freud, S. (1959). *Introductory lectures on psychoanalysis*. London: Hogarth (Original work published in 1917).

Gamborg, B. L., Elliott, W. S., & Curtis, K. W. (1992). Chronic disability syndrome. *Canadian Family Physician, 37*, 1966–1973.

Gardner, J. A. (1991). Early referral and other factors affecting vocational rehabilitation outcome for the workers' compensation client. *Rehabilitation Counseling Bulletin, 34*, 197–209.

Gatchel, R. J., McGeary, D. D., Peterson, A., Moore, M., LeRoy, K., Isler, W. C., et al. (2009). Preliminary findings of a randomized controlled trial of an interdisciplinary military pain program. *Military Medicine, 174*, 270–277.

Gatchel, R. J., & Okifuji, A. (2006). Evidence-based scientific data documenting the treatment and cost-effectiveness of comprehensive pain programs for chronic nonmalignant pain. *The Journal of Pain, 7*, 779–793.

Geerts, A., Kornblith, B., & Urmson, J. (1977). *Compensation for bodily harm*. Brussels: Fernand Nathan.

Giordano, J., & Schatman, M. E. (2008a). A crisis in chronic pain care: An ethical analysis; Part 2. Proposed structure and function of an ethics of pain medicine. *Pain Physician, 11*, 589–595.

Giordano, J., & Schatman, M. E. (2008b). A crisis in chronic pain care: An ethical analysis. Part 3: Toward an integrative, multi-disciplinary pain medicine built around the needs of the patient. *Pain Physician, 11*, 771–784.

Gironda, R. J., Clark, M. E., Ruff, R. L., Chait, S., Craine, M., Walker, R., et al. (2009). Traumatic brain injury, polytrauma, and pain: Challenges and treatment strategies for the polytrauma rehabilitation. *Rehabilitation Psychology, 54*, 247–258.

Greenberg, S. N., & Bello, R. P. (1996). The work hardening program and subsequent return to work of a client with low back pain. *The Journal of Orthopaedic and Sports Physical Therapy, 24*, 37–45.

Gross, D. P., Stephens, B., Bhambhani, Y., Haykowsky, M., Bostick, G. P., & Rashiq, S. (2009). Opioid prescriptions in Canadian workers' compensation claimants: Prescription trends and associations between early prescription and future recovery. *Spine, 34*, 525–531.

Guyton, G. P. (1999). A brief history of workers' compensation. *The Iowa Orthopaedic Journal, 19*, 106–110.

Guzmán, J., Esmail, R., Karjalainen, K., Malmivaara, A., Irvin, E., & Bombardier, C. (2002). Multidisciplinary bio-psychosocial rehabilitation for chronic low back pain. *Cochrane Database of Systematic Reviews, 1*, CD000963.

Habeck, R. V., Leahy, M. J., Hunt, H. A., Chan, F., & Welch, E. M. (1991). Employer factors related to workers' compensation claims and disability management. *Rehabilitation Counseling Bulletin, 34*, 210–226.

Habeck, R. V., Scully, S. M., VanTol, B., & Hunt, H. A. (1998). Successful employer strategies for preventing and managing disability. *Rehabilitation Counseling Bulletin, 42*, 144–161.

Hadler, N. M. (1995). The disabling backache: An international perspective. *Spine, 20*, 640–649.

Hanley, E. N., Jr., & Levy, J. A. (1989). Surgical treatment of isthmic lumbosacral spondylolisthesis. Analysis of variables influencing results. *Spine, 14*, 48–50.

Harden, R. N., & Cole, P. A. (1998). New developments in rehabilitation of neuropathic pain syndromes. *Neurologic Clinics, 16*, 937–950.

Harris, I., Mulford, J., Solomon, M., van Gelder, J. M., & Young, J. (2005). Association between compensation status and outcome after surgery: A meta-analysis. *JAMA: The Journal of the American Medical Association, 293*, 1644–1652.

Heilbronner, R. L., Sweet, J. J., Morgan, J. E., Larrabee, G. J., Millis, S. R., & Conference Participants. (2009). American Academy of Clinical Neuropsychology Consensus Conference Statement on the neuropsychological assessment of effort, response bias, and malingering. *The Clinical Neuropsychologist, 23*, 1093–1129.

Herbert, R., Janeway, K., & Schecter, C. (1999). Carpal tunnel syndrome and workers' compensation among an occupational clinic population in New York State. *American Journal of Industrial Medicine, 35*, 335–342.

Herron, L. D., & Mangelsdorf, C. (1991). Lumbar spinal stenosis: Results of surgical treatment. *Journal of Spinal Disorders, 4*, 26–33.

Hester, E. J., Decelles, P. G., & Gaddis, E. L. (1986). *Predicting which disabled employees will return to work: The Menninger RTW scale*. Topeka, KS: Menninger Foundation.

Hooten, W. M., Townsend, C. O., Sletten, C. D., Bruce, B. K., & Rome, J. D. (2007). Treatment outcomes after multidisciplinary pain rehabilitation with analgesic medication withdrawal for patients with fibromyalgia. *Pain Medicine, 8*, 8–16.

Huge, V., Schloderer, U., Steinberger, M., Wuenschmann, B., Schöps, P., Beyer, A., et al. (2006). Impact of a functional restoration program on pain and health-related quality of life in patients with chronic low back pain. *Pain Medicine, 7*, 501–508.

Hungerer, S., Trapp, O., Augat, P., & Buhren, V. (2011). Posttraumatic arthrodesis of the subtalar joint—Outcome in workers compensation and rates of non-union. *Foot and Ankle Surgery, 17*, 277–283.

Hunt, H. A. (Ed.). (2004). *Adequacy of earnings replacement in workers' compensation programs*. Kalamazoo, MI: W.E. Upjohn Institute for Employment Research and NASI.

Hunt, H. A. (2008) Total permanent disability in Washington. *W.E. Upjohn Institute for Employment Research Newsletter*. Available at: http://research.upjohn.org/cgi/viewcontent.cgi?article=1013&context=empl_research&sei-redir=1&referer=http%3A%2F%2Fscholar.google.com%2Fscholar%3Fstart%3D10%26q%3DWashington%2BL%2526I%26hl%3Den%26as_sdt%3D0%2C48%26as_ylo%3D2006#search=%22Washington%20 L%26I%22. Accessed on December 12, 2011.

Hunt, H. A., & Barth, P. S. (2010) Compromise and release settlements in workers' compensation: final report. *Report prepared for State of Washington, Department of Labor and Industries*. Available at: http://research.upjohn.org/cgi/viewcontent.cgi?article=1181&context=reports&sei-redir=1#search="comparison+of+"workers+compensation"+systems+United+States". Accessed on June 11, 2011.

Hunt, H. A., Barth, P., Grob, H., Harder, H., & Silverstein M. (n.d.). *Washington pension system review*. Available at: http://research.upjohn.org/cgi/viewcontent.cgi?article=1004&context=testimonies&sei-redir=1&referer=http%3A%2F%2Fscholar.google.com%2Fscholar%3Fhl%3Den%26q%3DWA%2BL%2526I%2B%2522vocational%2522%26as_sdt%3D0%252C48%26as_ylo%3D2005%26as_vis%3D0#search=%22WA%20L%26I%20vocational%22. Accessed on December 12, 2011.

Hunt, H. A. (n.d.). The evolution of disability management in North American workers' compensation programs. Available at: http://research.upjohn.org/cgi/viewcontent.cgi?article=1180&context=reports. Accessed on February 7, 2012.

Iezzi, T., Duckworth, M. P., Mercer, V., & Vuong, L. (2007). Chronic pain and head injury following motor vehicle collisions: A double whammy or different sides of a coin. *Psychology, Health & Medicine, 12*, 197–212.

Illinois State Medical Society. (2011) *Position paper related to proposed changes to the Illinois Workers' Compensation Act*. Available at: http://www.isms.org/govtaffairs/Documents/2011_workcomp.pdf. Accessed on February 11, 2012.

International Labour Organization. (2002). *ILO Code of Practice on managing disability in the workplace*. Geneva, Switzerland: International Labour Organization.

Jamison, R. N., Matt, D. A., & Parris, W. C. (1988). Effects of time-limited vs unlimited compensation on pain behavior and treatment outcome in low back pain patients. *Journal of Psychosomatic Research, 32*, 277–283.

Järvikoski, A., & Tuunainen, K. (1978). The need for early rehabilitation among Finnish municipal employees. *Scandinavian Journal of Rehabilitation Medicine, 10*, 115–120.

Kennedy, M. Q., Badger, E., Pompeii, L., & Lipscomb, H. J. (2003). The North Country on the job network: A unique role for occupational health nurses in a community coalition. *AAOHN Journal, 51*, 204–209.

Kidner, C. L., Mayer, T. G., & Gatchel, R. J. (2009). Higher opioid doses predict poorer functional outcome in patients with chronic disabling occupational musculoskeletal disorders. *The Journal of Bone and Joint Surgery. American Volume, 91*, 919–927.

King, S. (1994). Concept of secondary gain—How valid is it? *American Physical Society Journal, 3*, 279–281.

Kirsh, B. (2001). *Making the system better: Injured workers speak out on compensation and work issues in Ontario.* Toronto: University of Toronto.

Kleinke, C. L., & Spangler, A. S., Jr. (1988). Predicting treatment outcome of chronic back pain patients in a multidisciplinary pain clinic: Methodological issues and treatment implications. *Pain, 33*, 41–48.

Kramer, S. N. (1958). *History begins at Sumer.* London: Thames and Hudson.

Kwan, O., Ferrari, R., & Friel, J. (2001). Tertiary gain and disability syndromes. *Medical Hypotheses, 57*, 459–464.

Kwan, O., & Friel, J. (2002). Clinical relevance of the sick role and secondary gain in the treatment of disability syndromes. *Medical Hypotheses, 59*, 129–134.

LaDou, J. (2011). The European influence on workers' compensation reform in the United States. *Environmental Health, 10*, 103.

Lane, C. (1980). Motivational deficits in depression. *Journal of Clinical Psychology, 36*, 647–652.

Lax, M. L., & Manetti, F. A. (2001). Access to medical care for individuals with workers' compensation claims. *New Solutions, 11*, 325–348.

Leventhal, A. M., Gelernter, J., Oslin, D., Anton, R. F., Farrer, L. A., & Kranzler, H. R. (2011). Agitated depression in substance dependence. *Drug and Alcohol Dependence, 116*, 163–169.

Levine, S. E. (n.d.). Trends in medical specialist participation in workers' compensation systems—Implications for California. Available at: https://csims.org/system/pdfs/54/original/Trends%20in%20Medical%20Specialist%20Participation%20in%20Workers%20Compensation%20Systems.pdf. Accessed on February 11, 2012.

Lew, H. L., Otis, J. D., Tun, C., Kerns, R. D., Clark, M. E., & Cifu, D. X. (2009). Prevalence of chronic pain, posttraumatic stress disorder, and persistent postconcussive symptoms in OIF/OEF veterans: Polytrauma clinical triad. *Journal of Rehabilitation Research and Development, 46*, 697–702.

Lippel, K. (2003). Compensation for musculoskeletal disorders in Quebec: Systemic discrimination against women workers? *International Journal of Health Services, 33*, 253–281.

Lipscomb, H. J., Moon, S. D., Li, L., Pompeii, L., & Kennedy, M. Q. (2002). Evaluation of North Country on the job network: A model of facilitated care for injured workers in rural upstate New York. *Journal of Occupational and Environmental Medicine, 44*, 246–257.

Loeser, J. D., Henderlite, S. E., & Conrad, D. A. (1995). Incentive effects of workers' compensation benefits: A literature synthesis. *Medical Care Research and Review, 52*, 34–59.

MacEachen, E., Clarke, J., Franche, R.-L., Irvin, E., & The Workplace-Based Return to Work Literature Review Group. (2006). Systematic review of the qualitative literature on return to work after injury. *Scandinavian Journal of Work, Environment & Health, 32*, 257–269.

MacEachen, E., Kosny, A., Ferrier, S., & Chambers, L. (2010). The "toxic dose" of system problems: Why some injured workers don't return to work as expected. *Journal of Occupational Rehabilitation, 20*, 349–366.

Mahmud, M. A., Webster, B. S., Courtney, T. K., Matz, S., Tacci, J. A., & Christiani, D. C. (2000). Clinical management and the duration of disability for work-related low back pain. *Journal of Occupational and Environmental Medicine, 42*, 1178–1187.

Malloy, S. E. W. (2003). The interaction of the ADA, the FMLA, and workers' compensation: Why can't we be friends? *Brandeis Law Journal, 41*, 821–852.

Martelli, M. F., Zasler, N. D., Bender, M. C., & Nicholson, K. (2004). Psychological, neuropsychological, and medical considerations in assessment and management of pain. *The Journal of Head Trauma Rehabilitation, 19*, 10–28.

Mayer, T. G., Anagnostis, C., Gatchel, R. J., & Evans, T. (2002). Impact of functional restoration after anterior cervical fusion on chronic disability in work-related neck pain. *The Spine Journal, 2*, 267–273.

Mendelson, G. (1986). Chronic pain and compensation: A review. *Journal of Pain and Symptom Management, 1*, 135–144.

Mendelson, G. (1988). *Psychiatric aspects of personal injury claims.* Springfield: Charles C. Thomas.

Mendelson, G. (1991). Chronic pain, compensation and clinical knowledge. *Theoretical Medicine and Bioethics, 12*, 227–246.

Mendelson, G. (1995). 'Compensation neurosis' revisited: Outcome studies of the effects of litigation concluded that the label of "compensation neurosis" is an invalid one. *Journal of Psychosomatic Research, 39*, 695–706.

Mincer, J. (1962). On-the-job training: Costs, returns and some implications. *Journal of Political Economy, 70*, S50–S79.

Mnookin, R. H. (1998). Negotiation, settlement and the contingent fee. *DePaul Law Review, 47*, 363,365–369.

Mowla, A., Kianpor, M., Bahtoee, M., Sabayan, B., & Chohedri, A. H. (2008). Comparison of clinical characteristics of opium-induced and independent major depressive disorder. *The American Journal of Drug and Alcohol Abuse, 34*, 415–421.

Nampiaparampil, D. E. (2008). Prevalence of chronic pain after traumatic brain injury: A systematic review. *JAMA: The Journal of the American Medical Association, 300*, 711–719.

Nordström-Björverud, G., & Moritz, U. (1998). Interdisciplinary rehabilitation of hospital employees with musculoskeletal disorders. *Scandinavian Journal of Rehabilitation Medicine, 30*, 31–37.

OECD. (n.d.). Society at a glance 2011—OECD social indicators. Available at: http://www.oecd.org/document/24/0,3746,en_2649_37419_2671576_1_1_1_37419,00.html. Accessed on January 8, 2012.

Okawa, Y., Nakamura, S., Kudo, M., & Ueda, S. (2009). An evidence-based construction of the models of decline of functioning. Part 1: Two major models of decline of functioning. *International Journal of Rehabilitation Research, 32*, 189–192.

Ownsworth, T., Fleming, J. M., & Hardwick, S. (2006). Symptom reporting and association with compensation status, self-awareness, causal attributions, and emotional wellbeing following traumatic brain injury. *Brain Impairment, 72*, 95–106.

Patil, V. K., St Andre, J. R., Crisan, E., Smith, B. M., Evans, C. T., Steiner, M. L., et al. (2011). Prevalence and treatment of headaches in veterans with mild traumatic brain injury. *Headache, 51*, 1112–1121.

Perlin, M. L. (1985). The German and British roots of the American workers' compensation systems: When is an "intentional act" "intentional"? *Seton Hall Law Review, 15*, 849–879.

Pocius, J. (n.d.). Return to work—A forgotten aspect of workers compensation. IRMI.com. Available at: http://www.irmi.com/expert/articles/2002/pocius01.aspx. Accessed on January 8, 2012.

Proctor, T. J., Mayer, T. G., Gatchel, R. J., & McGeary, D. D. (2004). Unremitting health-care-utilization outcomes of tertiary rehabilitation of patients with chronic musculoskeletal disorders. *The Journal of Bone and Joint Surgery. American Volume, 86*, 62–69.

Reville, R. T., Boden, L. I., Biddle, J. E., & Mardesich, C. (2001). *An evaluation of New Mexico workers' compensation permanent partial disability and return to work*. Santa Monica, CA: RAND.

Richards, P., & Ruff, R. (1989). Motivational effects in neuropsychological functioning: Comparison of depressed versus nondepressed individuals. *Journal of Consulting and Clinical Psychology, 57*, 396–402.

Roberts-Yates, C. (2003). The concerns and issues of injured workers in relation to claims/injury management and rehabilitation: The need for new operational frameworks. *Disability and Rehabilitation, 25*, 898–907.

Robinson, J. P., Fulton-Kehoe, D., Franklin, G. M., & Wu, R. (2004). Multidisciplinary pain center outcomes in Washington State Workers' Compensation. *Journal of Occupational and Environmental Medicine, 46*, 473–478.

Robinson, J. P., Fulton-Kehoe, D., Martin, D. C., & Franklin, G. M. (2001). Outcomes of pain center treatment in Washington State workers' compensation. *American Journal of Industrial Medicine, 39*, 227–236.

Sander, R. A., & Meyers, J. E. (1986). The relationship of disability to compensation status in railroad workers. *Spine, 11*, 141–143.

Schatman, M. E. (2006). The demise of multidisciplinary pain management clinics? *Practical Pain Management, 6*, 30–41.

Schatman, M. E. (2007). The demise of the multidisciplinary chronic pain management clinic: Bioethical perspectives on providing optimal treatment when ethical principles collide. In M. E. Schatman (Ed.), *Ethical issues in chronic pain management* (pp. 43–62). New York: Informa Healthcare.

Schatman, M. E. (2009). Working to avoid collateral emotional harm to clients: Cases and recommendations for the personal injury attorney. *Psychological Injury and Law, 2*, 149–166.

Schatman, M. E. (2011). The role of the health insurance industry in perpetuating suboptimal pain management: Ethical implications. *Pain Medicine, 12*, 415–426.

Schatman, M. E., & Sullivan, J. (2010). Whither suffering? The potential impact of tort reform on the emotional and existential healing of traumatically injured chronic pain patients. *Psychological Injury and Law, 3*, 182–202.

Schlesinger, I., Hering-Hanit, R., & Dagan, Y. (2001). Sleep disturbances after whiplash injury: Objective and subjective findings. *Headache, 41*, 586–589.

Scholten-Peeters, G. G. M., Verhagen, A. P., Bekkering, G. E., et al. (2003). Prognostic factors of whiplash-associated disorders: A systematic review of prospective cohort studies. *Pain, 104*, 303.322.

Schultz, I. Z., Crook, J., Berkowitz, J., Milner, R., Meloche, G. R., & Lewis, M. L. (2008). A prospective study of the effectiveness of early intervention with high-risk back-injured workers—A pilot study. *Journal of Occupational Rehabilitation, 18*, 140–151.

Sengupta, I., Reno, V., & Burton, J. F. (2009). *Workers' compensation: Benefits, coverage, and costs, 2007*. Washington, DC: National Academy of Social Insurance.

Shin, T. H., Chang-Bong, G., Min-Su, K., et al. (2010). Development of a cognitive level explanation model in brain injury: Comparisons between disability and non-disability evaluation groups. *Journal of Korean Neurosurgical Society, 48*, 506–517.

Smith, J. M. P. (1931). *Origin & history of Hebrew law*. Chicago, IL: University of Chicago Press.

Social Security Online. (n.d.). The full retirement age is increasing. Available at: http://ssa.gov/pubs/ageincrease.htm. Accessed on December 12, 2011.

Spearing, N. M., & Connelly, L. B. (2010). Is compensation "bad for health"? A systematic meta-review. *Injury, 41*, 683–692.

Spieler, E., & Burton, J. F., Jr. (1998). Compensation for disabled workers: Workers' compensation. In T. Thomason, J. Burton Jr., & D. Hyatt (Eds.), *New approaches to disability in the workplace (p. 229)* (pp. 205–244). Madison, WI: Industrial Relations Research Association.

Sprehe, D. J. (1984). Workers' compensation: A psychiatric follow-up study. *International Journal of Law and Psychiatry, 7*, 165–178.

State of Minnesota Office of the Legislative Auditor, (2009) Oversight of workers' compensation. Available at: http://www.auditor.leg.state.mn.us/ped/pedrep/workcomp.pdf. Accessed on August 1, 2011.

State of Vermont Department of Labor. (n.d.). Medical case management in workers' compensation. Available at: http://www.labor.vermont.gov/Default.aspx?tabid=277. Accessed on February 11, 2012.

Stempel, J. W. (2009). The "other" intermediaries: The increasingly anachronistic immunity of managing general agents and independent claims adjusters. *Connecticut Insurance Law Journal, 15*, 599–722.

Stover, B., & Seixas, N. (2009). Occupational injuries and illnesses in OSHA region 10: Safety and health surveillance indicators 2000–2005. Available at: http://depts.washington.edu/nwcohs/documents/ohindicatorsregion10.pdf. Accessed on June 21, 2011.

Stover, B. D., Turner, J. A., Franklin, G., Gluck, J. V., Fulton-Kehoe, D., Sheppard, L., et al. (2006). Factors associated with early opioid prescription among workers with low back injuries. *The Journal of Pain, 7*, 718–725.

Sullivan, M. D., Von Korff, M., Banta-Green, C., Merrill, J. O., & Saunders, K. (2010). Problems and concerns of patients receiving chronic opioid therapy for chronic non-cancer pain. *Pain, 149*, 345–353.

Tarsh, M. J., & Royston, C. (1985). A follow-up study of accident neurosis. *The British Journal of Psychiatry, 146*, 18–25.

Tate, D. G. (1992). Workers' disability and return to work. *American Journal of Physical Medicine & Rehabilitation, 71*, 92–96.

Taylor, W., Simpson, R., Gow, D., & McNaughton, H. (2001). Rehabilitation that works—Vocational outcomes following rehabilitation for occupational musculoskeletal pain. *The New Zealand Medical Journal, 114*, 185–187.

Telles, C. A., Eccleston, S. M., Radeva, E., Yang, R., & Tanabe, R. P. (2009). *CompScope benchmarks, 9th ed: The data book*. Cambridge, MA: Workers Compensation Research Institute.

Tollison, C. D., Satterthwaite, J. R., Kriegel, M. L., & Hinnant, D. W. (1990). Interdisciplinary treatment of low back pain. A clinical outcome comparison of compensated versus noncompensated groups. *Orthopedic Reviews, 19*, 701–706.

Townsend, C. O., Kerkvliet, J. L., Bruce, B. K., Rome, J. D., Hooten, W. M., Luedtke, C. A., et al. (2008). A longitudinal study of the efficacy of a comprehensive pain rehabilitation program with opioid withdrawal: Comparison of treatment outcomes based on opioid use status at admission. *Pain, 140*, 177–189.

Trief, P., & Stein, N. (1985). Pending litigation and rehabilitation outcome of chronic back pain. *Archives of Physical Medicine and Rehabilitation, 66*, 95–99.

United States Department of Labor Bureau of Labor Statistics. (n.d.). *Occupational outlook handbook* (2010–11 edn.). Available at: http://www.bls.gov/oco/ocos125.htm#related. Accessed on February 11, 2012.

Volinn, E., Fargo, J. D., & Fine, P. G. (2009). Opioid therapy for nonspecific low back pain and the outcome of chronic work loss. *Pain, 42*, 194–201.

Vowles, K. E., Gross, R. T., & Sorrell, J. T. (2004). Predicting work status following interdisciplinary treatment for chronic pain. *European Journal of Pain, 8*, 351–358.

Washington Engrossed House Bill 2123. (n.d.). Available at: http://apps.leg.wa.gov/documents/billdocs/2011-12/Pdf/Bills/Session%20Law%202011/2123.SL.pdf. Accessed on January 20, 2012.

Washington State Legislature. (n.d.). *WAC 296-20-01002*. Available at: http://apps.leg.wa.gov/WAC/default.aspx?cite=296-20-01002. Accessed on January 21, 2012.

Webster, B. S., Cifuentes, M., Verma, S., & Pransky, G. (2009). Geographic variation in opioid prescribing for acute, work-related, low back pain and associated factors: A multilevel analysis. *American Journal of Industrial Medicine, 52*, 162–171.

Webster, B. S., Verma, S. K., & Gatchel, R. J. (2007). Relationship between early opioid prescribing for acute occupational low back pain and disability duration, medical costs, subsequent surgery and late opioid use. *Spine, 32*, 2127–2132.

Weil, D. (2001). Valuing the economic consequences of work injury and illness: A comparison of methods and findings. *American Journal of Industrial Medicine, 40*, 418–437.

Wood, R. L. I., & Rutterford, N. A. (2006). The effect of litigation on long term cognitive and psychosocial outcome after severe brain injury. *Archives of Clinical Neuropsychology, 21*, 239–246.

Wright, A., Mayer, T. G., & Gatchel, R. J. (1999). Outcomes of disabling cervical spine disorders in compensation injuries. A prospective comparison to tertiary rehabilitation response for chronic lumbar spinal disorders. *Spine, 24*, 178–183.

Part IV
Prevention and Intervention Methods

Health and Wellness Promotion in the Workplace

17

William S. Shaw, Silje E. Reme, and Cécile R.L. Boot

The Evolution of Worksite Wellness

Worksite wellness is a relative newcomer to the professional field of occupational health, and there is tremendous variability in employer programs and initiatives intended to support employee health and wellness across occupational settings and around the world. Many questions remain about the health benefits and cost effectiveness of these formal and informal strategies to improve employee health, but most of the research evidence so far has supported their effectiveness provided the programs are sufficiently comprehensive, far-reaching, and targeted to the specific needs of individual workers and occupational settings (Carnethon et al., 2009; Pelletier, 2011; Soler et al., 2010). Today, the concept of worksite wellness includes attention to both the physical and psychosocial well-being of workers (Levy, Wegman, Baron, & Sokas, 2011), and health promotion efforts fall within primary, secondary, and tertiary aspects of disease and disability prevention (Harris, Lichiello, & Hannon, 2009). With an aging workforce and proliferation of chronic health conditions among workers in the US and elsewhere (Caban-Martinez et al., 2011; Szinovacz, 2011), employers are likely to dedicate more attention and resources to preventing and dealing with serious health problems in the workplace of the future. While disability benefits and other health insurance programs are in place in most industrialized nations as a

---

W.S. Shaw, Ph.D. (✉)
Liberty Mutual Research Institute for Safety,
71 Frankland Road, Hopkinton, MA 01748, USA
e-mail: William.shaw@libertymutual.com

S.E. Reme, Ph.D.
Harvard School of Public Health and Liberty Mutual Research Institute for Safety,
71 Frankland Road, Hopkinton, MA 01748, USA
e-mail: siljee_reme@dfci.harvard.edu

C.R.L. Boot, Ph.D.
VU University Medical Center, EMGO Institute for Health and Care Research,
Van der Boechorststraat 7, 1081 BT, Amsterdam, The Netherlands
e-mail: CRL.Boot@vumc.nl

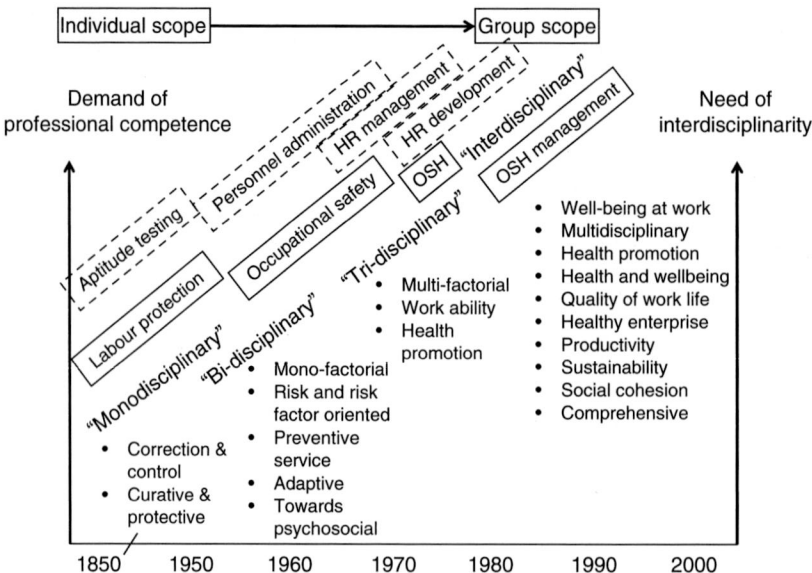

Fig. 17.1 Development of the concept of worksite wellness (from Anttonen & Pääkkönen, 2010; reprinted with permission)

safety net for ill workers, health promotion and early intervention programs may become more commonplace as an employer-supported or workplace-centered effort.

While employers have had a vested interest in worker health and well-being for centuries, formal systems to promote worker health have evolved substantially since the rapid industrialization of the late nineteenth century. Figure 17.1 shows a historical timeline developed by Anttonen and Pääkkönen (2010) as an illustration of how the concept of well-being at work has been transformed over the past 150 years in Finland. This timeline is representative of the changes in many industrialized nations during this time period. The early focus was on reengineering workplace processes, machinery, and environments to prevent deaths, amputations, and disabling injuries that came with industrialization. Few laws were in place to protect the health of the labor force, and hiring decisions often focused on whether candidates had sufficient physical strength and endurance to perform job tasks (Aldrich, 1997).

In the early twentieth century, many countries enacted laws governing workplace safety and enabling employers or government sectors to provide insurance, healthcare, and disability benefits to workers. In the decades that followed, there was growing scientific evidence of environmental and physical hazards in the workplace, and substantial improvements in workplace health and safety ensued. Around the 1980s, the concept of worksite wellness began to expand beyond worksite safety to include other issues as well. Problems like job stress, work-family conflict, sedentary work, second-hand smoke, and repetitive motion emerged as workplace issues, alongside physical force requirements and chemical and particulate exposures (Karasek & Theorell, 1990). More recently, researchers have focused on the more complex interactions between health and work: presenteeism; the negative health effects of job stress and low decision latitude; the benefits of job accommodation; return-to-work strategies; social support in the workplace; and employer support of healthy lifestyles (Akabas, Gates, & Galvin, 1992; Quick & Tetrick, 2003; Talmage & Melhorn, 2005). More research has documented the substantial employer and societal costs attributable to poor employee health (Institute of Medicine, 1997), and employers have begun to consider the economic and organizational benefits of having a healthier workforce (Koper, Moller, & Zwetsloot, 2009; Whitehead, 2001). All of these changes have led to a broader perspective of worksite wellness that addresses not just workplace safety, but issues of worker productivity and sustainability, well-being, organizational factors, lifestyle choices, home safety, and disease management. The number of employers offering workplace wellness programs with financial incentives to employees in the US has been steadily rising despite a recessionary economic environment (National Business Group on Health, 2012).

Although the concept of worksite wellness encompasses many domains and potential research questions, this chapter summarizes key research findings in six aspects of worksite wellness that have been the subject of multiple research studies: dietary and physical activity interventions; smoking cessation interventions; health-risk appraisal and tailored health advice; comprehensive wellness programs; integration of workplace health and safety policies and practices; and economic evidence. Each of these elements is summarized and discussed in the sections that follow.

Dietary and Physical Activity Interventions at the Workplace

Maintaining the balance between energy intake (nutrition) and energy expenditure (physical activity) is an increasing problem for workers worldwide. The prevalence of overweight and obesity is on the rise and, despite excessive attempts to reverse the trend, obesity is expected to become the main determinant of preventable burden of disease in the future (Peeters et al., 2003; Popkin, 2006). Recent estimates show that only 34% of U.S. workers are classified as normal weight compared to 44% in the late 1980s, while 29% are classified as obese (Hertz & McDonald, 2004). In the workplace, obesity accounts for costs associated with injuries, disability, absenteeism, sick leave, and healthcare claims (Ostbye, Dement, & Krause, 2007). In response to this, research on dietary and physical activity interventions has been expanding both in quantity and in quality the last decades. Also, there has been a shift of focus away from interventions aiming at reducing obesity and towards a focus on attempts to prevent obesity (Lemmens, Oenema, Klepp, Henriksen, & Brug, 2008). The preventive approach has proven to be less expensive and potentially more effective than treating a fully developed obesity problem.

Working adults spend a lot of their time at the workplace. Up to 60% of employees' waking hours are spent at the worksite, and the occupational setting has therefore been suggested as an opportunity to promote a healthy lifestyle among workers. A range of different worksite health promotion programs have been conducted and studied over the years, ranging in quality and efficiency. Recent developments have demonstrated that, in order to succeed in significant behavior change in the target populations, health promotion strategies need to go beyond education or communication alone, and add environmental modifications to the worksite as well (Engbers, van Poppel, Chin, & van Mechelen, 2005). Employees' dietary behavior is not only determined by conscious choices, but also by unconscious processes (or habits), which is why changes in the physical environment have proven to be so useful. Environmental strategies aim to make healthy choices easier (e.g., by access to healthy foods, enhancing opportunities to physical activity, etc.). They target the whole work force by modifying physical or organizational structures, as opposed to behavioral and societal strategies where the aim is to influence behaviors indirectly by targeting individual cognition believed to mediate behavior change (Anderson et al., 2009).

Several studies of workplace interventions have investigated the effects of targeting physical activity, dietary behavior, or both, in attempts of preventing weight gain. The overall findings from systematic literature reviews show favorable effects of both physical activity and dietary behavior on weight outcomes (Anderson et al., 2009) and on fruit, vegetable and fat intake (Engbers et al., 2005). The effect seems to be consistent, albeit somewhat modest. In the systematic review by Anderson et al. (2009), a net loss of 2.8 lb were seen at 6–12 months follow-up, with similar effects observed for the studies that could not be included in the meta-analysis. The evidence for potential differences between program components (information, behavioral skills, or environmental and policy) was limited, but the overall findings showed that more intensive modes of interventions were associated with increased program impact. That is, more structured programs were more effective than unstructured programs, and adding behavioral counseling to educational information was more beneficial than information alone (Anderson et al., 2009). This is further in line with studies finding that those health behavior interventions that are effective tend to involve more intensive and sustained interventions with longer-term coaching and follow-up (Lemmens et al., 2008).

Worksite interventions that focus exclusively on physical activity do not show very convincing effects, and they have yet to demonstrate a statistically significant increase in physical activity or fitness (Dishman, Oldenburg, O'Neal, & Shephard, 1998; Engbers et al., 2005). Most studies included in a systematic review concerning physical activity interventions were found to have serious design flaws, and the only moderating variable that significantly influenced the size of the intervention effects was research design, with quasi-experimental designs showing larger effects than randomized controlled designs (Dishman et al., 1998). Furthermore, few of the worksite health promotion programs included environmental modifications to stimulate physical activity, which could be one explanation for the lack of documented effects (Engbers et al.). However, whether an intervention is effective or not always depends on the outcome it is measured by. Hence, another systematic review on the same topic, but with different outcomes and criteria, concluded that there is strong evidence for a positive effect of worksite physical activity programs on physical activity and musculoskeletal disorders (Proper et al., 2003). The different conclusions are primarily the result of differences in methods of reviewing (qualitative in the latter; quantitative in the former), differences in included outcomes (other health outcomes besides fitness included in the latter), and different inclusion criteria for the studies that were included.

Worksite interventions that focus exclusively on promoting a healthy diet show moderate evidence of effect (Maes et al., 2011). Particularly effective are educational and multicomponent dietary interventions, with effects showing on dietary behaviors and determinants of such. This particular review found less positive results for nutrition and physical activity interventions combined. This is not quite in line with previous reviews, and this could be a result of systemic and methodological differences. Methodologically, the review included studies with a wide range of different research designs and, systemically, they included only studies from European countries, while most other reviews include studies from non-European countries (Maes et al.).

In recent years, there has been a gradual shift towards more primary preventive interventions, and less secondary and tertiary prevention efforts for overweight and obesity. While secondary and tertiary prevention is easier to accomplish because of more motivated and easily identified groups of people, primary prevention has proven to be more cost-effective and beneficial in the long run, and seems to be more efficient in addressing the obesity epidemic. Accordingly, a recent systematic review addressed the issue of primary prevention by excluding studies focusing primarily on weight loss, and studies among only overweight or obese populations (Verweij, Coffeng, van Mechelen, & Proper, 2011). The results showed moderate quality of evidence that workplace physical activity and dietary interventions significantly reduced body weight, body mass index (BMI) and body fat percentage. Subgroup analyses revealed that interventions that included an environmental component were more effective in reducing body weight than studies without such components, despite a wide variety of environmental components in the different studies (Verweij et al., 2011). For instance, in one of the studies, the worksite program included walking maps, team competitions, participation cards, and participation rewards, and every week a dietician would visit the worksite to give out new material, punch participation cards, give rewards and discuss individual health questions (Racette et al., 2009). In another study from Japan, a 4-days health promotion program conducted at a hot spring resort was followed by a follow-up program involving active participation

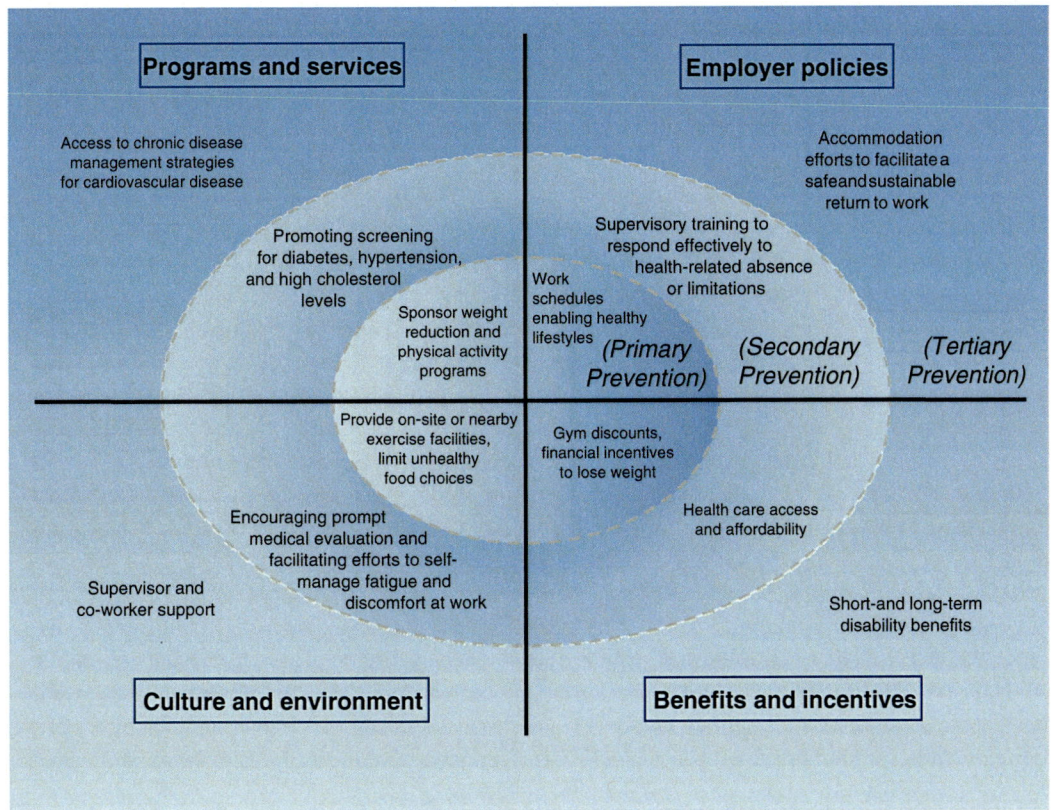

Fig. 17.2 Potential workplace health promotion activities related to diet and exercise

from the participant's supervisor and family (Muto & Yamauchi, 2001). Both these approaches produced good results that were long lasting. This indicates that future studies should look beyond personal components and also include environmental components in their worksite health promotion programs.

Most of the research focus on workplace interventions has focused on reducing risk factors for cardiovascular disease, but workplace health promotion activities may also encompass secondary and tertiary prevention efforts once disease processes have led to symptoms, clinical endpoints and diagnoses, and more severe health limitations. In the worksite context, primary prevention would include all of the means intended to protect workers from developing diseases or experiencing injuries. Secondary prevention is to halt or slow the progress of disease or reduce its disabling effects. Tertiary prevention is focused on managing complicated, long-term health problems. Figure 17.2 shows the multiple ways that workplace health promotion activities might impact workers with regard to cardiovascular disease. Primary prevention strategies might include sponsorship of weight reduction programs, changes in the work environment to support healthy lifestyles, adopting work schedules and other policies that enable healthy behaviors, and financial incentives or gym discounts. For workers with activity-limiting cardiovascular diseases, the employer may play a role by encouraging prompt medical attention, providing affordable health care access, and providing appropriate help from supervisors to manage sickness absence and any functional limitations at work. For workers with more severe cardiovascular events or complications, an employer may be influential by providing worksite accommodations, funding disability benefits, facilitating supervisor and coworker support, and by supporting disease management strategies.

The financial consequences of obesity involve reduced productivity, but also an increase in medical costs in countries with employer-provided health insurance. The financial return of worksite health promotion programs was extensively evaluated in a recent systematic review of programs that aimed to improve nutrition and/or increase physical activity in the workers (van Dongen et al., 2011). On average, the financial return was found to be positive; worksite health promotion programs generated financial savings in terms of reduced absenteeism costs, medical costs or both. This is also in line with previous reviews that generally conclude reduced employer-related expenses resulting from worksite health promotion programs (Aldana, 2001; Chapman, 2005; Soler et al., 2010). However, this is only the case for non-randomized studies. Subgroup analysis revealed that the effect was caused by the non-randomized studies in the review, while no significant effects on financial savings could be documented for the randomized controlled trials (van Dongen et al., 2011). This raises the issue of the general methodological quality of worksite health promotion studies, and the possibility of *selection bias*. Selection bias arises when allocation methods other than randomization are used, which means that the intervention and control group are unlikely to be comparable. That is probably why non-randomized studies of health care interventions in general tend to result in larger estimates of effect (Kunz, Vist, & Oxman, 2007). Several of the previously mentioned reviews also point to methodological flaws in the included studies, such as the lack of randomization procedures, blinding, co-interventions and intention-to-treat analysis, and suggest paying more attention to this in the future (Verweij et al., 2011). On the other hand, there seems to be increasing consensus about the fact that randomized controlled trials often are inappropriate, unachievable, and even irrelevant for public health interventions (Maes et al., 2011). The debate on grading of evidence for public health interventions is, in other words, still ongoing, and new frameworks for categorizing interventions have been proposed where certainty of effectiveness and potential population impact are combined in one and the same framework (Swinburn, Gill, & Kumanyika, 2005).

Workplace Interventions for Smoking Cessation

Probably no single negative health behavior has received as much research attention in the second half of the twentieth century as tobacco use. The negative health consequences of smoking are now commonly known and well documented (Bullen, 2008; U.S. Department of Health and Human Services, 2010), and the evidence of tobacco's negative effect on bodily systems, diseases processes, and population health continues to mount. Smoking rates have seen a slow, steady decline in the US from nearly 50% in 1965 to a current rate of 19.8% among working age adults (Syamlal, Mazurek, & Malarcher, 2011), but smoking rates are still elevated in some occupational groups (e.g., restaurant and construction workers; Syamlal et al., 2011), and the rate is as high as 40–50% in some other regions of the world (World Health Organization, 2011). The gold standard for smoking cessation is either individual or group behavioral intervention, often augmented with nicotine replacement or other pharmacotherapies (Tonnesen, 2009). These programs show a reasonable level of success, with a 1-year abstinence rate of about 25% (Tonnesen), but the majority of individuals quit smoking without any formal intervention. Still, smoking cessation is no simple matter, and like any lifestyle change, it requires motivation, support, and personal fortitude. Employer policies and programs can assist workers in these efforts.

In many countries, the problem of worksite tobacco use and second-hand smoke has been significantly mitigated by legislative and policy changes that prohibit smoking in indoor working environments and in public places such as stores, restaurants, and libraries. Such "smoke-free" policies have not only reduced second-hand smoke exposure, but also reduced smoking rates among employees who face a major inconvenience to smoke during working hours (Gadomski, Stayton,

Krupa, & Jenkins, 2010; Longo, Johnson, Kruse, Brownson, & Hewett, 2001). Despite these efforts, smoking continues to be a major health and mortality risk among working age adults in the US and elsewhere (U.S. Department of Health and Human Services, 2010), and the health consequences of smoking generate a significant financial burden to employers and social insurance systems due to increases in chronic medical conditions, increased mortality, more functional limitations, and higher healthcare and disability costs (Goetzel et al., 2009; U.S. Department of Health and Human Services). Such evidence has led the Centers for Disease Control to encourage employers to integrate smoking cessation programs with other worksite health promotion efforts (Syamlal et al., 2011).

Workplace interventions for smoking cessation can include both individual-level efforts (i.e., helping an individual employee quit smoking) and group-level programs (e.g., bans, restrictions, and health messaging). Eight types of workplace interventions were identified in a 2008 systematic review of 51 trials evaluating workplace interventions for smoking cessation (Cahill, Moher, & Lancaster, 2008). These included the following: (1) intensive group behavioral interventions, (2) individual counseling, (3) self-help interventions (typically of less intensity), (4) pharmacological therapies (typically nicotine replacement), (5) engaging social support (e.g., friend, coworker, or spouse), (6) environmental support (e.g., posters), (7) monetary incentives, and (8) comprehensive programs involving multiple components. The primary conclusion of the systematic review was that group programs, individual counseling and nicotine replacement were effective to increase smoking cessation rates, and this mirrors the results of programs outside of the workplace (Tonnesen, 2009). The review also concluded that more research was needed of incentive schemes and comprehensive worksite programs in order to conclude whether consistent benefits existed across studies. A meta-analysis of worksite smoking cessation programs conducted in 1990 (Smedslund, Fisher, Boles, & Lichtenstein, 2004) and repeated in 2004 (Lee et al., 2007) concluded initial effectiveness of worksite programs, but with waning effects beyond 12 months. Thus, the longevity of workplace intervention effects may be deserving of more research.

One question of importance to employers is whether incentives and/or competitions between working groups might improve enrollment or outcomes of smoking cessation programs. A recent systematic review of worksite-based incentives and competitions found 14 studies of sufficient quality to synthesize results across studies (Leeks et al., 2010). The reviewers concluded that incentives and competitions increased the effectiveness of programs by 67%, and this translated to an improvement in 1-year smoking cessation rates by an average of 4.4 percentage points. Thus, there is strong evidence that worksite-based incentives and competitions, in combination with additional interventions, are effective in increasing the number of workers who quit using tobacco. Also, studies have shown net cost savings to employers when program costs are adjusted for averted healthcare expenses and productivity losses (Serxner et al., 1993; Tanaka et al., 2006). There is no current evidence, however, that incentives and competitions alone are effective to reduce smoking rates when not combined with a formal smoking cessation program.

Most of the research focus on workplace interventions for tobacco use has focused on primary prevention (i.e., smoking cessation), but workplace health promotion activities for tobacco use may involve secondary and tertiary prevention efforts as well. Figure 17.3 shows the multiple ways that workplace health promotion activities might impact workers with regard to tobacco use and its longer-range health implications. Primary prevention strategies might include a media campaign to quit smoking, sponsorship of smoking cessation programs, financial incentives to quit smoking, and a property-wide ban on smoking. For workers with emerging respiratory symptoms related to tobacco use, the employer may play a role by encouraging prompt medical attention, providing affordable health care access, and providing appropriate help from supervisors to manage sickness absence and any functional limitations at work. For older workers with chronic obstructive pulmonary disease and other complicated smoking-related medical conditions, an employer may be influential by providing worksite accommodations, access to disability benefits, supervisor and coworker support, and by supporting disease management strategies.

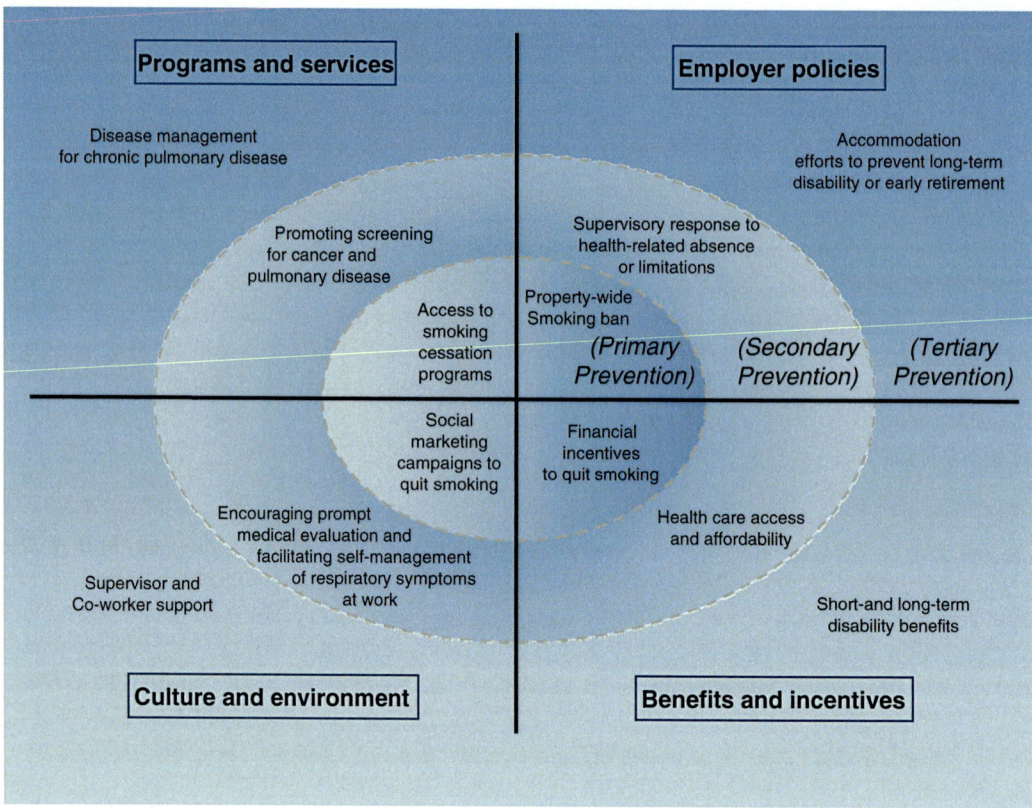

Fig. 17.3 Potential workplace health promotion activities related to tobacco use

For employers contemplating a more aggressive smoking cessation effort in the workplace, the most compelling evidence is the number of deaths and chronic health conditions attributed to smoking, and the high concomitant employer healthcare and disability costs. Smoking still accounts for 30% of all cancer deaths and 80% of deaths from chronic obstructive pulmonary disease in the US (Centers for Disease Control and Prevention, 2007). The U.S. Centers for Disease Control estimates an annual price tag of $97 billion in productivity losses, and $96 billion for healthcare costs attributable to tobacco use (Centers for Disease Control and Prevention). Workers who smoke have higher healthcare expenses, higher rates of absenteeism and presenteeism, and are more likely to use short-term disability benefits (Hill, Thompson, Shaw, Pinidiya, & Card-Higginson, 2009; Kowlessar, Goetzel, Carls, Tabrizi, & Guindon, 2011). For these reasons, providing employees with easy access to smoking cessation programs and promoting their use through incentives and competition is a very critical component to worksite wellness efforts.

Health Risk Appraisals and Tailored Health Advice

One wellness strategy applied in many employment settings is to conduct regular health risk appraisals (HRA), and to provide workers with tailored health advice based on HRA results. This secondary prevention strategy is typically focused on reducing cardiovascular risk factors, but HRAs can also cover issues related to safety practices, personal hygiene, mental stress, and overall fitness planning (Anderson & Staufacker, 1996; DeFriese & Fielding, 1990; Soler et al., 2010). In some work settings, an HRA might also address a potential workplace health concern (e.g., an audiogram for factory workers with significant noise exposures) or a potential public safety concern (e.g., vision tests for truck drivers). But typically, HRA participation is voluntary and confidential, and an HRA might include biometric screening from a single blood draw coupled with a brief self-report questionnaire describing health habits. HRAs may be recommended at regular intervals or periodic milestones (e.g., after every 5 years with the company) at relatively low cost to the employer (as low as $5–15 per worker), and results are typically delivered to employees in an automated written report with additional explanation or follow-up with a nurse available upon request. More elaborate HRAs can include a full physical exam, medical history, and face-to-face consultation. Cash incentives can increase rates of employee participation (Merrill, Hyatt, Aldana, & Kinnersley, 2011). Results of the 1999 National Survey of Worksite Health Promotion (Association for Worksite Health Promotion, 1999) indicated that 35% of companies (57% of large companies) offer HRAs either directly or through their health insurance carriers. Early reviews of the literature on workplace health promotion programs recommended a healthy skepticism given the entrepreneurial and rapid proliferation of prepackaged worksite wellness programs and the limited number of research studies (Alexander, 1988; Anderson & Staufacker; Warner, Wickizer, Wolfe, Schildroth, & Samuelson, 1988), but more recent evidence has supported the usefulness of HRA and tailored advice as a way to direct employees to available health resources and wellness activities (Soler et al., 2010).

The challenge of measuring the sole impact of HRA and tailored advice is that these represent "gateway" interventions that increase employee awareness and motivation to seek other health care services or engage in other worksite health promotion activities (e.g., smoking cessation). Thus, the multiple pathways by which an HRA might ultimately lead to improved health are complex, and it is difficult to separate the impact of HRA as a stand-alone intervention. Thus, there is evidence that HRAs increase employee awareness of possible health concerns (Rula & Hobgood, 2010), but health benefits are only evident after workers seek health advice, lifestyle counseling, or other forms of wellness support as a next step. Ethical and privacy considerations limit the breadth of HRA screening and the ability of employers to communicate directly with employees about follow-up care or counseling. Two systematic reviews of the effectiveness of worksite interventions, including health risk appraisal and feedback, have concluded no effect unless combined with broader employer efforts to provide health education and counseling (Anderson & Staufacker, 1996; Soler et al., 2010).

Although workers may be provided a list of available resources to address health risk factors identified in the HRA report, results are confidential, and a worker's decision to enroll in specific health promotion activities or lifestyle interventions is completely voluntary. However, rapidly escalating health care costs and the increasing number of chronic medical conditions among working adults are leading some employers to consider more effective methods to provide outreach to high-risk workers and encourage additional health screening and secondary prevention efforts (Loeppke et al., 2009; Nicholson, Taitel, Sweeney, Haufle, & Kessler, 2008). Thus, there has been emerging research of the ways that workers with chronic or recurring medical problems are able to manage their symptoms at work (Anderson, Mangen, Grossmeier, Staufacker, & Heinz, 2010; de Vries, Reneman, Groothoff, Geertzen, & Brouwer, 2012), and how workers and employers might effectively communicate to overcome or accommodate health-related functional limitations without violating worker privacy concerns or creating litigation risks for employers (Shaw et al., 2011).

Comprehensive Worksite Health Promotion Programs

Although HRA and feedback alone may not produce measurable health benefits, these methods can provide an important cornerstone for more large-scale comprehensive worksite wellness programs. These programs can encompass many different prevention and treatment strategies, and the large

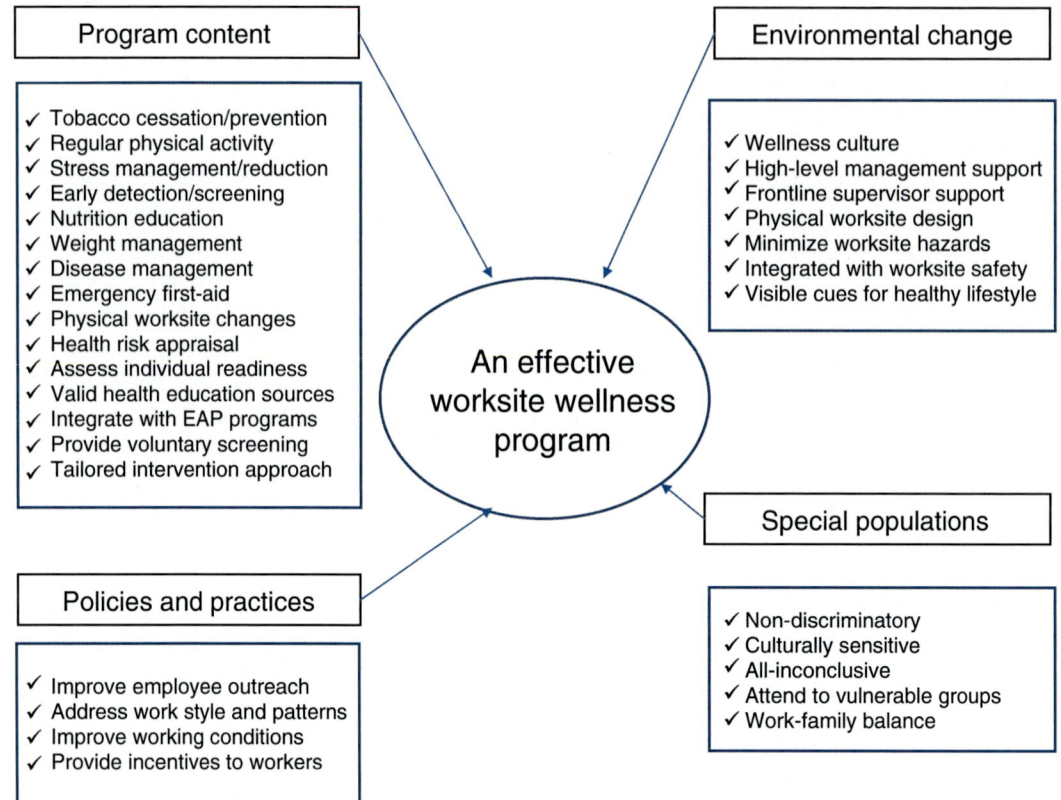

Fig. 17.4 Summary recommendations for an effective worksite wellness program (adapted from Carnethon et al., 2009)

heterogeneity of wellness programs (and heterogeneity in employment settings and occupations) has posed challenges for researchers and consensus panels who have attempted to synthesize the available studies evaluating their effectiveness. Components of a comprehensive wellness program might include tobacco cessation, physical activity promotion, stress management, health screening, weight management, nutritional guidance, first aid instruction, disease management, and environmental and administrative changes in the workplace that support healthy lifestyles. Summary recommendations from a policy statement of the American Heart Association (Carnethon et al., 2009) are shown in an abbreviated form in Fig. 17.4. In addition to being comprehensive in scope, it is important that wellness programs be well integrated into the normal practices, values, and culture of a workplace organization and legislative and societal frameworks (Carnethon et al.; Peltomäki et al., 2008). Despite these challenges, the accumulating evidence seems to support the health and productivity benefits of these more comprehensive efforts to improve employee health (Pelletier, 2011).

Most of the studies on multicomponent or comprehensive health promotion programs including HRA, tailored health advice and information, and worksite health seminars and workshops have been evaluated (without the benefit of a comparable control or comparison group), but their benefits can only be assessed among workers who actually take advantage of these offerings. Nevertheless, most studies have shown reductions in health risk factors (Colkesen et al., 2011; Hochart & Lang, 2011; Loeppke et al., 2008; Mills, Kessler, Cooper, & Sullivan, 2007), absenteeism (Mills et al., 2007), presenteeism (Cancelliere, Cassidy, Ammendolia, & Côté, 2011), health care costs (Merrill, Hyatt, et al., 2011), and improvements in work performance (Mills et al.). One of the best research summaries in this area is a series of periodic reviews published in the *Journal of Occupational and Environmental Medicine* of the clinical and cost-effectiveness of comprehensive health promotion and disease management programs (Pelletier, 2005, 2009, 2011). The most recent review in this series reported improvements in the number and quality of studies, also a fairly consistent positive effect on employee health and employer costs (Pelletier, 2011). A recent example is a controlled study of 266 workers completing a HRA and given access to tailored health information, wellness literature, and seminars and workshops focusing on identified health risks. There were statistically significant improvements in the reduction of health risk factors, reduced absenteeism, and improved work performance after 1 year (Mills et al.). In two larger studies involving multiple employer sites, a similar comprehensive worksite wellness program showed improvements in health risk factors that were sustained for 2–5 years (Hochart & Lang, 2011; Merrill, Anderson, & Thygerson, 2011).

Based on this evidence, we conclude that more comprehensive worksite promotion efforts can be effective to prevent disability and reduce health risks, especially with regard to metabolic and cardiovascular disorders. There is a current trend among comprehensive worksite health wellness programs to not only make improvements in healthy lifestyles, but to also provide more intensive support and assistance to workers with chronic diseases (Pelletier, 2011). Another research direction has been to develop and study worksite health promotion programs that are targeted to the needs of specific occupational settings or demographic groups; for example, construction workers (Groeneveld et al., 2011), female blue-collar workers (Campbell et al., 2002), and transportation workers (Olson, Anger, Elliot, Wipfli, & Gray, 2009). In general, researchers have emphasized the importance of social and cultural context that can impact on the design and feasibility of health promotion programs and the variable level of acceptance across settings and locations (Peltomäki et al., 2008). In the US, health promotion programs are typically offered only among larger employers (>500 employees), and these programs are over-represented among manufacturing and business/professional employers in comparison with retail, transportation, and warehousing (U.S. Department of Health and Human Services, 2000). Thus, worksite wellness programs provide important health benefits to employees, but they reach only a limited percentage of the total working-age population. Unfortunately, occupations representing workers with the greatest number of cardiovascular and behavioral health risk factors [e.g., firefighters (Soteriades, Smith, Tsismenakis, Baur, & Kales, 2011)], are among those least likely to encounter employer-sponsored health promotion programs.

The Business Case for Worksite Health Promotion

Apart from knowing that worksite health promotion efforts benefit the health of workers, another important question for employers has been whether program costs are sufficiently offset by reductions in disability and health care costs or concomitant improvements in worker productivity. Other economic questions are what minimum intensity of health promotion efforts are required to show an effect, and whether there is a consistent dose–response relationship between the cost of worksite health promotion efforts and their measurable benefits. Regardless of long-term economic benefits, some employers are still unwilling to invest in employee health programs due to immediate budgetary considerations. To address these questions and to build a business case for worksite health promotion programs, researchers have included economic evaluations alongside controlled or pragmatic trials of new or experimental health promotion programs. The purpose of economic evaluations is to identify, measure, and compare costs and health consequences of two or more programs or interventions (including comparison with nominal or usual practices). In most countries, employers would bear the financial consequences of lost worker productivity and the administrative burden of rehiring and training, but other costs associated with disability and health care expense may or may not be relevant to the employer depending on national differences in health insurance and disability systems. Thus, the financial benefits to employers may be greater where there is employer-subsidized healthcare (e.g., USA), and less where healthcare costs are born by a national health service (e.g., UK).

Four types of economic evaluations should be distinguished: cost analysis; cost-effectiveness analysis; cost-utility analysis; and cost-benefit analysis. Cost-analysis involves systematic collection and analysis of net costs associated with a program or intervention. Cost-effectiveness analysis (CEA) is applied to compare the costs of different interventions with a common health effect. A cost-effectiveness ratio is calculated by the difference in costs between the intervention and control intervention, divided by the difference in effects between the two interventions. CEA can be expressed as dollar value per kg weight loss. In Cost-Utility analysis (CUA), the effect of an intervention is expressed in utilities, such as Quality Adjusted Life Years (QALYs). CUA is beneficial to compare different interventions, and/or different groups. For example, a 1.0 QALY increase by a diabetes program may cost $20,000, and a 1.0 QALY increase for a chronic obstructive pulmonary disease (COPD) program may cost $40,000. CUA can be expressed as the dollar value per QALY saved or gained.

In a Cost-Benefit analysis (CBA), all effects and costs are expressed in monetary values (e.g., dollars). This is a useful analysis to investigate return on investment (e.g., for each dollar spent, over a 12-month period you will receive $10 in return [because productivity costs reduce because of the intervention]). For example, in a large-scale evaluation of a comprehensive worksite wellness program among municipal employees, a $3.85 return on investment was reported over 5 years for every dollar spent (Merrill, Hyatt, et al., 2011). In general, programs have achieved a return on investment from $3 to $15 for each dollar invested, with benefits offsetting costs within 12–18 months (Anderson, Serxner, & Gold, 2001). A systematic review applying meta-analytic techniques concluded an average 28% reduction in sick leave, 26% reduction in health care costs, and 30% decrease in workers' compensation claims costs (Aldana, 2001). These effect sizes can equate to considerable financial incentives for employers to invest in comprehensive wellness program.

Overall, economic evaluations of worksite wellness programs have analyzed the costs associated with worksite wellness programs in relation to the positive health benefits that they generate. In situations where resources are limited, economic evaluations give insight in how investments lead to effects over time. An important aspect of economic evaluations is the perspective that is used to determine which costs are included in the analyses. In the societal perspective, all relevant costs categories are included, regardless of who pays. Within the context of worksite wellness, where the employer is often the one deciding whether to invest, the employer return on investment (taking into account only those costs paid directly by the employer) are included, and an employer perspective becomes the guiding framework for comparing costs and benefits.

Worksite health promotion programs aiming at either improving diet or increasing physical activity, or a combination of both, have positive effects on workers' health, although the cost of such programs are not trivial (van Dongen et al., 2011). It depends on the willingness of employers to pay if these programs will be implemented. A recent review showed that the research design determined the outcomes of the economic evaluation. Worksite health promotion programs aimed at improving diet and/or increasing physical activity generate financial savings in terms of reduced absenteeism costs, medical costs or both according to non-randomized trials. However, according to randomized controlled trials, they do not generate financial savings (van Dongen et al., 2011). Economic evaluations regarding smoking cessation at the workplace are sparse. Some earlier published work indicates that smoking-cessation programs that rely on counseling are cost-effective in many settings (Brown & Garber, 1998). Some research has been conducted on the evaluation of a smoke-free policy, showing that smoke-free workplaces are more cost-effective compared to nicotine replacement therapy (Ong & Glantz, 2005). An important issue associated with economic evaluations of smoking cessation is that the benefits are particularly clear in the long term, which may exceed the working age (Warner, Smith,

Smith, & Fries, 1996). The results of economic evaluations have been very influential in persuading large employers to invest in vendor-based health promotion programs.

Apart from the potential economic benefits, implementation of large-scale employee wellness programs may have a less tangible but positive effect on employee life and job satisfaction, labor relations, job stress, and employee engagement (Duncan, Liechty, Miller, Chinoy, & Ricciardi, 2011; Grossmeier, Terry, Cipriotti, & Burtaine, 2010; Jasperson, 2010; Kimathi, Gregoire, Dowling, & Stone, 2009; Merrill, Anderson, et al., 2011; Schulte & Vainio, 2010; Tveito & Eriksen, 2009). Employers hoping to attract new talent in a competitive marketplace may invest more heavily in workplace health and wellness programs because positive health messages and healthy lifestyle benefits are enticing for young workers. Among existing workers, additional offerings in worksite health programs may improve overall perceptions of the company, engender a greater sense of trust and commitment, and improve retention. The positive financial impact to employers for maintaining strong labor relations has been well documented (Huselid, 1995), and this remains an important incentive for businesses to increase their investment in employee health and wellness programs.

One inherent source of tension that deserves mention is the potential conflict that an employer faces while trying to promote workforce health, on the one hand, and driving productivity, on the other. Thus, development of a worksite wellness program may require that employers revisit some of their existing policies regarding working hours, pay structure, productivity demands, working hours, shift work requirements, and overtime hours. Although healthy workers are likely to be more productive in the long run, employer support for a new wellness program might be undermined if high production demands are perceived as having negative health consequences. This may explain why some wellness programs have shown improved employee health and life satisfaction, but a concurrent decrease in job satisfaction (Merrill, Anderson, et al., 2011). The effectiveness of a comprehensive worksite wellness program, then, depends on the readiness of the organization, including compatibility with existing policies and procedures, and adequate labor relations. If workers perceive that employer support for health and wellness is not genuine, then a wellness program is not likely to generate a high level of participation or engagement. A number of authors have commented on the need to assess organizational readiness as a first step in launching a comprehensive wellness program (Grossmeier et al., 2010; Renaud et al., 2008; Seymour & Dupré, 2008).

Integration of Health and Wellness Promotion in the Workplace

Although research into worksite wellness programs has, by necessity, required evaluation of discrete elements and procedures that can be easily replicated, one universal observation from this research is that changing lifestyle habits and reducing health risks among workers can require a substantial shift in the organizational culture of the workplace, and this can only be accomplished with considerable management support, employee outreach, and benevolent persistence (Renaud et al., 2008; McLellan et al., 2009; Seymour & Dupré, 2008). Another observation is that considerable fragmentation of health and safety processes exist in the workplace: a safety professional provides training to reduce workplace hazards; a disability case manager coordinates return-to-work; an employee assistance program provides stress management and crisis intervention; a health care insurer coordinates disease management efforts; physicians direct medical care; an on-site nurse provides first aid; supervisors deal with work and family conflict, and so on. These "silos" of separate vendors, consultants, and individuals can make it difficult to communicate positive and uniform health messages in the workplace, and substantial efforts are needed to maintain consistent wide-scale health directives within the organization.

To address this problem, there is an emerging view in occupational health and safety that these programs should be more fully integrated to uniformly attend to issues of disease and injury prevention, health promotion, stress reduction, symptom management, and accommodations to age, family, and life stage (Cherniack et al., 2011). Many industrialized nations are experiencing a significant aging of the workforce with a greater number of chronic health conditions, and this has led some employers to embrace a more expanded view of workplace wellness beyond conventional safety and disability management practices. This new perspective suggests a greater interest in functional performance at work (not just absenteeism), a broader view of economic consequences (e.g., including medical costs), a prevention focus, and a concern for fitness and overall well-being, not just disease or injury. This integrated occupational wellness paradigm focuses attention on worker attitudes, job characteristics, and coping strategies in addition to biomedical diagnoses and functional capacities. This paradigm also suggests that some corporate reorganization may be necessary to unite health-related activities under fewer departmental divisions.

The real advantage of an integrated wellness approach is the ability to communicate a consistent message to employees about the high priority placed on employee health and safety. Though wellness efforts of the company may be housed in a number of separate departments, workers have a more singular view of the organization's overall commitment to their health and safety (Ribisl & Rieschl, 1993). Thus, there should be an overall set of corporate values guiding policies and practices around wellness whether it pertains to promoting healthy lifestyles, responding to workplace safety concerns, or helping workers manage chronic disorders. This is not easy to achieve when health-related practices are governed by different sets of legislative rules, insurance and healthcare systems, and financial considerations. Nevertheless, the concept of integrated wellness serves as an important guiding framework for the development of effective worksite health and wellness promotion programs.

Conclusions and Future Directions

Overall, there is growing evidence that worksite wellness programs can improve the health of workers with positive economic returns to employers. Worksite health and wellness promotion can be comprised of specific programs and services, employer policies and procedures, financial benefits and incentives, and changes in workplace culture or environment. Specific programs focusing on smoking cessation, weight reduction, or health risk appraisal have shown a moderate level of success and economic benefit, but the greatest impact has been for comprehensive wellness programs that include multiple initiatives, involve environmental and cultural changes in the workplace, and are tailored to meet the unique circumstances of organizations, employee health concerns, and work settings.

One emerging issue in the design of worksite wellness programs is the need to include environmental modifications and changes in employer policies and practices along with employee health risk appraisal, health education, and health behavior change programs. Thus, a comprehensive wellness program is more effective when employees perceive that the employer is not only sponsoring new health promotion programs but also reassessing the work environment and organizational culture in an effort to promote health and wellness. Another emerging issue in worksite health and wellness promotion is a need to better integrate health promotion efforts across different health and safety divisions within the organization. Otherwise, employees can receive confusing or mixed messages regarding the company's commitment to employee health and well-being. Also, worksite health promotion efforts may be ineffective in the presence of extreme production demands, lack of attention to basic safety concerns, poor labor relations, or failure to provide normative health and disability benefits.

Though worksite wellness is a relative newcomer to the professional field of occupational health and safety, there is mounting evidence that employers have a significant opportunity and economic incentive to improve employee health through comprehensive wellness programs. Such programs, however, are still uncommon among smaller employers and in many occupational settings, so the potential population-wide impact of these programs on public health has not been realized. Many questions remain unanswered about the specific elements of wellness programs that are most effective, but the current evidence suggests that a comprehensive program that reaches a larger number of employees will provide the greatest impact. In countries with an aging workforce and a growing number of chronic health conditions (e.g., USA), health and wellness promotion efforts within the workplace is likely to become more commonplace and more expansive in the coming years.

References

Akabas, S. H., Gates, L. B., & Galvin, D. E. (1992). *Disability management: A complete system to reduce costs, increase productivity, meet employee needs, and ensure legal compliance.* New York: American Management Association.

Aldana, S. G. (2001). Financial impact of health promotion programs: A comprehensive review of the literature. *American Journal of Health Promotion, 15*(5), 296–320.

Aldrich, M. (1997). *Safety first: Technology, labor, and business in the building of work safety, 1870–1939.* Baltimore: Johns Hopkins University Press.

Alexander, J. (1988). The ideological construction of risk: An analysis of corporate health promotion programs in the 1980s. *Social Science & Medicine, 26*, 559–567.

Anderson, D. R., Mangen, D. J., Grossmeier, J. J., Staufacker, M. J., & Heinz, B. J. (2010). Comparing alternative methods of targeting potential high-cost individuals for chronic condition management. *Journal of Occupational and Environmental Medicine, 52*(6), 635–646.

Anderson, L. M., Quinn, T. A., Glanz, K., Ramirez, G., Kahwati, L. C., Johnson, D. B., et al. (2009). The effectiveness of worksite nutrition and physical activity interventions for controlling employee overweight and obesity: A systematic review. *American Journal of Preventive Medicine, 37*(4), 340–357.

Anderson, D. R., Serxner, S. A., & Gold, D. B. (2001). Conceptual framework, critical questions, and practical challenges in conducting research on the financial impact of worksite health promotion. *American Journal of Health Promotion, 15*, 281–288.

Anderson, D., & Staufacker, M. (1996). The impact of worksite-based health risk appraisal on health-related outcomes: A review of the literature. *American Journal of Health Promotion, 10*(6), 499–508.

Anttonen, H., & Pääkkönen, R. (2010). Risk assessment in Finland: Theory and practice. *Safety and Health at Work, 1*(1), 1–10.

Association for Worksite Health Promotion. (1999). National Worksite Health Promotion Survey: William M. Mercer, Incorporated; and the US Department of Health and Human Services, Office of Disease Prevention and Health Promotion; 1999.

Brown, A. D., & Garber, A. N. (1998). Cost effectiveness of coronary heart disease prevention strategies in adults. *PharmacoEconomics, 14*(1), 27–48.

Bullen, C. (2008). Impact of tobacco smoking and smoking cessation on cardiovascular risk and disease. *Expert Review of Cardiovascular Therapy, 6*, 883–895.

Caban-Martinez, A. J., Lee, D. J., Fleming, L. E., Tancredi, D. J., Arheart, K. L., LeBlanc, W. G., et al. (2011). Arthritis, occupational class, and the aging US workforce. *American Journal of Public Health, 101*(9), 1729–1734.

Cahill, K., Moher, M., & Lancaster, T. (2008). Workplace interventions for smoking cessation. *Cochrane Database of Systematic Reviews, 4*, CD003440.

Campbell, M. K., Tessaro, I., DeVellis, B., Benedict, S., Kelsey, K., Belton, L., et al. (2002). Effects of a tailored health promotion program for female blue-collar workers: Health works for women. *Preventive Medicine, 34*, 313–323.

Cancelliere, C., Cassidy, J. D., Ammendolia, C., & Côté, P. (2011). Are workplace health promotion programs effective at improving presenteeism in workers? A systematic review and best evidence synthesis of the literature. *BMC Public Health, 11*, 395.

Carnethon, M., Whitsel, L. P., Franklin, B. A., Kris-Etherton, P., Milani, R., Pratt, C. A., et al. (2009). Worksite wellness programs for cardiovascular disease prevention: A policy statement from the American Heart Association. *Circulation, 120*, 1725–1741.

Centers for Disease Control and Prevention. (2007). Smoking-attributable mortality, years of potential life lost, and productivity losses—United States, 2000–2004. *Morbidity and Mortality Weekly Report, 57*(45), 1226–1228 [accessed 2011 Mar 11].

Chapman, L. S. (2005). Meta-evaluation of worksite health promotion economic return studies: 2005 update. *American Journal of Health Promotion, 19*(6), 1–11.

Cherniack, M., Henning, R., Merchant, J. A., Punnett, L., Sorensen, G. R., & Wagner, G. (2011). Statement on national worklife priorities. *American Journal of Industrial Medicine, 54*, 10–20.

Colkesen, E. B., Ferket, B. S., Tijssen, J. G. P., Kraaijenhagen, R. A., van Kalken, C. K., & Peters, R. J. G. (2011). Effects on cardiovascular disease risk of a web-based health risk assessment with tailored health advice: A follow-up study. *Vascular Health and Risk Management, 7*, 67–74.

de Vries, H. J., Reneman, M. F., Groothoff, J. W., Geertzen, J. H., & Brouwer, S. (2012). Factors promoting staying at work in people with chronic nonspecific musculoskeletal pain: A systematic review. *Disability and Rehabilitation, 34*, 443–458.

DeFriese, G. H., & Fielding, J. E. (1990). Health risk appraisal in the 1990s: Opportunities, challenges, and expectations. *Annual Review of Public Health, 11*, 401–418.

Dishman, R. K., Oldenburg, B., O'Neal, H., & Shephard, R. J. (1998). Worksite physical activity interventions. *American Journal of Preventive Medicine, 15*(4), 344–361.

Duncan, A. D., Liechty, J. M., Miller, C., Chinoy, G., & Ricciardi, R. (2011). Employee use and perceived benefit of a complementary and alternative medicine wellness clinic at a major military hospital: Evaluation of a pilot program. *Journal of Alternative and Complementary Medicine, 17*(9), 809–815.

Engbers, L. H., van Poppel, M. N., Chin, A. P. M. J., & van Mechelen, W. (2005). Worksite health promotion programs with environmental changes: A systematic review. *American Journal of Preventive Medicine, 29*(1), 61–70.

Gadomski, A. M., Stayton, M., Krupa, N., & Jenkins, P. (2010). Implementing a smoke-free medical campus: Impact on inpatient and employee outcomes. *Journal of Hospital Medicine, 5*, 51–54.

Goetzel, R. Z., Carls, G. S., Wang, S., Kelly, E., Mauceri, E., Columbus, D., et al. (2009). The relationship between modifiable health risk factors and medical expenditures, absenteeism, short-term disability, and presenteeism among employees at Novartis. *Journal of Occupational and Environmental Medicine, 51*, 487–499.

Groeneveld, I. F., van Wier, M. F., Proper, K. I., Bosmans, J. E., van Mechelen, W., & van der Beek, A. J. (2011). Cost-effectiveness and cost-benefit of a lifestyle intervention for workers in the construction industry at risk for cardiovascular disease. *Journal of Occupational and Environmental Medicine, 53*, 610–617.

Grossmeier, J., Terry, P. E., Cipriotti, A., & Burtaine, J. E. (2010). Best practices in evaluating worksite health promotion programs. *American Journal of Health Promotion, 24*(3), TAHP1–TAHP9. iii.

Harris, J. R., Lichiello, P. A., & Hannon, P. A. (2009). Workplace health promotion in Washington State. *Preventing Chronic Disease, 6*(1), A29. http://www.cdc.gov/ped/issues/2009/jan/07_0276.htm. Accessed February 17, 2012.

Hertz, R. P., & McDonald, M. (2004). *Obesity in the United States Workforce. Findings from the National Health and Nutrition Examination Surveys (NHANES) III and 1999–2000*. New York: Pfizer.

Hill, R. K., Thompson, J. W., Shaw, J. L., Pinidiya, S. D., & Card-Higginson, P. (2009). Self-reported health risks linked to health plan cost and age group. *American Journal of Preventive Medicine, 36*, 468–474.

Hochart, C., & Lang, M. (2011). Impact of a comprehensive worksite wellness program on health risk, utilization, and health care costs. *Population Health Management, 14*, 111–116.

Huselid, M. A. (1995). The impact of human resource management practices on turnover, productivity, and corporate financial performance. *Academy of Management Journal, 38*(3), 635–672.

Institute of Medicine. (1997). *Enabling America: Assessing the role of rehabilitation science and engineering*. Washington, DC: National Academy Press. pp. 40–61.

Jasperson, D. B. (2010). RadSurg wellness program: Improving the work environment and the workforce team. *Radiology Management, 32*(1), 48–53.

Karasek, R., & Theorell, T. (1990). *Healthy work: Stress, productivity, and the reconstruction of working life*. New York: Basic Books. pp. 1-30.

Kimathi, A. N., Gregoire, M. B., Dowling, R. A., & Stone, M. K. (2009). A healthful options food station can improve satisfaction and generate gross profit in a worksite cafeteria. *Journal of the American Dietetic Association, 109*(5), 914–917.

Koper, B., Moller, K., & Zwetsloot, G. (2009). The occupational safety and health scorecard—A business case example for strategic management. *Scandinavian Journal of Work, Environment & Health, 35*(6), 413–420.

Kowlessar, N. M., Goetzel, R. Z., Carls, G. S., Tabrizi, M. J., & Guindon, A. (2011). The relationship between 11 health risk and medical and productivity costs for a large employer. *Journal of Occupational and Environmental Medicine, 53*, 468–477.

Kunz, R., Vist, G., & Oxman, A. D. (2007). Randomisation to protect against selection bias in healthcare trials. *Cochrane Database of Systematic Reviews, 2*, MR000012.

Lee, D. J., Fleming, L. E., Arheart, K. L., LeBlanc, W. G., Caban, A. J., Chung-Bridges, K., et al. (2007). Smoking rate trends in U.S. occupational groups: The 1987 to 2004 National Health Interview Survey. *Journal of Occupational and Environmental Medicine, 49*, 75–81.

Leeks, K. D., Hopkins, D. P., Soler, R. E., Aten, A., Chattapadhyay, S. K., & Task Force on Community Preventive Services. (2010). Worksite-based incentives and competitions to reduce tobacco use: A systematic review. *American Journal of Preventive Medicine, 38*(2 Suppl), S263–S274.

Lemmens, V. E., Oenema, A., Klepp, K. I., Henriksen, H. B., & Brug, J. (2008). A systematic review of the evidence regarding efficacy of obesity prevention interventions among adults. *Obesity Reviews, 9*(5), 446–455.

Levy, B. S., Wegman, D. H., Baron, S. L., & Sokas, R. K. (2011). Occupational and environmental health: Twenty-first century challenges and opportunities. In B. S. Levy, D. H. Wegman, S. L. Baron, & R. K. Sokas (Eds.), *Occupational and environmental health: Recognizing and preventing disease and injury* (pp. 3–22). New York: Oxford University Press.

Loeppke, R., Nicholson, S., Taitel, M., Sweeney, M., Haufle, V., & Kessler, R. C. (2008). The impact of an integrated population health enhancement and disease management program on employee health risk, health conditions, and productivity. *Population Health Management, 11*, 287–296.

Loeppke, R., Taitel, M., Haufle, V., Parry, T., Kessler, R. C., & Jinnett, K. (2009). Health and productivity as a business strategy: A multiemployer study. *Journal of Occupational and Environmental Medicine, 51*, 411–428.

Longo, D. R., Johnson, J. C., Kruse, R. L., Brownson, R. C., & Hewett, H. E. (2001). A prospective investigation of the impact of smoking bans on tobacco cessation and relapse. *Tobacco Control, 10*, 267–272.

Maes, L., Van Cauwenberghe, E., Van Lippevelde, W., Spittaels, H., De Pauw, E., Oppert, J. M., et al. (2011). Effectiveness of workplace interventions in Europe promoting healthy eating: A systematic review. *European Journal of Public Health* [Epub ahead of print] doi 10.1093/eurpub/ckr098.

McLellan, R. K., Mackenzie, T. A., Tilton, P. A., Dietrich, A. J., Comi, R. J., & Feng, Y. Y. (2009). Impact of workplace sociocultural attributes on participation in health assessments. *Journal of Occupational and Environmental Medicine, 51*(7), 797–803.

Merrill, R. M., Anderson, A., & Thygerson, S. M. (2011). Effectiveness of a worksite wellness program on health behaviors and personal health. *Journal of Occupational and Environmental Medicine, 53*, 1008–1012.

Merrill, R. M., Hyatt, B., Aldana, S. G., & Kinnersley, D. (2011). Lowering employee health care costs through the Healthy Lifestyle Incentive Program. *Journal of Public Health Management and Practice, 17*, 225–232.

Mills, P. R., Kessler, R. C., Cooper, J., & Sullivan, S. (2007). Impact of a health promotion program on employee health risks and work productivity. *American Journal of Health Promotion, 22*, 45–53.

Muto, T., & Yamauchi, K. (2001). Evaluation of a multicomponent workplace health promotion program conducted in Japan for improving employees' cardiovascular disease risk factors. *Preventive Medicine, 33*(6), 571–577.

National Business Group on Health. (2012). *Performance in an era of uncertainty: 17th Annual Towers Watson/National Business Group on Health Employer Survey on Purchasing Value in Health Care*. Washington, DC: National Business Group on Health. pp. 25-29.

Nicholson, S., Taitel, M., Sweeney, M., Haufle, V., & Kessler, R. C. (2008). The impact of an integrated population health enhancement and disease management program on employee health risk, health conditions, and productivity. *Population Health Management, 11*, 287–296.

Olson, R., Anger, W. K., Elliot, D. L., Wipfli, B., & Gray, M. (2009). A new health promotion model for lone workers: Results of the safety & health involvement for truckers (SHIFT) pilot study. *Journal of Occupational and Environmental Medicine, 51*, 1233–1246.

Ong, M. K., & Glantz, S. A. (2005). Free nicotine replacement therapy programs vs implementing smoke-free workplaces: A cost-effectiveness comparison. *American Journal of Public Health, 95*(6), 969–975.

Ostbye, T., Dement, J. M., & Krause, K. M. (2007). Obesity and workers' compensation: Results from the Duke Health and Safety Surveillance System. *Archives of Internal Medicine, 167*(8), 766–773.

Peeters, A., Barendregt, J. J., Willekens, F., Mackenbach, J. P., Al Mamun, A., & Bonneux, L. (2003). Obesity in adulthood and its consequences for life expectancy: A life-table analysis. *Annals of Internal Medicine, 138*(1), 24–32.

Pelletier, K. R. (2005). A review and analysis of the clinical and cost-effectiveness studies of comprehensive health promotion and disease management programs at the worksite: Update VI 2000–2004. *Journal of Occupational and Environmental Medicine, 47*, 1051–1058.

Pelletier, K. R. (2009). A review and analysis of the clinical and cost-effectiveness studies of comprehensive health promotion and disease management programs at the worksite: Update VII 2004–2008. *Journal of Occupational and Environmental Medicine, 51*, 822–837.

Pelletier, K. R. (2011). A review and analysis of the clinical and cost-effectiveness studies of comprehensive health promotion and disease management programs at the worksite: Update VIII 2008–2010. *Journal of Occupational and Environmental Medicine, 53*, 1310–1331.

Peltomäki, P., Johansson, M., Ahrens, W., Sala, M., Wesseling, C., Brenes, F., et al. (2008). Social context for workplace health promotion: Feasibility considerations in Costa Rica, Finland, Germany, Spain, and Sweden. *Health Promotion International, 18*, 115–126.

Popkin, B. M. (2006). Global nutrition dynamics: The world is shifting rapidly toward a diet linked with noncommunicable diseases. *The American Journal of Clinical Nutrition, 84*(2), 289–298.

Proper, K. I., Koning, M., van der Beek, A. J., Hildebrandt, V. H., Bosscher, R. J., & van Mechelen, W. (2003). The effectiveness of worksite physical activity programs on physical activity, physical fitness, and health. *Clinical Journal of Sport Medicine, 13*(2), 106–117.

Quick, J. C., & Tetrick, L. E. (2003). *Handbook of occupational health psychology*. Washington, DC: American Psychological Association. pp. 1-97.

Racette, S. B., Deusinger, S. S., Inman, C. L., Burlis, T. L., Highstein, G. R., Buskirk, T. D., et al. (2009). Worksite opportunities for wellness (WOW): Effects on cardiovascular disease risk factors after 1 year. *Preventive Medicine, 49*(2–3), 108–114.

Renaud, L., Kishchuk, N., Juneau, M., Nigam, A., Téreault, K., & Leblanc, M. C. (2008). Implementation and outcomes of a comprehensive worksite health promotion program. *Canadian Journal of Public Health, 99*(1), 73–77.

Ribisl, K. M., & Rieschl, T. M. (1993). Measuring the climate for health at organizations. Development of the worksite health climate scales. *Journal of Occupational Medicine, 35*(8), 812–824.

Rula, E. Y., & Hobgood, A. (2010). The impact of health risk awareness on employee risk levels. *American Journal of Health Behavior, 34*, 532–543.

Schulte, P., & Vainio, H. (2010). Well-being at work—Overview and perspective. *Scandinavian Journal of Work, Environment & Health, 36*(5), 422–429.

Serxner, S., Adams, V. G., Hundahl, L. S., Lau, S., Adessa, C. J., Jr., & Hopkins, D. (1993). A smoking cessation pilot program. *Hawaii Medical Journal, 52*(10), 266–272.

Seymour, A., & Dupré, K. (2008). Advancing employee engagement through a healthy workplace strategy. *Journal of Health Services Research & Policy, 13*(Suppl 1), 35–40.

Shaw, W. S., Tveito, T. H., Geehern-Lavoie, M., Huang, Y. H., Nicholas, M. K., Reme, S. E., et al. (2011). Adapting principles of chronic pain self-management to the workplace. *Disability and Rehabilitation, 34*(8), 694–703.

Smedslund, G., Fisher, K. J., Boles, S. M., & Lichtenstein, E. (2004). The effectiveness of workplace smoking cessation programmes: A meta-analysis of recent studies. *Tobacco Control, 13*, 197–204.

Soler, R. E., Leeks, K. D., Razi, S., Hopkins, D. P., Griffith, M., Aten, A., et al. (2010). A systematic review of selected interventions for worksite health promotion. The assessment of health risks with feedback. *American Journal of Preventive Medicine, 38*(Suppl 2), S237–S262.

Soteriades, E. S., Smith, D. L., Tsismenakis, A. J., Baur, D. M., & Kales, S. N. (2011). Cardiovascular disease in US firefighters: A systematic review. *Cardiology in Review, 19*, 202–215.

Swinburn, B., Gill, T., & Kumanyika, S. (2005). Obesity prevention: A proposed framework for translating evidence into action. *Obesity Reviews, 6*(1), 23–33.

Syamlal, G., Mazurek, J. M., & Malarcher, A. M. (2011). Current cigarette smoking prevalence among working adults—United States, 2004–2010. *Morbidity and Mortality Weekly Report, 60*(38), 1305–1309.

Szinovacz, M. E. (2011). Introduction: The aging workforce: Challenges for societies, employers, and older workers. *Journal of Aging & Social Policy, 23*(2), 95–100.

Talmage, J. B., & Melhorn, J. M. (2005). How to think about work ability and work restrictions: Risk, capacity, and tolerance. In J. B. Talmage & J. M. Melhorn (Eds.), *A physician's guide to return to work* (pp. 7–18). Chicago, IL: American Medical Association.

Tanaka, H., Yamato, H., Tanaka, T., et al. (2006). Effectiveness of a low-intensity intra-worksite intervention on smoking cessation in Japanese employees: A three-year intervention trial. *Journal of Occupational Health, 48*(3), 175–182.

Tonnesen, P. (2009). Smoking cessation: How compelling is the evidence? A review. *Health Policy, 91*(Suppl 1), S15–S25.

Tveito, T. H., & Eriksen, H. R. (2009). Integrated health programme: A workplace randomized controlled trial. *Journal of Advanced Nursing, 65*(1), 110–119.

U.S. Department of Health and Human Services. (2000). *Healthy People 2010. Volume II: Objectives for improving health (Part B)*. Washington, DC: US Government Printing Office.

U.S. Department of Health and Human Services. (2010). *How tobacco smoke causes disease: The biology and behavioral basis for smoking-attributable disease: A report of the Surgeon General*. Atlanta, GA: U.S. Department of Health and Human Services, Centers for Disease Control and Prevention, National Center for Chronic Disease Prevention and Health Promotion, Office on Smoking and Health.

van Dongen, J. M., Proper, K. I., van Wier, M. F., van der Beek, A. J., Bongers, P. M., van Mechelen, W., et al. (2011). Systematic review on the financial return of worksite health promotion programmes aimed at improving nutrition and/or increasing physical activity. *Obesity Reviews, 12*(12), 1031–1049.

Verweij, L. M., Coffeng, J., van Mechelen, W., & Proper, K. I. (2011). Meta-analyses of workplace physical activity and dietary behaviour interventions on weight outcomes. *Obesity Reviews, 12*(6), 406–429.

Warner, K. E., Smith, R. J., Smith, D. G., & Fries, B. E. (1996). Health and economic implications of a work-site smoking-cessation program: A simulation analysis. *Journal of Occupational and Environmental Medicine, 38*(10), 981–992.

Warner, K. E., Wickizer, T. M., Wolfe, R. A., Schildroth, J. E., & Samuelson, M. H. (1988). Economic implications of workplace health promotion programs: Review of the literature. *Journal of Occupational Medicine, 30*, 106–112.

Whitehead, D. A. (2001). A corporate perspective on health promotion: Reflections and advice from Chevron. *American Journal of Health Promotion, 15*(5), 367–369.

World Health Organization. (2011). *WHO Report on the global tobacco epidemic, 2011: Warning about the dangers of tobacco*. Geneva, Switzerland: World Health Organization.

Stress Reduction Programmes for the Workplace

Tores Theorell

Overview

The theoretical basis for stress reduction in the workplace—psychosocial and physiological aspects—forms the first part of this chapter. A distinction is made between improvement of "good" forces and reduction of "evil" forces. The physiological counterparts of "good" (regeneration) and "bad" (energy mobilization) are presented. Furthermore, a distinction between organization-based and individual stress reduction programmes is made.

Several examples of intervention approaches and evaluation of their effects on employee health are presented. Many studies have shown that stress reduction programmes for the workplace can be effective in health promotion. There are many difficulties, however, that encounter the researcher who wants to do evaluation of the effects of such programmes on employee health, and these difficulties are particularly pronounced for those who evaluate organizational interventions.

When workplace-based stress interventions are discussed in relation to employee health, a frequent assumption is that such interventions should be confined to individual stress management programmes. Such programmes have indeed proved to be fruitful when applied skilfully. Reviews of scientific evaluations of stress management programmes on employee health—including both individual and more collective organizational approaches—even point out that the benefits of individual stress management are easier to prove than are those of organizational approaches. Part of this, however, may be due to the fact that it is more difficult to scientifically examine beneficial employee health effects of an organizational stress reduction strategy than to design evaluations of an individual approach—when each individual's health promotion is dealt with separately and each one's health is also followed separately without reference to the group (Kristensen, 2005). Practitioners involved in anti-stress health promotion programmes often point out, however, that beneficial effects of an individual stress management programme may turn out to have a short duration if the individual teaching it is not joined with an organizational approach at the same time. This complicates the theoretical analysis of stress reduction approaches in the workplace. As a consequence, the present review includes individual as well as organizational approaches to workplace stress prevention. Most of the organizational approaches will relate to work organization and to education of managers, factors that are crucial for the well-being of employees.

T. Theorell, M.D., Ph.D. (✉)
Karolinska Institutet and Stockholm University, 106 91, Stockholm, Sweden
e-mail: tores.theorell@stressforskning.su.se

Individual Versus Organizational Stress Reduction Approaches

Figure 18.1 shows schematically the interplay between structural and individual factors in workplace stress reactions. There are three levels in the diagram—*stressors and regenerative factors, coping and stress/regeneration reactions*. Each level theoretically represents a level for intervention efforts. The diagram illustrates that the processes are dealing both with positive (anabolism or regeneration) and energy mobilization (stress) aspects of the interplay. The black parts represent energy mobilization and the white parts regeneration. The floating border between black and white illustrates that stressors can become anti-stressors and vice versa; that destructive patterns of coping can become constructive and that catabolic reactions could change to anabolic reactions. First I shall briefly introduce the three levels, and then discuss each one of them in more detail. What this model adds to previously published similar models is that it combines the positive and the negative aspects. For each box in the diagram, there is a positive white upper part and a negative black lower part, with a grey zone between them indicating that some factors may be protective in some situations and damaging in others.

Figure 18.1 Schematic presentation of the interplay between environment, individual coping and reactions to the environment. The black parts represent energy mobilization and the white parts regeneration. The floating border between black and white illustrates that stressors could become anti-stressors and vice versa, that destructive patterns of coping could become constructive and that catabolic reactions could change to anabolic *Stressors and anti-stressors, the environmental level—positive and negative aspects.*

Factors in the environment that cause, trigger or sustain stress reactions or their positive counterparts are labelled *stressors and anti-stressors (or regenerative factors), respectively*. These are positioned to the left in the diagram. Work organization is a very important prerequisite for the working individual's stressors, but also for his/her positive reactions to the job situation. The theoretical stress chapter (see Chap. 2, Cooper et al.) in this text describes the many aspects of work organization that have to be taken into account in the understanding of workplace stressors. Stressor reduction in the workplace could be based upon work with key groups, such as managers or company leadership, union representatives, or the whole organization. Most of the experience in this field points at the importance of dialogue in the application of stressor reduction, between employees and management, between work units and between different specialist groups. Moreover, most of the literature on work organization interventions is devoted to the reduction of negative stressors. An important observation, however, is that the worksite also has responsibility for creating a positive atmosphere that stimulates creativity and social support. A label for these factors could be *anti-stressors*. Anti-stressors are likely to stimulate regenerative "healing" and health promotion processes in the employees. This pertains to both psychosocial and bodily processes. In the diagram, stressors are black and anti-stressors white. There is a grey zone between them indicating that the border between positive and negative stressors may sometimes be floating, and that one circumstance may change from being positive to negative and vice versa.

Coping: The Individual Stress Management Level

The individual programme for *coping* with stress is in the middle of the diagram. This level theoretically represents stress reduction aimed at changes in the attitudes and strategies for dealing with stressors in the workplace, rather than changing the stressors themselves. This type of stress management is mostly based on behavioural therapy principles (for instance, "mindfulness", "heart math" or other similar systems for stimulating the individual to systematically analyze his/her own situation in relation

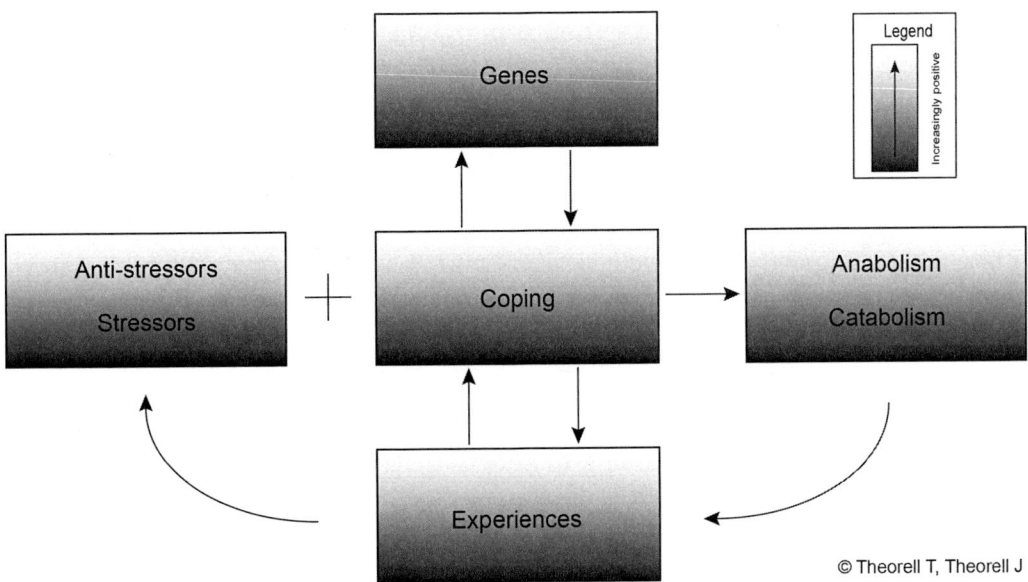

Fig. 18.1 Schematic presentation of the interplay between energy mobilization (*right hand side*) and regeneration (*left hand side*) from the hypothalamus through the pituitary to the endocrine end organs. The two sides influence one another (Tores Theorell and Jakob Theorell)

to stressors). The individual's coping programme is shaped by an interaction between genetic and environmental factors. The individual's coping strategy, however, is subjected to continuous change. New experiences throughout life influence coping strategies, in both old as well as young subjects. Accordingly, the individual is not a static machine which has been built in the beginning of life by genes and childhood. Also, as quite old individuals, we may change our coping patterns when the environment changes. We have seen this in psychosocial intervention studies performed on elderly subjects (Arnetz, Theorell, Levi, Kallner, & Eneroth, 1983; Lökk, Theorell, Arnetz, & Eneroth, 1991; Wikström, Theorell, & Sandström, 1993). These studies show that coping patterns may change also in old subjects when psychosocial intervention programmes are introduced. This also means that educational approaches could influence coping patterns. This is the basis for individual stress management.

Negative stress reactions and their positive counterpart, regenerative positive reactions, arise in an interplay between stressors and anti-stressors on one hand, and the individual coping programme on the other hand. The "interpretation" of the stressors and the subsequent handling of them (coping) is a result of genes and previous experiences. According to CATS (Cognitive Activation Theory of Stress) formulated by Ursin and Eriksen (2004), the coping pattern is to a great extent formed by the expectancies that the individual has on the consequences of his/her actions. A *positive expectancy* of outcome is likely to be associated with an active coping pattern. According to this terminology, negative expectancies could be labelled either *helplessness* (actions will not help) or—even worse—*hopelessness* (actions will make things worse). The experiences that the individual may have had from similar situations in the past will partly determine how the interplay between stressor and coping will develop, and how the physiological and psychosocial reaction will be. An important goal in worksite-based stress management programmes is, accordingly, to increase the likelihood that an employee will have positive outcome expectancies—a way of reducing individual stress reactions. The CATS theory, however, illustrates how interwoven the three levels (stressors, coping and stress reactions) are. In order to influence outcome expectancy in employees, one probably has to work more broadly with other aspects of coping as well and, in order to sustain effects, it may be necessary to influence stressors.

The Stress Reaction and Its Positive Counterpart, Regeneration

The psychophysiological background of stress reactions has been discussed elsewhere (e.g., Theorell, 2009). One of the central parts of the stress reaction is the Hypothalamic Pituitary Adrenocortical (HPA) axis, extending from the hypothalamus to the adrenal cortex (see Fig. 18.2). If the organism interprets the situation as energy demanding, a chain of reactions starts resulting in raised blood concentration of corticosteroids. In a number of ways, these corticosteroids help the organism sustain its fight in a stressful situation. In the acute situation, this is purposeful since the release of energy is facilitated by mobilization of fuel for energy requiring actions (carbohydrates and free fatty acids), and there is retention of salt and fluid which may otherwise get lost in an uncontrollable way in a physically-demanding situation. There is also inhibition of acute inflammatory reactions. However, if the stressor is long-lasting (for instance, lasting for weeks or months), those same effects may be damaging to health. There are other components in the immediate stress reaction, some of which occur more immediately (within seconds or parts of seconds) than the reactions of the HPA system (which take place within minutes), such as those taking place in the sympatho-adrenergic system (noradrenalin) and in the sympathomedullary system (adrenalin).

There is also a "good" counterbalancing system an anti-stress system which protects from adverse effects of long lasting stress. This HPG (Hypothalamo Pituitary Gonadal) axis has the same levels as the HPA axis, ranging from the hypothalamus to the gonadal glands. The balance between the HPA and HPG axes is illustrated by Fig. 18.2. The HPG axis represents the "regenerative" or "anabolic" part of metabolism. The male testes and the female ovaries are the end organs of this axis, and they represent the extremes of this activity, namely, reproduction. "Building a new human individual" is of course the most pronounced "anabolic/regenerative activity" that the body can be involved in. Building new cells and repairing worn-out tissues, is closely related to this. Some of the production of anabolic corticosteroids takes place in the adrenal cortex. Accordingly, some of the release of these regenerative hormones takes place in the adrenal cortex (for instance, testosterone in women), together with the corticosteroids that are important for energy mobilization. This means that the separation in the left and right side of Fig. 18.2 is theoretical and not anatomical. Cells producing hormones that are mainly active in regeneration are located in the adrenal cortex, which is mainly producing and releasing hormones that are active in energy mobilization. The diagram illustrates that the two forces, "energy mobilization" and "regeneration", are balancing one another on all levels of the HPA and HPG axes.

In all bodily organs, cells are being worn out and have to be repaired or replaced. In some cell systems, this is a rapid process (days or weeks, such as in mucosa, skin and white blood cells) whereas, in other systems, it is slow (years, such as in the skeleton). Of particular interest in the discussion regarding effects of long lasting stress is the fact that connective tissues and muscles depend on regeneration, and otherwise there will be increasing fragility in muscles and tendons. Similarly, white blood cells have to be replaced when they are worn out. If not, increased resistance against infections may arise. A third example is the brain with its own support system, the glia cells. These cells are constructed like connective tissue cells, and they also depend on sufficient regenerative activity. It this is not sustained, the glial cells will be dysfunctional. This affects the brain function, possibly resulting for instance in deteriorating short memory function. Testosterone and oestrogen, as well as their precursor DHEA-s (dehydroepiandrosterone sulphate), are examples of corticosteroids with mainly anabolic/regenerative function. Also, other hormones participate in this, such as the pituitary growth hormone. There is a balance between the HPA axis and the HPG axis. This means that the HPG axis tends to lower its activity when the HPA axis has maximal activity (in stressful situations). But it also means that damaging effects of long lasting stress can be dampened by a high activity in the HPG axis. The balance between HPA and HPG activity is an important principle in health promotion.

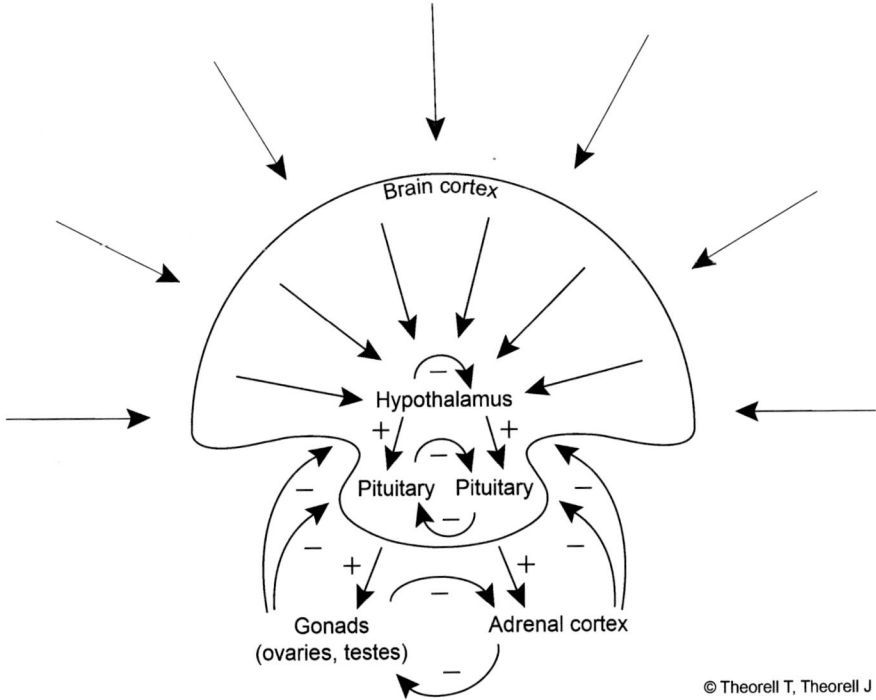

Fig. 18.2 Schematic presentation of the interplay between energy mobilization (right hand side) and regeneration (left hand side) from the hypothalamus through the pituitary to the endocrine end organs. The two sides influence one another (Tores Theorell and Jakob Theorell)

We are constructed for a life in "swings between the two". We need challenges and periods with energy mobilization in order to "train" all our biological systems, but periods or energy focus have to be interspaced with periods of regeneration and recuperation. This balance theory has been developed previously by several authors. See for instance Karasek and Theorell (1990). Karasek has recently published an interesting theoretical framework for the analysis of psychosocial work environments. Using the second law of thermodynamics from physics he describes the dynamic needs—in both individuals and organizations—of energy storage and energy release periods. Ideally it should be one of the responsibilities of occupational health care organizations to monitor these dynamics in the work place (Karasek, 2008).

The Workplace and Balance Between Energy Mobilization and Regeneration

In Chap. 2, working conditions (both stressors and health promoting factors) were described. Factors that increase energy mobilization in employees include factors such as excessive demands (both physical and psychological), repeated frequent reorganizations, lack of support from superiors and co-workers, lack of possibilities to exert control, lack of reward, negative feedback and bullying (Siegrist 1996). All these factors could be turned into their opposites; that is to say, *reasonable challenges* adapted to the resources in terms of number of employees and knowledge in the organization, *well-planned reorganizations* rooted in the needs of the worksite activity, a good organizational structure for *employee influence*, social, psychological and material *reward* for hard work, *good emotional and instrumental support* from superiors and co-workers and *good emotional climate* preventing bullying. All of these now positive factors could, in turn: reduce the number of negative factors (stressors); strengthen the ability for the individuals and the organization to handle the stressors; and turn some of the negative biological reactions into positive ones. In addition, all of them could be influenced by organizational work. Such organizational work has been described by several researchers (e.g., Israel, Schurman, & House, 1989; Rosskam, 2009; Semmer, 2006).

There are several ways in which a workplace could introduce health-promoting activities in the organization. The general rule is always that there has to be dialogue between employees and management for any such intervention to have sustained effects. A reorganization that is introduced with a "top-down" perspective (with directives from management and no dialogue with employees) is likely to fail in the long run. Barbara Israel and co-workers have developed "participatory action research" (PAR) which builds upon active participation of researchers and stimulating employees to act as researchers in the dialogue between management and employees in improvement of work organization (Israel et al., 1989; for more recent discussions, see Rosskam, 2009; Semmer, 2006). Although not always explicitly stated, the goal in such processes is always to both identify and reduce the prevalence of destructive stressors and to identify, introduce and strengthen anti-stressors in the organization.

Although it is always preferable to work with the whole organization, it could sometimes be feasible to work with the managers in the organization—in order to convince them that they need to take psychosocial factors into account when the work organization is designed. Financial arguments are often important in such discussions. It has been shown that organizations that produce ill health in employees loses large amounts of money, much more than managers actually realize, in the form of indirect costs (see Jauregui & Schnall, 2009). I describe two scientific evaluations of manager education effects on employee health, both of which had an explicit goal of improving working climate. From these examples, I discuss possibilities and difficulties in these types of efforts, and I also discuss the extent to which these intervention programmes have influenced stressors and anti-stressors, respectively.

Manager Education in the Troubled Swedish Insurance Company

This evaluation study (Theorell, Emdad, Arnetz, & Weingarten, 2001) was planned during the Spring, 1998. During that period, Sweden was in the final part of a financial crisis that started in 1990. During the late 1990s, the economy had started to recuperate and unemployment rates had decreased. The crisis had started a new era in Swedish business life, however, with a high pressure for reorganization of worksites, privatization of several parts of the public sector, increased competition and lively discussions about management models. The insurance company in the study had a monopoly for a specific kind of insurances, but politicians were now demanding more competition. During the study period, no pronounced change in the company's market conditions took place, but there was a constant discussion about such a change for the company and this created organizational anxiety. The leaders of the company argued that psychosocial education for the managers could be of benefit. For instance, one argument was that managers who have psychosocial knowledge would be more able to handle employee anxiety and, accordingly be able to prevent dysfunction in the organization during the turmoil. A consulting agency was contacted and, at the same time, a team of researchers was contacted taking responsibility for evaluation.

The manager education that was launched was founded in organizational research, and had the following structure:

- It was mandatory for all managers in the organization (13% of the employees) to participate.
- There were meetings every second week during two semesters (Fall, 1998 and Spring, 1999), lasting for 2 h each time. The meetings consisted of a lecture lasting for half an hour, followed by group discussions with seven participants in each group. An expert from the external consulting group participated in all group discussions. The gatherings took place in the workplace during work hours.
- An important aspect of the design of this intervention was that all managers in this part of the organization took part in the meetings. This meant that they could support one another during the intervention year. They could discuss with one another about themes that had been discussed during the meetings. Another important aspect was that they could use the 2 weeks between the meetings for practical applications of what they had been discussing. There were four themes, each one occupying one fourth of the period, namely, *individual stress, group stress, organizational stress and ways for instituting and maintaining beneficial change.*

A condition for a meaningful evaluation was that there was a control group. This was a similar part of the same insurance company. The control group had similar numbers of employees and similar work tasks. Both groups were geographically located in the central part of Stockholm. The evaluation was a *quantitative* one, with emphasis on work environment and employee health. Standardized questionnaires were distributed, and morning blood samples (for the measurement of cortisol and liver enzymes, as well as lipids in serum) were collected before start, as well as after 1 year. There was no *qualitative* evaluation of the intervention programme. The researchers even deliberately avoided extensive qualitative interviewing because it was felt that this could have had an adverse effect on the course of the psychosocial process. However, interviews with the personnel management after the end of the intervention year showed that the managers in the psychosocial intervention group were more orientated towards the psychosocial needs of their employees, so some effect of the programme was clearly visible. The results from the questionnaires showed that there was a significantly more favourable development of reported decision authority in the experimental group than in the control group during the intervention year. In the control group, decision authority deteriorated, whereas in the intervention group, it improved. This significant difference in development was observed both in the managers themselves (approximately 20 in each group) and in their respective subordinates (about 100 in each group). In the examination of 260 employees who provided blood sample collections (130 in each group), morning serum cortisol remained unchanged during the study year in the control group, but decreased in the experimental group (with a significant Group×Time interaction effect). Similarly, gamma glutamyl transferase (a liver enzyme sensitive to excessive alcohol consumption, but also to long-lasting negative stress) developed significantly more favourably in the experimental group. This latter finding did not correspond to any difference in development of alcohol consumption in the two groups, and the interpretation was therefore that both these changes (not only the decreased cortisol concentration) were related to decreased stress levels in the experimental group's employees. There was also a significant decrease in serum cholesterol in both groups, a likely consequence of the blood tests and the individual information about the results in both groups. This information helped the employees focus on diet and healthy lifestyle more than before the study. Of course, the results of one single intervention study do not unequivocably prove anything, and more studies with similar designs are needed. Important characteristics in the design and interpretation were the following:

- Initiative came from management, not from the employees or union. Although the target of the intervention was the manager group, one of the specific aims of the programme was to increase managers' awareness of the employees' psychosocial needs. This means that, although the design could imply a top-down perspective, the contents of several lectures and group discussions aimed at an increase in bottom-up processes. Interestingly, analyses of changes in decision authority showed a favourable development in the experimental group, both in the managers themselves and in employees. Indeed, improved decision authority has been shown to be an important mediator of improved employee health in successful psychosocial job site interventions (Bond & Bunce, 2001; Jackson, 1983). Our results could be interpreted to mean that increased power sharing could be perceived at the same time in both managers and employees during a successful psychosocial intervention.

- The biological stress reduction following the intervention was more significant in the employees than in managers, although it is important to emphasize that the statistical power of the analyses in the managers was much smaller in the manager group due to smaller numbers.
- Stress reduction was visible after a whole year of the intervention, not before that (data not published)—no significant difference was observed after half a year. This is logical since psychosocial processes may take a long time and, in this case, there had to be effects first on the attitudes and knowledge of the managers, and then subsequently on the whole employee group.
- The educational principles in the intervention programme for the managers followed present theory and are, therefore, representative of psychosocial interventions for managers in the Nordic countries.
- From an evaluation point of view, it is interesting that it was not feasible to follow the study groups in this examination longer than during the intervention year. After the intervention year, a major reorganization took place, which made interpretation of subsequent follow-up data impossible, at least from an intervention point of view.
- It could be argued, since there was only one intervention group and one control group, that irrelevant factors that were not recorded could explain the difference in development. While this may theoretically be true, we found no competing processes in the two halves of the organization that were likely to explain the difference.

To summarize, there were both preventive (eliminating stressors by improving the work organization and improving the managers' knowledge of psychosocial factors) and promoting components (stimulating anti-stressors by improving the working climate) in the intervention programme. There was no effect on work load or work tempo. The significant psychosocial effect that was observed was a more favourable development of decision authority in the intervention group than in the other group during the study year. This was associated with a reduced morning cortisol concentration which, in this relatively healthy working population, is an indication of reduced energy mobilization. The most likely interpretation is that the intervention programme had reduced the stressors by improved influence over decisions and, thereby, decreased their level of energy mobilization.

"Artistic Manager Education", an Effort to Strengthen Anti-stressors

The second evaluation study (Romanowska, Larsson, Eriksson, et al., 2011; Romanowska, Larsson, & Theorell, 2011) was based upon a different educational principle than the first one. In addition, the framework was different because the participants in the study did not represent whole organizations. They came more or less randomly from many companies/agencies, and represented themselves only. Therefore, they did not enjoy the support from other managers who had taken part in the same education concomitantly. The participating managers were recruited from a larger group of managers who had applied for manager education. They were informed that they would be randomly allocated into two different groups, and that examinations (including questionnaires and blood samples) would be collected from them during the process (before start, after 1 year and after 18 months). If they did not accept these conditions before randomization had taken place, they were not recruited for the study. Accordingly, the participants had no possibility to choose between the educational groups.

The basic new educational idea of this study was that managers need training in empathy and emotional competence when they communicate with their employees. Aesthetic experiences may give important educational triggers in such a learning process and, therefore, the managers in the "artistic training" group were subjected to a collage of poems with adjacent emotionally-adapted music—Schibbolet performances. The topics in the Schibbolet performances were related to human suffering, and also related to the responsibility that human beings may have in situations that are dangerous for their colleagues. The topics were not necessarily related to work situations but, rather, to more general situations in human history (such as the holocaust). They were, however, certainly translatable into situations that managers encounter in their employee contacts (e.g., when bullying arises against an employee in a work place). There were ten Schibbolet performances during the intervention year, and the performances were always systematically followed up with group discussion (in the large group and in smaller groups) led by experts. In addition, the participating managers were asked to write diaries after each performance. Notes from the diaries were used in follow-up talks.

The educational programme in the comparison condition was similar to the programme in the previous study. Like the Schibbolet programme, it had ten meetings during a year, but the participants were asked to perform activities ("home lessons" according to CBT [cognitive behaviour therapy]) principles and not diaries as in the Schibbolet group between the sessions. The time allotted to joint activities in the educational programmes was the same for the two study groups. The comparison programme contained lectures with subsequent group discussions. There was no artistic component. In the comparison programme, the participants introduced themselves to one another and presented their own solutions to problems after listening to lectures. Thus, mutual sharing of experiences was an important component. The final study evaluation was performed on the participating managers, as well as on a group of subordinates (4 for each manager) for a total of 136 subjects. The results from the subordinates showed that the cortisol concentration changes did not differ significantly between the groups. There was a tendency (similar to the results in the first intervention study) for the cortisol concentration in the non-artistic group subordinates to decrease compared to the corresponding other group after 1 year. This was an expected finding, although it failed to reach statistical significance and the difference had decreased half a year after the end of the interventions. A positive finding was that the concentration of the anabolic hormone DHEA-s (dehydroepiandrosterone sulphate)—which is a precursor of both male and female sex hormones and which has anabolic effects on its own—developed significantly more favourably after 18 months in the Schibbolet than in the corresponding control group subordinates. The expected winter decrease in DHEA-s concentration (seasonal effect that is "normal") was significantly less pronounced in the Schibbolet subordinates. One interpretation of this is that the changes induced by the manager intervention were able to dampen the winter deterioration in health in the subordinates—a positive "anabolic effect".

The development of a psychosocial work environment (as assessed by standardized questionnaires) did not differ between the two employee groups. The development of mental health in the subordinates, on the other hand, had developed significantly more favourably in the Schibbolet subordinates up to the end of the study 18 months after start. Accordingly, there was a more favourable development in the Schibbolet subordinate group with regard to a total mental health score (including emotional exhaustion, sleep disturbance and depressive symptoms), covert coping (tendency not to deal with problems arising in relation to work mates and superiors) and performance based self-esteem. This combination of findings suggest a climate increasingly allowing employees to talk about problems and solving them jointly, not only with increased individual effort. The finding that there was no significant group difference in development of the psychosocial work environment is consistent with the fact that the participating managers were not from the same organization. Accordingly, in neither of the study groups could they support one another throughout the process. Therefore, the effects of the programmes are likely to have been more individualistic manager effects than collective organizational ones. However, if the managers' attitudes to psychosocial problems have changed, this is likely to have had an effect on the psychosocial climate. The lack of group support may have been particularly deleterious to the effects of the comparison group intervention since that intervention depends to a great extent on joint follow-up discussions of the seminars and group activities. The control group intervention was similar to the intervention in the insurance company study described above. However, in the previous study, the participating managers could support one another. If it is true that, in the more recent study, the effects of the interventions have been more individualistic, then the next question will be how the managers themselves were influenced by the two intervention programmes.

The managers were followed by means of two different psychological dimensions—"sense of coherence" according to Antonowsky, and "agreeableness" as it is assessed on the NEO-PIR. The findings indicated that there was no change in the comparison group managers, whereas the Schibbolet mangers showed an increase in both sense of coherence and agreeableness which resulted in a significant group development difference after 18 months. However, it was not significant after 12 months. This was consistent with the employee changes in health which showed no significant group differences after 12 months, but did so after 18 months. Accordingly, there was a delay in effect which is consistent with the idea that it takes time before the programme with artistic components has an observable effect on the managers, and that it then takes additional time before this becomes observable in the employees due to changes in the working climate. However, if the managers become more agreeable and feel a greater sense of coherence, they are also likely to improve their ability to handle conflicts and to realize when they have to actively deal with conflict situations rather than stay passive. In summary, the analysis of this study may show that the artistically-flavoured manager intervention has had a positive influence in the direction of health promotion, rather than on a reduction of stressors (strengthening HPG rather dampening HPA influence). The results also confirm that it may take more than a year before differences are observable.

Cultural Participation in Work Places

Above, I have described an experiment indicating that a manager intervention with artistic components, if handled professionally, may have a beneficial effect on the working climate. If we extend this to the whole workplace, what do we know about the extent to which workplaces organize cultural activities for their employees? And, do such activities in general have any beneficial effect on employee health? An epidemiological survey of a random selection of more than 5,000 working Swedish men and women (SLOSH) was used in order to examine relationships between work-based cultural activities and mental employee health. The hypothesis was that we would find a positive relationship between frequent cultural activity organized at work and good employee health. The participants were asked to answer the same questions on three occasions over 2-year intervals (2006, 2008 and 2010). The average participation rate was 60%. A postal questionnaire was used to ask questions, on one hand, about cultural activities organized for employees (Are cultural activities such as movies, theatre performances, concerts or exhibitions organized for the employees in your work place? Never/some time per year/some time per month/some time per week and more often), and, on the other hand, questions about emotional exhaustion and depressive symptoms. Employee assessments of the manager function and work environment (psychological demands and decision latitude), as well as socioeconomic variables were covariates. The results indicated that only 50% of Swedish employees reported that there had been any cultural activity in their workplace during the past year. However, there was some variation during the three study years 2006, 2008 and 2010 (Fig. 18.3). A statistically significantly lower frequency of cultural activities at work was reported during the period of the highest unemployment rate of 8.5% (2010)—than during the other measurement periods—with unemployment rates

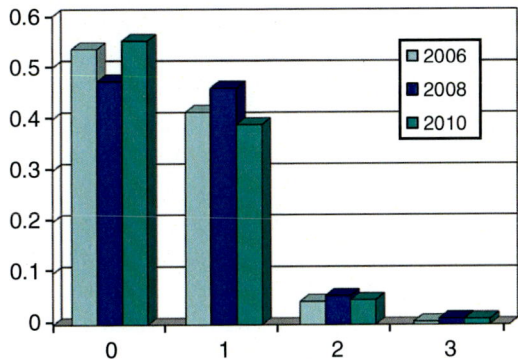

Fig. 18.3 Prevalence of cultural activities at work reported during the three study years in Are cultural activities such as movies, theatre performances, concerts or exhibitions organized for the employees in your work place? (From Theorell et al., 2011). 0=No activities, 1=Some time per year, 2=Some time per month, 3=Some time per week or more often. Swedish Longitudinal Occupational Study of Health, 2006 n=5,037, 2008 n=9,623, 2010 n=8,912

Table 18.1 Cross-sectional multiple linear regression coefficients (B) for independent statistical "protective contribution" of cultural activities in relation to ill health in the different steps

Year	2006	2008	2010
Alternative a (adjusted for age, gender and income only)			
Exhaust	0.61*** (n=4,955) T=4.44	0.68*** (n=9,381) t=7.26	0.58*** (n=8,671) t=6.09
Depr	0.27* (n=4,946) t=2.28	0.41*** (n=9,414) t=4.96	0.34*** (n=8,729) t=3.98
Alternative b (adjusted for same as a plus "Does your boss listen?")			
Exhaust	0.30* (n=4,826) t=2.20	0.44*** (n=8,564) t=4.53	0.27*** (n=7,964) t=2.73
Depr	0.06 NS (n=4,816) t=0.47	0.17* (n=8,586) t=1.96	0.11 NS (n=8,020) t=1.27
Alternative c (adjusted for same as b plus demands and decision latitude at work) (n=3,420)			
Exhaust	0.22(*) (n=4,660) t=1.70	0.27** (n=8,297) t=3.07	0.09 NS (n=7,677) t=0.97
Depr	0.05 NS (n=4,655) t=0.42	0.03 NS (n=8,318) t=0.30	0.00 NS (n=7,721) t=0.05

(*)$p<0.10$, *$p<0.05$, **$p<0.01$, ***$p<0.001$
Each year has been analyzed separately. (From Theorell et al., 2012)

varying between 6 and 6.5%. Statistically, there was a significant "protective effect" of cultural activities in relation to emotional exhaustion (Table 18.1). In 2008 (the best year in this particular study with the lowest unemployment rate), this relationship remained significant, even after statistical adjustment had been made for perceived management (Does your manager listen to you?) and two central psychosocial work environment dimensions (psychological demands and decision latitude). During the other study years, the protective effect of cultural activity on emotional exhaustion prevalence became non-significant after this statistical adjustment. The conclusion was that the relationship between cultural activity at work and likelihood of emotional exhaustion may have been partly mediated by a listening manager and a good work environment, particularly during the more problematic years of 2006 and 2010.

However, even in 2008, when the relationship was significant after adjustment, the introduction of these variables reduced the magnitude of the association. Formulated in other words, a listening management and a good psychosocial work environment increase the likelihood that there are cultural activities organized at work. However, during the good period, the cultural activities had an independent statistical effect in the direction of lowered likelihood of emotional exhaustion over and above the effect of the good management and good work environment. This should be regarded as an anabolic, regenerative effect of the cultural activities (see Figs. 18.1 and 18.2 presented earlier), although this is speculative since no physiological examinations were performed in this study. No independent statistical effect of cultural activity was found during the periods with a lower cultural activity at work, although the unadjusted relationship was significant also during those years. Prospective analyses indicated that cultural activities at work had a statistically independent value for predicting beneficial change in emotional exhaustion scores 2008-2010. This indicated that cultural activity at work might sometimes protect against emotional exhaustion. It should be pointed out that most of the cultural activities that were offered were vaguely defined and, therefore, long-lasting effects may have been unlikely for most of them. For depressive symptoms, no significant relationships were observed. Depressive symptoms could be regarded as a more serious ill health outcome than emotional exhaustion, and it could therefore be that even stronger and more frequent activity levels would have been required.

Thus, the question on cultural activity at work was a vague and superficial one without specification of type of cultural activity. When the responses indicated that some activity had taken place, they may have been an indication of a social indirect "caring" emphasis in the work environment. However, most of the activities reported were infrequent. Other research (Bygren, Konlaan, & Johansson, 1996 and Bygren, Johansson, et al., 2009) has indicated that social activities should take place at least once a week to have an effect on health indicators (mortality), and there is no reason to assume that this would not apply to cultural activity in the workplace. Still the findings do show a "dose response pattern" with decreasing evidence of emotional exhaustion among employees with increasing cultural activity at work. That no effects lasting for as long as 2 years were shown could be explained by the low intensity and heterogeneous nature of this exposure. An important observation was that these positive activities decreased during a period of high unemployment rate and, that during that period, the effects of cultural activity were not statistical significant (after adjustment for psychological demands, decision latitude and the degree to which the manager listened or not). Perhaps the recommendation should be the opposite one: the more unemployment, the more cultural activity at work because such activities could promote both health and creativity in employees.

Very few studies have been published from interventions specifically designed to improve employee health by means of cultural activity. An experiment performed by Bygren, Weissglas, et al. (2009) was designed as a randomized control trial, in which employees in a municipality in northern Sweden were offered the possibility to participate in the experiment which comprised cultural activities once a week (the participants could select films, concerts, or art exhibition visits, or singing in a choir), lasting for 2 months. Half of the participants were randomized to the experimental group ($n=51$), while the other group ($n=50$) served as a control group. Standardized questionnaires were used before and after the intervention period. The results indicated a statistically more favourable development of vitality, social functioning and somatic health (composite score) in the experiment group than in the other group.

A subsequent study by our group (Theorell, Hartzell, & Näslund, 2009) was performed in order to illuminate the possible significance of collective effects of cultural activities at work. There was no control group. The experiment took place in four work places in which employees had the possibility to participate in cultural activities organized at the workplace during working hours, once a week during 3 months. The activities were organized by regional groups (theatre, classical music, jazz, interactive theatre, dance, Chinese and Scottish dance, bingo lottery after art exhibition etc.). Ten participants were selected from each workplace for observations. These key participants had a high presence in the cultural activities throughout the experimental period, but the presence of other employees varied substantially and, therefore, collective effects on whole worksites could not be studied. Employees who did not belong to the observation group could attend, but did so only when other conditions at work allowed this. The subjects in the observation group were asked to fill out visual analogue scales before and after each activity Changes from before to after performance in emotional states were calculated from these scales. This allowed us to calculate the average activity related to increases in joy, relaxation, and alertness for each person during the 3 months. Participants were asked before and after the 3 months period to fill out standardized questionnaires relating to health (emotional exhaustion, depressive symptoms and sleep disturbance), and blood specimens were also collected before and after the study period. Because there was no control group, no conclusions can be drawn regarding possible effects of the cultural activities. Another complication was that the start of the study was in August, when most subjects had just come back from summer vacation, and the end was in late November with darkness, cold weather and deteriorating atmosphere at work. As a result, there was a significant worsening both in subjective well-being and in biological stress indicators that could be assessed in the blood samples in the total study group. However, those subjects who, on average, felt more than other participants that they were vitalized and became more joyful and relaxed after the cultural activities had a better health development than other participants. There was, however, also a negative result which we considered important: Those who benefited the most with regard to emotional states also reported that their social support became worse during the study period. This could be interpreted as a "jealousy" effect. Many of their work mates were not allowed to leave their work for the cultural activity. When the "beneficiaries" came back, these work mates may have been irritated and angry.

This above "jealousy" finding raises an important point. If cultural activities in the work place should have optimal effects it is necessary to: provide a diversity of activities so that everyone can find something of interest in the cultural activity; and allow an equal possibility for everybody to participate. Otherwise, the cohesiveness effects are unlikely to arise, the social climate is not likely to improve, and the beneficial "regenerative" effects will also be unlikely.

Other Organizational Changes That Have Been Evaluated in Relation to the Employee Health Change Organization

Improvement in work organization could in general have beneficial effects on employee health. In the examples produced above, specific goals were formulated, such as improved psychosocial competence in managers and increased cultural activity at work. There are, however, many other possible targets. A few examples should be mentioned.

In 1983, Orth Gomer (Orth Gomér, 1983) described an experiment in which 45 policemen were randomly allocated to two groups (22 and 23 subjects, respectively) with different shift work schedules. In one group, they started working in a counter clock-wise schedule (essentially condensing shifts) for 4 weeks, and then continued working in a clock-wise schedule (spreading shifts) for 4 weeks. In the other group, the order between these schedules was reversed. The number of working hours was exactly the same in the two alternatives. After clock-wise rotation, sleep was reported to be longer and systolic blood pressure and urinary catecholamine excretion became lower than after the counter clock-wise rotation. These findings indicate that an improvement in shift work scheduling is associated with improved employee health, mainly because of decreased HPA axis activity (mirrored in reduced blood pressure and catecholamine excretion). The example is interesting from another point of view. Spreading of shifts (clock-wise) had been less popular than condensing them. The reason for this was that a condensed shift work schedule allowed the policemen to have longer free periods between their shift cycles. Accordingly, from a social point of view, the health improving schedule was less popular. However, when the participants had experienced the difference and realized how the counter clock-wise schedule increased their "stress" level, many of them changed their mind. This discussion also tended to differ with age; older participants were more interested in health promotion, whereas younger participants favoured the social aspects and regarded the health aspects as less interesting.

Working with the whole organization is to be recommended whenever this is possible. A British group of researchers (Bond & Bunce, 2001) examined how the method originally described by Israel et al. (1989)—Participation Activation Research (PAR)—affected the health of employees. Six office worksites (that all reported some problem with the work environment) were recruited. Three of them were randomly allocated to the experimental group in which PAR was applied. The other worksites served as comparison groups. These worksites had to wait for a year before they were allowed to participate in PAR. PAR takes many months. It builds upon the general idea that employees should be stimulated to examine their own work organization. Through a series of discussions and structured efforts to improve the organization, improved working climate is likely to arise. Self-rated psychological symptoms, sick leave and self-rated effectiveness were assessed before the start and after 1 year. With regard to all three measures, improvement was observed in the experimental group, and a worsened condition in the comparison group. There was a statistically significant interaction between time and group for all of them. Most of the improvement in the experimental group was shown statistically to be due to improved decision authority for the employees.

A similar experiment was performed by Orth Gomer, Eriksson, Moser, Theorell, and Fredlund (1994). By means of random allocation, four office worksites were selected as the experimental group, and one worksite as the comparison group. Group discussions regarding individual stress mechanisms and organizational stress factors were instituted, and proposals for improvement were structured during 8 months. Stimulation from, and control over, work was reported to improve significantly in the experimental group, and this was paralleled by an improved serum lipid pattern in the same group. No such changes were observed in the comparison group. The other classical coronary risk factors (smoking, eating, exercise, relative weight) did not change differently in the two groups. The interpretation of these results was that there was a reduced stress level (reduced HPA activity) in the experimental group mirrored by improved serum lipids.

Improved HPG activity has also been observed after improvement of the psychosocial work environment, as described earlier in this chapter in the study of the "Schibbolet programme". One other example is the study (Theorell, Liljeholm-Johansson, Björk, & Ericson, 2007) of two symphony orchestras that were followed every 6 months during 2 years. The psychosocial work environment was examined by means of standardized questionnaires, and physiological assessments of the musicians were made by means of saliva specimens (six tests on every test day on five occasions during the 2-year period) and 24-h ECG recordings. In one of the orchestras, the atmosphere was seriously disturbed by the fact that one of the wind blowers became unconscious during two concerts in front of the audience. He also fainted during two rehearsals during this period. This resulted in a reduced sense of social support and the mean concentration of testosterone (regenerative hormone) was very low in the musicians during this period. However, the fainting musician was treated medically. As a consequence, his fainting stopped. In addition, group therapy was arranged for the musicians. The psychosocial atmosphere improved and the saliva testosterone levels became normalized after half a year. Similar findings were found for the ECG analyses (indicating normalization of parasympathetic activity). These results show that a destroyed feeling of control and support may lower the regenerative activity (HPG) but, also, that a normalization can occur relatively rapidly if collective action is taken.

That there is a need for increasing research efforts in the field of psychosocial manager competence and its relevance for work-family interaction is illustrated by the fact that the Centers for Disease Control and Prevention (CDC), in collaboration with the National Institutes for Health, in the United States have sponsored the Work, Family and Health Network (WFHN) to implement a workplace intervention and to evaluate the effect of this on employee health. The intervention is designed to increase supervisor and co-worker support for employees' families and their personal lives. The intervention includes participatory work redesign activities that identify new work practices and processes that increase employees' control over work time, while still meeting business needs. There are no results published from this research yet, but other research has indicated that this may be a fruitful area for interventions (Brough & O'Driscoll, 2010; Kelly et al., 2008)

Frequently, actions oriented towards improved production in general have the spin-off effect that employee health improves. Arnetz et al. (1983) have described an experiment in which staff working in a home for the elderly tenants were stimulated to participate in cultural activities. The effects of this were evaluated by means of a controlled study, with pre- and post-assessments in an experimental and a control group. During the process, the staff participated in the construction of assessment tools and in stimulating the tenants to participate in the activities. Pronounced beneficial health effects were found in the experimental group's elderly participants. The psychosocial work environment for the staff in the two groups was followed as well. Although the number of staff was small for this kind of study ($n = 13$ in both groups), the development of the rates of absenteeism recorded during the 6 months that the experiment lasted, and during the 3 months that followed, merits attention. The numbers developed differently in the two staff groups. The recorded absenteeism in the staff was identical at start. Whereas staff in the control group (with no particular added stimulation for the elderly during the 6 months) had increasing numbers of worker absences per tour (by approximately 50%) during the 9 months from start, the staff in the experimental group decreased absenteeism (personal communication, June 1984, see figure 5.2, page 196, Karasek & Theorell, 1990).

Karasek and Theorell (1990) have described an experiment (without a control group) in which employees in six different occupations participated in repeated explorations of their own health (blood tests, blood pressure measurements and questionnaire measures of health), and their own work environment. These assessments were performed on four occasions during a year. At the end of the experimental period, feedback of all the data collected was given at a group session for each worksite, as well as individually. In terms of discussions regarding the psychosocial work environment, the participants reported a significant increase in such discussions after, compared to before, the data collection period. Before the study, 27% of them ($n = 133$) reported that such discussions took place whereas, after feedback, the corresponding number was 44% (Table 6.3, page 212, Karasek & Theorell, 1990).

Participatory Action Research (PAR, see above, Rosskam, 2009) is an organizational technique for making this happen in a structured and constructive way. Through a series of meetings, identification of strengths and difficulties, scheduled group activities, goal formulations and other collective activities for all employees, it is possible to improve the psychosocial conditions. For instance, successful improvements of health, well-being and working conditions for hotel room cleaners and bus drivers in San Francisco have been described after PAR processes (Antonio, Fisher, & Rosskam, 2009; Casey & Rosskam, 2009).

As another example, long-term effects of a successful intervention on the health of Canadian health-care personnel have been described by Bourbonnais, Brisson, and Vezina (2011). The intervention programme was very similar to PAR, as it is described above. The health-care settings were subjected to a work environment exploration (based upon structured telephone interviews), followed by interviews and goal-directed group meetings. For the evaluation, a quasi-experimental design with a control group was used. Assessments were made before the intervention and 3 years later. The results showed that all adverse psychosocial factors, except one, were reduced in the experimental group, and the improvement was statistically significant for 5 of 9 factors, namely, psychological demands, effort–reward imbalance, quality of work, physical load and emotional demands. In addition, all health indicators improved—2 of 5 significantly, namely, work-related stress and personal burnout. In the control hospital, decision latitude and social support deteriorated significantly during the same period. In addition, decision latitude and social support deteriorated in the control hospital. This study shows that a reduction of stressors is an achievable goal using psychosocial intervention techniques, and that the significant effects are not only temporary, but may last for 3 years.

In yet another study, physiological and psychological effects of a change from conventional assembly-line work to group-based work were evaluated (Melin, Lundberg, Söderlund, & Granqvist, 1999). A total of 36 male and 29 female assembly-line workers were examined during and after work at a car engine factory. The two ways of organizing assembly-line work were: a traditional assembly line, with fixed work stations organized as a chain and involving short repetitive work cycles; and a new and more flexible work organization, with small and autonomous groups having greater opportunity to influence the pace and content of their work. During both conditions, the workers were studied during two consecutive days of normal working and during a corresponding work-free period at home. In the flexible organization, the workers reported significantly more variation, independence and possibility to learn new skills at work. Successive self-reports of tiredness increased significantly more at the assembly line, compared to the flexible work organization. Along with this, systolic blood pressure, heart rate and epinephrine excretion increased significantly during the work shift at the assembly line, but not during work in the flexible organization. In addition, analyses of urinary catecholamine excretion revealed that subjects were able to "unwind" more rapidly after work in the flexible organization. This study showed that it is possible to influence worker health by means of flexible work redesign, resulting in reduced HPA activity.

Individual Stress Management

Individual stress management refers to a number of techniques that aim to improve coping with stress. The concept "stress inoculation training" has been used. This relates to the discussion above regarding improved individual coping strategies and builds upon principles formulated in behavioural therapy (Meichenbaum, 1989). Several controlled evaluation studies of the effects of individual stress management programmes have been published and the field has been subjected to several reviews (see for instance Deborah, Tanigawa, & Stephen, 2003; Murphy, 1996 and Van der Klink, Blonk, Schene, & van Dijk, 2001). Our own research group has performed a study of the employee health effects of individual stress management, 303 white collar workers in 22 units in 4 information technology and 2 media companies were randomized into an intervention and a control group (Hasson, Anderberg, Theorell, & Arnetz, 2005). Web-based tools for health promotion and stress management were introduced. These were developed for this intervention, and were building upon principles established in web-based intervention research and in cognitive behavioural therapy. All participants (in both the intervention and comparison groups) received a short web-based questionnaire for repeated monitoring of current health and stress status, a diary and information about stress and health. In addition, the participants in the intervention group were offered web-based exercises aiming at decreasing unwanted stress. These exercises included techniques for relaxation, time management, cognitive reframing and a chat. For the evaluation, a structured questionnaire with 100 "mostly" questions (most of them based upon visual analogue scales) was delivered before the start of the programme and 6 months later. Venous blood samples were collected from all participants during these data collection periods in both groups. The dropout rate was small and very similar in the two groups. At the end of the 6-month intervention period, the means in the intervention group had developed significantly better than the comparison group with regard to "ability to manage stress", "sleep quality", "mental energy", " concentration ability", "social support" and "competence usage at work". Correspondingly, the intervention group's means had developed significantly better with regard to the hormone DHEA-s, Neuropeptide Y (also a protective "anti-stress" hormone) and TNF alpha (a marker of immune activity). These results were very encouraging since they pointed at beneficial effects in the form both of reduced HPA and increased HPG activity. However, when the participants were followed for an additional 6 months, all of the significant differences between intervention and comparison group participants had disappeared (partly reported in Hasson, Arnetz, Theorell, & Anderberg, 2006). This illustrates the difficulty that is encountered in several evaluations of individual stress management programmes: That the effects of these programmes depend on continuous use of them for long periods of time, and that individuals may tend to attend to them initially and then abandon them. Motivation is the key concept: Individuals must have motivation to continue. Increased motivation can be facilitated if individuals themselves see that programme participation continues to be meaningful. This is only one part of the equation, however. If only a small proportion of employees have participated in the stress management programme, the surrounding employees will not have a good tolerance for the activities and may even try to prevent their colleagues from participating. On the other hand, if the majority of employees have participated and, therefore, have developed an accepting tolerance, this may increase the likelihood that structures facilitating participation will arise. Returning to Fig. 18.1 in this chapter, individual stress management represents interventions focused on individual coping. If such a programme is entirely individually focused and no attention is paid to work organization (stressors and anti-stressors), it is very likely that there will be no lasting effects. A poor work organization may in itself create obstacles for participation. Conversely, it could be argued that an intervention that is entirely organization-focused may lack components that motivate individuals to participate. Monitoring of the individuals' health and their work environment raises the interest in organizational conditions. Semmer (2006), in a review of job stress interventions summarizing evaluations of interventions, has concluded that "a combination of person-focused and organization-focused approaches is the most promising".

In addition to the "real" difficulties that are encountered in interventions, both organizational and individual-focused, there are often other potential barriers that researchers encounter in such evaluations. Kristensen (2005) has discussed those. Random trials are preferred in scientific evaluations. The rationale behind this is that groups should be comparable from the start. In the ideal case, participants in the groups to be followed in the evaluation should not have influence over the choice of group since this could introduce error—those who prefer one of two interventions might be more healthy/ill or more willing/reluctant to institute change than those in the comparison group. When the intervention is focused on individuals in the work place, a difficulty may also arise if participants in the two groups work at the same worksite since they might influence one another during the process. This is likely to reduce possible differences. In addition, the longer the intervention lasts, the greater risk that the groups will contaminate one another, or that they will both be contaminated by irrelevant external factors. In organizational interventions, it is preferable to randomize whole worksites rather than individuals since the intervention to be evaluated is "collective" in its nature. This could sometimes be very difficult for practical reasons. One additional difficulty, particularly in organizational interventions, is that, although those planning the intervention may have very distinct ideas about the contents of the intervention, they will have to negotiate and sometimes compromise in order to make the final product only remotely similar to the initial plans; what is being evaluated in that situation may be a tiny fraction of the ideal intervention.

Several authors have pointed out that researchers tend to focus their evaluation efforts on the effects of individual stress management programmes for employees rather than on interventions with an organizational focus. This is regrettable although it is understandable in view of the difficulties encountered in evaluating organizational interventions. In a review published in Australia Caulfield, Chang, Dollard, and Eishaug (2004) summarize their findings stating: "Most interventions were individually focused, despite the preponderance of research identifying risky work environment stressors. Results suggest a paucity of published information regarding what works with occupational stress interventions in Australia".

Interventions of a physical nature that could reduce stress in the workplace are also of interest. One example is improvement of acoustics. Blomkvist, Eriksen, Theorell, Ulrich, and Rasmanis (2005) performed an evaluation of the effects of a change in ceiling tiles (one period with sound reflecting, and one period with sound absorbing tiles) in an intensive coronary care ward. The results showed that reverberation time (echo) and speech intelligibility improved significantly when sound was absorbed. Staff were asked to rate work environment factors at the start and end of each shift during a period with sound absorbing and sound reflecting ceiling, respectively. Differences in psychosocial ratings between start and end of shifts were calculated, and these differences were regarded as "accumulated effects" of the environment. In results comparing the sound reflecting and sound absorbing period revealed the following: during the afternoon shift (which is characterized by a more lively atmosphere), significant improvement in such accumulated effects were reported (lower demands and less pressure and strain; despite a higher intake of patients during the sound absorbing period). In addition, the patients rated higher scores for care quality during the sound absorbing period. This is of course not unexpected, although the magnitude of the effect was stronger than expected. When sounds reverberate in the room, many statements and instructions have to be repeated. In addition, there is increased risk of wrong-doing since signals may be misinterpreted. All of this increases the level of irritation, and psychological demands rise. Thus, an improved sound environment provides a method to decrease the HPA axis activity.

Summary and Conclusions

Psychosocial interventions for dealing with excessive stress levels at work could be designed either to reduce the level of stressor exposure or to strengthen the resistance against adverse reactions. Some interventions do both—they aim at reduction of negative and strengthening of positive factors at the same time. Regardless of the positive/negative framework, the target could be either the work organization or the individuals—or both. Physiological stress research has advanced our knowledge regarding the physiological and endocrinological counterparts of energy mobilization and regeneration, the bodily representatives of negative long lasting stress and anabolism respectively. The first part of this chapter summarizes the role of interventions in worksites. The physiological levels from the brain to the body periphery with competition between energy mobilization (mirrored for instance in the hypothalamo pituitary adrenocortical, HPA, axis) and regeneration/anabolism (mirrored in the hypothalamo pituitary gonadal, HPG, axis) are described since they are important in understanding change processes. In the intervention process three levels, the environment, the individual and the psychophysiological reaction are identified.

The chapter then describes several "stress prevention" projects in which health consequences for employees are evaluated. On the organizational level, a wide range of approaches have been used in many different countries—Scandinavia, USA, Canada, Great Britain, western central Europe and Australia. Organizational approaches with beneficial effects on employee stress levels include such diverse things as changes in shift work schedules, improved acoustics, reorganized assembly lines, psychosocial education of managers, cultural activities for the employees and improved employee participation in work organization planning (Participation Activation Research, PAR). Drawing on several projects from the author's research group, details related to the execution and interpretation of evaluations are discussed.

First of all, failure or success of an intervention in relation to employee health depends on how the intervention is presented/introduced in the organization, whether the intervention really affects a large proportion of the employees or not, whether it is relevant for employee health, whether the efforts are sufficiently sustainable and long lasting to have any health effect.

Secondly, researchers may fail to show an employee health effect although there may be such an effect. This may be due to shortcomings of the evaluation design such as too small study samples, irrelevant health measures, factors not measured that mask an effect and too short follow-up periods—if effects are delayed. In the opposite way, evaluations may present positively biased results, for instance when there is no comparison group, and when there is too short a follow up—if effects are transitory and therefore of marginal importance. Poorly planned and instituted interventions which have been designed for the benefit of employee health could even have adverse effects.

Despite all these difficulties there are several published studies which show that well planned organizational interventions aiming at reduced stress levels and/or strengthened resistance against long lasting stress do have beneficial effects on variables or relevance to employee health. This shows that there is a great potential in these kinds of interventions. Outcome variables have included various aspects of mental health assessed by means of standardized questionnaires but also physiological variables such as cortisol and regenerative hormones. There is also a growing literature on qualitative aspects of the intervention process itself. This is of central importance for practical application.

In organizational intervention research there is also a discussion regarding the level of intervention. It is preferable to work with the total organization (such as PAR, see above) but in some circumstances it is also beneficial to improve the psychosocial competence of managers. Managers who are knowledgeable in the area of the organization's psychosocial needs are likely to be of benefit to the health of the employees.

There is a growing literature on the benefit of individual stress management programmes. Such programmes have been proved to be of benefit to human beings wherever they are applied and workplaces are no exception. Therefore it is a good idea for workplaces to stimulate and facilitate the use of such programmes. It should be emphasized however that many evaluations of employee health effects of such programmes have been based upon short follow-up periods. And in studies using longer follow-up the effects are attenuated. Part of this may be due to the fact that employees who lack organizational support for the practice of individual stress management find it difficult to sustain practice in the workplace. The conclusion is that individual and organizational interventions mutually strengthen one another.

Directions for future research: It is evident that publications of good scientific evaluations of interventions against adverse effects of stressors in the work place are rare. There is urgent need for such studies. This review shows that stress prevention programmes in the workplace could have substantial beneficial effects. There is a great potential and more evaluation research is warranted.

References

Antonio, R., Fisher, J., & Rosskam, E. (2009). The MUNI health and safety project: A 26-year union-management research collaboration. In P. Schnall, M. Dobson, & E. Rosskam (Eds.), *Unhealthy work: Causes, consequences, cures*. New York: Baywood.

Arnetz, B., Theorell, T., Levi, L., Kallner, A., & Eneroth, P. (1983). An experimental study of social isolation of elderly people: Psychoendocrine and metabolic effects. *Psychosomatic Medicine, 45*(5), 395–406.

Blomkvist, V., Eriksen, C. A., Theorell, T., Ulrich, R., & Rasmanis, G. (2005). Acoustics and psychosocial environment in intensive coronary care. *Occupational and Environmental Medicine*. doi:10.1136/oem.2004.017632.

Bond, F. W., & Bunce, D. (2001). Job control mediates change in work organization intervention for stress reduction. *Journal of Occupational Health Psychology, 6*, 290–302.

Bourbonnais, R., Brisson, C., & Vezina, M. (2011). Long-term effects of an intervention on psychosocial work factors among healthcare professionals in hospital setting. *Occupational and Environmental Medicine, 68*, 479–486.

Brough, P., & O'Driscoll, M. P. (2010). Organizational interventions for balancing work and home demands: An overview. *Work and Stress, 24*(3), 280–297.

Bygren, L. O., Johansson, S. E., Konlaan, B. B., Grjibovski, A. M., Wilkinson, A. V., & Sjöström, M. (2009). Attending cultural events and cancer mortality: A Swedish cohort study. *Arts & Health, 1*, 64–73.

Bygren, L. O., Konlaan, B. B., & Johansson, S. E. (1996). Attendance at cultural events, reading books or periodicals, and making music or singing in a choir as determinants for survival: Swedish interview survey of living conditions. *British Medical Journal, 313*, 1577–1580.

Bygren, L. O., Weissglas, G., Wikström, B. M., Konlaan, B. B., Grjibovski, A., Karlsson, A. B., et al. (2009). Cultural participation and health: A randomized controlled trial among medical care staff. *Psychosomatic Medicine, 71*, 469–473.

Casey, M., & Rosskam, E. (2009). Organizing and collaborating to reduce hotel workers' injuries. In P. Schnall, M. Dobson, & E. Rosskam (Eds.), *Unhealthy work: Causes, consequences, cures*. New York: Baywood.

Caulfield, N., Chang, D., Dollard, M., & Eishaug, C. (2004). A review of occupational stress interventions in Australia. *International Journal of Stress Management, 11*, 149–166.

Deborah, L. J., Tanigawa, T., & Stephen, M. W. (2003). Stress management and workplace disability in the US, Europe and Japan. *Journal of Occupational Health, 45*, 1–7.

Hasson, D., Anderberg, U. M., Theorell, T., & Arnetz, B. B. (2005). Psychophysiological effects of a web-based stress management system: A prospective, randomized controlled intervention study of IT and media workers (ISRCTN54254861). *BMC Public Health*. doi:10.1186/1471-2458-578.

Hasson, D., Arnetz, B. B., Theorell, T., & Anderberg, U. M. (2006). Predictors of self-rated health: A twelve month prospective study of IT and media workers. *Population Health Metrics*. doi:10.1186/14787954-4-8.

Israel, B. A., Schurman, S. J., & House, J. S. (1989). Action research on occupational stress: Involving workers as researchers. *International Journal of Health Services, 19*, 135–155.

Jackson, S. (1983). Participation in decision making as a strategy for reducing job related strain. *The Journal of Applied Psychology, 68*, 3–19.

Jauregui, M., & Schnall, P. (2009). Work, psychosocial stressors and the bottom line. In P. Schnall, M. Dobson, & E. Rosskam (Eds.), *Unhealthy work: Causes, consequences, cures*. New York: Baywood.

Karasek, R. A. (2008). Low social control and physiological deregulation—The stress disequilibrium theory, towards a new demand-control model. *Scandinavian Journal of Work, Environment & Health, 6*, S117–S135.

Karasek, R. A., & Theorell, T. (1990). *Healthy work: Stress, productivity and the reconstruction of working life*. New York: Basic Books.

Kelly, E. L., Kossek, E. E., Hammer, L. B., Durham, M., Bray, J., Chermack, K., et al. (2008). Getting there from here: Research on the effects of work family initiatives on work-family conflict and business outcomes. *Academy of Management Annals, 2*, 305–349.

Kristensen, T. S. (2005). Intervention studies in occupational epidemiology. *Occupational and Environmental Medicine, 62*, 205–210.

Lökk, J., Theorell, T., Arnetz, B., & Eneroth, P. (1991). Physiological concomitants of an "autonomous day care programme" in geriatric day care. *Scandinavian Journal of Rehabilitation Medicine, 23*, 41–46.

Meichenbaum, D. H. (1989). *Stress inoculation training*. New York: Plenum Press.

Melin, B., Lundberg, U., Söderlund, J., & Granqvist, M. (1999). Psychophysiological stress reactions of male and female assembly workers: A comparison between two different forms of work organization. *Journal of Organizational Behavior, 20*, 47–61.

Murphy, L. R. (1996). Stress management in work settings: A critical review of the health effects. *American Journal of Health Promotion, 11*, 112–135.

Orth Gomér, K. (1983). Intervention on coronary risk factors by adapting a shift work schedule to biological rhythmicity. *Psychosomatic Medicine, 45*, 407–415.

Orth Gomer, K., Eriksson, I., Moser, V., Theorell, T., & Fredlund, P. (1994). Lipid lowering through work stress reduction. *International Journal of Behavioral Medicine, 1*, 204–214.

Romanowska, J., Larsson, G., Eriksson, M., Wikström, B. M., Westerlund, H., & Theorell, T. (2011). Health effects on leaders and co-workers of an art-based leadership development program. *Psychotherapy and Psychosomatics, 80*, 78–87.

Romanowska, J., Larsson, G., & Theorell, T. (2011). *Individual pro-social psychological effects of an art-based leadership development program*. Stockholm: Stress Research Institute, Stockholm University.

Rosskam, E. (2009). Using participatory action research methodology to improve worker health. In P. Schnall, M. Dobson, & E. Rosskam (Eds.), *Unhealthy work: Causes, consequences, cures*. New York: Baywood.

Semmer, N. (2006). Job stress interventions and the organization of work. *Scandinavian Journal of Work, Environment & Health, 32*, 515–527.

Siegrist, J. (1996). Adverse health effects of high-effort/low-reward conditions. *J Occ Health Psychol 1*, 27–41.

Theorell, T. (2009). Anabolism and catabolism. In S. Sonnentag, P. L. Perrewé, & D. C. Ganster (Eds.), *Research in occupational stress and wellbeing* (Current perspectives on job-stress recovery, Vol. 7, pp. 249–276). UK: Emerald Group Publishing Limited.

Theorell, T., Emdad, R., Arnetz, B., & Weingarten, A.-M. (2001). Employee effects of an educational program for managers at an insurance company. *Psychosomatic Medicine, 63*, 724–733.

Theorell, T., Hartzell, M., & Näslund, S. (2009). Brief report. A note on designing evaluations of health effects of cultural activities at work. *Art & Health, 1*, 89–92.

Theorell, T., Osika, W., Leineweber, C., Hanson Magnusson, L., Bojner Horwitz, E., & Westerlund, H. (2011). Is cultural activity at work related to mental health in employees? *International Archives of Occupational and Environmental Health* DOI 10.1007/s00420-012-0762-8, 2012

Theorell, T., Osika, W., Leineweber, C., Hanson Magnusson, L., Bojner Horwitz, E., & Westerlund, H. (2012). *Is cultural activity at work related to mental health in employees?* Stockholm: Stress Research Institute, Stockholm University.

Ursin, H., & Eriksen, H. R. (2004). The cognitive activation theory of stress. *Psychoneuroendocrinology, 29*, 567–592.

Van der Klink, J. J. L., Blonk, R. W., Schene, A. H., & van Dijk, F. J. H. (2001). The benefits of interventions for work related stress. *American Journal of Public Health, 91*, 270–276.

Wikström, B. M., Theorell, T., & Sandström, S. (1993). Medical health and emotional effects of art stimulation in old age. *Psychotherapy and Psychosomatics, 60*, 195–206.

Primary and Secondary Prevention of Illness in the Workplace

19

Brian R. Theodore

Overview

Illnesses and injuries in the workplace have a considerable impact that go beyond the ill-health and suffering of the affected individual. The broader socioeconomic impact of workplace illnesses and injuries include reduced workplace productivity, creating a dangerous work environment, increasing healthcare costs, and potentially increased liability assessments through workers' compensation premiums. This chapter discusses primary and secondary prevention strategies suitable for implementation at the workplace. An overview of the principles of preventive medicine is presented, with a description and broad goals for primary, secondary, tertiary, and quaternary prevention strategies. Following this, a review of the theoretical framework that was developed to address prevention strategies and health promotion behaviors is discussed, with a focus on the *Health Belief Model*, the *Theory of Reasoned Action and Planned Behavior*, the *Precaution Adoption Process Model*, and the *Transtheoretical Model*. Finally, overviews of primary and secondary prevention strategies are discussed for common diseases and illness prevalent in the workplace, including prevention of occupational injuries and disability, smoking, cardiovascular disease, cancer, and mental health disorders.

At the outset, it should again be noted that illnesses and injuries in the workplace have a considerable impact that go beyond the affected individual. There are broader socioeconomic impacts of such workplace illnesses and injuries as have been discussed in other chapters of this handbook. For example, in the United States, the Department of Labor's Bureau of Labor Statistics (BLS) compiles annual reports of workplace illnesses and injuries across all public and private organizations nationwide. The most recent statistics from the BLS indicate that approximately 3.8 cases of nonfatal workplace injuries and illness per 100 full-time workers were recorded for the 2010 fiscal year, including 1.8 cases (per 100 workers) that involved days away from work, job transfers, or job restrictions (Bureau of Labor Statistics, 2011). Among the total reported cases, 95% of these cases

B.R. Theodore, Ph.D. (✉)
Department of Anesthesiology and Pain Medicine, University of Washington,
Box 356540, Seattle, WA 98195, USA
e-mail: brianrt@uw.edu

involved workplace injuries, while the remaining 5% were due to occupational-related illness (the majority being skin diseases/disorders, respiratory conditions, poisonings, and hearing loss). Over the last decade, statistics have also identified mental health disorders as another significant contributor to workplace disability, and also potentially as a risk factor for injuries and illnesses (The World Health Organization, 2004). In the United States, the population prevalence of mental health disorders for adults over the age of 18 is approximately 26%, with nearly half these affected individuals suffering from comorbid mental health disorders (i.e., two or more mental health diagnoses) (Kessler et al., 2005).

The financial impact of workplace injuries and illnesses are also quite immense. The total annual cost of workplace injuries and illnesses were estimated to be $250 billion (Leigh, 2011). Of this figure, only 27% of the costs were attributed to medical costs, while the remaining 73% of costs were associated with indirect costs (e.g., lost productivity, indemnity payments, litigation). Furthermore, a significant portion of medical costs are associated with medications, especially narcotic analgesics, at a cost of approximately $13.8 billion annually (Krueger & Stone, 2008). Narcotic analgesics such as opioids, especially, may result in further complications, such as dependence disorders, prescription misuse, medication diversion, and deaths from overdose, further adding to the long-term costs of the injury or illness (Paulozzi et al., 2012). However, despite these relatively high incidence rates and associated costs, it is worth noting that, between the years 2003 and 2010, the United States has seen a decreasing trend in the incidence of workplace injuries and illnesses, corresponding to approximately a 30% reduction in incidence rate (Bureau of Labor Statistics, 2011). One contributing factor to this decrease is the greater emphasis on the efficacy and cost-effectiveness of prevention strategies in reducing the risks of injuries and illnesses. Recently, the US Department of Labor's Occupational Safety and Health Administration (OHSA) published a "white paper" documenting the positive results from a decade's worth of promoting injury and illness prevention programs across the US (Occupational Health and Safety Administration, 2012).

The present chapter will aid in understanding exactly why such prevention programs are effective in reducing the risks of injuries and illnesses in the workplace, with a specific focus on primary and secondary prevention strategies. A discussion of the levels of prevention strategies provides an overview of primary, secondary, tertiary, and quaternary prevention strategies. This is followed by a review of the prevailing theoretical models that account for the effectiveness of such prevention strategies, and their effect on an individual's behavior in successfully complying and adhering to prevention programs. Finally, the chapter reviews several effective strategies and programs for primary and secondary prevention applicable to a broad list of medical conditions and health-related issues, with recommendations for future directions using novel technology and strategies.

Prevention Strategies

The field of preventive medicine underscores four strategies, differing in level of services, that can be broadly classified as primary prevention, secondary prevention, tertiary prevention, and quaternary prevention. Each of these preventive strategies target individuals who are at different stages of disease progression, and require different strategies for managing the disease state (or risk of disease). Central to understanding these strategies of preventive medicine is the distinction between *disease* versus *illness*. In the broadest sense, *disease* corresponds to the specific medical or physiological state that defines a deviation from healthy functioning, whereas *illness* corresponds to the individual's response set of behaviors to the underlying symptoms of the disease (Helman, 1981). In this regard, it is possible for one to manifest itself without the other although, in most chronic stages of disease progression, both *disease* and *illness* co-occur.

Primary Prevention

Primary prevention strategies target individuals who currently have no disease or illness present. This is a proactive prevention strategy at the most basic level, and is targeted to the general population. The goal here is to preempt the development of disease, by promoting healthy lifestyles, behaviors and strategies. Interventions, in the broadest sense, may include health education programs, policies and guidelines, and immunizations. Specific examples include smoking cessation programs, nutritional guidelines, and workplace guidelines on physical exertion associated with activities such as lifting heavy objects. Generally, these primary prevention strategies are low-cost with little-to-none in terms of potential to cause harm or side-effects (Leutwyler, 1995). In addition, primary prevention strategies are highly effective in maintaining healthy lifestyles, and are associated with lower risk of developing diseases and increased lifespan (Fraser & Shavlik, 2001). As discussed by Brannon and Feist (Brannon & Feist, 2007), there is also a significant multiplier effect obtained from primary prevention strategies (pp. 478–497). For example, a combination of healthy behaviors (e.g., smoking cessation, balanced diet, regular exercise) can decrease the risk of developing several types of disorders such as cancer, diabetes, and cardiovascular diseases.

Secondary Prevention

Secondary prevention strategies are designed to screen for potential signs of diseases at its extant stages, so that a proper diagnosis can be determined and treatment be administered at an early stage to prevent further morbidity. The underlying strategy here is to target individuals who have one or more risk factors for the disease. For example, individuals who have higher than normal blood sugar levels should screen themselves routinely to ensure that they keep blood sugar levels in check. At this stage, illness behaviors are not apparent, and the disease is often treatable or successfully managed if discovered early. Interventions at this stage often consist of specific screening to determine a diagnosis, and to subsequently treat the condition at its acute stage. It should be noted that secondary prevention is much more costly, and therefore appropriately targeted to individuals in high-risk groups for developing a disease (Brannon & Feist, 2007). Nevertheless, it is an important component in the healthcare system, because detecting and treating diseases at an early stage would likely prevent further development into a chronic illness, which will have far more costly consequences (due to deteriorating health and increased use of healthcare resources that are required to treat or manage the resulting complex sequelae of disease progression).

Tertiary Prevention

The tertiary level of prevention strategies are needed when both primary and secondary strategies have either failed or were not implemented. The tertiary stage is the first stage at which both disease and illness are present (Norman & Tesser, 2009). Tertiary prevention strategies are designed to manage the disease and illness by preventing the further exacerbation of the disease, restoring normal function to the patient where applicable, and preventing further complications. Oftentimes, specific modalities to treat the disease are part of the tertiary prevention strategy, but it can also include greater surveillance and monitoring of the patient's condition, as well as more intensive levels of patient education and engagement by the healthcare provider to ensure that the patient adheres to the recommended treatment plan. Examples of tertiary prevention strategies can include prescription medications, invasive interventions such as surgery, or non-invasive interventions such as structured rehabilitation and exercise regimens. Needless to say, the cost factor is considerably elevated at this stage of disease and illness management, relative to primary and secondary prevention strategies.

Quaternary Prevention

The final type of prevention strategy differs from the previous three, in that it is designed to reduce excessive utilization of healthcare resources and interventions. The focus is primarily on stemming any negative consequences that can arise from unnecessary interventions, such as side effects of medications or complications from procedures (Norman & Tesser, 2009). Patients targeted at this stage often manifest illness behaviors, but with no corresponding disease states as determined by healthcare providers. In these cases, the "usual care" modalities fail to achieve satisfactory outcomes (for example, among patients who suffer from chronic pain). Examples of quaternary prevention for such cases include recent guidelines on chronic opioid therapy, requiring a taper-down from excessively high-doses of prescription opioids if adequate pain relief and functional improvements are not observed (Agency Medical Directors Group, 2010).

Factors and Barriers to Modifying Health Behaviors: The Theoretical Framework

The successful modifying of health behaviors is the central concept in prevention strategies, especially in primary and secondary stages of prevention. There are several prevailing theoretical models that account for some of the variation observed in health behaviors, and that reliably explain the factors that contribute towards, as well as barriers against, modifying health behaviors to ensure a healthy lifestyle and prevention of diseases and illness. These models, all of which emphasize biopsychosocial factors that influence behavior, include the following: the *Health Belief Model*, the *Theory of Reasoned Action and Planned Behavior*, the *Precaution Adoption Process Model*, and the *Transtheoretical Model*. Following an overview of each of these models, a brief discussion on the success of these models in predicting health behaviors is presented.

The Health Belief Model

The *Health Belief Model* underscores the importance of *beliefs* and *common sense* in an individual's health-seeking and health-promoting behaviors (Hochbaum, 1958; Becker & Rosenstock, 1984). Four beliefs are identified in the model that, in combination, predicts an individual's health behavior. These are (1) perceived susceptibility to disease, (2) perceived severity of the disease, (3) perceived benefits of health-enhancing behaviors, and (4) perceived barriers to health-enhancing behaviors. The *Health Belief Model* predicts that individuals should actively modify their behavior accordingly, or seek appropriate healthcare, when they perceive susceptibility for a disease, and believe that they can benefit from overcoming barriers to effecting healthy behaviors. The model assumes a linear progression from one component of belief to the next, across the four categories of health beliefs. Although this would imply a common sense approach to effecting modified behavior for the better, research has indicated that behavioral outcomes often do not comply very well with the "theory of action" that the model predicts.

Several major factors account for the mismatch between the hypothesized course of action, and the actual behavior observed. First, barriers may arise due to perceived health risks or potential discomfort from engaging in the behavior predicted. A common example of this would be fear of a suffering from a heart attack (the risk) due to engaging in any physical activity or exercise regimen (the predicted healthy behavior) (O'Brien Cousins, 2003, 2000). A second contributing factor is that individuals may also be inhibited to action by an unrealistic sense of optimism or invulnerability, by assuming that they have a lower-than-average risk for developing the disease. Therefore, despite recognizing the benefits of a course of action towards modifying their behavior, they are lulled into a false sense of security, and this perpetuates any high risk behaviors they are engaging in. This inflated sense of optimism is also correlated with age, with younger individuals more likely to assume a sense of invulnerability (Madey & Gomez, 2003). Third, socioeconomic and demographic factors, specifically poverty and ethnic/cultural background, may also play a role in countering the assumption of the *Health Belief Model*, when issues such as costs of healthcare, access to healthcare, and subjective norms about treatment-seeking may dictate whether or not an individual adheres to the linear progression of endorsing the four beliefs and subsequently modifying their behavior (Brannon & Feist, 2007) (pp. 47–49). Finally, another significant contributing factor is an individual's sense of personal control; the *Health Belief Model* posits external factors as guiding the individual's behavior, but does not account for the fact that an individual may ultimately make a choice whether or not to engage in a course of action towards beneficial behavior (Brannon & Feist, 2007) (pp. 47–49).

Although founded on the assumption of common sense, the *Health Belief Model* is weakened by individuals' succumbing to the effect of *irrational beliefs*, the effect of *reasoned action* guided by their own attitudes in weighing risks and benefits, and subjective norms that guide health-seeking behaviors. Therefore, a more complex formulation was needed to account for the variance observed in individuals' health-related behaviors that were counter to the predictions of the *Health Belief Model*. The following theories discussed below build upon the *Health Belief Model*, especially by accounting for an individual's level of self-efficacy in effecting the required changes in behavior.

Theory of Reasoned Action and Planned Behavior

The *Theory of Reasoned Action* incorporated several of the elements not accounted for by the *Health Belief Model*. Departing from the notion that beliefs alone direct behavior, this theory emphasizes an individual's *intention* to engage in a course of action as the primary determinant of behavior (Ajzen & Fishbein, 1980; Fishbein & Ajzen, 1975). That intention itself is moderated by two additional factors, specifically one's attitude towards the desired behavior, as well as subjective norms (e.g., cultural, societal, or peer pressure) that may influence an individual's intention to engage in the desired behavior. In turn, each of these is moderated by two other higher order factors. The theory predicts that attitude is shaped by the individual's underlying beliefs about the benefits of the desired course of action. Subjective norms, on the other hand, are shaped by societal influence and endorsement of the desired course of action. Figure 19.1 illustrates the interaction among all these different components of the *Theory of Reasoned Action*.

A further refinement of this model was subsequently presented, adding an additional factor that influenced both an individual's attitude, as well as the subjective norm towards the course of action leading to the desired health outcome. This modified model, the *Theory of Planned Behavior*, incorporated perceived behavioral control as a moderator of attitude and norms (Ajzen, 1985, 1991). This theory predicted that perceived behavioral control increases an individual's intention to engage in the desired course of action, if that individual believes they can easily achieve the desired behavior. This model predicts both direct and indirect effects of perceived control on intention, with the indirect effects achieved through moderating attitude (more positive attitude with increased perceived control) and subjective norms (override norms that discourage the desired course of action). Figure 19.2 illustrates the interaction among all these different components of the *Theory of Planned Behavior*.

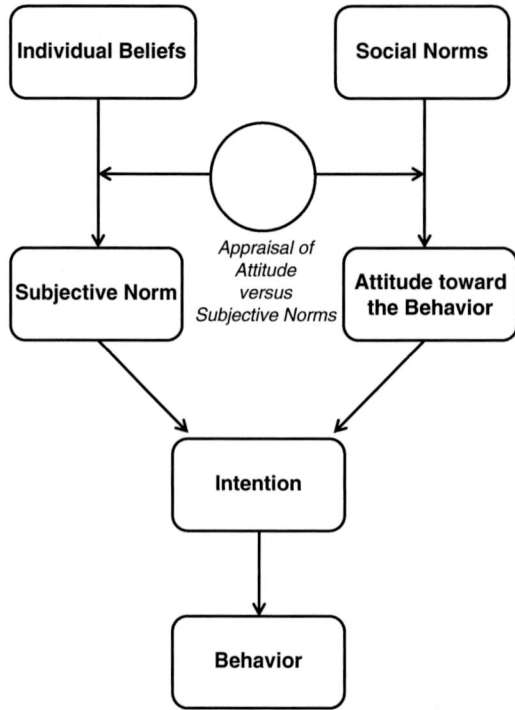

Fig. 19.1 The theory of reasoned action. Adapted from: Ajzen I. and Fishbein M., *Understanding attitudes and predicting social behavior*, 1980, Englewood Cliffs, NJ: Prentice-Hall

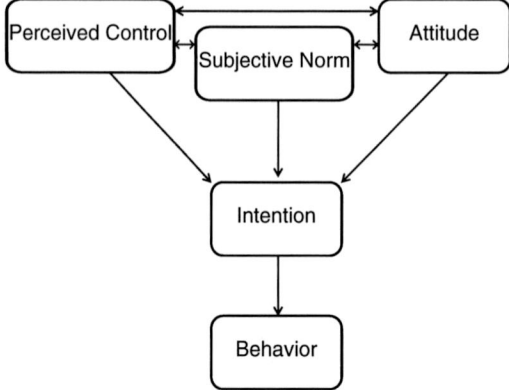

Fig. 19.2 The theory of planned behavior. Adapted from: Ajzen I., *The theory of planned behavior*. Organizational Behavior and Human Decision Processes, 1991. 50: p. 179–211

The Precaution Adoption Process Model

The *Precaution Adoption Process Model* (Weinstein, 1988) departs from the previous ones in two major ways. First of all, this is the first of the models to predict that individuals do not progress from stage to stage in the cycle of health behavior modification, but can even move backwards in stages and situations of relapse. Second of all, the model posits that the presence of an optimistic bias moderates an individual's response to engaging in behavior modification. The entire model

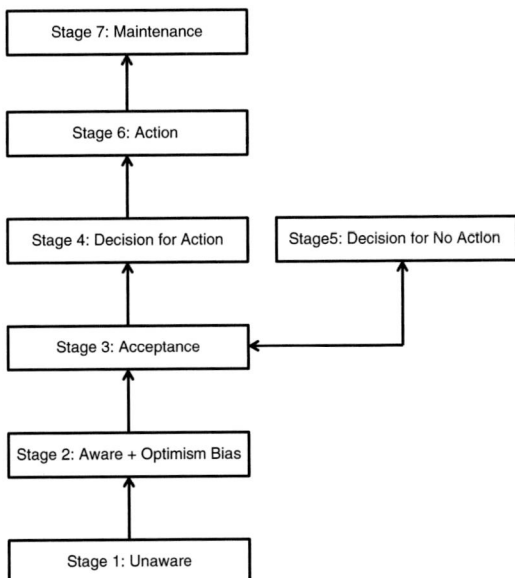

Fig. 19.3 The precaution adoption process model. Adapted from: Weinstein N.D., *The precaution adoption process.* Health Psychology, 1988. 7: p. 355–386

consists of seven stages of belief about an individual's perceived susceptibility to developing a disease. Figure 19.3 illustrates these stages of belief, with a brief description of the nature of beliefs that individuals hold at each stage. While *Stage 1* describes a situation where an individual is unaware of the risk factors for developing a disease, *Stage 2* beliefs emphasize the presence of the optimism bias among those individuals who are aware of the risk present in their lives. At this second stage, however, individuals do not believe that the disease would befall them, although they are aware of the risk factors present and acknowledge that the risk factors can predispose one to developing the disease. *Stage 3* consists of individuals' acceptance that risk factors present in their lives do pose a risk for developing disease, but have not decided on taking action to modify health behaviors. *Stages 4 and 5* denote a decision point, where individuals' decide and make a commitment to modify their health behavior by engaging in a particular activity or treatment (*Stage 4*), or they may decide against taking any actions due to some other perceived ill effect of undergoing any treatment (*Stage 5*). It is possible for individuals in *Stage 5* to go backwards in the process of formulating beliefs. Specifically, the model proposes the possibility that an individual may decide to undergo a process of behavioral modification and go back to *Stage 4*. Finally, *Stages 6 and 7* involve individuals who recognize their risk and susceptibility to disease and are actively engaging in behavior modification (*Stage 6*), or have advanced even further and are now in the process of maintenance (i.e., sustaining their new course of action towards a healthier lifestyle; *Stage 7*).

The Transtheoretical Model

The *Transtheoretical Model* (Prochaska, DiClemente, & Norcross, 1992; Prochaska, Norcross, & DiClemente, 1994), named such for its adoption of concepts from the previously discussed models, describes an individual's progression in a spiraling fashion through five stages of behavior modification. The model also accounts for the possibility of relapse by allowing a reverse flow through these differ-

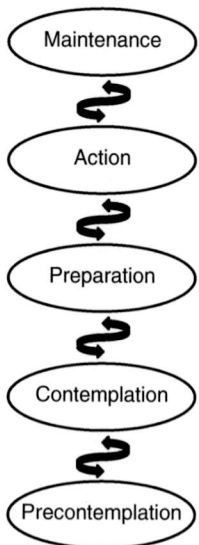

Fig. 19.4 The transtheoretical model. Adapted from: Prochaska J.O., DiClemente C.C., and Norcross J.C., *In search of how people change: Applications to addictive behaviors.* American Psychologist, 1992. 47: p. 1102–1114

ent stages of an individual's cycle through the process of change. The five stages correspond to different levels of engagement throughout the behavior modification process, and include the following: *Precontemplation, Contemplation, Preparation, Action,* and *Maintenance* (see Fig. 19.4).

The *Precontemplation Stage* denotes an individual's baseline level of engagement in the behavioral modification process (i.e., there is no inherent intention on the part of individuals to effect any changes in their behavior). Once individuals progress to the *Contemplation Stage*, they now accept that there is a problem or risk factor associated with their present behaviors, and have thoughts (but no actions yet) about effecting a change. This is followed by the *Preparation Stage*, where individuals begin the process of effecting change by developing structured plans and engaging in preparatory actions to achieve their goal. Once sufficient preparation has been achieved, the individual enters the *Action Stage*, where overt efforts are made to modify behavior, and remove barriers to change. Finally, when successful, individuals adopt a *Maintenance Stage* strategy to sustain their modified healthy behaviors, and to avoid or manage "triggers" for potential relapse.

As mentioned previously, the *Transtheoretical Model* accounts for relapse by recognizing that individuals do often cycle among the various stages, before finally achieving a successful outcome. The model also recognizes relapse as a learning process that can be used to strengthen further efforts to progress through the stages. Additionally, the model also explicitly recognizes that individuals at different stages will require different methods of intervention to help them achieve their goals (Armitage et al., 2004). Therefore, targeted interventions, taking into account an individual's own history, beliefs, and motivation, would likely yield the best outcomes in effecting successful change in behavior.

The Success of the Theoretical Models

How well does the theoretical framework account for behaviors observed in clinical practice? Brannon and Feist (Brannon & Feist, 2007) provide a useful discussion and critique of each of these models (pp. 53–55). In sum, there is moderate evidence for these models. However, where these models fall short are in their exclusion of significant contributing factors, such as secondary gain, socioeconomic

Table 19.1 Summary of Primary and Secondary Prevention Strategies for the Workplace

Primary Prevention	Secondary Prevention
Goal: • Prevent onset of disease, injury and illness	*Goal*: • Prevent progression of disease and illness
Methods: • Informational and educational material • Workplace safety training and compliance • Organizational policies promoting healthy workplace • Conduct health promotion programs • Provide access to or information about support and counseling services	*Methods*: • Partner with managed care organizations to provide comprehensive health promotion services • Provide higher intensity healthy lifestyle programs where feasible • Provide employee support services at the workplace to address common underlying risk factors (e.g., smoking cessation programs, counseling services)

disparities, and lack of access to quality healthcare. Furthermore, systematic reviews of the literature have also noted that such models often vary in their predictive ability across disease states (Rosen, 2000), and therefore should not be relied upon too heavily without proper understanding of the mechanisms underlying the illness behaviors associated with any given unique disease. However, the theoretical framework does provide useful concepts to guide effective interventions for Primary and Secondary Prevention strategies. The following section discusses several different disease states/illnesses, and some useful methods for prevention that are grounded in the theoretical frameworks discussed above.

Primary and Secondary Prevention Methods for Changing Health-Relevant Beliefs and Behaviors

The successful application of the theoretical models described in the previous section has resulted in effective primary and secondary prevention strategies and interventions that are routinely deployed in the clinical setting. When used within the primary care setting, these prevention strategies are able to reach a wide population of individuals who seek routine care. Incorporating prevention strategies within occupational settings provide an even larger target population that may benefit from the principles of preventive medicine. This section provides a brief overview of several prevention methods used in the clinical and occupational settings, with an emphasis on preventing and managing unintentional injuries that could lead to pain and disability, consumption of tobacco, risk factors for cardiovascular disease, risk factors for cancer, and risk factors for mental health disorders. The underlying philosophy in primary and secondary prevention strategies involves modification of behavior using a multifaceted method, as summarized in Table 19.1. These themes recur throughout the remaining discussion of various diseases and illness that commonly impact the occupational setting.

Prevention Strategies for Occupational Injuries

Occupational injuries resulting in workers compensation claims and time off work are primarily caused by overexertion. In a survey conducted by Liberty Mutual, slightly more than 25% of all compensable workplace injuries fall under this category, and are due to excessive lifting, pushing, pulling, holding, carrying or throwing of an object (Michael, 2001). These injuries also account for approximately $9.8 billion (in 1998 US $) in direct healthcare costs. Primary prevention strategies suitable for the workplace should therefore ideally consist of a combination of a safe and conducive workplace environment, workplace policies and guidelines on safety, and training and support provided to the worker. The goal here is to elevate the individual worker's attitudes and beliefs about workplace safety from knowledge to action and finally to maintenance, in as rapid a manner as possible. However, it is often the case that, even with adequate attention to these factors, workplace risks are not adequately controlled. Complicating the matter further is the fact that there is little knowledge about the causal factors that lead to chronic disability resulting from workplace injuries, even relatively minor ones (Frank & Cullen, 2006). Therefore, designing truly comprehensive and targeted primary prevention methods for occupational injuries is often not feasible for any given organization beyond very broad policies, training material, and ergonomic improvements. However, there are at least two principles that can help enhance the effectiveness of primary injury prevention strategies in the occupational setting. First, a key component to increase compliance to safety protocols and to adhere to principles of training programs is to provide feedback about performance to the individual worker (Schultz, 2004). Second, but most importantly, the principles of primary prevention should be a "top-down approach" (i.e., the literature on occupational disability shows evidence that individual behavior at the workplace is strongly influenced by the attitude towards safety cultivated by management) (DeJoy et al., 2004; Mullen, 2004).

Secondary prevention for workplace injuries has been relatively well developed over the past few decades. The key here is to prevent the emergence of chronic disability once a worker has already sustained an injury. This should be a multipronged approach designed to control symptoms, reduce disability, and optimize functional status (Frank & Cullen, 2006). Therefore, the major component of secondary prevention is to ensure the availability of effective disability management interventions. Treatment modalities at this level include the following: structured exercise programs, functional training for improving general health and work capacity, and cognitive-behavioral interventions designed to address psychosocial barriers to recovery that play a role in the development of chronicity. These are often accomplished through structured work conditioning and work hardening programs, with low-intensity psychosocial interventions to help with coping skills and identifying barriers to recovery (Mayer & Press, 2005; Mayer et al., 2006). In addition, it is also a benefit to the worker if organizational policies incorporate temporary modified work protocols, or even vocational retraining to accommodate any permanent levels of disability, if feasible (Frank & Cullen, 2006).

Presently, it is common for primary and secondary prevention strategies to be fragmented in terms of delivery. For example, organizations are often only mandated to be responsible for primary prevention strategies, while secondary prevention is outsourced to healthcare delivery organizations often dictated by third-party payors (Frank & Cullen, 2006; Gatchel & Okifuji, 2006). However, the literature indicates that an integrated primary-secondary prevention approach at the organizational level is often more effective (Yassi et al., 1995a, 1995b). This combined strategy should incorporate not only ergonomic improvements, policies and training, but also the establishing of workplace committees on disability management and to negotiate with insurance carriers for the availability of multidisciplinary care teams to provide a comprehensive, biopsychosocial oriented treatment approach to prevent development of chronic disability (Frank & Cullen, 2006).

Prevention Strategies for Consumption of Tobacco

The primary mode for consumption of tobacco is through smoking of cigarettes. Although there has been a sharp decline of approximately 42% in the prevalence of cigarette smoking in the United States since the 1960s, that rate has been at a relatively standstill pattern between 2005 and 2010 (Center for Disease Control, 2011). The prevalence rate of cigarette smoking among the working adult population in the United States stands at approximately 19% (Center for Disease Control, 2011). The importance of prevention strategies against smoking is underscored by the link between smoking and a myriad of undesirable and serious health outcomes, such as developing a variety of cancers, cardiovascular disorders, respiratory disorders, and increased susceptibility to mental health and other substance abuse problems (Brannon & Feist, 2007) (pp. 358–360). The major factors that can benefit from targeted prevention strategies include addiction to nicotine, the habitual effect of smoking, the optimistic bias that causes one to underestimate their personal health risks, and the fear of weight gain from quitting (Brannon & Feist, 2007) (pp. 355–357).

Primary prevention strategies against smoking are based on the goal of deterring smoking in the first place. In the workplace, this is usually not feasible, since the initial choice to smoke may have been made far earlier in the life of the working adult. However, certain primary prevention strategies that may deter smoking at the workplace can include a total ban on smoking anywhere around the workplace. Such policies have often gone into effect at universities and medical centers, which are designated as "smoke-free areas," and include the outdoor areas of the property in question. This method may be effective as it replicates some of the relatively more successful strategies employed to deter smoking. For example, while information alone about the health risks of smoking has been totally ineffective for deterrence (Siegel & Biener, 2000), information in combination with community-wide antismoking campaigns have demonstrated favorable long-term outcomes in avoiding that habit-forming first step of lighting up a cigarette (Vartiainen et al., 1998).

Secondary prevention techniques are more suitable for a workplace setting, especially when combined with a "smoke-free" organizational policy. The goal here should be multifaceted by combining information along with support mechanisms and interventions that can be provided within healthy lifestyle programs within the organization itself, or through the managed healthcare organization that is partnered with through the organization's healthcare benefits program. Secondary interventions may include information and successful self-management strategies for quitting without therapy (i.e., "cold turkey"), and information and support for quitting with various types of interventional therapies. The latter may include nicotine replacement therapy (patches, gum, lozenges, nasal sprays), psychosocial interventions (motivational interviewing techniques, enhancing self-efficacy), and workplace community campaigns that provide the required social support for maintenance of successful cessation of smoking and prevention of relapse (Brannon & Feist, 2007) (pp. 363–368). The ultimate goal in such strategies should be multipronged. Based on the framework of the *Transtheoretical Model*, dissemination of information should be designed to move smokers from the *Precontemplation Stage* to the *Contemplation Stage*. Once achieved, the goal is to direct the individuals to the necessary resources (often the healthcare delivery organization responsible for the workplace) to initiate action, and then to successfully maintain the successful outcome. Most importantly, especially for smokers, is the enhancement of self-efficacy throughout the process of quitting, as relapse is a common occurrence (Fiore et al., 1996). The goal here is to then utilize the occurrence of relapse as a learning strategy to identify weaknesses, reshape the event to focus on enhancing self-efficacy to the previously successful attempt (no matter how brief), and to chart a modified behavioral strategy to successfully quit (Brannon & Feist, 2007) (pp. 367–368).

Prevention Strategies for Cardiovascular Diseases

Cardiovascular disease (CVD; which has also been reviewed in another chapter of this handbook) is the leading cause of death, accounting for 37% of all deaths in the United States (Hoyert, Kung, & Smith, 2005). This is despite the fact that that there has been a dramatic reduction in deaths due to CVD since the 1960s, from a peak of 522 deaths per 100,000 in the 1960s down to 317 per 100,000 in 2002 (Brannon & Feist, 2007) (p. 226). Risk factors for CVD include the following: biological/genetic (advancing age, family history, gender, ethnic background), physiological (hypertension, serum cholesterol level), and behavioral and psychosocial factors (smoking, diet, physical activity, social support, stress, anxiety, depression, anger, and hostility) (Brannon & Feist, 2007) (pp. 228–240). Prevention strategies targeting behavioral risk factors and promoting surveillance of physiological risk factors for CVD, when employed at the workplace, are beneficial in terms of improving worker's health, promoting healthy lifestyles, reducing time lost from work due to illness, preventing worker mortality due to CVD, and keeping organizational healthcare premiums down. Therefore, both primary and secondary prevention strategies targeted for the occupational setting can be mutually beneficial for both the individual workers, as well as the organization.

Primary prevention strategies for CVD are designed with the goal to prevent the first heart attack, whereas secondary prevention strategies for CVD are designed to rehabilitate cardiac patients and to prevent subsequent CVD events such as a heart attack (Brannon & Feist, 2007) (pp. 241–245). While secondary prevention strategies, specifically cardiac rehabilitation, are best managed at the healthcare delivery organization responsible for the patient, the goal of enhancing and maintaining healthy lifestyle choices for the CVD patient can benefit from primary prevention strategies already well-developed and suitable for promotion at the workplace. Both primary and secondary prevention strategies suitable to implement at the workplace are healthy lifestyle programs designed to modify behaviors that impact the three most potent risk factors for CVD (i.e., smoking, blood cholesterol levels, and blood pressure) (Stamler et al., 1999). As with all behavioral modification programs that are consistent with the theoretical framework previously discussed, the most important components of any prevention strategies are to remove the optimistic bias that serves as a barrier to lifestyle changes, and engaging the individual through the stages of *Precontemplation/Contemplation* through the stages of *Action* and *Maintenance*.

As discussed in the previous section, programs that promote the prevention and cessation of smoking have a multiplier effect across several disease states, with CVD being one of the major preventable diseases linked to smoking. The methods previously discussed for smoking apply here as well. Although cholesterol and blood pressure levels constitute physiological risk factors for CVD, they can be indirectly impacted by behavioral factors and lifestyle choices. Promoting healthy lifestyle choices on appropriate nutrition, balanced diet, maintaining optimal weight, managing stress, and engaging in physical activity and exercise are optimal strategies that can be incorporated into the workplace setting. These can be promoted through informational media about risk factors and benefits of healthy lifestyle (e.g., brochures), but also through workplace activity programs and interest groups incorporating physical and/or relaxation activities (Marcus et al., 1998; Plotnikoff et al., 2005). Promoting routine screening for cholesterol, blood pressure, and stress-related mental health should also be encouraged as part of the overall workplace healthy lifestyle program, so that early signs of CVD (e.g., high cholesterol or blood pressure) and psychosocial risk factors (unmanaged stress) can be addressed and treated before progressing to later stages of CVD. For more detailed resources on designing such workplace programs, the Centers for Disease Control and Prevention provide useful toolkits and suggested programs suitable for enhancing physical activity and promoting healthy lifestyles in the workplace as part of the Healthier Worksite Initiative (Centers for Disease Control and Prevention, 2010).

Prevention Strategies for Cancer

Cancer has been addressed in another chapter of this handbook. The overall incidence and death rates from cancers have significantly declined in the United States, specifically from between 1990 and 2003 (Brannon & Feist, 2007) (p. 251). However, certain types of cancers have seen an increase in incidence and mortality over the last decade and account for approximately 13% of cancer cases and related deaths in the United States (Brannon & Feist, 2007) (p. 254). These include non-Hodgkin's lymphoma, liver cancer, melanoma, cancer of the esophagus, leukemia, and cancers of the soft connective tissue, thyroid, small intestine, and vulva (Brannon & Feist, 2007) (p. 254). Despite lower incidence rates, cancer, like other diseases and illness, has a negative impact on the worker's health, causes lost time from work due to illness, may cause worker mortality, and negatively impacts workplace productivity. Similarly to CVD, cancers are also linked to risk factors that are both within and beyond the control of the individual and the workplace. Risk factors beyond an individual's control include family history, genetics, ethnic background, and age. However, certain risk factors are within the control of the workplace and the individual worker and include environmental factors at the workplace and behavioral factors. Therefore, prevention strategies targeting these latter two risk factors are suitable to be implemented as part of the overall workplace wellness and health promotion strategies.

Primary prevention strategies against cancer in the workplace should target both environmental factors of the occupational setting, as well as modifiable behavioral factors for the individual worker. Depending on the type of occupational setting and nature of the work, environmental risk factors may include exposure to asbestos, pesticides, carbon-based fumes from exhausts and motors, pesticides, carcinogenic chemicals, and radiation (Brannon & Feist, 2007) (pp. 256–257). Detailed safety guidelines and mandatory protection equipment must be a part of the primary prevention strategy. As similarly described in the previous section on workplace injuries, comprehensive training programs should be part of the primary prevention strategy, and compliance with safety protocols should be monitored, with adequate and timely feedback provided for any deviations towards unsafe practices. Detailed procedures for how to report and respond to any exposure to carcinogenic environmental risk factors must be part of the workplace primary prevention procedures.

The major behavioral risk factors with moderate to strong evidence for causing cancer include smoking, diet and nutrition, sedentary lifestyle, excessive consumption of alcohol, and exposure to ultraviolet light. Promoting healthy lifestyle choices, such as smoking cessation, a balanced diet, and physical activity, has a multiplier effect across health states, including cancer. Therefore, the same strategies described in the previous section on CVD apply to primary prevention of cancer as well. Although there is mixed evidence for the causal link between excessive alcohol consumption and cancer (Singletary & Gapstur, 2001), it is worth noting that the combination of alcohol consumption and smoking greatly increases the risk for developing some types of cancers, in some cases by up to 50% (Flanders & Rothman, 1982; Garavello et al., 2005). Therefore, educational material advising against excessive consumption of alcohol, along with its associated risks for increasing susceptibility to cancer, should be incorporated as part of any materials or programs for smoking prevention or cessation. Similarly, information and educational material should be provided on the risk of excessive exposure to ultraviolet light, and the steps one can take to mitigate such exposure through the use of adequate clothing as well as sun-block products (Moyal & Fourtanier, 2008).

Secondary prevention for cancer involves helping the patient navigate through the complexity of the diagnosis, treatment, outcome of treatment, and potentially living with cancer. Secondary prevention strategies suitable for the workplace may include two important components for helping an individual worker with cancer cope with his/her present health state. First, it is crucial that cancer patients be provided adequate social support to cope with their condition. While this may not be under the purview of the workplace, it will be beneficial to provide general information about cancer patient and cancer survivor support groups, and how to get in touch with such groups or organizations. Second, it will be beneficial to provide access to stress-reduction and management strategies within the overall workplace health promotion program. The effect of stress-management psychosocial interventions show some evidence for obtaining successful outcomes among cancer patients that, in turn, improve immune function. These include improved mood, increase in perceived social support, and adoption of healthy behaviors such as cessation of smoking and adopting a healthy diet (Andersen et al., 2004). In addition, poorer psychosocial states, especially depression, is linked to progression of the cancer as well as mortality (Spiegel & Giese-Davis, 2003). This underscores the importance of providing an organizational-level program for stress-reduction and management, not only for cancer, but in terms of its benefits as a multiplier effect for other diseases and illnesses discussed in the previous sections.

Prevention Strategies for Mental Health Disorders

Again, the topic of mental health issues has been addressed in another chapter of this handbook. Indeed, stress in the workplace, and its resulting psychological toll, has a significant impact on workers' well-being and the productivity of the organization. In a 2009 survey conducted by the American Psychological Association, 69% of employees report that work is a significant source of stress, 41% report that they feel tense during the workday, and 51% report being less productive at work as a result of stress (American Psychological Association, 2009). Mood disorders, a frequent result of unmanaged stress, are estimated to result in 321 million lost days annually, at a cost of $50 billion in productivity losses (Kessler et al., 2006). Although stress has been identified as a risk factor for some of the illnesses discussed above, it also has its own unique effect on well-being in the workplace, as well as an underlying cause for psychological disorders such as depression and anxiety (Brannon & Feist, 2007) (pp. 152–155). Other associated mental health and psychosocial comorbidities associated with unmanaged stress in the workplace include interpersonal strain in family relationships, workplace violence, and substance abuse disorders (Gabriel & International Labour Office, 2000). Therefore, prevention strategies targeting mental health would also contribute a multiplier effect towards prevention of risk factors for the onset and progression of other illnesses.

The most basic primary prevention strategy makes available educational information about stress-management and coping, with resources to community providers for counseling services. However, with increasing recognition of the impact of stress in the workplace and its link to associated illnesses, many employers now provide a more comprehensive bundle of services as part of the organizational healthy lifestyle promotion programs. These services include both facets of primary and secondary prevention strategies. Some examples of effective primary prevention, in addition to information and educational material, include lunchtime talks by professional counselors on stress-management techniques, as well as strategies for maintaining a healthy work-life balance (Gabriel & International Labour Office, 2000). Broader scope of services that incorporate secondary prevention strategies are now also commonplace as part of the organizational healthy lifestyle promotion programs. Some examples have been reported in a survey conducted by the United States Bureau of National Affairs over the last decade. For example, in partnership with managed care organizations, more than 90% of 120 employers surveyed have expanded the scope of preventive mental health programs that included counseling on alcohol and substance abuse, mental health counseling, and family and marital counseling (Gabriel & International Labour Office, 2000).

However, it should be noted that, when mental health services are provided as part of an overall healthy lifestyles program that incorporates a biopsychosocial approach to preventing onset of diseases and their progression into illnesses, the multiplier effect will be broad and benefits both employees as well as the employer. In a survey on the effectiveness and usefulness of workplace health programs, an overwhelming 85% of employees who participated in such programs endorsed them for being effective in promoting good health (Towers Perrin, 2008). The beneficial impact for employers and workplace productivity were also similarly pronounced, as reported in a systematic review of 56 journal articles on worksite health promotion programs. That study reported the following: an average 26.8% reduction in sick leave absenteeism, 26.1% reduction in healthcare costs. 32% reduction in workers' compensation and disability management claims costs. and an average $5.81 in savings for every dollar invested in workplace health promotion programs (Chapman, 2005).

Conclusions and Future Directions

Primary and secondary prevention programs should be an essential component of the occupational setting. As discussed above, prevention strategies targeting even a few of the more common risk factors or lifestyle behaviors will provide a multiplier effect that promotes prevention of multiple other diseases. In addition to maintaining a healthy workforce, there is documented evidence on the benefits reaped by employers when such programs are well-designed and implemented as part of organizational policy. The United States Occupational Safety and Health Administration's (OHSA) recent report on the effectiveness of mandatory prevention programs in several States estimate that occupational injuries and illness can be reduced by between 15 and 35% when implemented, translating to a cost-savings of between $9 billion to $23 billion annually in direct healthcare costs alone (Occupational Health and Safety Administration, 2012). Further accounting of indirect costs, such as lost productivity, retraining of temporary or replacement employees, and the potential increase in workers compensation premiums, would yield an even more substantial amount. Additionally, a 2010 report published by the human resources consulting firm, Towers Watson, noted that companies with the most effective health and productivity programs achieved 11% more revenue per employee, delivered 28% higher shareholder returns and had lower medical trends and fewer absences per employee (Towers Watson 2010) (p. 2).

According to the OSHA, all States have made some level of effort in promoting injury and illness prevention programs among the employers within their jurisdiction. These include 35 States that have laws and regulations covering prevention programs (mandatory in 15 of these States), while the remaining States promote prevention programs through financial incentives for employers, for example, through discounts on workers' compensation premiums (Occupational Health and Safety Administration, 2012). It should be noted, that such laws and regulations do not necessarily cover all employers in all cases; in some States, the focus may only be on employers who are classified as "hazardous" due to the nature of the business and its associated occupational risks. Ideally, some level of prevention program should be a part of every organization, even if it only means low-cost primary prevention strategies. Future directions in the fields of occupational health and preventive medicine should more aggressively promote the efficacy and cost-effectiveness of prevention programs to small businesses (<50 employees), who often lack prevention programs due to cost-restrictions on providing healthcare benefits, maintaining medical and disability committees, and designing and implementing large-scale programs. Oftentimes, all it would take is to guide the employers to the available resources that would help them achieve the goal of implementing prevention programs in the workplace. For example, the United Nations' International Labour Office provides recommendations for implementing low-cost prevention programs at small businesses (<50 employees), including partnering with community resources such as State and local rehabilitation agencies and support groups that impose little-to-none in terms of financial burden to the organization (Gabriel & International Labour Office, 2000).

With increased penetration of broadband internet service nationwide, it is also possible to leverage new technologies and applied clinical solutions to meet occupational health needs, especially among small businesses in rural and underserved areas. One such example is the University of New Mexico's Project ECHO (Extension for Community Healthcare Outcomes), that utilizes low-cost, telemedicine-based provider-to-provider consultation designed to bridge the gap between primary care providers in rural or underserved regions with medical specialists who may not be available in that particular rural area (Arora et al., 2011a, 2011b). Although initially developed to provide specialty consultation for chronic medical conditions, this low-cost model of service delivery may also be adapted for delivery of secondary prevention to the community provider who manages the disease or illness of the affected employee. Such a model of care can also be combined with Web-based cognitive behavioral therapy interventions to increase self-efficacy and enhance existing coping skills for the affected employee (Ruward et al., 2009; Grover et al., 2011).

In conclusion, employers should incorporate comprehensive primary and secondary prevention programs as part of their overall organizational mission. Efforts to plan and implement such programs are today much easier, given the wealth of existing material in the medical and occupational health literature as well as the resources and recommendations provided by large organizations, State and local governments, academia, managed care organizations, insurers, and unions. Furthermore, the rapid development of new technologies should provide low-cost applied clinical solutions that can alleviate some employers' fears on the cost-prohibitions of implementing comprehensive prevention programs. No doubt, the evidence shows that a healthy workforce translates into a more productive organization, and mutual benefit is accorded to both the employee and the employer when there is organizational investment in well-designed disease prevention and health promotion programs.

References

Agency Medical Directors Group. (2010). *Interagency guideline on opioid dosing for chronic non-cancer pain: An educational aid to improve care and safety with opioid therapy. 2010 update* [cited 12 Jan 2012]. Available from http://www.agencymeddirectors.wa.gov/Files/OpioidGdline.pdf

Ajzen, I. (1985). From intentions to actions: A theory of planned behavior. In J. Kuhland & J. Beckman (Eds.), *Action-control: From cognitions to behavior* (pp. 11–39). Heidelberg, Germany: Springer.

Ajzen, I. (1991). The theory of planned behavior. *Organizational Behavior and Human Decision Processes, 50*, 179–211.

Ajzen, I., & Fishbein, M. (1980). *Understanding attitudes and predicting social behavior*. Englewood Cliffs, NJ: Prentice-Hall.

American Psychological Association. *Stress in America 2009*. 2009 [cited 10 Feb 2012]. Available from http://www.apa.org/news/press/releases/stress-exec-summary.pdf.

Andersen, B. L., Farrar, W. B., Golden-Kreutz, D. M., Glaser, R., Emery, C. F., Crespin, T. R., et al. (2004). Psychological, behavioral, and immune changes after a psychological intervention: A clinical trial. *Journal of Clinical Oncology, 22*(17), 3570–3580.

Armitage, C. J., Sheeran, P., Conner, M., & Arden, M. A. (2004). Stages of change or changes of stage? Predicting transitions in transtheoretical model stages in relation to healthy food choice. *Journal of Consulting and Clinical Psychology, 72*(3), 491–499.

Arora, S., Thornton, K., Murata, G., Deming, P., Kalishman, S., Dion, D., et al. (2011a). Outcomes of treatment for hepatitis C virus infection by primary care providers. *The New England Journal of Medicine, 364*(23), 2199–2207.

Arora, S., Kalishman, S., Dion, D., Thornton, K., Bankhurst, A., Boyle, J., et al. (2011b). Partnering urban academic medical centers and rural primary care clinicans to provide complex chronic disease care. *Health Affairs, 30*(6), 1176–1184.

Becker, M. H., & Rosenstock, I. M. (1984). Compliance with medical advice. In A. Steptoe & A. Mathews (Eds.), *Health care and human behavior*. London: Academic.

Brannon, L., & Feist, J. (2007). *Health psychology: An introduction to behavior and health*. Belmont, CA: Thomson Wadsworth.

Bureau of Labor Statistics. (2011). *News release: Workplace injuries and illnesses—2010*. U.S. Department of Labor, Editor.

Center for Disease Control. (2011). Current cigarette smoking prevalence among working adults—United States, 2004–2010. *Morbidity and Mortality Weekly Report, 60*(38), 1305–1309.

Centers for Disease Control and Prevention. (2010). *Healthier worksite initiative: Toolkits* [cited 12 Feb 2012]. Available from http://www.cdc.gov/nccdphp/dnpao/hwi/toolkits/index.htm.

Chapman, L. S. (2005). Meta-evaluation of worksite health promotion economic return studies: 2005 update. *American Journal of Health Promotion, 19*(6), 1–11.

DeJoy, D. M., Schaffer, B. S., Wilson, M. G., Vandenberg, R. J., & Butts, M. M. (2004). Creating safer workplaces: Assessing the determinants and role of safety climate. *Journal of Safety Research, 35*(1), 81–90.

Fiore, M. C., Bailey, W. C., Cohen, S. J., Dorfman, S. F., Goldstein, M. G., Gritz, E. R., et. al. (1996). *Smoking cessation: Clinical practice guideline No. 18*. Rockville, MD: Department of Health and Human Services.

Fishbein, M., & Ajzen, I. (1975). *Belief, attitude, intention, and behavior: An introduction to theory and research.* Reading, MA: Addison-Wesley.

Flanders, W. D., & Rothman, K. J. (1982). Interaction of alcohol and tobacco in laryngeal cancer. *American Journal of Epidemiology, 115*(3), 371–379.

Frank, J., & Cullen, K. (2006). Preventing injury, illness and disability at work. *Scandinavian Journal of Work, Environment & Health, 32*(2), 160–167.

Fraser, G. E., & Shavlik, D. J. (2001). Ten years of life: Is it a matter of choice? *Archives of Internal Medicine, 161*(13), 1645–1652.

Gabriel P., & International Labour Office. (2000). *Mental health in the workplace: Situation analyses, United States.* GLADNET collection (Paper 228) [cited 10 Feb 2012]. Available from http://digitalcommons.ilr.cornell.edu/gladnetcollect/228

Garavello, W., Negri, E., Talamini, R., Levi, F., Zambon, P., Dal Maso, L., et al. (2005). Family history of cancer, its combination with smoking and drinking, and risk of squamous cell carcinoma of the esophagus. *Cancer Epidemiology, Biomarkers & Prevention, 14*(6), 1390–1393.

Gatchel, R. J., & Okifuji, A. (2006). Evidence-based scientific data documenting the treatment and cost-effectiveness of comprehensive pain programs for chronic nonmalignant pain. *The Journal of Pain, 7*(11), 779–793.

Grover, M., Naumann, U., Mohammad-Dar, L., Glennon, D., Ringwood, S. Eisler, I., et al. (2011). A randomized controlled trial of an internet-based cognitive-behavioural skills package for carers of people with anorexia nervosa. *Psychological Medicine, 41*, 2581–2591.

Helman, C. G. (1981). Disease versus illness in general practice. *The Journal of the Royal College of General Practitioners, 31*(230), 548–552.

Hochbaum, G. (1958). *Public participation in medical screening programs, in DHEW Public Health Service.* Washington, DC: U.S. Government Printing Office.

Hoyert, D. L., Kung, H. C., & Smith, B. L. (2005). Deaths: Preliminary data from 2003. *National Vital Statistics Reports, 53*(15), 1–48.

Kessler, R. C., Chiu, W. T., Demler, O., Merikangas, K. R., & Walters, E. E. (2005). Prevalence, severity, and comorbidity of 12-month DSM-IV disorders in the National Comorbidity Survey Replication. *Archives of General Psychiatry, 62*(6), 617–627.

Kessler, R. C., Akiskal, H. S., Ames, M., Birnbaum, H., Greenberg, P., Hirschfeld, R. M., et al. (2006). Prevalence and effects of mood disorders on work performance in a nationally representative sample of U.S. workers. *The American Journal of Psychiatry, 163*(9), 1561–1568.

Krueger, A. B., & Stone, A. A. (2008). Assessment of pain: A community-based diary survey in the USA. *Lancet, 371*(9623), 1519–1525.

Leigh, J. P. (2011). Economic burden of occupational injury and illness in the United States. *The Milbank Quarterly, 89*(4), 728–772.

Leutwyler, K. (1995). The price of prevention. *Scientific American, 272*(4), 124–129.

Madey, S. F., & Gomez, R. (2003). Reduced optimism for perceived age-related medical conditions. *Basic and Applied Social Psychology, 25*, 213–219.

Marcus, B. H., Emmons, K. M., Simkin-Silverman, L. R., Linnan, L. A., Taylor, E. R., Bock, B. C., et al. (1998). Evaluation of motivationally tailored vs. standard self-help physical activity interventions at the workplace. *American Journal of Health Promotion, 12*(4), 246–253.

Mayer, T. G., & Press, J. M. (2005). Musculoskeletal rehabilitation. In A. Vaccaro (Ed.), *Orthopedic knowledge update* (pp. 655–661). Chicago, IL: AAOS Press.

Mayer, T. G., Gatchel, R. J., Porter, S., & Theodore, B. R. (2006). Postinjury rehabilitation/management. In W. S. Marras & W. Karwowski (Eds.), *The occupational ergonomics handbook: Interventions, controls, and applications in occupational ergonomics.* Boca Raton, FL: CRC Press.

Michael R. (2001). *Liberty Mutual releases workplace injury and cost data.* Ergonomics Today [cited 2 Oct 2012]. Available from http://www.ergoweb.com/news/detail.cfm?id=395

Moyal, D. D., & Fourtanier, A. M. (2008). Broad-spectrum sunscreens provide better protection from solar ultraviolet-simulated radiation and natural sunlight-induced immunosuppression in human beings. *Journal of the American Academy of Dermatology, 58*(5 Suppl 2), S149–S154.

Mullen, J. (2004). Investigating factors that influence individual safety behavior at work. *Journal of Safety Research, 35*(3), 275–285.

Norman, A. H., & Tesser, C. D. (2009). Quaternary prevention in primary care: A necessity for the Brazilian Unified National Health System. *Cadernos De Saude Publica, 25*(9), 2012–2020.

O'Brien Cousins, S. (2003). Grounding theory in self-referent thinking: Conceptualizing motivation for older adult physical activity. *Psychology of Sport and Exercise, 4*, 81–100.

O'Brien Cousins, S. (2000). "My heart couldn't take it": Older women's beliefs about exercise benefits and risks. *The Journals of Gerontology. Series B, Psychological Sciences and Social Sciences, 55*(5), P283–P294.

Occupational Health and Safety Administration. (2012). *Injury and illness prevention programs: White paper* [cited 3 Feb 2012]. Available from http://www.osha.gov/dsg/InjuryIllnessPreventionProgramsWhitePaper.html

Paulozzi, L., Baldwin, G., Franklin, G., Kerlikowske, R. G., Jones, C. M., Ghiya, N., & Popovic, T. (2012). CDC grand rounds: Prescription Drug overdoses—A U.S. epidemic. *Morbidity and Mortality Weekly Report, 61*(1), 10–13.

Plotnikoff, R. C., McCargar, L. J., Wilson, P. M., & Loucaides, C. A. (2005). Efficacy of an E-mail intervention for the promotion of physical activity and nutrition behavior in the workplace context. *American Journal of Health Promotion, 19*(6), 422–429.

Prochaska, J. O., DiClemente, C. C., & Norcross, J. C. (1992). In search of how people change: Applications to addictive behaviors. *The American Psychologist, 47*, 1102–1114.

Prochaska, J. O., Norcross, J. C., & DiClemente, C. C. (1994). *Changing for good*. New York: Avon Books.

Rosen, C. S. (2000). Is the sequencing of change processes by stage consistent across health problems? A meta-analysis. *Health Psychology, 19*, 593–604.

Ruward, J., Schrieken, B., Schrijver, M., Broeksteeg, J., Dekker, J., Vermeulen, H., & Lange, A. (2009). Standardized web-based cognitive behavioural therapy of mild to moderate depression: A randomized controlled trial with long-term follow-up. *Cognitive Behaviour Therapy, 38*(4), 206–221.

Schultz, D. (2004). Employee attitudes—A must have. *Occupational Health & Safety, 73*(6), 66–72.

Siegel, M., & Biener, L. (2000). The impact of an antismoking media campaign on progression to established smoking: Results of a longitudinal youth study. *American Journal of Public Health, 90*(3), 380–386.

Singletary, K. W., & Gapstur, S. M. (2001). Alcohol and breast cancer: Review of epidemiologic and experimental evidence and potential mechanisms. *JAMA: Journal of the American Medical Association, 286*(17), 2143–2151.

Spiegel, D., & Giese-Davis, J. (2003). Depression and cancer: Mechanisms and disease progression. *Biological Psychiatry, 54*(3), 269–282.

Stamler, J., Stamler, R., Neaton, J. D., Wentworth, D., Daviglus, M. L., Garside, D., et al. (1999). Low risk-factor profile and long-term cardiovascular and noncardiovascular mortality and life expectancy: Findings for 5 large cohorts of young adult and middle-aged men and women. *JAMA: Journal of the American Medical Association, 282*(21), 2012–2018.

The World Health Organization. (2004). *The world health report 2004: Changing history, annex table 3: Burden of disease in DALYs by cause, sex, and mortality stratum in WHO regions, estimates for 2002*. Geneva: WHO.

Towers Perrin. (2008). *Closing the engagement gap: A road map for driving superior business performance*, In: *Towers Perrin global workforce study 2007-2008*. [cited 6 Feb 2012]. Available from http://www.towersperrin.com/tp/getwebcachedoc?webc=HRS/USA/2008/200803/GWS_Global_Report20072008_31208.pdf.

Towers Watson. (2010). *2009/2010 Staying@work report: The Health and productivity advantage* [cited 6 Feb 2012]. Available from http://www.towerswatson.com/assets/pdf/648/TW_NA_2010_16703_SatW.pdf.

Vartiainen, E., Paavola, M., McAlister, A., & Puska, P. (1998). Fifteen-year follow-up of smoking prevention effects in the North Karelia youth project. *American Journal of Public Health, 88*(1), 81–85.

Weinstein, N. D. (1988). The precaution adoption process. *Health Psychology, 7*, 355–386.

Yassi, A., Khokhar, J., Tate, R., Cooper, J., Snow, C., & Vallentyne, S. (1995a). The epidemiology of back injuries in nurses at a large Canadian tertiary care hospital: Implications for prevention. *Occupational Medicine, 45*(4), 215–220.

Yassi, A., Tate, R., Cooper, J. E., Snow, C., Vallentyne, S., & Khokhar, J. B. (1995b). Early intervention for back-injured nurses at a large Canadian tertiary care hospital: An evaluation of the effectiveness and cost benefits of a two-year pilot project. *Occupational Medicine, 45*(4), 209–214.

Organizational Aspects of Work Accommodation and Retention in Mental Health

Izabela Z. Schultz, Terry Krupa, E. Sally Rogers, and Alanna Winter

Introduction

Mental health problems and disorders constitute an escalating challenge in the workplace. Another chapter in this handbook by Dewa and colleagues has also addressed this important topic. According to the World Health Organization (WHO, 2001a), mental health disorders comprise 40% of the leading causes of disability worldwide, and they account for 10.5% of the total global burden of disease. About 450 million people, most of them of working age, are affected by at least one mental health disorder. Importantly, mental health disorders are projected to account for 15% of the disability burden internationally by the year 2020. Depression alone is projected to account for the second highest burden of disease, following only cardiovascular disease (Scott & Dickey, 2003; WHO, 2001b). Furthermore, mental health disabilities are becoming increasingly common in the workplace. According to the Canadian Community Health Survey, in 2002, approximately one in every five individuals over the age of 15 experienced psychological symptoms over the course of the year, including

---

I.Z. Schultz, Ph.D. (✉)
Department of Educational and Counselling Psychology, and Special Education,
The University of British Columbia, Vancouver, BC Canada
e-mail: ischultz@telus.net

T. Krupa, Ph.D.
Department School of Rehabilitation Therapy, Queen's University,
31 George Street, Kingston, ON K7L 3N6, Canada
e-mail: krupat@queensu.ca

E.S. Rogers, Sc.D.
Department—Center for Psychiatric Rehabilitation,
Boston University, 940 Commonwealth Ave, Boston, MA 02215, USA
e-mail: erogers@bu.edu

A. Winter
BC Women's Hospital & Health Centre,
Vancouver, BC Canada

depression, anxiety disorders, and alcohol or drug dependence (CCHS; Statistics Canada, 2003). Estimates exist that approximately 10% of the working population has at least one mental health disorder (Dewa, Lin, Kooehoorn, & Goldner, 2007). Given these numbers, it is not surprising that the societal costs of mental health disorders are so high. In North America, the annual societal costs are estimated at $83.1 billion (Greenberg et al., 2003) and, in the European Union, at EU$320 billion (Andlin-Sobocki, Jonsson, Wittchen, & Olesen 2005). Between 30 and 60% of the costs are losses associated with reduced productivity. In Canada, this cost has been estimated to be C$17.7 billion annually (Lim, Jacobs, Ohinmaa, Schopflocher, & Dewa, 2008). Absenteeism (to be discussed later in this chapter) related to mental health problems accounts for about 7% of the total payroll (Watson Wyatt Worldwide, 2000). Stephens and Joubert (2001) suggested that the costs to Canadian employers in lost productivity arising from presenteeism (i.e., less than optimal job performance) and absenteeism due to mental health problems are in the billions of dollars each year. Overall, mental health problems have a multifold impact on work, including diminished productivity, absenteeism, presenteeism and short-term disability, increased unemployment rates, early retirement, as well as decreased productivity related to spillover effects on coworkers and supervisors (Dewa & McDaid, 2010). It therefore seems there are significant economic, social and humanitarian reasons to implement workplace initiatives which will reduce the incidence of mental health distress in the workplace, as well as to facilitate the rehabilitation of those employees affected by mental health disabilities (Dewa & McDaid, 2010).

However, Goldner and colleagues (2004) reported that there is limited research to guide disability management practices for mental health disorders. Furthermore, despite an emerging consensus on the importance of integration of clinical treatment and vocational rehabilitation, the current literature is still fragmented, focused on selected diagnoses, and weak at identifying functional limitations cross-diagnostically. While there is an accumulated evidentiary support for employment interventions for individuals with severe mental illness, there is less of an evidence base for individuals with more common mental health problems, including anxiety and mood disorders. A recent survey conducted by Schultz and colleagues (Schultz, Milner, Hanson, & Winter, 2010) investigated the attitudes of Canadian employers towards workers with mental health disorders. The results indicated that over 50% of the 80 Canadian employers surveyed (mid-size to large companies) had significant concerns about workers with mental health disability. The most significant concerns included mental instability (83.1%), bizarre behaviors (80.7%), inability to tolerate work pressure and stress (79.5%), becoming violent (75.9%), and being unable to tolerate working conditions (74.7%). Clearly, the improved societal attitudes and increased acceptance of workers with physical disabilities are not paralleled by workplace inclusion of individuals with mental health disorders. Social stigmatization continues to be a more salient barrier to employment than actual disability (Baldwin & Marcus, 2010; Corrigan, Larson, & Kuwabara, 2007; Goldner et al., 2004; Haslan, Atkinson, Brown, & Haslan, 2005)

Of particular concern in this present chapter is the lack of an overarching conceptual model and a satisfactory evidentiary basis for best practices to support work accommodation and retention of individuals with mental health disorders. Work accommodations are defined as efforts to modify any element of a job so that it can be accomplished by a qualified person with a disability. This intervention can include accommodation aspects of the hiring process, the actual performance of the job, or the individual's ability to enjoy the full benefits of the job (US Equal Opportunity Commission, 2002). The goal of this chapter is to provide readers with an understanding of current models and interventions, in both research and practice, regarding work accommodation in mental health, and to address the unresolved issues and barriers to the integration and transfer of this knowledge to practice. This chapter also reviews and integrates the themes presented in the literature, as well as highlights future research, policy, and practice directions.

Towards an Integrative Conceptual Framework for Work Accommodation in Mental Health

There is a gap between the predominance of medical and treatment-focused models for persons with mental health problems and the reality of the workplace environment. Medical models, while useful for optimizing treatment and controlling symptoms, are not useful as a framework for maximizing work capacity or job accommodations in the workplace (Schultz, Stowell, Feuerstein, & Gatchel, 2007). A system-based, social model of mental health disability, with service and research emphases on function and functional accommodations, would seem more suitable (Gates & Akabas, 2010), especially in combination with the biopsychosocial model integrating clinical and occupational interventions. The mismatch between the worker with mental health problems and the workplace organization is likely at the core of poor employment outcomes of persons with mental health disorders (Akabas, 1994; Bond, 2004; Gates & Akabas, 2010; Spataro, 2005; Stone & Colella, 1996). Workplace policies and practices often do not match the needs of qualified workers with mental health problems. Occupational stress, now inherent in the workplace, tends to compound functional problems individuals with mental health disorders might have with specific task and interpersonally related aspects of the work environment. As Gates and Akabas aptly emphasize, "Inclusion into the workplace is not just a function of reducing the extent to which individual characteristics and symptoms interfere with workplace policies and practices, but also a function of organizational responsiveness to these individuals as expressed through the attitudes and behaviors of management, supervisors and coworkers." (2010, p. 375). Therefore, work accommodation needs to be understood as a strategy for inclusion and social process. It involves dynamic multiparty interactions in the workplace leading, in the context of organizational readiness, to an improved match between the job and relationship requirements in the workplace on the one hand, and individual skills and needs on the other.

Currently, no guidelines for job accommodations and employment retention for persons with mental health disabilities have been published, despite the mounting research worldwide on similar interventions for individuals with physical and pain-related disabilities. Yet, societal, professional and economic concerns are escalating over the low rates of employment of persons with mental health disabilities, decreased productivity, "presenteeism," premature job terminations, and lower rates of job retention. These factors, together with what some refer to as a spiraling "mental health disability epidemic" in the workplace (Dewa & McDaid, 2010; Lerner et al., 2010), indicate a problem of significant magnitude. Research evidence to date shows a high, and increasing, prevalence of mental health disorders, accompanied by a strongly negative economic impact for society, the workplace, health care and compensation systems, and for persons with mental health disorders themselves (Baldwin & Marcus, 2010; Dewa & McDaid, 2010; Gnam, 2005).

To compound the problem, health care for persons with mental health disorders, despite recent advances in psychiatric vocational rehabilitation, still bears the burden of the medical model that separates mind and body and focuses on psychopathology rather than on preserved strengths and functional capacity (Schultz, Crook, Fraser, & Joy, 2000; Schultz & Gatchel, 2005; Schultz, Stowell, Feuerstein, & Gatchel, 2007). Such models are ill-equipped to provide occupationally relevant and effective interventions that facilitate long term employment. The growing movement towards mental health systems based on a recovery vision may hold the promise of shifting the paradigm of mental health services from one based largely on pathology, to one that focuses on realizing potential. Recovery has gained strength internationally as an orientation to care that focuses on enabling people to move beyond the limits that are associated with mental illness, and to enjoy meaningful and valued lives in the community. A recovery-oriented vision could lead to a growing awareness of participation in work as an important outcome, along with the development of strengths-based approaches to support this outcome. (Mental Health Commission of Canada, 2009).

The provision of appropriate work accommodations, with the goal of enhancing employment retention for individuals with mental health disorders and preventing work disability, is challenging for many reasons. The complex and episodic nature of mental health disorders can be exacerbated by a wide range of stressors inherent in daily life and work environments. When planning workplace interventions in mental health, the specific nature of organizational, task-related and interpersonal stressors needs to be clearly identified, with a view to evolving strategies to reducing stressors and their impact, and to developing personal illness and impairment management strategies in response to these stressors. Furthermore, societal stigma and employers' negative attitudes and fears often lead to a lack of awareness and preparation for employees with mental health disorders (Baldwin & Marcus, 2010; Schultz, Milner, et al., 2010). In an attempt to avoid stigma, individuals with mental health disorders often try to conceal their problems, resulting in adverse consequences for the workplace. The following workplace consequences of unidentified and unaddressed mental health problems in the workplace were enumerated by Harnois and Gabriel (2000): absenteeism (increase in overall sickness absence, particularly frequent short periods of absence); poor health, depression, stress, and burnout; physical conditions including high blood pressure, heart disease, ulcers, sleeping disorders, skin rashes, headache, neck- and backache, and low resistance to infections; changes in work performance, also known as presenteeism (reduction in productivity and output, increase in error rates, increased amount of accidents, poor decision-making, and deterioration in planning and control of work); staff attitude and behavior problems (loss of motivation and commitment, burnout, staff working increasingly long hours but for diminishing returns, poor timekeeping, labor turnover); and difficulties with relationships at work (tension and conflicts between colleagues, poor relationships with clients, increase in disciplinary problems).

The development of strategies to address these barriers and limitations that individuals with mental health disorders face once employed are important given the high estimates of unemployment among these workers. Figures for the United States show that between 75 and 85% of people with severe mental illness are unemployed while, in the United Kingdom, estimates range from 61 to 73% (Crowther, Marshall, Bond, & Huxley, 2001a, 2001b). Individuals with less severe disorders still experience a 26% unemployment rate (New Freedom Commission on Mental Health, 2003). Depression alone, although underdiagnosed, has been estimated to have a prevalence of approximately 10% among employees (Berndt et al., 1998). A growing body of research literature into the effectiveness of work accommodations and employment retention initiatives attests to the need for accommodations. Compounding the challenge of the provision of job accommodations in the workplace is the absence of an integrative conceptual model of employment interventions in mental health, and the paucity of solid research evidence informing workplace policies and disability prevention practices for employees with mental health disorders.

A recent series of studies on work accommodation in mental health (Schultz, Duplassie, Hanson, & Winter, 2010; Schultz, Milner, et al., 2010; Schultz, Winter, & Wald, 2010) proposed a broader ecological, person-environment conceptualization of work accommodations. Figure 20.1 illustrates optimization of work performance of workers with mental health problems affecting their cognitive, emotional, and social functioning, through job accommodation, leading to ability to meet work demands.

Multisystem Interventions in Occupational Mental Health

Work accommodations and interventions for persons with mental health disorders show promise for improving employment outcomes. To be maximally effective, these interventions should be offered in an integrated and multi-systemic manner, as well being consistent with the biopsychosocial model of

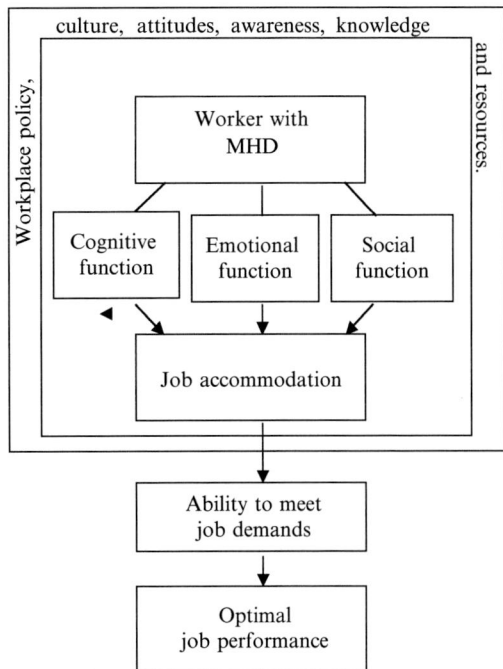

Fig. 20.1 Optimizing work performance of workers with mental health disability (MHD) through job accommodation

occupational disability, which postulates the integration of vocational and clinical services and emphasizes the worker's strengths and abilities rather than psychopathology and diagnosis (Goldner et al., 2004; Loisel et al., 2001; Schultz, 2008; Schultz et al., 2007). Interventions and accommodations for persons with mental health disorders can be conceptualized at the following three system levels: macrosystem interventions, focusing on society, culture, legislation, and policies; employer-level (mesosystem) interventions; and employee-level (microsystem) interventions. The current chapter focuses on macrosystem and mesosystem interventions, as they best inform organizational policy and practice.

Macrosystem Interventions

Macrosystem interventions can be defined as large scale interventions that aim to change societal attitudes at large, generally involving legislative, policy, cultural, or systemic changes in both the public and private sectors. Barriers to the employment of persons with mental health disorders best addressed at the macrosystem level include the negative societal attitudes, stigma, fears and lack of knowledge. Negative attitudes, fears and lack of knowledge permeate society and, consequently, inform the expectations held by employers, coworkers, disability compensation and management systems, and society at large. As well, social stigma, thought by some to be more disabling than the primary mental health condition, itself, is a major barrier in the workplace for persons with mental health disorders (Baldwin & Marcus, 2010; Haslan et al., 2005; Wang, 2010). Indeed, it has been suggested that interventions directed at reducing stigma need to understand how negative attitudes and discrimination operate within specific life domains, such as employment. A recent study by Krupa and colleagues (2010), for example, suggested that a range of assumptions about people with mental illness (e.g., competence dangerousness, the legitimacy of mental illness, the impact of work on mental health and work as charity), is particularly salient in the work context, and that the impact of these assumptions depends on the positions of key people holding these assumptions. While society-wide public awareness campaigns utilizing a social marketing approach could benefit this field (Schultz, Krupa & Rogers, 2010), focusing efforts in particular social contexts such as employment may prove particularly fruitful. For example, the *Opening Minds Initiative* of the Mental Health Commission of Canada has included the workforce as one of the key foci for anti-stigma initiatives. A key element of this initiative is to include the promising practice of contact-based education (Couture & Penn, 2003), which involves developing opportunities for key stakeholders in the workforce to have meaningful and positive exchanges with people who have lived the experience of mental illness (Mental Health Commission of Canada, 2011). Another important macrosystem intervention involves *legislative and public policy support* for parity for persons with mental health conditions in health care, insurance, compensation and rehabilitation systems, as well as fairness in employment practices (Baldwin & Marcus, 2010; Black, 2008; Center, 2010; Commission of European Communities, 2008; Department of Work and Pensions and Department of Health, 2008; Gallie, Schultz, & Winter, 2010; Standing Senate Committee, 2006; World Health Organization, 2005). In addition, studies of public policy have suggested that policy documents are weakened by inconsistent representations of mental illness, vague descriptions of the functional implications of mental illness, and few concrete and positive examples of work accommodations (Cockburn et al., 2006). Developing meaningful legislation and policy related to employment equity and workplace accommodation, as well as processes for promoting employer buy-in, is essential. Stuart (2006) noted that research suggests that employer compliance with legislation has been problematic, as demonstrated by the high number of complaints submitted for charges of discrimination based on the *U.S. Americans with Disabilities Act*.

In order to prevent occupational disability in general, a *multisystem interaction*, involving the integration of clinical and vocational rehabilitation services, is essential. There is strong and growing evidence demonstrating the effectiveness of integrated clinical and occupational interventions, using a biopsychosocial model in the field of musculoskeletal pain (Schultz & Gatchel, 2005; Schultz, Krupa, & Rogers, 2010; Schultz et al., 2007). Integration of mental health and vocational services has been found effective in enhancing employment retention of persons with mental health disorders (Arthur, 2000; Berndt et al., 1998; Bishop, 2004; Holzberg, 2001; Johnstone, Vessell, Bounds, Hoskins, & Sherman, 2003; Macias, DeCarlo, Wang, Frey, & Barreira, 2001; Means, Stewart, & Dowler, 1997; Scheid, 1998; Sherbourne et al., 2001; Smith et al., 2002). However, practical implementation of this approach in the workplace has been lagging behind. Moreover, the high profile *Canadian Global Business and Economic Roundtable on Mental Health* (2005) highlighted the importance of addressing the occupational stress experienced by employees in workplaces, and the accompanying need to support their intellectual and emotional capacities and thereby meet growing business demands for innovation and global competition. The idea of developing a psychologically safe and healthy workplace has gained traction as the legal basis for protecting employee mental health (Shain, 2009). Efforts have been directed at identifying key psychosocial risk factors and creating associated tools for workplaces (Shain, 2009). The Guarding Minds@Work strategy is one such example (www.guardingmindsatworks.ca). *Guarding Minds* provides employers with strategies and tools to identify and address 12 psychosocial risk factors. Indeed, organizational infrastructure to facilitate communication among various mental health stakeholders is much needed. Involving the health care system, compensation system, employer, union and the worker in reciprocal multisystem interactions, with a common goal of promoting job retention, is essential to effect lasting paradigm changes in attitudes, organizational structure, policy and practices.

Employer-Level (Mesosystem) Interventions

Mesosystem interventions can be defined as workplace organization-based interventions focusing on the extent to which the workplace itself can be constructed to facilitate job retention and health.

An optimal environment for work accommodations and retention interventions is found in a workplace culture that embraces the following: opportunities for control and decision-making; the full utilization of worker capacities and skills; the opportunity for a variety of workplace activities; employee involvement; reasonable and well-integrated job demands; clear and predictable work expectations and conditions; interpersonal contacts; valued social positions in the workplace; and productivity connected to gains and rewards. These all seem to be associated with greater psychosocial benefits for employees (Kirsh & Gewurtz, 2010; Krupa, 2007; Vézina, Bourbonnais, Brisson, & Trudel, 2004; Warr, 1987). It should also be noted that employer-level interventions can be divided into Level and Level II interventions. Those interventions focusing on *primary prevention* of occupational disability and disease, and the promotion of health and wellness in the workplace, comprise Level I interventions. Those focusing on *secondary prevention* of occupational disability, including early detection, identification, and intervention with mental health problems in the workplace to prevent or reduce emerging disability, comprise Level II interventions.

Level I Intervention: Primary Prevention

A recent series of studies (Gallie et al., 2010; Krupa, 2010a, 2010b; Schultz, Duplassie, et al., 2010; Schultz, Milner, et al., 2010), and a synthesis of the literature (Schultz, Winter, & Wald, 2010), converge to suggest that the following employer-based interventions may facilitate employment outcomes for persons with mental health disabilities.

Organizational Restructuring

A workplace organizational structure that integrates and synchronizes employer resources in occupational health and safety, health and wellness, disability management, return-to-work, corporate training and Employee Assistance Programs (EAPs), in service of health promotion and disability prevention, and in a climate of inclusion of workers with mental health disabilities, is likely to be beneficial according to the emerging literature (Gallie et al., 2010). Experts seem to concur that the provision of EAPs is a hallmark of a caring employer. Unfortunately, as presently constructed, EAPs are an insufficient means for retention of employees with mental health disorders. While helpful in addressing life issues and emotional concerns, EAPs often do not focus on employment problems and job accommodations. A multifaceted intervention should include EAPs that address *both* the clinical and occupational needs of employees.

Written Policies on Health and Wellness

Specific policies and practices aiming to attach an employer to his or her employees is the ultimate translation of work attitudes. In turn, these policies and practices affect the attitudes of management and employees. Written company policies should demonstrate a commitment to the well-being and productivity of employees with mental health disorders. Together with expressing policies on health, wellness, stigma, discrimination and employee privacy/confidentiality protection in writing, developing policies on diversity (inclusive of mental health disability), is one additional way of showing commitment to greater workplace tolerance (Kirsh & Gewurtz, 2010).

Budgeting for Costs of Accommodations

The cost of a job accommodation provision is a necessary consideration for employers. Thus, it is important to have specific policies regarding the payment and costs of providing these accommodations. While the research in this area is scant, it suggests that costs to employers may not be large out-of-pocket expenses; rather, accommodations in mental health often rely on creative and flexible solutions (MacDonald-Wilson, Rogers, Massaro, Lyass, & Crean, 2002). Examples include: extending additional paid and unpaid leave during a hospitalization or other absence; allowing additional time for workers to reach performance milestones; extending probationary periods; allowing an employee to make phone calls during the day to personal and professional supports; providing a private space in which to make such phone calls; providing a private space to rest or talk to supportive coworkers; allowing an employee to work at home; and allowing workers to consume fluids at their workstation (e.g., due to medication side effects; as cited by Bruyere, 2000). The costs of such accommodations may be relatively low, but research in this area is needed. For example, a recent study of employers' experiences of intermittent work capacity in the context of episodic health conditions, such as those associated with mental illness, suggested that providing coverage, (particularly when absences are not anticipated, there is little warning of the absence, or where there are expectations related to return-to-work) can pose significant organizational challenges for workplaces, that may translate into increased costs if ineffectively managed (Lysaght, Krupa, & Gregory, 2011).

Training of Management
The literature suggests that training of management and supervisory staff in early detection and intervention for mental health-related performance difficulties, as well as the nature and importance of job accommodations, is of critical importance (Gallie et al., 2010; MacDonald-Wilson et al., 2002). Ideally, this training would be combined with awareness raising, stigma reduction, and developing the best organizational conditions for a mentally healthy workplace (Gallie et al., 2010). Several training and educational programs have recently been developed in response to the need to: address stigma in the workplace; promote early identification of mental illness and early access to treatment; and develop the capacity of the workplace to effectively support people who experience mental illness in the workplace (see for example, Canadian Mental Health Association, 2008; Canadian Mental Health Association, 2011). Research into the effectiveness of these interventions is still pending.

Levell II Interventions: Enhancing Employment Outcomes

In light of the growing recognition, in both research and practice, of the complexity of supporting the employment of individuals with mental health conditions, an integrated organizational framework is required to ensure that interventions are provided in a comprehensive, coordinated, fair, and cost-effective manner. There are two well-developed and disseminated organizational frameworks for meeting the employment needs of people with mental health disorders. The first, for those already work-attached, is disability management. The second framework is supported employment approaches, generally used for those with more severe mental health disabilities, and those who have had histories of no, or little, labor market attachment for a significant duration of time. Job-employee matching, a human resource strategy designed to enhance employment retention in mental health, could be incorporated into either of these frameworks.

Disability Management
Disability management programs are employer-directed programs and practices focused on prevention of work disability and facilitation of quick return-to-work (Currier, Chan, Berven, Habeck, & Taylor, 2001; Habeck & Hunt, 1999; Harder, Hawley, & Stewart, 2010). Typically, such programs involve a single management plan designed to ensure implementation of key disability management practices (Westmorland & Buys, 2002). By balancing both economic and productivity needs with the sustained health and well-being of the workforce, these approaches can support labor and management relationships (Scully, Habeck, & Leahy, 1999). While promising, this approach is restricted to those already

in the workforce. Other noted limitations to disability management programs are the potential lack of sensitivity to the complexity of interactions between an individual's mental health and organizational practices, as well as employers' inadequate preparation for dealing with employees with mental health disabilities, and privacy and confidentiality risks.

Supported Employment

Supported employment refers to models of service delivery designed to secure employment for individuals with a disability who are currently unemployed. The focus is on rapid job placement with "wrap around supports" rather than long periods of training and preparation prior to employment (Anthony & Blanch, 1989). The *Individual Placement and Support Model* (IPS) is an example of supported employment. The goal of this program is to help individuals with severe mental illness rapidly enter into competitive jobs in the community. The IPS model has repeatedly demonstrated effectiveness in reaching this goal (Bond, Drake, & Becker, 2008; Bond, McHugo, Becker, Rapp, & Whitley 2008). However, it has not yet been validated outside of the spectrum of severe mental illness, intellectual disability (McInnes, Orgul, McDermott, & Mann, 2010), and brain injury (Fadyl & McPherson, 2009; Kirsh et al., 2009; McInnes et al., 2010. Further research regarding efficacy, with more prevalent mental health conditions such as mood and anxiety disorders, would be useful.

Job-Employee Matching

A number of studies indicate that improved job retention results when workers' interests and abilities are matched with the appropriate job (Haffey & Abrams, 1991; Mueser, Becker, & Wolfe, 2001). The importance of determining functional limitations and capacity to provide more effective job accommodations has already been underscored in the literature (MacDonald-Wilson, Rogers, & Massaro 2003), and is likely to be even more critical for individuals with mental health disorders. An ecological approach to job matching, utilizing a "person-environment fit" that attends to the goals of the individual, as well as the workplace and organizational culture, is a hallmark of effective job matching (Szymanski & Vancollins, 2003).

Targeting Barriers to Job Accommodation

Negatively held attitudes and fears, often arising from a lack of education, knowledge and awareness among employers, coworkers and individuals with mental health disorders, can act as barriers to implementing job accommodations in the workplace. Not only are many employers lacking in understanding about mental health symptoms and their impact on work performance, they are also minimally aware of accommodation needs of employees with mental health conditions and what accommodation options exist (Schultz, Milner, et al., 2010). It is imperative to recognize organizational, policy and resource-related challenges that exist at the employer level. Systemic and contextual factors that limit employers' willingness and ability to implement such initiatives are behind most barriers to job accommodations. Research suggests that size of company and type of industry are key factors in whether employers provide job accommodations (Schultz, Milner, et al., 2010). Due to greater financial and structural resources, larger companies (as compared to small and mid-size companies) have the ability to offer such services and, as a result, more often have established policies regarding hiring persons with mental health disabilities and offering job accommodations. Furthermore, the use of job accommodations tends to be predicted by the existence of a company policy about hiring individuals with disabilities. Findings from Schultz and colleagues (Schultz, Duplassie, et al., 2010; Schultz, Milner, et al., 2010) indicate that systemic limitations faced by employers are key barriers to provision of these services, even more critical than holding positive attitudes and a willingness to hire persons with mental health disorders.

An employer's sole reliance on a narrow understanding of the disability management model is also of concern. Under this model, the necessity of coordination of services with direct intervention with the employee may be lost. Likewise, recognition of the clinical and psychosocial complexities of the workplace may not be sufficient. Similarly, excessive reliance on traditional external Employee Assistance Programs for counseling is problematic due to the absence of occupational interventions with attention to system-related factors (Gallie et al., 2010). Often of concern is the fact that effective relationship-based accommodations, including natural supports in the workplace (e.g., using coworkers), are often under-utilized by employers. Recent research has suggested that workplace support from coworkers, supervisors and others on the job is associated with the existence of positive relations between workers, and the sense that the worker requiring accommodations is committed to the goals of the workplace (Lysaght et al., 2011). Where there is existing unresolved conflict between workers, support for accommodation and job retention is compromised (Williams-Whitt & Taras, 2010). Employers also seem least aware of job accommodations for persons with mental health disorders that require flexibility in redesigning or reorganizing work processes (e.g., working from home, job sharing, establishing distraction-free work space and the appropriate use of work scheduling and breaks; Schultz, Winter, & Wald, 2010). Workplaces that have strong leadership to support inclusive work practices, and communication structures that promote information sharing about workplace accommodations and local problem solving, offer an organizational culture of practice that enables flexibility in the design of work processes that balance the accommodation needs of workers with the productivity goals of the employer (Krupa & Lysaght, 2011)

Towards Best Evidence-Informed Work Accommodations

Research to validate various interventions and accommodations in mental health is in its early stages, and emphasis should be placed on those interventions and accommodations that have the best evidentiary support to date. Nonetheless, a range of useful "best practices" have emerged from a research literature synthesis (Schultz, Winter, & Wald, 2010), expert interviews (Schultz, Duplassie, et al. 2010), and an employer survey (Schultz, Milner, et al., 2010). The following interventions and accommodations have been suggested by the research to be useful in ameliorating the social, emotional or cognitive limitations associated with mental health conditions:
- Modified work duties
- Flexible scheduling
- Modified work environment
- Job sharing
- Assistive technologies

Research, however, is still lacking in a number of areas: (1) the characteristics of those who are most likely to benefit from these accommodations; (2) what organizational circumstances are needed to optimize the outcomes of accommodations; (3) at what point in time, by whom, and how specific work accommodations are to be introduced in the workplace; and (4) the effectiveness of work accommodations involving social interactions and processes rather than technology and changes in organization,

Where Are We Headed? Conclusions and Best Practices

The design, implementation and evaluation of job accommodations and interventions for persons with mental health problems are more complex and multidimensional than the development of analogous interventions and job accommodations for persons with physical limitations. Such interventions are evolving from legislative, policy, attitudinal, employer and disability stakeholder perspectives, as well as from a research perspective. Despite the compilation of a seemingly comprehensive list of job accommodations by the US Department of Labor Job Accommodation Network (2007), research and evidentiary support for most accommodations is just emerging. Even though there is considerable stigma surrounding mental health conditions, employers' awareness of job accommodations depends less on their attitudes and more on the size of the company, the existence of written policies in regards to accommodations, and prior experience in hiring a person with mental health disability (Schultz, Milner, et al., 2010). Solutions to the problem of poor awareness and under-utilization of job accommodations are multi-systemic and multi-layered, involving the need for a significant paradigm shift, among the key stakeholders, in conceptualizing and accommodating mental health problems in the workplace.

Systemic solutions center around the issues delineated below:

1. The need for macro-level interventions to change public attitudes towards persons with mental health problems, as well as changes in legislative health and employment policies.
2. The enhancement of multi-system interactions among employer, health care, rehabilitation systems, and the insurance and compensation system in order to bridge the chasm between medical model-based mental health services and employer-based vocational services.
3. At the employer level, key interventions need to be performed from both primary and secondary prevention perspectives.
   (a) Primary prevention in the workplace should focus on: the promotion of the health and wellness of a diverse work force; awareness-raising and anti-stigma initiatives, combined with the development of written policies reflective of management commitment; appropriate organizational restructuring to integrate various health, human resource and occupational services within the company; and early detection and intervention with employees with mental health disorders.
   (b) Secondary prevention should target both supported employment for employees with persistent and serious mental health disabilities, and an expanded disability management approach combined with modern, proactive, and biopsychosocial-based vocational rehabilitation approaches.

In addition to the above, in the workplace, accommodation-focused interventions should be integrated with clinical interventions at the individual level in order to enhance a person's work readiness and work retention, and should include the steps noted below:

4. Conducting assessments: Following disclosure of a mental health disability, utilize qualified individuals to conduct workplace-based functional ("ecological") assessments, collaboratively with workers, management and unions, to identify job accommodation needs using an individualized, worker-centered approach that emphasizes the employee's capacities, strengths and compensatory skills that promote job performance and retention.
5. Staff training: In addition to training of direct line supervisors and coworkers on how to best promote mental health through social relations in the workplace, orientation, training and supervision for new employees with mental health disorders, including training in giving feedback, problem-solving and realistic goal-setting.
6. Enhancing social support: Increase workplace social support and utilize natural supports at work (coworkers) by engaging coworkers as trainers and mentors; recognize negative workplace attitudes; improve awareness and educational opportunities about mental health disabilities for coworkers and management; when appropriate, provide employees with sensitivity training on mental health issues and how to work with individuals who may be exhibiting overt symptoms or have cognitive difficulties, such as distractibility, short term memory problems and impairments in organization.
7. Promoting flexibility: Be flexible with job accommodations that involve modification of work-task requirements, changes to the work environment and location, scheduling and hours of work, use, frequency and duration of breaks, time to complete work, work organization and the application of assistive technology.

8. Use of an employment specialist: In the case of complex or unfamiliar work conditions, or challenging labor-relations situations, engage an internal or external employment/return to work/ vocational rehabilitation/case management specialist familiar with accommodations and job retention issues among persons with mental health conditions.
9. Use of multidisciplinary resources: in complex cases, particularly for serious mental illness, it is important to ensure that the employee has access to multidisciplinary resources to help manage work performance and changes at work, and is actively engaged in an illness and symptom management process. Furthermore, assessing the effectiveness of accommodations and identification of other treatment and occupational needs (including expanded EAP interventions), requires considerable workplace attention. It is also important to ensure that workers are collaborating with the employer in the process of maintaining both their physical and psychological wellness and developing self-management strategies.
10. Protecting privacy and confidentiality: Be sensitive to employees' possible guardedness around mental health issues and the need to protect their privacy and confidentiality (MacDonald-Wilson et al., 2010). The employer is not entitled to know the worker's diagnosis, but should understand the functional capacities and limitations that arise from the diagnosis and that affect work performance. Workers experiencing mental illness can benefit from disclosure-related counseling.
11. Performance evaluations and feedback: Recognize functional problems arising from the employee's mental health difficulties and differentiate them from true under-performance that requires a disciplinary approach. Identify environmental, management and social factors in the workplace that may help the employee enhance performance and implement desired changes. Recognize the role of stress in reduced function among persons with mental health problems, and the types of stressors that are problematic. Provide regular supportive feedback to the employee and use both supervisors and peers as coaches. Ensure access to special skills training, for example organizational skills, assertiveness or conflict resolution skills that the employee may require to augment the utility of job accommodations and their overall job performance (Schultz, Duplassie, et al., 2010).

Future Research

The literature review on work accommodations in mental health has identified significant research gaps in the following areas:
- *Methodology*: There is a lack of well-developed transdisciplinary methodologies for research on multisystem interactions affecting job retention and accommodations among workers with mental health disorders.
- *Research Paradigms*: Most of the existing research is based upon a psychopathology/medical model. There is no consistent research funding with a mandate for bridging clinical and occupational paradigms.
- *Scope of Diagnostic Categories*: Serious mental illness, anxiety and mood disorders, intellectual disability, and brain injury are some of the most researched diagnoses; very little relevant research has been conducted in highly prevalent pervasive neuropsychological conditions affecting both cognitive and emotional functioning in adults, such as Learning Disorders and autism-spectrum disorders, although some literature on Attention Deficit Disorder is emerging.
- *Predictors of Work Disability*: Research on predictors of occupational disability in mental health, except for emerging studies in brain injury, post-traumatic stress disorder and depression, has been limited. Research does suggest that diagnoses along the schizophrenia-spectrum are associated

with poorer vocational outcomes; likewise, cognitive difficulties and low educational attainment also predict poorer vocational outcomes (Rogers & MacDonald-Wilson, 2010).

- *Functional Assessment*: There is a paucity of validated assessment instruments that measure functional work capacity; existing psychosocial and neuropsychological tests are diagnostically, rather than functionally, oriented. Yet, standardized and validated functional "ecological" assessments are critical for the development of job accommodations and to facilitate future research (Rogers & MacDonald-Wilson, 2010).
- *Organizational Interventions and Job Accommodations*: There is a lack of research on which primary and secondary workplace prevention programs are associated with improved job retention and accommodations, and under what conditions (who, where, when and what) they are effective. Moreover, there is no consensus on how to best measure clinical, occupational and employment outcomes.
- *Effectiveness of Job Accommodations*: Research on effectiveness of job accommodations is in the emerging stage; methodological difficulties include small sample sizes, the use of samples of convenience, a lack of tools for pooling data from several studies, a lack of control groups and randomized designs, difficulties in standardizing protocols for job accommodations in workplace environments, and the multitude of extraneous ("environmental noise") factors affecting outcomes, together with difficult-to-capture organizational and clinical treatment factors. Moreover, multivariate and multilevel analysis models are underutilized. In addition, the effectiveness of accommodations is likely dependent on the type and stability of functional work limitations, timing of interventions, consistency of application, a variety of employer-related and coworker-related support factors, as well as task demands and worker control over the work tasks. Such conditions and factors demand difficult, labor-intensive, and costly-to-execute research designs. A combination of qualitative and quantitative research studies, using a mixed design, undertaken by teams of researchers in different geographic locations, yet using the same methodology, is likely to be the most promising approach.
- *Voice of the Consumer*: There is a need to develop more understanding of the living experience of working with a mental health disability. Attention needs to be directed at how peer support and social interaction-related approaches and strategies can be effectively used in the workplace context.

In conclusion, despite major societal, clinical, employer, and research advances in the area of mental health in the workplace, a major gap continues to exist between health care services and the occupational needs of workers with mental health disorders on the one hand, and research evidence on what works with whom, where and when in the workplace, on the other. A new research paradigm for mental health disabilities in the workplace, integrating multisystem research with combined clinical and occupational approaches, is needed. Only by integrating the efforts of researchers, policy-makers, health-care practitioners, employers, educators, disability compensation systems, and persons with mental health disorders can the challenge of mental health in the workplace be addressed.

Acknowledgment Parts of this chapter were informed by research reports prepared for a Social Development Canada funded project "Towards Evidence-Informed Best Practice Guidelines for Job Accommodations for Persons with Mental Health Disabilities" and published in Work Accommodation and Retention in Mental Health, Schultz I.Z. & E.S. Rogers (eds) 2011; Springer.

References

Akabas, S. H. (1994). Workplace responsiveness: Key employer characteristics in support of job maintenance for people with mental illness. *Psychosocial Rehabilitation Journal, 17*(3), 91–101.

Andlin-Sobocki, P., Jonsson, B., Wittchen, H. U., & Olesen, J. (2005). Cost of disorders of the brain in Europe. *European Journal of Neurology, 12*(Suppl 1), 1–27.

Anthony, W. A., & Blanch, A. K. (1989). Research on community support services: What have we learned? *Psychosocial Rehabilitation Journal, 12*(3), 55–81.

Arthur, A. R. (2000). Employee assistance programs: The emperor's new clothes of stress management. *British Journal of Guidance and Counselling, 28*(4), 549–559.

Baldwin, M. W., & Marcus, S. C. (2010). Stigma, discrimination, and employment outcomes among persons with mental health disabilities. In I. Z. Schultz & E. S. Rogers (Eds.), *Work accommodation and retention in mental health*. New York: Springer.

Berndt, E. R., Finkelstein, S. N., Greenberg, P. E., Howland, R. H., Keith, A., Rush, A. J., et al. (1998). Workplace performance effects from chronic depression and its treatment. *Journal of Health Economics, 17*, 511–535.

Bishop, M. (2004). Determinants of employment status among a community-based sample of people with epilepsy: Implications for rehabilitation interventions. *Rehabilitation Counseling Bulletin, 47*(2), 112–120.

Black, C. (2008). *Working for a healthier tomorrow*. London: TSO.

Bond, G. R. (2004). Supported employment: Evidence for an evidence-based practice. *Psychiatric Rehabilitation Journal, 27*(4), 345–359.

Bond, G., Drake, R., & Becker, D. (2008). An update on randomized controlled trials of evidence-based supported employment. *Psychiatric Rehabilitation Journal, 31*, 280–290.

Bond, G. R., McHugo, G. J., Becker, D. R., Rapp, C. A., & Whitley, R. (2008). Fidelity of supported employment: Lessons learned from the national evidence-based practice project. *Psychiatric Rehabilitation Journal, 31*, 300–305.

Bruyere, S.M. (Ed.) (2000). *Employing and accommodating workers with psychiatric disabilities* (Brochure). Ithaca, NY: Cornell University (Originally written in 1994, and updated in 2000 by L.L. Manusco). http://digitalcommons.ilr.conrnell.edu/edicollect/5

Canadian Mental Health Association. (2011). *Mental health works*. Retrieved from http://www.mentalhealthworks.ca/

Canadian Mental Health Association, Calgary Region. (2008). *The copernicus project*. Retrieved from http://www.cmha.calgary.ab.ca/programs/PDFs/Biff

Center, C. (2010). Law and job accommodation in mental health disability. In I. Z. Schultz & E. S. Rogers (Eds.), *Work accommodation and retention in mental health*. New York: Springer.

Cockburn, L., Krupa, T., Bickenbach, J., Kirsh, B., Gewurtz, R., Chan, P., et al. (2006). Work and psychiatric disability in Canadian Public Policy. *Canadian Public Policy, XXXII*(2), 197–211.

Commission of the European Communities. (2008). *European pact for mental health and wellbeing*. Commission of the European Communities. http://ec.europa.eu/health/ph_determinants/life_style/mental/docs/pact_en.pdf

Corrigan, P. W., Larson, J. E., & Kuwabara, S. (2007). Mental illness stigma and the fundamental components of supported employment. *Rehabilitation Psychology, 52*, 451–457.

Couture, S. M., & Penn, D. L. (2003). Interpersonal contact and the stima of mental illness: A review of the literature. *Journal of Mental Health, 12*(3), 291–305.

Crowther, R. E., Marshall, M., Bond, G. R., & Huxley, P. (2001a). Helping people with severe mental disorder obtain work: Systematic review. *British Medical Journal, 322*, 204–208.

Crowther, R. E., Marshall, M., Bond, G. R., & Huxley, P. (2001b). Vocational rehabilitation for people with severe mental illness (Cochrane Review). *The Cochrane Library, 4*. Oxford: Update Software.

Currier, K. F., Chan, F., Berven, N. L., Habeck, R. V., & Taylor, D. W. (2001). Functions and knowledge domains for disability management practice: A delphi study. *Rehabilitation Counseling Bulletin, 44*(3), 133–143.

Department of Work and Pensions and Department of Health. (2008). *Improving health and work: Changing lives*. London: Department of Work and Pensions.

Dewa, C. S., Lin, E., Kooehoorn, M., & Goldner, E. (2007). Association of chronic work stress, psychiatric disorders and chronic physical conditions with disability among workers. *Psychiatric Services, 58*(5), 652–658.

Dewa, C. S., & McDaid, D. (2010). Investing in the mental health of the labour force: Epidemiological and economic impact of mental health disabilities in the workplace. In I. Z. Schultz & E. S. Rogers (Eds.), *Work accommodation and retention in mental health*. New York: Springer.

Fadyl, J. K., & McPherson, K. M. (2009). Approaches to vocational rehabilitation after traumatic brain injury: A review of the evidence. *The Journal of Head Trauma Rehabilitation, 24*(3), 195–212.

Gallie, K. A., Schultz, I. Z., & Winter, A. (2010). Company-level interventions in mental health. In I. Z. Schultz & E. S. Rogers (Eds.), *Work accommodation and retention in mental health*. New York: Springer.

Gates, L. B., & Akabas, S. H. (2010). Inclusion of people with mental health disabilities into the workplace: Accommodation as a social process. In I. Z. Schultz & E. S. Rogers (Eds.), *Work accommodation and retention in mental health*. New York: Springer.

Global business and economic roundtable on addiction and mental health, (2005). Retrieved September 12, 2005, from http://www.mentalhealthroundtable.ca/about_us.html

Gnam, W. H. (2005). The prediction of occupational disability related to depressive and anxiety disorders. In I. Z. Schultz & R. J. Gatchel (Eds.), *Handbook of complex occupational disability claims: Early risk identification, intervention and prevention* (pp. 371–384). New York: Springer.

Goldner, E., Bilsker, D., Gilbert, M., Myette, L., Corbière, M., & Dewa, C. S. (2004). Disability management, return to work and treatment. *Healthcare Papers, 5*(2), 76–90.

Greenberg, P. E., Kessler, R., Birnbaum, H. G., Leong, S. A., Lowe, S. W., Bergland, P. A., et al. (2003). The economic burden of depression in the United States: How did it change between 1990 and 2000? *The Journal of Clinical Psychiatry, 64*(12), 1465–1475.

Habeck, R. V., & Hunt, H. A. (1999). Disability management perspectives. Developing accommodating work environments through disability management. *American rehabilitation, 25*, 18–25.

Haffey, W. J., & Abrams, D. L. (1991). Employment outcomes for participants in a brain injury work re-entry program: Preliminary findings. *The Journal of Head Trauma Rehabilitation, 6*(3), 24–34.

Harder, H., Hawley, J., & Stewart, A. (2010). Disability management approach to job accommodation for mental health disability. In I. Z. Schultz & E. S. Rogers (Eds.), *Work accommodation and retention in mental health*. New York: Springer.

Harnois, G., & Gabriel, P. (2000). *Mental health work: Impact, issues and good practices*. Joint publication of the World Health Organization [WHO] and the International Labour Organization [ILO], (pp. 1–66). Geneva, Switzerland: WHO/ILO.

Haslan, C., Atkinson, S., Brown, S. S., & Haslan, R. A. (2005). Anxiety and depression in the workplace: effects on the individual and organization (a focus group investigation). *Journal of Affective Disorders, 88*, 209–215.

Holzberg, E. (2001). The best practice for gaining and maintaining employment for individuals with traumatic brain injury. *Work, 16*, 245–258.

Johnstone, B., Vessell, R., Bounds, T., Hoskins, S., & Sherman, A. (2003). Predictors of success for state vocational rehabilitation clients with traumatic brain injury. *Archives of Physical Medicine and Rehabilitation, 84*, 161–167.

Kirsh, B., & Gewurtz, R. (2010). Organizational culture and work issues for individuals with mental health disabilities. In I. Z. Schultz & E. S. Rogers (Eds.), *Work accommodation and retention in mental health*. New York: Springer.

Kirsh, B., Stergiou-Kita, M., Gewurtz, R., Dawson, D., Krupa, T., Lysaght, R., et al. (2009). From margins to mainstream: What do we know about work integration for persons with brain injury, mental illness and intellectual disability. *Work, 32*, 391–405.

Krupa, T. (2007). Interventions to improve employment outcomes for workers who experience mental illness. *Canadian Journal of Psychiatry, 52*(6), 339–345.

Krupa, T. (2010a). Approaches to improving employment outcomes for people with serious mental illness. In I. Z. Schultz & E. S. Rogers (Eds.), *Work accommodation and retention in mental health*. New York: Springer.

Krupa, T. (2010b). Employment and serious mental health disabilities. In I. Z. Schultz & E. S. Rogers (Eds.), *Work accommodation and retention in mental health*. New York: Springer.

Krupa, T., Kirsh, B., Cockburn, L., & Gewurtz, R. (2010). Understanding the stigma of mental illness in employment. *Work, 33*, 413–425.

Krupa, T., & Lysaght, R. (2011). *Case studies on information rich, inclusive workplace: How employers, co-workers, unions, employer associations, occupational health professionals and disability organizations can work together to create an environment that supports people with disabilities who have intermittent work capacity*. Ottawa: Human Resources and Skill Development Canada

Lerner, D., Adler, D., Hermann, R. C., Rogers, W. H., Change, H., Thomas, P., et al. (2010). Depression and work performance: The Work and Health Initiative Study. In I. Z. Schultz & E. S. Rogers (Eds.), *Work accommodation and retention in mental health*. New York: Springer.

Lim, K. L., Jacobs, P., Ohinmaa, A., Schopflocher, D., & Dewa, C. S. (2008). A new population-based measure of the economic burden of mental illness in Canada. *Chronic Diseases in Canada, 28*(3), 92–98.

Loisel, P., Durand, M., Berthelette, D., Vézina, N., Baril, R., Gagnon, D., et al. (2001). Disability prevention: New paradigm for the management of occupational back pain. *Disease Management and Health Outcomes, 9*(7), 351–360.

Lysaght, R., Krupa, T., & Gregory, A. (2011). *Employers' perspectives of intermittent work capacity: What can qualitative research tell us?* Ottawa: Human Resources and Skill Development Canada.

MacDonald-Wilson, K. L., Rogers, E. S., & Massaro, J. (2003). Identifying relationships between functional limitations, job accommodations, and demographic characteristics of persons with psychiatric disabilities. *Journal of Vocational Rehabilitation, 18*, 15–24.

MacDonald-Wilson, K. L., Rogers, E. S., Massaro, J., Lyass, A., & Crean, T. (2002). An investigation of reasonable workplace accommodations for people with psychiatric disabilities: Quantitative findings from a multi-site study. *Community Mental Health Journal, 38*(1), 35–50.

MacDonald-Wilson, K. L., Russinova, Z., Rogers, E. S., Lin, C. H., Ferguson, T., Dong, S., et al. (2010). Disclosure of mental health disabilities in the workplace. In I. Z. Schultz & E. S. Rogers (Eds.), *Work accommodation and retention in mental health*. New York: Springer.

Macias, C., DeCarlo, L. T., Wang, Q., Frey, J., & Barreira, P. (2001). Work interest as a predictor of competitive employment: Policy implications for psychiatric rehabilitation. *Administration and Policy in Mental Health, 28*(4), 279–297.

McInnes, M., Orgul, D., McDermott, S., & Mann, J. (2010). Does supported employment work? *Journal of Policy Analysis and Management, 29*, 506–525.

Means, C. D., Stewart, S. L., & Dowler, D. L. (1997). Job accommodations that work: A follow-up study of adults with attention deficit disorder. *Journal of Applied Rehabilitation Counseling, 28*(4), 13–16.

Mental Health Commission of Canada. (2009). *Toward recovery and well-being: A framework for a mental health strategy for Canada*, Retrieved from http://www.mentalhealthcommission.ca/SiteCollectionDocuments/boarddocs/15507_MHCC_EN_final.pdf.

Mental Health Commission of Canada. (2011). *Opening minds program*, Retrieved from http://www.mentalhealthcommission.ca

Mueser, K. T., Becker, D. R., & Wolfe, R. (2001). Supported employment, job preferences, job tenure and satisfaction. *Journal of Mental Health, 10*(4), 411–417.

New Freedom Commission on Mental Health (2003). Achieving the promise: transforming mental health in America. Final report. Rockville, MD. US Department of Health and Human Services, Publication SMA-03-3832

Rogers, E. S., & MacDonald-Wilson, K. L. (2010). Vocational capacity among individuals with mental health disabilities. In I. Z. Schultz & E. S. Rogers (Eds.), *Work accommodation and retention in mental health*. New York: Springer.

Scheid, T. L. (1998). The ADA, mental disability, and employment practices. *The Journal of Behavioral Health Services and Research, 25*(3), 312–325.

Schultz, I. Z. (2008). Disentangling disability quagmire in psychological injury and law. Part II Evolution of disability models: Conceptual, methodological and forensic issues. *Psychological Injury and Law, 1*(2), 103–121.

Schultz, I. Z., Crook, J., Fraser, K., & Joy, P. (2000). Models of diagnosis and rehabilitation in pain-related occupational disability. *Journal of Occupational Rehabilitation, 10*(4), 271–293.

Schultz, I. Z., Duplassie, D., Hanson, D., & Winter, A. (2010). Systemic barriers and facilitators to job accommodations in mental health: Experts' consensus. In I. Z. Schultz & E. S. Rogers (Eds.), *Work accommodation and retention in mental health*. New York: Springer.

Schultz, I. Z., & Gatchel, R. J. (2005). Research and practice directions in risk for disability prediction and early intervention. In I. Z. Schultz & R. J. Gatchel (Eds.), *Handbook of complex occupational disability claims: Early risk identification, intervention and prevention*. New York: Springer.

Schultz, I. Z., Krupa, T., & Rogers, S. E. (2010). Best practices in accommodating and retaining persons with mental health disabilities at work: Answered and unanswered questions. In I. Z. Schultz & E. S. Rogers (Eds.), *Work accommodation and retention in mental health*. New York: Springer.

Schultz, I. Z., Milner, R., Hanson, D., & Winter, A. (2010). Employer attitudes towards accommodations in mental health disability. In I. Z. Schultz & E. S. Rogers (Eds.), *Work accommodation and retention in mental health*. New York: Springer.

Schultz, I. Z., Stowell, A. W., Feuerstein, M., & Gatchel, R. J. (2007). Models of return to work for musculoskeletal disorders. *Journal of Occupational Rehabilitation, 17*, 327–352.

Schultz, I. Z., Winter, A., & Wald, J. (2010). Evidentiary support for best practices in job accommodation in mental health: Macrosystem, employer-level and employee-level interventions. In I. Z. Schultz & E. S. Rogers (Eds.), *Work accommodation and retention in mental health*. New York: Springer.

Scott, J., & Dickey, B. (2003). Global burden of depression: The intersection of culture and medicine. *The British Journal of Psychiatry, 183*, 92–94.

Scully, S. M., Habeck, R. V., & Leahy, M. J. (1999). Knowledge and skill areas associated with disability management practice for rehabilitation counselors. *Rehabilitation Counseling Bulletin, 43*(1), 20–29.

Shain, M. (2009). Psychological safety at work: Emergence of a corporate and social agenda in Canada. *International Journal of Mental Health Promotion, 11*(3), 42–48.

Sherbourne, C. D., Wells, K. B., Duan, N., Miranda, J., Unutzer, J., Jaycox, L., et al. (2001). Long-term effectiveness of disseminating quality improvement for depression in primary care. *Archives of General Psychiatry, 58*, 696–703.

Smith, J. L., Rost, K. M., Nutting, P. A., Libby, A. M., Elliott, C. E., & Pyne, J. M. (2002). Impact of primary care depression intervention on employment and workplace conflict outcomes: Is value added? *The Journal of Mental Health Policy and Economics, 5*, 43–49.

Spataro, S. E. (2005). Diversity in context: How organizational culture shapes reactions to workers with disabilities and others who are demographically different. *Behavioral Science and Law, 23*, 21–38.

Standing Senate Committee on Social Affairs, Science and Technology. (2006, May). *Out of the shadows at last. Transforming mental health, mental illness and addiction services in Canada* (Final Report, pp. 1–484). Ottawa, ON: Government of Canada Printing Office.

Statistics Canada (2003). Canadian Community Health Survey [CCHS] - *Mental health and well-being* (Rep. No. Catalogue no.82-617-XIE).

Stephens, T., & Joubert, N. (2001). The economic burden of mental health problems. *Chronic Diseases in Canada, 22*(1), 18–23.

Stone, D., & Colella, A. (1996). A model of factors affecting the treatment of disabled individuals in organizations. *Academic Management Review, 21*, 352–401.

Stuart, H. (2006). Mental illness and employment discrimination. *Current Opinion in Psychiatry, 19*, 522–526.

Szymanski, E., & Vancollins, J. (2003). Career development of people with disabilities: Some new and not-so-new challenges. *Australian Journal of Career Development, 12*, 9–16.

US Department of Labor Job Accommodation Network. (2007). *Accommodation information by disability*. Morgantown, WV. [JAN is a contracted service funded by the U.S. Government, Department of Labour, Office of Disability Employment Policy under agreement J-9-M-2-0022]. Electronic version retrieved from http://www.jan.wvu.edu/media/atoz.htm

US Equal Employment Opportunity Commission. (2002). *Enforcement guidance: Reasonable accommodation and undue hardship under the Americans with disabilities act*. Retrieved from http://www.eeoc.gov/policy/docs/accommodation.html

Vézina, M., Bourbonnais, R., Brisson, C., & Trudel, L. (2004). Workplace prevention and promotion strategies. *Healthcare Papers, 5*(2), 32–44.

Wang, J. L. (2010). Mental health literacy and stigma associated with depression in the working population. In I. Z. Schultz & E. S. Rogers (Eds.), *Work accommodation and retention in mental health*. New York: Springer.

Warr, P. B. (1987). *Work, unemployment and mental health*. Oxford: Oxford University Press.

Watson Wyatt Worldwide. (2000). *Staying at work 2000/2001—the dollars and sense of effective disability management*. Vancouver: Watson Wyatt Worldwide.

Westmorland, M., & Buys, N. (2002). Disability management in a sample of Australian self-insured companies. *Disability and Rehabilitation, 24*(14), 746–754.

Williams-Whitt, K., & Taras, D. (2010). Disability and the performance Paradox: Can social capital bridge the divide? *Brithish Journal of Industrial Relations, 48*, 534–559.

World Health Organization. (2005). *Mental health action plan for Europe. Facing the challenges, building solutions*. Copenhagen: World Health Organization.

World Health Organization [WHO]. (2001a). *International classification of functioning, disability and health*. Geneva: World Health Organization.

World Health Organization [WHO]. (2001b). *The world health report 2001—Mental health: New understanding, new hope*. Geneva: World Health Organization.

Employee Assistance Programs: Evidence and Current Trends

21

Mark Attridge

Introduction

Many employees suffer from emotional issues, family and home life conflicts, mental health concerns, substance abuse problems, and other health disorders that can interfere with doing their work effectively. The nature of work itself can also sometimes contribute to employee performance problems. In addition, societal changes and community problems (such as natural disasters, violence, economic distress) can influence employee health and behavior. Whether the source is from the individual, the workplace itself or greater society, many employers have turned to employee assistance programs (EAPs) to help respond to these kinds of problems. This chapter addresses the topic of EAPs, and their role in occupational health and wellness. It is organized into three main parts. The first part presents an overview of the EAP. The middle part reviews the research evidence for EAPs. The final part describes major trends in the field of EAP. Global expansion is also examined as a future direction for EAPs.

Overview of EAP

Before examining the evidence for EAPs and the current trends in the field, it is necessary to first understand the nature of EAPs. Thus, this part of the chapter provides an overview of EAP (Attridge, 2009a). It includes a brief history of the field, the primary activities of an EAP, the unique qualities that distinguish an EAP, the contemporary business models and major market types, the promotion and use of EAPs, and the professional standards that guide the industry.

M. Attridge, Ph.D., M.A. (✉)
Attridge Consulting, Inc., 1129 Cedar Lake Road South,
Minneapolis, MN 55405, USA
e-mail: mark@attridgeconsulting.com

Definition of EAP

EAPs are defined as employer- or group-supported programs designed to alleviate employee issues (Employee Assistance Society of North America [EASNA], 2009). Most employees use EAP services on a voluntary basis through self-referrals. Most often, the EAP is used for assistance with mild to moderate problems that cause acute stress (e.g., family/marital relationship issues, work problems, and legal or financial concerns), rather than for the treatment of more serious mental health and substance abuse disorders. The goal of these programs is to have a positive effect on restoring the health and well-being of the employee which, in turn, results in a return to higher productivity and improves overall organizational performance. Modern EAPs are complex programs that often feature interaction with work/life and other behavioral health services to address a host of mental health and, substance abuse issues, as well as workplace performance problems among employees and their family members. EAPs can reach employees through a combination of different channels, including face-to-face visits with counselors, 24/7 telephone calls, Internet resources, and onsite workplace events. Several kinds of operating models are available for EAPs—those that involve staff who work as employees of the same organization where they provide EAP services, programs that rely on external staff who work for a different company (a vendor of EAP services), and a combination of internally staffed services and externally provided resources.

Brief History of EAP

EAP services initially arose out of a need for a stable and skilled workforce during World War II. During the 1940s, companies in the United States figured that it might be more cost-effective to rehabilitate problem drinkers than to have a "revolving door" employment policy of repeatedly hiring and firing impaired workers (Trice & Schonbrunn, 1981). Thus, these early EAPs focused largely on alcohol issues of employees by providing outreach to, identification of, and early intervention for employees struggling with alcohol-related problems. This approach led to the emergence of Occupational Alcoholism Programs. These workplace-based programs grew in acceptance and number throughout the 1950s and 1960s. Since then, the EAP field has grown significantly and now addresses employee health and behavioral health problems, as well as work/life challenges in addition to retaining a specialization of supporting employees with addiction problems. In recognition of this wider scope of services, most EAPs are considered "broad-brush" programs that are designed to support multiple kinds of employee, family and workforce performance issues.

EAP Industry Today

Today, EAP services are benefits offered by tens of thousands of employers and used by millions of employees in North America and across the globe.

EAP in the United States. As the birthplace of the EAP, the United States has the greatest coverage of EAP services. The majority of large employers provide EAP benefits to their employees and often their family members too (Mercer, 2008). According to a national benefits survey of private sector companies conducted in 2008, EAPs are provided by 89% of large employers (500+ staff), 76% of medium employers (100–499 staff) and 52% of small employers (1–99 staff) (Society for Human Resources Management, 2009). As it is a challenge to directly serve smaller employers, collectives representing many small businesses in certain geographic locations, or through trade group associations, can now purchase EAPs.

Table 21.1 Primary services offered by employee assistance programs

1	Services for individuals	Counseling for emotional, mental health, addiction, and other issues with a focus on restoring job-performance; Clinical assessment, referral, and follow-up; and Assistance for legal, financial, and work/life family issues
2	Services for managers and supervisors, union leaders	Management consulting/coaching; Assistance in referring individual employees to the EAP; and Trainings on resolving intergroup conflict, understanding behavioral health issues, and improving interpersonal skills
3	Services for the organization	Violence prevention, Crisis response and trauma management; Work team interventions; Organizational culture of health, and Educational trainings and resources
4	Liaison services to support other programs and services	Integration with other areas to conduct risk screening, cross-referral and case management support for other workplace health and employee support programs, including Work/Life, Wellness, Absence Management, Disease Management, and Disability/Return to Work
5	Administrative services for the sponsor/purchaser	development of EAP policies and procedures, outreach, evaluation, and referral resources development

Source: Adapted from EASNA (2009)

EAP in Canada. Similar to the United States, EAPs have become the primary channel for many Canadian workers to get their first access to mental health care and addiction treatment services. In Canada, these programs are called EFAPs—Employee and Family Assistance Programs—and are particularly popular in unionized environments, and medium to larger size organizations (Csiernik, 2002). A national survey found that EFAPs were present in 68% of Canadian employers with at least 100 employees (Macdonald, Csiernik, Durand, Rylett & Wild, 2006). Although similar in most regards, EFAPs in Canada tend to emphasize services to the organization (see next section) more so than programs in the United States, and to also provide more extensive clinical counseling services to individuals.

EAP in Europe. Survey data from 2007 indicates that approximately 10% of organizations in the UK, Germany, Switzerland, and Denmark have EAP services (Buon & Taylor, 2007). Anecdotal evidences notes that the present day rates of EAP service offerings in this region are now somewhat higher (Athanasiades, 2011). EAP services in Europe are delivered mostly by external EAP providers who offer a broad array of counseling and other services designed to help employees with personal and work problems (Grange, 2005). As with EAPs in North America, an important focus of the EAPs in the UK is maintaining and improving workplace effectiveness and performance.

EAP Services

EAPs differ greatly in the level of workplace support, the degree of program integration, and the range of services provided to the organization, management, union and employees. However, there are five kinds of activities that are performed to varying degrees by all EAPs (see Table 21.1). These primary activities include: (1) Services for individuals; (2) Services for managers and supervisors; (3) Services for the organization; (4) Liaison services to support other programs and services; and (5) Administrative services for the sponsor/purchaser. Arguably, the most essential function of a successful EAP is its ability to provide confidential counseling services, free of charge, when it is needed on a 24/7 basis to employees, management and their family members. A recent survey of EAP professionals in the United States found that this aspect of EAP services was ranked first in its importance to defining "what an EAP should be" (Attridge & Burke, 2011). Similarly, a recent survey of human resources professionals in Europe found that various kinds of individual counseling were the kinds of services they wanted most to be provided by the EA programs at their organizations (Buon & Taylor, 2007).

Having quick and easy access to professionally trained and licensed counselors from an EAP is a very important benefit to organizations, as mental health and substance abuse disorders are among the most common and most costly problems affecting the workplace and yet they are profoundly undertreated. According to national epidemiologic surveys in the United States, about 1 in 4 people each year in the general population have symptoms that meet clinical criteria for having mental and substance use disorders, and yet two-thirds of them do not receive any treatment at all for their condition (Kessler, Chiu, Demler, Merikangas & Walters, 2005; Wang et al., 2005). Similarly high prevalence rates for mental health and addiction disorders and lack of treatment are found throughout the world (World Health Organization, 2011).

To appreciate the "assess and refer" role of EAPs, consider that on a covered population basis, roughly 10% of all employees in the United States have claims each year for use of some form of outpatient or inpatient mental health or substance abuse treatment services (Dentzer, 2009). However, most of these outpatient "treatments" are delivered by primary care doctors and tend to feature a medication only approach. For example, in the United States in year 2007, of the patients who used outpatient mental health care services, 57% received only medications, 32% received both medications and psychotherapy, and only 11% received psychotherapy alone (Olfson & Marcus, 2010). Based upon the thousands of studies supporting the clinical effectiveness of psychotherapy (Lipsey & Wilson, 1993), a superior response would be for more primary care doctors to encourage the use of mental health professionals who can provide effective "talk therapy" types of treatments. And, yet, this is precisely what EAPs do every day, when an EAP counselor makes a referral to outpatient counseling benefits for the 10–25% of clients who have issues serious enough to merit further treatment.

Unique Qualities of EAP: The Core Technology

Although EAPs share some similarities with other providers of mental health and addiction counseling and with consultation to the workplace, the field of EAP is grounded in its own core technology. The EAP Core Technology represents a set of practices that defines the distinguishing properties of delivering employee assistance programming (Roman & Blum, 1985, 1988; Roman, 1990). The key elements of these components are presented in Table 21.2, and described below.

Work Focus. The primary reason for an organization to purchase an EAP service is to improve the at-work performance of their employees. This focus on restoration of work function is important because personal and work problems can impair an individual's ability to carry out their work effectively and efficiently (Grange, 2005). EAP counselors are expert at the identification of employees' behavioral problems, and it includes assessment of job performance issues (tardiness, absence, productivity, work relationships, safety, etc.). Consequently, the EAP service should be judged primarily on the basis of the success of the service to positively influence client improvement in job performance. As seen later in this chapter in the section on outcomes, EAPs often have positive results in the area of improving employee work performance.

Manager Training. For the EAP to be successful, the program must be understood by key employees at the organization. Given the important role of supervisors and managers in noticing problems

Table 21.2 Components of EAP original core technology

1	The identification of employees' behavioral problems includes assessment of job performance issues (tardiness, absence, productivity, work relationships, safety, etc.)
2	The evaluation of employee's success with use of EAP service is judged primarily on the basis of improvement in job performance issues
3	Provision of expert consultation to supervisors, managers, and union stewards on how to use EAP policy and procedures for both employee problems and for management issues
4	Availability and appropriate use of constructive confrontation techniques by EAP for employees with alcohol or substance abuse problems to encourage treatment
5	The creation and maintenance of micro-linkages with counseling, treatment, and other community resources (for successful referral of EAP cases)
6	The creation and maintenance of macro-linkages between the work organization and counseling, treatment, and other community resources (for appropriate role and use of EAP)
7	EAP has a focus on employees' alcohol and other substance abuse problems

Source: Adapted from Roman and Blum (1985, 1988) and Roman (1990)

among their staff and making an informal or formal (for cause) referral to the EAP counselor for assistance, another core technology component is the provision of expert consultation to supervisors, managers and union stewards on how to use EAP policy and procedures for both employee problems and for management issues.

Linkages and Referral. The EAP should know the range of resources available to assist employees from within the company (called micro-linkages) and also from the surrounding local communities as well (called macro linkages). The EAP should be able to offer direction to troubled employees for what to learn about, where to go and what to do in order to improve their situation. Offering this kind of information that is tailored to the individual's problem and local environment is empowering and spurs the feelings of confidence and self-efficacy that is needed to effectively respond to the situation and to make behavioral lifestyle changes. Most EAPs use a thorough initial assessment process, and maintain a database of current and accurate resources appropriate for referral to fulfill this core component.

Alcohol and Drug Abuse. Harking back to its early roots, EAPs have always had a substance abuse and addiction focus. The workplace offers a useful context for the identification and referral for individuals with drinking and drug abuse problems (Roman & Blum, 2002). Most EAPs provide confidential services to management and workers with substance abuse and misuse problems. A 2003 survey of over 800 professionals in the EAP field (Attridge, 2003a) found that 89% of EA programs offered alcohol or drug screenings. Another finding from this survey was that 92% of the alcohol and drug cases identified were employees of the organizations they supported, compared to only 8% who were nonemployees. Of these employees with alcohol or drug issues, about two-thirds were self-referrals, with the remaining one-third referred to the EAP by their supervisors due to performance or safety problems.

While almost all EAPs offer alcohol and drug screenings and referral, the higher-quality EAPs also have staff specifically trained and certified in providing clinical assessments and case management for people with substance abuse problems (Malain, 2010). For example, in the 2003 survey, about half of EAPs (54%) offered EAP Substance Abuse Professional (SAP) services. As a result of the expertise of the SAP specialists (over half in the study had 15 years or more experience), and the required use of long-term follow-up services, the vast majority of clients (89%) working with SAP specialists from EAPs went on to complete substance abuse treatment. Although used infrequently today, the appropriate use of constructive confrontation techniques by EAP counselors can lead some employees to get past their denial and agree to enter treatment for their alcohol or substance abuse problems.

Contemporary EAP Business Models and Markets

While the types of services offered through the EAP may vary in breadth from organization to organization, they are typically delivered through one of three basic staffing models. The *internal model* is defined by EAP staff who are employees of the organization. The *external model* is when the sponsoring company or organization has entered into a contract for EAP services with an outside vendor. The *blended or hybrid model* shares elements of both of the other models, and it usually has a full-time EAP staff resident at the host organization, and also has external contract personnel involved in the delivery of EAP services (such as a network of affiliate counselors, specialist for crisis event support, and so on). These EAPs operate in a range of market contexts that reflect these different delivery models. Seven markets for EAP business have been identified based on model, organizational context and size (Amaral, 2010). These market types include internal programs for private sector organizations, internal programs for public sector organizations, internal programs for universities and colleges, internal programs for unions and other member-based groups, external programs serving national and/or international markets, external programs serving specific regions or smaller markets, and hybrid programs resident in one organization but also selling EA services to other local organizations (these are often in hospital or health care systems). According to a recent industry report (Open Minds, 2011), significant consolidation exists at the provider level in the United States, with three-fourths of the total market for external EAP services being controlled by only 10 firms.

EAP Promotion and Use

According to industry norms, the number of employee and family members who use EAP counseling services in a year for clinical support represents about 3–5% of the total number of all covered employees (Amaral, 2008; EASNA, 2009). When one also includes use of the nonclinical kinds of services, then the overall EAP usage rate is higher (often doubled). However, this metric depends on how the EAP counts the many services they provide—such as clinical counseling services, management consultations, organizational services, crisis support services, information and referral assistance, education/training, and other services it provides. Even so, this level of EAP service utilization is relatively small when compared against the 100% of an employee population (and their family members) that has access to potentially using the service. However, a more realistic usage target may be the segment of the working population each year who have some form of mental health and/or addiction problem that interferes with their ability to function properly at work or home. A recent national survey in Canada found that 12% of employees met this definition as having a mental health issue in the past year (Thorpe & Chenier, 2011)

In practice, EAP utilization varies widely from company to company. It is determined largely by how it is set up and promoted. At the high end is the full-service traditional EAP that is staffed with a core group of EAP professionals (likely with Certified Employee Assistance Professional (CEAP) status) who are employees within the organization it serves. These kinds of programs tend to have the highest levels of use (in the range of 10–20% rate) due to their high visibility and the ability of EAP personnel to interact frequently on-site with management at the organization to collaborate on workplace health and risk issues. At the other extreme is the external EAP that is given away as a "perk" when the organization purchases a comprehensive health or risk insurance benefit package (the EAP fees are rolled into the total cost and hidden from the purchaser). These so-called free EAP programs are typically under-promoted (if at all) and consequently have very little usage (less than 1%). But this low level of use can be acceptable to the organization when the business goal is limited to providing risk-management coverage by having crisis incident support services on call if needed and to at least "offer" its employees access to a counselor (Burke & Sharar, 2009). In this regard, the phrase "you get what you pay for" certainly applies to EAP services.

Research has shown higher levels of EAP use when company policy specifically features the EAP (Weiss, 2003). Indeed, part of an effective implementation process for the EAP involves formalizing the availability and role of the EAP by including it in the written HR practices and policies for the organization and then including it in regular promotional communications to the employees at work and at home (Csiernik, 2003b). Regular and ongoing promotion of the EAP within the organization is also important because some users of services come to the EAP as referrals given by others in the organization, such as supervisors, union stewards, human resources staff, safety officers, medical personnel, disability case managers, and staff in other areas. Despite frequent communication and promotion for the EAP, stigma and discrimination against people with mental health and addiction problems can dampen EAP use, even though it is convenient and available at no cost. The result is that many employees who could potentially benefit from using the EAP do not because of their fears of discrimination or shame from others where they work (Mood Disorders Society of Canada, 2009). EAPs have attempted to counter this stigmatization issue through offering services at private clinic office locations away from the worksite, over the telephone and online via the Internet (Butterworth, 2001). Some EAPs have also folded the entry point into the program under the umbrella of larger and less stigmatized workplace services, such as Work/Life programs or corporate health and wellness departments. The *EY Assist* program at global financial services firm Ernst & Young is an example of this approach (Turner, Weiner & Keegan, 2005). When they combined the EAP, Work/Life and HR/benefits Web sites into one central function, the result was a higher use rate of 25% annually for the combined new program, compared to the 8% for the EAP separately, and 12% for the Work/Life program separately as stand-alone programs the year before.

EAP Professional Standards

The EAP industry offers voluntary certification of individual professionals and accreditation of provider companies. The Employee Assistance Professional Association (EAPA) is the largest professional organization for EAPs, with over 6,000 members worldwide. It offers the (CEAP) designation. The CEAP is a voluntary credential that identifies individuals as EAP professionals who have met established standards for practice (EAPA, 2010), and who adhere to the code of ethics (EAPA, 2009). Over 5,000 individuals have earned the CEAP designation (EAPA, 2006). It should also be noted that the accreditation process for EA programs was designed to ensure that providers meet specific minimum standards for quality practice and that clinical staff possesses the required qualifications and experience needed in order to provide high quality service (Maiden, 2003). In partnership with the Council on Accreditation (COA), the Employee Assistance Society of North America first created the accreditation standards in 2001 (Stockert, 2004). The accreditation process provided by the COA includes a comprehensive self-study program followed by an on-site review conducted by trained and experienced EAP peer reviewers. The COA accreditation standards are now in their eighth edition, and include 12 primary components with over 50 sub-areas. To date, there are 57 EAP programs that have been accredited by COA (Attridge, Tannenbaum, Wolinsky, Slater & Goehner, 2009). Note that this number represents only a small fraction of the more than 1,000 external providers who sell EA services in Canada and the United States (Amaral, 2010). Finally, those interested in learning more about EAPs are encouraged to get the recently published guide to EAP, called *Selecting and Strengthening Employee Assistance Programs: A Purchaser's Guide* (EASNA, 2009). This 62-page document is available at no cost as a download from the Web site of the Employee Assistance Society of North America. Also, this guide and other related resources for employers are reviewed in a journal article (Attridge, 2010d).

EAP Evidence

This part of the chapter examines the state of the empirical evidence for EAP services. More specifically, it discusses the applied nature of EAP research, the historical themes of research in the field over the last 25 years, typical research findings for EAP clinical effectiveness, client satisfaction and outcomes, the cost-benefit of EAP services and some calculation issues in determining return on investment or ROI based on workplace outcomes.

Nature of EAP Evidence

The EAP field is grounded in a body of empirical and clinical evidence generated from hundreds of studies of individual, group and organizational-level EAP services. There are several research-based books and texts specifically on EAP services (e.g., Attridge, Herlihy & Maiden, 2005; Masi, 1984; Oher, 1999; Richard, Emener & Hutchison, 2009; Shain & Groeneveld, 1980; Sonnenstuhl & Trice, 1990; Wrich, 1980) and one scholarly journal dedicated to the field of EAP (*Employee Assistance Quarterly*; which changed its name in 2005 to the *Journal of Workplace Behavioral Health: Employee Assistance Practice and Research*). Over the past 25 years, over 500 peer-review articles on EAP have appeared in this journal alone, with the collected works from special issues also published separately as 13 edited books. In addition to this scholarly influence, as an applied industry, technical knowledge about EAP has been developed and shared over the years through participation at regular professional meetings and articles in several trade industry publications. EAPA hosts an annual conference (often drawing over 1,000 attendees) and publishes the *Journal of Employee Assistance*. EASNA also holds an annual institute and its' members receive the *Journal of Workplace Behavioral Health*.

The applied nature of the service delivery context for EAP being enacted within complex and changing organizations, however, has limited the rigor of research in this area (Attridge, 2001a). The result is that the vast majority of EAP studies have been conducted with nonexperimental research designs (Arthur, 2000; Attridge, 2001b; Csiernik, 1995, 2005a). More typical of EA research are studies that use a single-group design based on within-person changes over-time on clinical and work performance indicators, assessed by counselors and other similar outcomes assessed at follow-up from self-report surveys of clients. The quality level of research has waned, though, since major government funding for alcohol-related programs involving EAPs dried up after the heyday years of the 1980s. A chronic lack of funding to support more sophisticated research has led to debates within the field about whether it should be regarded as a true profession (based on open sharing of evidence and research) or an industry driven by commercial interests (Masi, 2011; Roman, 2007). Of course, to be fair, the field of EAP has elements of both of these identities.

Historical Themes of EAP Research

A recent 25-year retrospective analysis was prepared that discerned the most prevalent themes among the 545 articles published during this span in the *Employee Assistance Quarterly/Journal of Workplace Behavioral Health* (Maiden, Kurzman, Amaral, Stephenson & Attridge, 2010). The "Top 10" topics, in order by frequency, are provided in Table 21.3. The range of themes is representative of the major issues of how EAPs are established, operated and evaluated. The most common clinical issues during this period included alcohol abuse, drug abuse, psychological/emotional problems, critical incidents/trauma and relationship issues. The global growth of the field is also noted. The topic area of health

Table 21.3 Top 10 themes in 25 years of EAP research

Rank	Topic area
1	Alcohol Problems (330) & Alcohol Abuse Treatment (193)
2	EAP Models and Design (189) & Professional Roles and Dilemmas (97)
3	Drug Problems (160) & Drug Abuse Treatment (96)
4	EAP Effectiveness and Outcomes (129) & EAP Evaluation Design and Methods (102)
5	Psychological & Emotional Problems (171)
6	International Programs (127)
7	Health Promotion Program Design (123) & Health Care Benefits Costs (105)
8	Supervisory Referrals (120)
9	Critical Incident Stress Debriefing (CISD), Trauma Response, and Posttraumatic Stress Disorder (PTSD) (112)
10	Family/Marital/Relationship Issues (102)

Source: Adapted from Maiden et al. (2010)
Note: Inside the parentheses indicate the number of specific articles for that topic area that appeared in 25 years of *Employee Assistance Quarterly/The Journal of Workplace Behavioral Health: Employee Assistance Practice and Research*

promotion and health benefits—the one most closely related to the larger theme of this Handbook on occupational health and wellness—is also among the top areas of concern for the field.

EAP Clinical Effectiveness

The evidence shows that EAPs are often effective in improving the personal and clinical issues that prompted using the service. A review of over 30 workplace counseling research studies found varying levels of methodological rigor among the investigations, but came to the conclusion that there was consistent evidence for the effectiveness of EAP clinical counseling services (McLeod & McLeod, 2001). Improvements due to individual level EAP interventions have been measured from counselor assessments conducted at "case open" and "case close" points in time for each client user of the service, and also through self-report surveys of clients after their use of the EAP (Csiernik, 2003a; Csiernik, Hannah & Pender, 2007; Dersch, Shumway, Harris & Arredonondo, 2002; Harris, Adams, Hill, Morgan & Soliz, 2002; Philips, 2004). For example, results from a follow-up survey of 1,050 clients of an external model telephonic-based EAP service found that 75% of users reported reduced stress, and 73% reported improved health and well-being (Attridge, 2001c).

Basic clinical indicators of mental health and well-being, such as the *Global Assessment of Functioning* (GAF; Jacobson, Jones & Bowers, 2011), are also commonly used in evaluating EAP clinical services. For example, a study by the largest internal EAP in the world (Federal Occupational Health), with data from over 59,000 employees of the US government, found that GAF scores improved over 10% on average from "case open" to "case close" (Selvik & Stephenson, 2003). Other measures of patient functioning have been incorporated with similar success into counselor-based assessments and follow-up surveys (Greenwood, DeWeese & Inscoe, 2005; Harris et al., 2002).

EAP Outcomes

Research on the experience of individual users of EAP services has consistently found high levels client satisfaction (Attridge, 2003b; Csiernik, 2003b; Csiernik et al., 2007; Dersch et al., 2002; Harris et al., 2002; McLeod, 2010; Philips, 2004). Satisfaction levels are routinely at the 95% level or higher for the percentage of users being satisfied overall with the EAP services (Sealy, 2011; Selvik & Bingaman, 1998; Siddell, 2007). As EAPs serve organizations, it is no surprise that the literature also shows that they have a positive impact on a variety of organizational level outcomes. Numerous studies have found positive effects for crisis incident response services (Attridge & VandePol, 2010), consultation to managers for workgroup problems (Bidgood, Boudewyn & Fasbinder, 2005), support for workplace changes like mergers and lay-offs (Ginzberg, Kilburg & Gomes, 1999), and more synergistic support of other employee health programs through integration of services (Csiernik, 2005b). EAPs also routinely show positive outcomes for employers in areas of job performance, such as reductions in absence days and improvements in work productivity. In his recent review of the literature in this area, McLeod concluded that EAP "counselling has a consistent and significant impact on important dimensions of work behaviour" (2010, p. 245). Given the primacy of this outcome area as the most common value generated from EA services, three examples of workplace improvement for individual clients of EAP are presented below:

Workplace Outcome Study 1—Workplace performance outcome data were collected from over 26,000 cases during a 9 year period from a large external EAP. The results revealed that the average rating on a 1–10 scale of the level of work productivity had rebounded significantly from 4.8 at before use of the EAP to 8.3 after use of the EAP (Attridge, Otis & Rosenberg, 2002). The after EAP use rating of 8.3 is just under to the normative productivity level rating of 8.9 on the same scale that was obtained in a nationally representative sample of employees in the United States who had *not* used an EAP (Attridge, 2004). This study also found that almost half of the cases (48%) reported that they had been able to avoid taking time off from work because of their use of the EAP. The duration of this effect was an average of 1.8 days of absenteeism avoided per case.

Workplace Outcome Study 2—The EAP for the US government collected counselor-assessed ratings of employee productivity and absence over a several year period on over 59,000 EAP clinical cases (Selvik, Stephenson, Plaza & Sugden, 2004). The results showed that the percentage of employees using the EAP that had difficulty performing their work due to mental health factors was reduced from 30% of all cases to just 8%. There was also a significant reduction in work absenteeism days and tardiness, with absenteeism changing from an average among all EAP cases from 2.4 days to 0.9 days, respectively, for the 30 days before use of the EAP, compared to the 30 days after EAP use concluded.

Workplace Outcome Study 3—Another study featured the analysis of before and after data obtained from over 3,500 employee users of a national external EAP in the United States (Baker, 2007). Among the approximately 40% of cases who had work performance problems before the use of the EAP, the average number of days with impaired work productivity was reduced from 8.0 before use to 3.4 after EAP use. This study also found that, 25% of all EAP cases reported missing at least a half day or more of work before their use of the EAP. Among this group, the average level of work absenteeism was reduced from 7.2 days to 4.8 days, respectively, for the 30 days before EAP use versus the 30 days after EAP use concluded.

The effects obtained in these three large-scale research studies, when averaged together, indicate that for employee users of EAP counseling services: (1) the number of days being absent from work in the past month improved by 1.00 day; and (2) there was a 22% improvement in their work productivity over the past month.

EAP Cost-Benefit

As with other areas of occupational health and wellness, it is important to be able to show the value of providing services beyond just user satisfaction and clinical outcomes (Attridge, 2008a). Over the past 20 years, several dozen studies have demonstrated the financial cost-benefit of EAPs (see reviews by Attridge, 2010b; Attridge & Amaral, 2002; Blum & Roman, 1995; Christie & Harlow, 2007). These studies have examined savings from a range of outcomes, including health care claims costs, disability claims costs, avoided employee turnover, and workplace performance costs due to lost productivity and days at work. The common finding is that use of EAPs by employees with more severe clinical issues have contributed to long-term net reductions in overall health care costs for individual employees and their families that far exceed the cost of the EAP services, even when including the short-term increases in the costs of providing appropriate professional treatment for alcohol/drug and mental health disorders. Several of the best examples of this research are the cost-benefit studies of the internal EAPs at Abbott Laboratories (Dainas & Marks, 2000), Chevron (Collins, 1998) and Southern California Edison (Conlin, Amaral & Harlow, 1996). The landmark cost-benefit study of the EAP at the McDonnell Douglas Corporation (Smith & Mahoney, 1990; see critique by Attridge, 2010a) was replicated a year later at the company's helicopter division. Again, the analysis of objective company data revealed net cost savings from several areas over a multiyear period for the employees with alcohol/substance abuse and psychiatric problems who experienced EAP-directed behavioral health case management services, compared to other cases without EAP support (Alexander & Alexander Consulting Group, 1990). A key mechanism behind the positive results in these studies is that the EAPs were effective at helping employees with substance abuse issues to navigate successfully through the many treatment options available, and with providing follow-up support and case-management assistance after treatment to reduce relapse issues and improve return-to-work efforts (Attridge, 2010b). Indeed, sometimes the "leverage" that comes from the EAP counselor being affiliated with the employer or union can help an employee with substance abuse troubles to finally get into treatment in order to keep his job or union member status (Attridge & Bennett, 2011).

With regard to calculating a specific dollar figure from a cost-benefit analysis, researchers have documented Return-on-Investment (ROI) estimates of $3 or more (up to $10) return for every $1 dollar invested in the EAP (Blaze-Temple & Howat, 1997; Dainas & Marks, 2000; Hargrave & Hiatt, 2005; Hargrave, Hiatt, Alexander & Shaffer, 2008; Jorgensen, 2007; McClellan, 1990; Yamatani, Santangelo, Maue & Heath, 1999). It is important to note that the source of the cost-benefit examined in the these studies is limited to the small subset of the total EAP counselor caseload that has more serious addiction or mental health issues and that the cost savings are only realized over a multiyear period of time. In contrast, the financial benefits from improved work performance (i.e., reduced presenteeism and absenteeism) are present in many more EAP cases (both mild and more severe) than are cost-savings from health care claims or disability claim cases and they are evident soon after EAP use (Attridge, 2010c). Because of these factors, workplace-based cost savings from EAP usually comprise the largest part of the total dollar return to the employer when it has been included in ROI analyses with several other sources of cost savings (Goetzel, 2007; Goetzel & Ozminkowski, 2006).

ROI Calculation Example for EAP Workplace Outcomes

Even though it is a common and consistently positive outcome, some EAPs are hesitant to present an ROI to their customer organizations that includes workplace outcomes. Perhaps this reluctance is due to concerns of how to best convert the workplace outcomes into financial metrics that employers will believe (Gallagher & Morgan, 2002). However, consulting experience in this area shows that this "dollarzing" problem can be overcome (Attridge, 2002, 2007, 2008b; Fuller, Attridge & Doherty, 2001). The following math example illustrates the steps involved in this kind of ROI calculation.

Hourly Compensation Rate. To start, one needs to asign a dollar amount to an hour of work. Let's assume a company has an average hourly wage of $20 paid to the employee directly (i.e., what is paid in their paycheck). Using the hourly paid wage rate is adequate, but incomplete in most circumstances that involve other company-sponsored benefits as part of the total compensation to employees. For full-time employees, the dollar value of company-paid benefits is thus added to the hourly wage rate to yield the full compensation rate. For example, it is customary to add 25% of the paid wage rate as an estimate of the additional compensation value of benefits (i.e., health, disability, retirement) paid by the employer on behalf of the employee ($20 wage rate X 25%=$5 benefit load value; so $20 wage+$5 benefit load=$25 total compensation rate). One could further adjust this rate for the mix of employees with and without benefits.

Assigning Dollar Value to Work Absence Outcome. What is a day of work worth in dollars? Some analysts treat absence days as worth only the sum of the hourly compensation rate applied to a typical day of work (Trogdon, Finkelstein, Reyes & Deitz, 2009). But this ignores the value of the lost productivity when the employee is not at work. Intsead, what more advanced researchers do is to add in the financial estimate of the dollar value of work productivity (see below) as part of the dollar value of an absence (Goetzel et al., 2004). While this approach creates a much larger dollar value, it is actually more realistic from a business perspective. Why have a worker at all if all he returns in financial value back to the business is a dollar amount that is equal to his level of compensation? This break-even logic is not used by the business to justify hiring a new worker; therefore, it should not be used in a ROI analysis.

Assigning Dollar Value to Work Productivity Outcome. What is an hour of productive work worth in dollars? Although this qustion can be answered in many ways, one simple approach has been to apply what is called a "Revenue Capacity Factor" (RCF) as a mathematical mutliplier to the rate of employee compensation to reflect the capacity that an employee has to generate revenue or financial benefit (broadly considered) to the organization from their work. The RFC for each employee varies due to many factors, such as job grade and role within the organization, as more senior and more skilled employeyss are worth more (as this is usually reflected in their having higher compensation relative to other less tenured or less skilled staff). A conserative default RCF is 2.0. Thus, assuming a $25 per hour compensation rate X 2.0 RCF=$50 productivity value per hour for an employee working at normal productivity. For an employee who is at work but only working at 50% of his normal level of productivity (called presenteeism), this is a dollarized loss of $25 per hour ($50 per hour compensation X 50%). Applying this to the dollar value of work absence, missing one full day of work (at an 8 h work shift) is a productivity loss to the employer of $400 (8 h X $50 per hour as all of the productivity is lost). The loss of the compensation is then added to this lost productivity total as well (assuming the employee has a certain number of paid days off from work per year).

EAP Outcome Return. The estimated financial value of work productivity and work absence can now be applied to the outcomes data from the EAP. The financial value of the avoided further work productivity loss from EAP is $1,750 per case. This is based on 20 work days of 8 h per day in a month for a full-time employee (160 h) at 22% improvement per hour in productivity. This results in 35 h of productivity return at $50 value per hour. The financial value of avoided further work absence is $600 per case. This is based on a combination of two parts: Part 1=8 h for one day of avoided absence X paid compensation, which is 8 h X $25 per hour=$200; and Part 2=the lost productivity that was due to missing work altogether and having zero productivity=8 h of full productivity loss X $50 value of productivity per hour=$400; combined these two parts are worth $600.

EAP Outcome ROI. These two savings metrics are used to calculate the summary ROI figure, using the math below:
- Workplace Return per EAP clinical case = $1,750 productivity + $600 absence = $2,350
- Workplace Return Total = $2,350 per case X number of total clinical cases
- Assume annual clinical case use rate = 4% of covered employees
- Assume covered employee base of 1,000 lives
- EAP clinical case count = 4% X 1,000 = 40 cases at EAP relevant to outcomes
- Total Return = $2,350 per case X 40 cases = $94,000
- EAP fee = $30 per employee per year (PEPY)
- Total Investment in EAP = $30 X 1,000 employees = $30,000
- ROI = $94,000 Return/$25,000 Investment
- ROI = $3.1:$1

Thus, for every $1.00 invested in the EAP, the return is $3.13 dollars. In practice, this figure can be adjusted, if needed, depending on if employees have paid time off from work or not (or if one contends that lost productivity during work absence is made up again in the future through extra unpaid overtime work), what is the appropriate RCF rate, what is the most relevant period of outcome effect duration (only 1 month in this example), and so forth. But regardless of how it is adjusted, considering that this ROI figure of $3.1:$1 is derived *only* from the financial value of two kinds of workplace outcomes, it is undervaluing the true ROI from the totality of all of the services provided by the EAP. For example, it would be higher if the dollar value of EAP outcomes representing other areas of return, such as from health care cost savings, disability claims savings, avoided employee turnover cases, and so forth—were added to the full ROI analysis model.

EAP Trends

This part of the chapter examines various trends in the field of EAP. Current initiatives are occurring for EAPs and alcohol issues, disability cases, work/life, wellness and prevention, employee engagement, and technology. Also presented are the findings of a new research study of EAP Trends from the perspectives of professionals in the field.

Trend 1: EAP and Alcohol Issues

The last several years have seen renewed interest in the early core technology EAP focus on alcohol and addictions (Attridge & Wallace, 2009). EAPs are being asked to do more in the area of early identification and encouraging access into professional treatment. The Screening, Brief Intervention and Referral to Treatment (SBIRT) approach is being used by many EAPs to identify and manage risky and hazardous alcohol use and dependence within the workplace (McPherson et al., 2009). EAPs are also providing training to other staff at partner programs (such as wellness and work/life) on how to use scientifically validated brief screening tools that can help identify mental health and substance abuse problems among clients of their programs (Bray et al., 2009; Goplerud & McPherson, 2011). These screening tools can be added to population health risk assessments, to intake processes in other health management or coaching programs, and at primary care settings. A driver of this trend for SBIRT activity by EAPs is that most experts now consider addiction to be a chronic, relapsing brain disease with a complex etiology and clinical course (Gearhardt et al., 2011; Saitz, Larson, Labelle, Richardson & Samet, 2008). This view of addiction demands a more sophisticated approach to treatment. Most addiction treatment providers offer patients with mild or moderate severity symptoms brief and episodic care, with little or no long-term follow-up (McLellan & Meyers, 2004). In contrast, chronic disease management care approaches—such as the Physician Health Plan addiction care programs in Canada (Brewster, Kaufmann, Hutchison & MacWilliam, 2008) and the United States (McLellan, Skipper, Campbell & DuPont, 2008)—have more than doubled the typical success rates of the best episodic addiction service programs. PHP has seen success rates for abstinence from alcohol and drug use as high as 85% of all program participants over 5 years. These PHP programs use a holistic model that includes qualified service providers, a progression from more intensive to less intensive care settings, case management, family centered care, and long-term monitoring to manage relapse. The success of this approach indicates that it is possible to improve outcomes in addiction treatment by adopting elements of the chronic care approach and strengthening linkages across the continuum of care (Norlien Foundation, 2011).

Trend 2: EAP and Disability

Another trend is for more EAP support of employees on disability leave for mental health and addiction disorders (Attridge & Wallace, 2010, 2011). Mental health disability affects between 1 and 2% of working adults each year, and is the fastest growing health-related disability in the United States and Canada over the past 20 years (Sroujian, 2003; Williams, 2006). The past decade has seen a dramatic rise in the costs of disability-related claims (Carruthers, 2010). Once an employee has a disability, employers and unions are required to make every reasonable effort, short of undue hardship to the company, to accommodate these workers. Implementing a Return-to-Work (RTW) program meets the employer's legal duty to accommodate. The goal of RTW is to facilitate the return of disabled workers to safe, meaningful, and productive work. These programs are based on the philosophy that people can safely perform progressively more demanding levels of work while also participating in the process of recovery and getting medical and/or mental health care for their problem. These programs must be collaborative and sensitive to the particular challenges in preparing the employee to return to work after treatment for addictions in order to avoid a relapse (Pomaki et al., 2010).

An ally for disability case managers can be the EAP (Brunnelle & Lui, 2003). For the employee who is on disability leave, the EAP can provide RTW support services, such as preparing the supervisor and employee for reentry into the workplace. EAPs can also assist with psychological job analysis and provide supervisory consultation and educational services on an ongoing basis to assist those at the work site while the employee is away on leave. Due to the frequent comorbidity of mental disorders with other medical conditions, some employers now mandate a psychological clinical assessment as part of the requirement of anyone applying for disability benefits—not just those with mental disorder as the primary cause (The Hartford Group, 2007). The EAP may be able to perform these assessments or assist with making referrals to others who can provide it. Thus, the EAP can provide a valuable role in coordinating such care and supporting the employee and their family through this transitional period.

Trend 3: EAP and Work/Life

Collaboration with other benefits programs has been a growth area for EAPs in the past decade. Many EAPs now partner with a wide range of other workplace-based programs and benefits. The number of EAPs with "integration activity" increased from about 1 in 4 in 1994, to over 1 in 3 in 2002, and it is now present at the majority of all EAPs (Herlihy & Attridge, 2005). The most common integration partner has been with work/life programs and services. Work/Life programs include a wide range of services (Gornick, 2002). Typically, these services include: workplace flexibility policies; paid and unpaid time off; childcare; eldercare; financial education and support; and community involvement (Lingle, 2004). Work/Life services focus on normal life experiences, such as finding appropriate care for aging parents and attempts to prevent more serious problems developing due to personal or work stressors an individual may be facing. Often, the focus of these services is saving the employee time by carrying out time-consuming research rather than tackling problems that the employee could not manage as effectively own her own. Part of the reason for this growth in integrated programming is a natural development response to the rise in the popularity of work/life programs and the benefits to the organization from greater collaboration between EAP and work/life (Attridge et al., 2005; Csiernik, 2005a). The EAP and work/life fields often share similar goals of supporting employees and working families, while also supporting the needs of the employer and the broader workplace (Jacobson & Attridge, 2010). Both fields have a work focus and embrace the notion that one's work life and personal life influence each other. Both fields also typically report to HR or another department within the work organization, with services being managed internally but having most of their client-contact services provided by a network of external contractors. In many companies, EAPs and work/life services are provided by the same program or sold under the same contract; however, they may actually be business arrangements in which one program partners with another program to meet the needs of an organization. The 2011 *Open Minds Industry Report* noted a large increase since 2002 in these kinds of integrated models, with EAPs now being routinely bundled with providers of work/life services as a "one-stop shop" program for employer purchasers.

Trend 4: EAP and Wellness/Prevention

Although EAP and work/life are already closely aligned, EAP's also have a growing role in supporting wellness and health prevention programs (Goetzel & Ozminkowski, 2006). According to (Mulvihill, 2003), the core practices of these programs include the following: (1) strategic planning to prevent disease, decrease health risks, and contain rising health care costs, (2) conducting health screenings and risk stratification, (3) providing risk-related health management interventions (exercise, behavior change programs, health coaching, educational materials, nurse advice lines, and disease management), and (4) ongoing evaluation and metrics. Wellness programs reach employees and their family members through many different channels, including office visits, phone calls, Internet resources, and onsite workplace events (such as wellness fairs and health risk screenings). Many EAPs now support employee in making lifestyle behavioral changes after learning the results of health risk appraisal (HRA) screenings (Birkland & Birkland, 2005). Employees struggling to change chronic behaviors related to weight loss, diet and nutrition, and smoking cessation particularly value this kind of encouragement and practical advice. EAPs also are playing an increasing role in identifying and treating chronic behavioral health conditions (such as depression and anxiety) that negatively affect productivity and quality of life (Caggianelli & Carruthers, 2007).

A recent survey of 200 professionals in the EAP field provides evidence of the role of EAP in supporting prevention and wellness (Bennett & Attridge, 2008). The study assessed the percentage of respondents that provided eight different types of "prevention services" at their EAP at least on a quarterly basis. The results revealed that the most frequently offered prevention services were alcohol screening/training (41%) or drug screening/training (40%). Other findings were that about 1 in 4 EAPs regularly conducted screening and training for depression (25%), for workplace violence/bullying (23%), and for other health management issues (such as anxiety; 17%). EAPs also conducted prevention-oriented trainings on fostering better relationships among work teams (32%), and at home in the area of personal/marital relationships (15%). In contrast, few EAPs conducted cardiovascular screening/training (9%). Thus, in this study, roughly a third of EAPs delivered prevention services on mental health, substance abuse, and workplace behavioral risk issues.

Trend 5: EAP and Employee Engagement

EAPs can also get involved with company-wide efforts to improve the overall health of the organization by increasing employee engagement (Pugh & Dietz, 2008; Seidl, 2007). *Work engagement* is a term used to describe the extent to which employees are involved with, committed to, enthusiastic and passionate about their work (Macey & Schneider, 2008). Many organizations now engage in company-wide measurement of employee engagement levels and related constructs (Attridge, 2009b). The results of these measurement programs can then be used to improve HR practices and employee benefit services and other training programs, all of which are activities that EAPs can help to coordinate and implement as changes at the organizational level (Hyde, 2008). EAPs could add specific items on engagement to their intake and follow-up clinical assessment processes to measure changes in employee engagement for individual users of the EAP. The finding that strength-based styles of management and supervisory communication can improve employee engagement is good for the EAPs that have staff experienced at providing training in this area of positive psychology (Taranowski, 2009). Thus, the engagement movement has created a greater potential role for EAP to better serve their employer clients through offering assistance in measurement and training areas that support improved engagement at both the individual and the organizational levels.

Trend 6: EAP and Technology

There is an increasing use of new technological modalities to assist employees to better manage their health and to get access to related services. Web sites for EAPs are becoming more elaborate and now typically offer access to lists of counselors and other care providers, tip sheets, educational webinars, and a wide range of self-assessment tools (Richard, 2009). The use of Internet-based tools for the delivery of clinical services is less common, but is advancing as a new practice model (Klion, 2011). The early adopters of online clinical services have been more prevalent among Canadian EFAPs (Parnass et al., 2008; Wittes & Speyer, 2009) than among EAPs in the United States. In general, the technology for providing online therapeutic services for mental health and addiction treatment is widely available. This kind of clinical care is called a variety of names, including online therapy, cybercounseling, e-counseling, Internet-based therapy, among others (Christensen & Hickie, 2010). The majority of online therapy today takes place via exchanges of e-mail between the client and counselor. Less popular is the practice of online therapy that takes place in "real time," often using chat-based computer interfaces (e.g., via Instant Messaging—IM) or specialized Web site tools for live videoconferencing sessions between client and counselor (Richardson, Frueh, Grubaugh, Egede & Elhai, 2009). Other applications in this area feature the interaction of multiple clients at the same time for supportive group therapy, with the interaction managed by a counselor (Griffiths, Crisp, Christensen, Mackinnon & Bennett, 2010).

One reason for the trend in techno-therapy is that the stigma associated with addressing addictions and delivering prevention programs is reduced when using the Internet, where it can be accessed at anytime, from anywhere with relative anonymity and privacy. Another reason is that these services are appealing to people who may otherwise go untreated because they do not like certain aspects of in-person therapy. In addition, many people already trust and use online technologies as an everyday part of their lives for banking, health care, social networking and other purposes and extending this use to get help for psychological issues is a reasonable next step (Leibert & Archer, 2006; Young, 2005). A growing body of international research indicates that Internet-based delivery of mental health psychotherapy services for many common mental health conditions is as effective as traditional face-to-face treatment conducted in clinical offices (Attridge, 2011). More than a dozen high quality studies using a randomized control trial (RCT) experimental research design have tested the general clinical effectiveness of Internet-based psychotherapy (Griffiths & Christensen, 2006), and many more studies have been done using a variety of less rigorous research designs. All combined, the general finding is for positive clinical outcomes from online therapy (see reviews by Barak, Hen, Boniel-Nissim & Shapira, 2008; Reger & Gahm, 2009; Rochlen, Zack & Speyer, 2004). Thus, e-therapy has strong research support that provides evidence of its clinical effectiveness, particularly for common kinds of mental health cases with mild or moderate severity that typify EAP counseling services.

New Study on EAP Trends

A new research study explored the trends in EAP from the perspective of those in the EAP field (Attridge & Burke, 2011). This study surveyed senior level EAP professionals to explore trends in the use, importance, business value, and perceived viability of key kinds of EA services. The potential for providing more strategic consulting by EAPs at the organizational level was also examined. A final issue of interest was to determine which societal trends are shaping the future of the industry. Before getting to the results, the study procedures and sample are noted.

Study Methodology. Survey data were collected via a secure Web site from 150 professionals in the EAP industry from the United States and Canada. Most of these people were in senior management or clinical leadership roles, and were associated with the EAP field in a variety of ways, including working for external vendors of EAP services (51%), working for internal programs (23%), being an individual provider of clinical services (11%), being a consultant or academic (5%), or "other" (9%). Seven EAP services were included: (1) counseling with assessment, brief clinical support and referral, (2) management consultations and organizational support, (3) critical incident response, (4) integration of EAP with work/life and wellness, (5) high-risk case finding and long term case management, (6) support for employees on STD/LTD disability leave, and (7) technology and Web-enabled services. These services were rated on three issues: (a) estimated frequency of use, (b) importance to defining what EAP should be, and (c) trend in business value in the marketplace.

Study Results. The study identified three major groupings of services (see Table 21.4). The first cluster of services is called the Core EAP Services. These include counseling and referral for individual employees, manager consultations and organizational support, and critical incident response. The second cluster of services is called the "Pareto" EAP Services. The services involve using the EAP to find and support individuals in need of behavioral health expertise for treating high-risk conditions, and for assistance with return-to-work for mental health and addiction disability. The term "pareto" refers to the economic concept of a small segment of a population that is associated with a large share of an outcome of interest (in this case, a few cases that create a large annual cost in health care expenses and work performance losses). The third cluster of services is called Connecting EAP Services. These services use the Internet and other new technologies to connect employees to counselor and other resources, and also the benefits of integration of the EAP with Wellness and Work/Life programs to better engage individuals in self-care, prevention and family support services.

The Proactive EAP. While acknowledging the need to continue to provide the EAP core services and to expand the pareto and connecting kinds of services, there is also merit in adding a new set of services through which the EAP has a more proactive and strategic role within the organization (Burke & Paul, 2011). Many organizations are hungry for services that can help them address more complex

Table 21.4 Results of Survey of 150 EAP industry professionals

Service type	Outcome measure		
	Estimated level of use[a]	Importance to defining EAP[b]	Business value trend[c]
Sample Size	118	147	147
Rating	NO–L–M–H	L–M–H	F–S–R
Core EAP			
Counseling	01–01–25–73	01–08–91	18–61–21
Consultations	01–12–51–36	04–12–84	24–39–37
Crisis	01–15–49–35	01–21–78	09–47–44
Pareto EAP			
MH/SA Cases	08–40–30–22	16–37–47	31–39–30
Disability	13–43–28–16	13–39–48	24–39–37
Connecting EAP			
Technology	04–38–39–19	13–47–40	12–21–68
Integration	04–23–37–36	05–41–54	12–28–60

Source: Adapted from Attridge and Burke (2011)
Note: Numbers in the table are the percentage of the relevant total sample for each outcome measure. The figures in the rows for each service type within each column add up to 100%
[a]*NO* not offered, *L* low use, *M* medium use, *H* high use
[b]*L* low importance, *M* moderate importance, *H* high importance
[c]*F* fading value, *S* stable value, *R* rising value

issues at the organizational level. Issues at the top of this wish list include how to foster greater employee engagement and productivity, how to retain talent and develop their executives, how to comprehensively support employees with high-risk complex health conditions, and how to create a healthy and psychologically safe work culture for all employees. This issue was examined in the study with a qualitative question: *Given your knowledge of the marketplace, can the value of an EAP be enhanced by also offering services that provide more of a strategic, proactive and consultative approach to the organization?*

The results found that 91% of the sample responded favorably to this question. Thus, more than 9 in 10 EAP professionals recognized the opportunity for EAPs to become more proactive and strategic in focus. Many of the respondents lamented the limitations of having a largely "reactive model" of EAP practices with use of the EAP being dependent upon self-referrals. Others felt that the basic model of service should be reengineered. EAPs could take better advantage of their positive reputation as being experts in handling psychological and behavioral issues in the workplace. Some commented that EAPs are too isolated and need to be more deeply integrated into wellness and other workplace sponsored employee and family support programs. This would mean that assessments and referrals could be done more rapidly and more systematically via shared technological tools and by more regular interaction between the staff in different programs. However, a caveat is in order because roughly 1 in 4 of the respondents—although still positive in general—also expressed some reservations about making this kind of proactive service offering a reality for their EAP business.

Influences on the Future of EAP. A second qualitative item asked about which societal trends are shaping the future of the industry: *In the bigger picture, what societal or business trend do you think will contribute most to the viability and success of the employee assistance industry in the future?* The results for this item yielded the following four themes. Technology was the most commonly cited influence, with social media, online services, instant access, and self-management via technology as key aspects. For example, a 67-year-old female clinical consultant had the comment that "Technology and web-enabled services for education, self-care and clinical support from EAP counselors [is needed] because of the societal focus on quick, easy 24×7 access that's self initiated to address issues or secure information." The second theme was of workplace change. Examples of change included health care reform and parity laws in the United States, the poor economy, increasing social and domestic violence, employee retention issues, an aging population, and globalization. For example, a 56-year-old male professor commented that: "We need more clarity about the role of the EAP in the medical insurance industry. Some health insurance plans offer EAP-type counseling as part of their services, although at no extra costs, but also without having the necessary EAP expertise." The influence of the health and productivity movement on EAP was the third theme. This included issues of EAP partnering with other workplace programs and benefits, the impact of behavioral health issues on work performance, and creating a culture of health at the organization. A 52-year-old male CEO of an EAP commented that: "Promotion of employee mental health is just as important as physical health, which can lead to innovation and increased competitiveness." The last theme for this item focused on concerns for the future viability of the industry. Examples included a need to restate the value proposition for EAP, changing the name from EAP to something else, and the need for more research and industry benchmarks to guide operational practices in order to avoid becoming a non-profession.

Summary

This chapter presents a research-based overview of employee assistance programs. The first part of the chapter provides an overview of EAP, with sections on the following: the history of the field, the primary activities of EAP, the unique qualities of EAP, the main models and markets, the promotion and use of EAPs, and the professional standards for the industry. This second part of the chapter examines the state of empirical evidence for EAP services. EAP is an applied field with active participation in various professional associations and meetings and it has an applied methodology to most of its research. The historical themes of research in the field over the last 25 years have focused on clinical issues of alcohol and drug abuse, psychological/emotional problems, and critical incidents/trauma and relationship issues. The research literature supports the clinical effectiveness of EAP and finds high levels of client satisfaction and positive outcomes in areas of health care costs and workplace performance. This final part of the chapter highlights several trends in the field of EAP, including renewed interest in EAP support for alcohol issues, disability cases, work/life, wellness and prevention, employee engagement, and technology. These themes were replicated and put into a more coherent interpretive model from the findings of a study of trends in EAP.

Conclusions

In conclusion, EAPs currently provide assistance to employees and their dependents for a variety of work-related and personal issues. These programs are found in most large and medium-sized organizations in North America. Individual counseling is shown by research to be the flagship of employee assistance, and is its most popular service component. EAP services are generally effective for the individuals who use them, and they tend to produce a positive financial ROI for the organization. But the present day version of EAPs is underpriced and underutilized, which suggests a need to change with the times and to innovate in ways that can bring more value to the organizations they serve. Several trends are driving EAPs to reexamine and redefine themselves. The 2011 trend study revealed strong agreement among EAP professionals concerning the opportunity for EAPs to play a more proactive and consultative role in the workplaces they serve.

Along these lines, it may now be instructive to review how EAPs can support other aspects of occupational health and wellness. This is done by noting how EAPs fit into the topics of some of the other chapters in this Handbook:

- Chapter 6, on *Challenges Related to Mental Health in the Workplace* (by Dewa and colleagues), emphasizes the prevalence, variety, and deleterious impact of psychosocial issues common to working populations. This evidence supports why the need for EAP services in order to assist employees in the workplace with these kinds of problems.
- Chapter 8, on *The Problem of Absenteeism and Presenteeism in the Workplace* (by Howard and colleagues), goes into detail on the nature and extent of workplace performance problems of employees, which is a core technology focus for EAPs. Indeed, one of the most common positive effects for clients who use the EAP is a rebound in their work productivity levels and reduction in work absence.
- Chapter 10, on *Self-medication and Illicit Drug Use in the Workplace/Workforce* (by Fong), is devoted to the issue of drugs in the workplace. Alcohol and drug problems are an area that is the hallmark of what EAPs are good at supporting. Many EAPs today are involved with drug testing processes and offer case management to employees who self-refer for alcohol and drug problems.
- Chapter 11, on *Bullying and Violence in the Workplace* (by Jensen-Campbell and colleagues), examines a topic that is being addressed by most EAPs. How to best respond to bullying behavior of coworkers and to the issue of violence at work and at home is a frequent training issue, and a source of referrals to EAPs for consultation with managers and for counseling with affected individuals.
- Chapter 12, on *Mental Health Issues Related to Healthy vs. Non-Healthy Workplaces* (by Kirsh and colleagues), describes the organizational level issues concerning a positive work culture. This too is an area that some EAPs (particularly internal model EAPs) are getting more involved in supporting. This is a trend that likely will get more attention from EAPs.
- Chapter 13, on *Safety Issues and Enforcement in the Workplace* (by Sesek and colleagues), addresses areas that can involve the EAP, as well through the provision of worksite trainings, alcohol and drug testing support, and response for trauma resulting from serious safety incidents such as accidental deaths at the worksite.
- Chapter 15, on *Work-Family Balance Issues and Work-Leave Policies* (by King & Hammer), reviews a service area that is the most common integration partner for EAPs.
- Chapter 17, on *Health and Wellness Promotion in the Workplace* (by Shaw & Silje), focuses on the other major integration partner for EAPs in the last decade. EAPs have also become more involved with prevention goals through providing behavioral health risk assessments and related worksite trainings.
- Chapter 18, on *Job-stress Reduction Programs for the Workplace* (by Theorell and colleagues), examines issues of job stress and how to prevent and reduce the problems associated with stress at work. Many employees who seek out support from EAP counselors do so because of job stress. Similarly, many managers who consult with EAP staff are interested in learning how to reduce the stress from dysfunctional work team dynamics and corporate actions.
- Chapter 19, on *Primary and Secondary Prevention of Illness in the Workplace* (by Main and colleagues), is relevant to EAPs due to the growing recognition of the comorbid and exacerbating role of mental health and addictions in many medical illnesses. Some EAPs are also directly involved in supporting individuals to take effective action in their work and personal lives in ways that strive to reduce risks for mental health and physical health problems. Through the multidimensional assessment processes used at most EAPs, counselors can also help identify health risks that employees may not have been aware of and then direct the person to available resources.
- Chapter 20, on *Organizational Aspects of Work Accommodations in Mental Health* (by Schultz), one of the trend areas for EAPs who support employees on disability for mental health and

addictions issues. These EAPs often get involved in tailoring the return to work plans and interacting with the employee and the supervisor to encourage more effective accommodations are made once the employee is back at work so that they can stay at work.

Future Directions

Another significant trend that has only briefly been noted so far in this chapter is how EAP is going global. Due to its success, there is now market saturation, with many companies already having EAP services (at least among large and medium size employers) and also a mature product life cycle stage for traditional EA services in the United States and Canada. However, there remains significant growth for the EAP industry in other countries. This exciting developmental trend for the field is now reviewed. Indeed, various forms of EAPs are now active in many countries around the world (Maiden, 2001). As expected, the specifics of how EAP is defined and used varies based on the country's legal system, culture healthcare system, treatment resources for mental health and substance abuse and views toward behavioral health and work/life balance issues. A recent book profiles EAPs in 50 different countries (Masi & Tisone, 2010). There are member chapters of the EAPA organization located in Australia, Canada, Greece, Ireland, Japan, South Africa, and the UK, and recent development activity for new member chapters in Chile and China. Over a hundred research articles have examined aspects of international EAPs (see Table 21.3). There has also been qualitative research on the progress of EAP development in many countries and regions, including Argentina (Lardani & Lorenzo, 2010), Australia (Kirk, 2008; Kirk & Brown, 2005), China (Yin, 2011) Europe (Hoskinson & Beer, 2005; Nowlan, 2006; Malhomme, 2008; Quinlan, 2005), Germany (Barth, 2006; Gehlenborg, 2001), India (Baskar, 2011; Henry, 2011; Siddiqui & Sukhramani, 2001), Ireland (Powell, 2001), Israel (Katan, 2001), and South Africa (Maiden, 1992).

In the European region a new professional association for EAP providers, called The Employee Assistance European Forum, was initiated in 2002 (Buon & Taylor, 2007). The activity of the EAPs in this part of the world is also the topic of new research project funded by a grant from the Employee Assistance Research Foundation (EARF, 2011). The study is entitled "EAP in Continental Europe: State of the Art and Future Challenges." It will survey employers and employees in six European countries to examine the characteristics of existing EAPs and discover future needs of providers and customer organizations in the European region. A similar research project, also funded by EARF (2011), is now in progress by the US-based National Behavioral Consortium. It will survey EAP providers in North America to profile the operational characteristics and core business metrics that represent the current state of employee assistance programs. Thus, globalization offers many new opportunities for EAP (Burke, 2008). But there are also many contextual and cultural factors that must to be appreciated for it to be successful. Indeed, as global EAP vendors have branched out into other countries, it has been necessary to use local counselors and other staff in order to provide services that match the language, cultural identity, and logistical needs of their customers. It is hoped that this indigenous staffing model will ultimately result in new innovations in EAP practices and products (Pompe, 2011). Alternatively, for the home-grown EAP programs that have started up recently in other countries that are trying to adapt aspects of existing EAP models and services from other places, it is a challenge to determine which elements of the core technology and primary services apply to their environment and will be effective (Masi, 2011). Just as each country is different, so must be the manifestation of EAP that supports the organizations in each country. Along with the escalating worldwide interest in EAP, the field is moving in several directions to enhance their value to organizations and better reach employees in distress. The evidence and trends reviewed in this chapter indicate that EAPs are uniquely connected to the workplace, and are able support organizational health and wellness in multiple ways.

References

Alexander & Alexander Consulting Group. (1990). *The financial impact of the "ASSIST" managed behavioral health care program (1989) at the McDonnell Douglas Helicopter Company*. Unpublished report, Author, Westport, CT.

Amaral, T. (2008, April). *Global benchmarking: Implications of research data for EAP best practices*. Paper presented at the Employee Assistance Society of North America Annual Institute, Vancouver, BC, Canada.

Amaral, T. (2010, October). *The seven market segments of the EAP industry*. Presented at the Employee Assistance Professionals Association Annual Conference, Tampa, FL.

Arthur, A. R. (2000). Employee assistance programmes: The emperor's new clothes of stress management? *British Journal of Guidance and Counselling, 28*(4), 549–559.

Athanasiades, C. (2011). Employee assistance programmes: Past, present and future. *Counselling at Work Journal, Spring*, 20–21.

Attridge, M. (2001a). Can EAPs experiment in the real world? *EAPA Exchange, 31*(2), 26–27.

Attridge, M. (2001b). Inside the numbers: How organizations conduct EA research. *EAPA Exchange, 31*(4), 27–29.

Attridge, M. (2001c, June). *Outcomes of telephonic employee assistance services in a national sample: A replication study*. Presented at the American Psychological Society Annual Conference, Toronto, ON, Canada.

Attridge, M. (2002). *EAP outcomes and ROI*. Boston, MA: A full-day workshop for the Employee Assistance Professionals Association Professional Development Institute.

Attridge, M. (2003a, November). *EAPs and the delivery of alcohol and drug services: Results of the EAPA/Join Together 2003 survey of EAPA members*. Presented at the Employee Assistance Professionals Association Annual Conference, New Orleans, LA.

Attridge, M. (2003b, November). *Optum EAP client satisfaction and outcomes survey study 2002*. Presented at the Employee Assistance Professionals Association Annual Conference, New Orleans, LA.

Attridge, M. (2004, November). *Measuring employee productivity, presenteeism and absenteeism: Implications for EAP outcomes research*. Paper presented the Employee Assistance Professionals Association Annual Conference, San Francisco, CA.

Attridge, M. (2007). *Customer-driven ROI for EAPs*. Advanced Training Institute Audio-conference workshop. Yreka, CA: EAP Technology Systems, Inc.

Attridge, M. (2008a). *A quiet crisis: The business case for managing employee mental health*. Vancouver, BC, Canada: Homewood Human Solutions, from http://www.homewoodhumansolutions.com/docs/HSreport_08.pdf

Attridge, M. (2008b, March). *Return-on-investment (ROI) calculations for behavioral health: Development and application*. Presented at the Work Stress & Health Conference (APA/NIOSH), Washington, DC.

Attridge, M. (2009a). Employee assistance programs: A research-based primer. In J. C. Quick, C. Cooper, & M. Schbracq (Eds.), *The Handbook of Work and Health Psychology* (3rd ed., pp. 383–407). New York, NY: Wiley.

Attridge, M. (2009b). Measuring and managing employee work engagement: A review of the research and business literature. *Journal of Workplace Behavioral Health, 24*(1), 1–16.

Attridge, M. (2010a). EAP cost-benefit research: 20 years after McDonnell Douglas. Part 1 of 3. *Journal of Employee Assistance, 40*(2), 14–16.

Attridge, M. (2010b). Taking the pareto path to ROI. Part 2 of 3. *Journal of Employee Assistance, 40*(3), 12–15.

Attridge, M. (2010c). 20 years of EAP cost-benefit research: Taking the productivity path to ROI. Part 3 of 3. *Journal of Employee Assistance, 40*(4), 8–11.

Attridge, M. (2010d). Resources for employers interested in employee assistance programs: A summary of EASNA's *Purchaser's Guide* and *Research Notes*. *Journal of Workplace Behavioral Health, 25*(1), 34–45. doi:10.1080/15555240903538840.

Attridge, M. (2011). The emerging role of e-therapy: Online services proving to be effective. *Journal of Employee Assistance, 41*(4), 10–13.

Attridge, M., & Amaral, T. M. (2002, October). *Making the business case for EAPs with the core technology*. Paper presented at the Annual Conference of the Employee Assistance Professionals Association, Boston, MA.

Attridge, M., & Bennett, J. (2011). Workplace: Role, prevention, and programs. In M. A. R. Kleiman & J. E. Hawdon (Eds.), *Encyclopedia of drug policy* (Vol. 2, pp. 856–864). Thousand Oaks, CA: Sage.

Attridge, M., & Burke, J. (2011). Trends in EAP services and strategies: An industry survey. *EASNA Research Notes, Vol. 2, No. 3*, from http://www.easnsa.org/publications

Attridge, M., Herlihy, P., & Maiden, P. (Eds.). (2005). *The integration of employee assistance, work/life and wellness services*. Binghamton, NY: Haworth Press.

Attridge, M., Otis, J., & Rosenberg, T. *(2002). The impact of Optum counselor services on productivity and absenteeism: Survey results from 30,000+ employees.* Unpublished report. Optum Research Brief No. 22. Golden Valley, MN: Optum.

Attridge, M., Tannenbaum, E., Wolinsky, D., Slater, S. & Goehner, D. (2009, May). *Tools for demonstrating the value of EAPs: The EASNA 2009 purchaser's guide, industry resources, and accreditation*. Presented at the Employee Assistance Society of North America Annual Institute, Denver, CO.

Attridge, M., & VandePol, B. (2010). The business case for workplace critical incident response: A literature review and some employer examples. *Journal of Workplace Behavioral Health, 25*(2), 132–145. doi:10.1080/15555241003761001.

Attridge, M., & Wallace, S. (2009). *Hidden hazards: The business response to addictions in the workplace.* Vancouver, BC, Canada: Homewood Human Solutions, from http://www.homewoodhumansolutions.com/docs/HSreport_09.pdf

Attridge, M., & Wallace, S. (2010). *Able-minded: Return to work and accommodations for workers on disability leave for mental disorders.* Vancouver, BC, Canada: Homewood Human Solutions, from http://www.homewoodhumansolutions.com/docs/HSreport_10.pdf

Attridge, M., & Wallace, S. (2011, October). *Research based practices for supporting mental health disability*. Presented at the Provincial Minister of Health's Action On Wellness Conference, Banff, AB, Canada.

Baker, E. (2007, October). *Measuring the impact of EAP on absenteeism and presenteeism*. Presented at the Employee Assistance Professionals Association Annual Conference, San Diego, CA.

Barak, A., Hen, L., Boniel-Nissim, M., & Shapira, N. (2008). A comprehensive review and a meta-analysis of the effectiveness of internet-based psychotherapeutic interventions. *Journal of Technology in Human Services, 26*(2), 109–160. doi:10.1080/15228830802094429.

Barth, J. (2006). Germany: A difficult market for EAPs. *Journal of Employee Assistance, 36*(1), 26.

Baskar, K. (2011, October). *Shiftworkers in India: EAP response to the 24/7 workforce*. Paper presented at the Employee Assistance Professionals Association Annual Conference, Denver, CO.

Bennett, J. B., & Attridge, M. (2008). Adding prevention to the EAP core technology. *Journal of Employee Assistance, 38*(4), 3–6.

Bidgood, R., Boudewyn, A., & Fasbinder, B. (2005). Wells Fargo's employee assistance consulting model: How to be an invited guest at every table. *Journal of Workplace Behavioral Health, 20*(3/4), 325–350. doi:10.1300/J490v20n03_07.

Birkland, S. P., & Birkland, M. S. (2005). Integrating employee assistance services with organization development and health risk management at the state government of Minnesota. *Journal of Workplace Behavioral Health, 20*(3/4), 325–350. doi:10.1300/J490v20n03_07.

Blaze-Temple, D., & Howat, P. (1997). Cost benefit of an Australian EAP. *Employee Assistance Quarterly, 12*(3), 1–24. doi:10.1300/J022v12n03_01.

Blum, T. C., & Roman, P. M. (1995). *Cost effectiveness and preventive impact of employee assistance programs.* Washington DC: Center for Substance Abuse Prevention Monograph No. 5, Department of Health and Human Services.

Bray, J., Mills, M., Bray, L. M., Lennox, R., McRee, B., Goehner, D., & Higgins-Biddle, J. (2009). Evaluating web-based training for employee assistance program counselors on the use of screening and brief intervention for at-risk alcohol use. *Journal of Workplace Behavioral Health, 24*(3), 307–319. doi:10.1080/15555240903188372.

Brewster, J. M., Kaufmann, I. M., Hutchison, S., & MacWilliam, C. (2008). Characteristics and outcomes of doctors in a substance dependence monitoring programme in Canada: Prospective descriptive study. *British Medical Journal, 337*, a2098.

Brunnelle, A., & Lui, J. (2003). Disability management programs and EAP. *Journal of Employee Assistance, 33*(2), 7–8.

Buon, T., & Taylor, J. (2007). *A review of the employee assistance program (EAP) market in the UK and Europe.* Aberdeen, England: The Robert Gordon University, from http://www.buon.net/files/RGUEAEF.pdf

Burke, J. (2008, April). *The current global view of EAPs and the opportunity for tomorrow*. Paper presented at the Annual Institute of the Employee Assistance Society of North America, Vancouver, BC, Canada.

Burke, J., & Paul, R. (2011, October). *Creating a culture of health: The role of EAP*. Paper presented at the Employee Assistance Professionals Association Annual Conference, Denver, CO.

Burke, J., & Sharar, D. (2009). Do 'free' EAPs offer discernable value? *Journal of Employee Assistance, 39*(6), 6–9.

Butterworth, I. E. (2001). The components and impact of stigma associated with EAP counseling. *Employee Assistance Quarterly, 16*(3), 1–8. doi:0.1300/J022v16n03_01.

Caggianelli, P., & Carruthers, M. (2007). An integrated approach to behavioral health. *Journal of Employee Assistance, 37*(3), 16–18.

Carruthers, M. (2010). DMEC 2010 employer behavioral risk survey. DMEC white paper series. San Diego, CA: Disability Management Employers Coalition, from http://www.workplacementalhealth.org/2010dmec

Christensen, H., & Hickie, I. B. (2010). E-mental health: A new era in delivery of mental health services. *Medical Journal of Australia, 192*(11), S2–S3.

Christie, J., & Harlow, K. (2007). Presenting the business case. *Journal of Employee Assistance, 37*(3), 21–23.

Collins, K. R. (1998). Cost/benefit analysis shows EAPs value to employer. *EAPA Exchange, 28*(6), 16–20.

Conlin, P., Amaral, T. M., & Harlow, K. (1996). The value of EAP case management. *EAPA Exchange, 26*(3), 12–15.

Csiernik, R. (1995). A review of research methods used to examine employee assistance program delivery options. *Evaluation and Program Planning, 18*(1), 25–36.

Csiernik, R. (2002). An overview of employee and family assistance programming in Canada. *Employee Assistance Quarterly, 18*(1), 17–34.

Csiernik, R. (2003a). Employee assistance program utilization: Developing a comprehensive scorecard. *Employee Assistance Quarterly, 18*(3), 45–59.

Csiernik, R. (2003b). Ideas on best practices for employee assistance program policies. *Employee Assistance Quarterly, 18*(3), 15–32. doi:10.1300/J022v18n03_02.

Csiernik, R. (2005a). A review of EAP evaluation in the 1990s. *Journal of Workplace Behavioral Health, 19*(4), 21–34. doi:10.1300/J022v19n04_02.

Csiernik, R. (2005b). What we're doing in EAP: Meeting the challenge of an integrated model of practice. *Journal of Workplace Behavioral Health, 21*(1), 11–22. doi:10.1300/J490v21n01_02.

Csiernik, R., Hannah, D., & Pender, J. (2007). Change, evolution, and adaptation of a university EAP: Process and outcome at the University of Saskatchewan. *Journal of Workplace Behavioral Health, 22*(2/3), 43–56.

Dainas, C., & Marks, D. (2000). Abbott Laboratories' EAP demonstrates cost-effectiveness through two studies and builds the business case for program expansion. *Behavioral Health Management, 20*(4), 34–41.

Dentzer, S. (2009). Mental health care in America: Not yet good enough. *Health Affairs, 28*(3), 635–636. doi:10.1377/hlthaff.28.3.635.

Dersch, C. A., Shumway, S. T., Harris, S. M., & Arredonondo, R. (2002). A new comprehensive measure of EAP satisfaction: A factor analysis. *Employee Assistance Quarterly, 17*(3), 55–60. doi:10.1300/J022v17n03_04.

Employee Assistance Professionals Association. (2006). *EAPA standards and professional guidelines for employee assistance programs—Addendum: Toward the standardization of employee assistance measures.* Arlington, VA: Author, from http://www.eapassn.org/files/public/utilization06.pdf

Employee Assistance Professional Association. (2009). *EAPA code of ethics.* Arlington, VA: Author, from: http://www.eapassn.org/files/public/EAPAcodeofethics0809.pdf

Employee Assistance Professionals Association. (2010). *EAPA standards and professional guidelines for employee assistance programs.* Arlington, VA: Author, from http://www.eapassn.org/files/public/EAPASTANDARDS10.pdf

Employee Assistance Research Foundation. (2011). Employee Assistance Research Foundation announces winners of its first grant awards program. *EASNA Research Notes, Vol. 2, No.2,* from http://www.easna.org/publications-research-notes/

Employee Assistance Society of North America. (2009). *Selecting and strengthening employee assistance programs: A purchaser's guide.* Washington, DC: Author, from http://www.easna.org/publications-research-notes/

Fuller, J., Attridge, M., & Doherty, W. (2001, October). *You've got ROI: AOL's winning initiatives.* Presented at the Benefits Management Forum and Expo, Atlanta, GA.

Gallagher, P. A., & Morgan, C. L. (2002). Defining the intangible: Measuring the indirect costs related to workers' absence. *Health and Productivity Magazine, 1*(3), 26–27.

Gearhardt, A. N., Yokum, S., Orr, P. T., Stice, E., Corbin, W. R., & Brownell, K. D. (2011). Neural correlates of food addiction. *Archives of General Psychiatry, 4,* 2011. doi:10.1001/archgenpsychiatry.2011.32.

Gehlenborg, H. (2001). Occupational social work in Germany: A continuously developing field of practice. *Employee Assistance Quarterly, 17*(1–2), 17–41.

Ginzberg, M. R., Kilburg, R. R., & Gomes, P. G. (1999). Organizational counseling and the delivery of integrated human services in the workplace: An evolving model for employee assistance theory and practice. In J. M. Oher (Ed.), *The Handbook of Employee Assistance* (pp. 439–456). New York, NY: Wiley.

Goetzel, R. Z. (2007, May). *What's the ROI for workplace health and productivity management programs?* Presented at the Employee Assistance Society of North America Annual Institute, Atlanta, GA.

Goetzel, R. Z., Long, S. R., Ozminkowski, R. J., Hawkins, K., Wang, S., & Lynch, W. (2004). Health, absence, disability and presenteeism cost estimates of certain physical and mental health conditions affecting US employers. *Journal of Occupational and Environmental Medicine, 46*(X), 398–412.

Goetzel, R. A., & Ozminkowski, R. J. (2006). Integrating to improve productivity. *Journal of Employee Assistance, 36*(4), 25–28.

Goplerud, E., & McPherson, T. (2011, October). *Every EAP Purchaser's dream: Evidence-based SBIRT value.* Paper presented at the Employee Assistance Professionals Association Annual Conference, Denver, CO.

Gornick, M. E. (2002). Work/Life core competencies. *EAPA Exchange,* May/June, 11.

Grange, C. (2005). *The development of employee assistance programmes in the UK: A personal view* (pp. 2–5). Summer: Counselling at Work Journal.

Greenwood, K. L., DeWeese, P., & Inscoe, P. S. (2005). Demonstrating the value of EAP services: A focus on clinical outcomes. *Journal of Workplace Behavioral Health, 21*(1), 1–10. doi:10.1300/J490v21n01_01.

Griffiths, K. M., & Christensen, H. (2006). Review of randomized controlled trials of Internet interventions for mental disorders and related conditions. *Clinical Psychology, 10*(1), 16–29.

Griffiths, K. M., Crisp, D., Christensen, H., Mackinnon, A. J., & Bennett, K. (2010). The ANU Well Being study: A protocol for a quasi-factorial randomised controlled trial of the effectiveness of an Internet support group and an automated Internet intervention for depression. *BMC Psychiatry, 10*(20). Online publication. doi:10.1186/1471-244X-10-20

Hargrave, G. E., & Hiatt, D. (2005). The EAP treatment of depressed employees: Implications for return on investment. *Employee Assistance Quarterly, 19*(4), 39–49. doi:10.1300/J022v19n04_03.

Hargrave, G. E., Hiatt, D., Alexander, R., & Shaffer, I. A. (2008). EAP treatment impact on presenteeism and absenteeism: Implications for return on investment. *Journal of Workplace Behavioral Health, 23*(3), 283–293. doi:10.1080/15555240802242999.

Harris, S. M., Adams, M., Hill, L., Morgan, M., & Soliz, C. (2002). Beyond customer satisfaction: A randomized EAP outcome study. *Employee Assistance Quarterly, 17*(4), 53–61. doi:10.1300/J022v17n04_05.

Herlihy, P., & Attridge, M. (2005). Research on the integration of employee assistance, work/life and wellness services: Past, present and future. *Journal of Workplace Behavioral Health*, 20 (1/2), 67–93. doi:10.1300/J490v20n01_04.

Henry, J. (2011). A case for EAP in the Indian workplace. *Journal of Employee Assistance, 41*(4), 26–27.

Hoskinson, L., & Beer, S. (2005). Work-Life and EAPs in the United Kingdom and Europe: A qualitative study of integration. *Journal of Workplace Behavioral Health, 20*(3–4), 367–379. doi:10.1300/J490v20n03_09.

Hyde, M. (2008, April). *EAPs as workplace behavior experts: Do you share the dream?* Paper presented at the Employee Assistance Society of North America Annual Institute, Vancouver, BC, Canada.

Jacobson, J. M., & Attridge, M. (2010). Employee Assistance Programs (EAPs): An allied profession for Work/Life. In S. Sweet & J. Casey (Eds.), *Work and family encyclopedia*. Sloan Work and Family Research Network: Chestnut Hill, MA.

Jacobson, J. M., Jones, A. L., & Bowers, N. (2011). Using existing employee assistance program case files to demonstrate outcomes. *Journal of Workplace Behavioral Health, 26*(1), 44–58. doi:10.1080/15555240.2011.540983.

Jorgensen, D. G. (2007). Demonstrating EAP value. *Journal of Employee Assistance, 37*(3), 24–26.

Katan, J. (2001). Occupational social work in Israel. *Employee Assistance Quarterly, 17*(1–2), 81–95. doi:10.1300/J022v17n01_05.

Kessler, R. C., Chiu, W. T., Demler, O., Merikangas, K. R., & Walters, E. E. (2005). Prevalence, severity, and comorbidity of 12-month DSM-IV disorders in the National Comorbidity Survey Replication. *Archives of General Psychiatry, 62*(6), 617–627.

Kirk, A. K. (2008). Employee assistance program adoption in Australia: Strategic human resource management or 'knee-jerk' solutions? *Journal of Workplace Behavioral Health, 20*(3–4), 79–95. doi:10.1300/J490v21n01_07.

Kirk, A. K., & Brown, D. F. (2005). Australian perspectives on the organizational integration of employee assistance services. *Journal of Workplace Behavioral Health, 20*(3–4), 351–366.

Klion, R. E. (2011). Making clinical assessments online. *Journal of Employee Assistance, 41*(4), 14–15.

Lardani, A., & Lorenzo, P. (2010). Telephonic counseling: The experience in Argentina. *Journal of Employee Assistance, 40*(1), 19–20.

Leibert, T., & Archer, J. (2006). An exploratory study of client perceptions of Internet counseling and the therapeutic alliance. *Journal of Mental Health Counseling, 28*(1), 69–83.

Lingle, K. M. (2004). Work-Life. *Benefits and Compensation Solutions, 28*(12), 36–37.

Lipsey, M. W., & Wilson, D. B. (1993). The efficacy of psychological, educational, and behavioral treatment confirmation from meta-analysis. *The American Psychologist, 48*(12), 1181–1209. doi:10.1037/0003-066X.48.12.

Macdonald, S., Csiernik, R., Durand, P., Rylett, M., & Wild, T. C. (2006). Prevalence and factors related to Canadian workplace health programs. *Canadian Journal of Public Health, 97*(2), 121–125.

Macey, W., & Schneider, B. (2008). The meaning of employee engagement. *Industrial and Organizational Psychology: Perspectives on Science and Practice, 1*(1), 3–30.

Maiden, R. P. (Ed.). (1992). *Employee assistance programs in South Africa*. Binghamton, NY: Haworth.

Maiden, R. P. (Ed.). (2001). *Global perspectives of occupational social work*. Binghamton, NY: Haworth.

Maiden, R. P. (Ed.). (2003). *Accreditation of employee assistance programs*. Binghamton, NY: Haworth.

Maiden, R. P., Kurzman, P., Amaral, T., Stephenson, D., & Attridge, M. (2010, May). *25 years of EAP research: EASNA salutes the Employee Assistance Quarterly and the Journal of Workplace Behavioral Health*. Plenary presented at the Employee Assistance Society of North America Annual Institute, Montreal, QC, Canada.

Malain, A. (2010, June). *Substance abuse expert assessment*. Presented at the Health Care Working Group Special Session on Mental Health and Addictions in the Workplace, Pacific Northwest Economic Region (PNWER) Annual Meeting, Calgary, AB, Canada.

Malhomme, N. (2008, April). *The global workforce: EAP risk and reward in Europe*. Paper presented at the Employee Assistance Society of North America Annual Institute, Vancouver, BC, Canada.

Masi, D. A. (1984). *Designing employee assistance programs*. New York, NY: American Management Associations.

Masi, D. A. (2011). Redefining the EAP field. *Journal of Workplace Behavioral Health, 26*(1), 1–9. doi:10.1080/15555240.2011.540971.

Masi, D., & Tisone, C. (2010). *Fourth international employee assistance compendium*. Masi Research Consultants: Boston. MA.

McClellan, K. (1990). Cost-benefit analysis of the Ohio EAP. *Employee Assistance Quarterly, 5*(2), 67–85. doi:10.1300/J022v05n02 05.

McLellan, A. T., & Meyers, K. (2004). Contemporary addiction treatment: A review of systems problems in the treatment of adults and adolescents with substance use disorders. *Biological Psychiatry, 28*, 345–361.

McLellan, A. T., Skipper, G. S., Campbell, M., & DuPont, R. L. (2008). Five year outcomes in a cohort study of physicians treated for substance use disorders in the United States. *British Medical Journal, 337*, a2038. doi:10.1136/bmj.a2038.

McLeod, J. (2010). The effectiveness of workplace counselling: A systematic review. *Counselling and Psychotherapy Research, 10*(4), 232–248.

McLeod, J., & McLeod, J. (2001). How effective is workplace counseling? A review of the research literature. *Counselling and Psychotherapy Research, 1*(3), 181–191.

McPherson, T. L., Goplerud, E., Olufokunbi-Sam, D., Jacobus-Kantor, L., Lusby-Treber, K. A., & Walsh, T. (2009). Workplace alcohol screening, brief intervention and referral to treatment (SBIRT): A survey of employer and vendor practices. *Journal of Workplace Behavioral Health, 24*(3), 285–306. doi:10.1080/15555240903188372.

Mercer. (2008). *Mercer 2007 national survey of employer-sponsored health plans*. New York, NY: Author. Retrieved from: http://www.mercer.com/home.htm

Mood Disorders Society of Canada. (2009). Stigma research and anti-stigma programs: From the point of view of people who live with stigma and discrimination everyday. Guelph, ON: Author, from http://www.mooddisorderscanada.ca

Mulvihill, M. (2003). The definition and core practices of wellness. *Journal of Employee Assistance, 33*(3), 13–15.

Norlien Foundation. (2011). *Recovery from addiction: A science in society symposium. Summary report*. Calgary, AB, Canada: Author, from http://www.albertafamilywellness.org/resources/publication/2010-recovery-addiction-summary-report

Nowlan, K. (2006). The United Kingdom: Practical support and expert assessment. *Journal of Employee Assistance, 36*(2), 25.

Oher, J. M. (Ed.). (1999). *The employee assistance handbook*. New York, NY: Wiley.

Olfson, M., & Marcus, S. C. (2010). National trends in the use of outpatient psychotherapy. *The American Journal of Psychiatry, 167*(12), 1456–1463.

Open Minds. (2011). *US behavioral health management industry report: OPEN MINDS executive summary of the largest organizations in managed behavioral health, employee assistance and disease management, 2011-2012 Edition*. Gettysburg, PA: Author, from http://www.openminds.com/e-store/mbho.htm

Parnass, P., Mitchell, D., Seagram, S., Wittes, P., Speyer, C., & Fournier, R. (2008, April). *Delivering employee eCounseling programs: Issues and experiences*. Paper presented at the Employee Assistance Society of North America Annual Institute, Vancouver, BC, Canada.

Philips, S. (2004). Client satisfaction with university employee assistance programs. *Employee Assistance Quarterly, 19*(4), 59–70. doi:10.1300/J022v19n04_05.

Pomaki, G., Franche, R.-L., Khushrushahi, N., Murray, E., Lampinen, T., & Mah, P. (2010). *Best practices for return-to-work/stay-at-work interventions for workers with mental health conditions*. Vancouver, BC: Occupational Health and Safety Agency for Healthcare in BC (OHSAH), from http://www.ccohs.ca/products/webinars/best_practices_rtw.pdf

Pompe, J. (2011). The state of global EAP: A purchaser's perspective. *Journal of Workplace Behavioral Health, 26*(1), 10–24. doi:10.1080/15555240.2011.540973.

Powell, M. A. G. (2001). Occupational social work in Ireland. *Employee Assistance Quarterly, 17*(1–2), 65–79. doi:10.1300/J022v17n01_04.

Pugh, S. D., & Dietz, J. (2008). Employee engagement at the organizational level. *Industrial and Organizational Psychology, 1*(1), 44–47. doi:10.1111/j.1754-9434.2007.00006.x.

Quinlan, M. (2005). A social partnership approach to work-life balance in the European Union. *Journal of Workplace Behavioral Health, 20*(3–4), 381–394. doi:10.1300/J490v20n03_10.

Reger, M. A., & Gahm, G. A. (2009). A meta-analysis of the effects of internet- and computer-based cognitive-behavioral treatments for anxiety. *Journal of Clinical Psychology, 65*(1), 53–75. doi:10.1002/jclp. 20536.

Richard, M. A. (2009). Cyberspace: The new frontier for employee assistance programs. In M. A. Richard, W. G. Emener, & W. S. Hutchison Jr. (Eds.), *Employee assistance programs: Wellness/enhancement programming* (4th ed., pp. 288–292). Springfield, IL: Charles C Thomas.

Richard, M. A., Emener, W. G., & Hutchison, W. S., Jr. (Eds.). (2009). *Employee assistance programs: Wellness/enhancement programming* (4th ed.). Springfield, IL: Charles C Thomas.

Richardson, L. K., Frueh, B. C., Grubaugh, A. L., Egede, L., & Elhai, J. D. (2009). Current directions in videoconferencing tele-mental health research. *Clinical Psychology: Science and Practice, 16*(3), 323–338. doi:10.1111/j.1468-2850.2009.01170.x.

Rochlen, A. B., Zack, J. S., & Speyer, C. (2004). Online therapy: Review of relevant definitions, debates, and current empirical support. *Journal of Clinical Psychology, 60*(3), 269–283.

Roman, P. M. (1990). Seventh dimension: A new component is added to the EAP 'core technology.' *Employee Assistance*, February, 8–9.

Roman, P. M. (2007, May). *Underdeveloped workplace opportunities for Employee Assistance Programs*. Plenary presented at the Employee Assistance Society of North America Annual Institute, Atlanta, GA.

Roman, P. M., & Blum, T. C. (1985). The core technology of employee assistance programs. *The ALMACAN, 15*(3), 8–9. 16–19.

Roman, P. M., & Blum, T. C. (1988). Reaffirmation of the core technology of employee assistance programs. *The ALMACAN, 19*(8), 17–22.

Roman, P. M., & Blum, T. C. (2002). The workplace and alcohol problem prevention. *Alcohol Research & Health, 26*(1), 49–57.

Saitz, R., Larson, M. J., Labelle, C., Richardson, J., & Samet, J. H. (2008). The case for chronic disease management for addiction. *Journal of Addictive Medicine, 2*(2), 55–65. doi:10.1097/ADM.0b013e318166af74.

Sealy, R. (2011). We can all prove it! *Counselling at Work Journal, Autumn*, 25–27.

Seidl, W. (2007, October). *Employee engagement and presenteeism: Two new variables in ROI calculations*. Presented at the Employee Assistance Professionals Association Annual Conference, San Diego, CA

Selvik, R., & Bingaman, D. B. (1998). EAP outcomes from the client's point of view, *EAP Digest, September/October*, 21–23.

Selvik, R., & Stephenson, D. (2003). *EAP outcomes demonstrate value*. New Orleans, LA: Paper Presented at the Employee Assistance Professionals Association Annual Conference, New Orleans, LA.

Selvik, R., Stephenson, D., Plaza, C., & Sugden, B. (2004). EAP impact on work, relationship, and health outcomes. *Journal of Employee Assistance, 34*(2), 18–22.

Shain, M., & Groeneveld, J. (1980). *Employee assistance programs: Philosophy, theory, and practice*. Lexington, MA: D. C. Heath and Company.

Siddell, E. D. (2007, October). *Using control charts to enhance EAP satisfaction*. Paper presented at the Employee Assistance Professionals Association Annual Conference, San Diego, CA.

Siddiqui, H. Y., & Sukhramani, N. (2001). Occupational social work in India. *Employee Assistance Quarterly, 17*(1–2), 43–63. doi:10.1300/J022v17n01_03.

Smith, D. C., & Mahoney, J. J. (1990). *McDonnell Douglas Corporation employee assistance program financial offset study: 1985-1988*. Bridgeton, MI: McDonnell Douglas Corporation.

Society for Human Resources Management. (2009). *2008 employee benefits*. Washington, DC: Author.

Sonnenstuhl, W. J., & Trice, H. (1990). *Strategies for employee assistance programs: The crucial balance* (2nd ed.). Ithaca, NY: IRL Press/Sage House.

Sroujian, C. (2003). Mental health is the number one cause of disability in Canada. *The Insurance Journal*, (Aug. 7), 8.

Stockert, T. J. (2004). The Council on Accreditation employee assistance program accreditation process. *Employee Assistance Quarterly, 19*(1), 35–44. doi:10.1300/J022v19n01_03.

Taranowski, C. (2009). Advocating for a positive workplace. *Journal of Employee Assistance, 39*(1), 7–9.

The Hartford Group. (2007). *Healthier, more productive employees: A report on the real potential of employee assistance programs (EAP)*. Hartford, CT: Author.

Thorpe, K., & Chenier, L. (2011). *Building mentally healthy workplaces: Perspectives of Canadian workers and frontline managers*. Ontario, ON, Canada: Conference Board of Canada, from http://www.conferenceboard.ca/documents.aspx?did=4287

Trice, H., & Schonbrunn, M. (1981). A history of job-based alcoholism programs 1900-1955. *Journal of Drug Issues, 11*(1), 171–198.

Trogdon, J., Finkelstein, E. A., Reyes, M., & Deitz, W. H. (2009). W return-on-investment simulation model of workplace obesity interventions. *Journal of Occupational and Environmental Medicine, 51*(7), 751–758. doi:10.1097/JOM.0b013e3181a86656.

Turner, S., Weiner, M., & Keegan, K. (2005). Ernst & Young's Assist: How internal and external service integration created a 'single source solution'. *Journal of Workplace Behavioral Health, 20*(3–4), 243–262. doi:10.1300/J490v20n03_03.

Wang, P. S., Lane, M., Olfson, M., Pincus, H. A., Wells, K. B., & Kessler, R. C. (2005). Twelve month use of mental health services in the United States: Results from the National Comorbidity Survey Replication. *Archives of General Psychiatry, 62*, 629–640.

Weiss, R. M. (2003). Effects of program characteristics on EAP utilization. *Employee Assistance Quarterly, 18*(3), 61–70. doi:10.1300/J022v18n03_05.

Williams, C. (2006). *Disability in the workplace* (pp. 16–24). Perspectives (February): Statistics Canada.

Wittes, P., & Speyer, C. (2009, May). *Online counseling: A key component of 21st century EAP in a global economy*. Presented at the Employee Assistance Society of North America, Annual Institute, Denver, CO..

World Health Organization. (2011). *Mental health atlas 2011*. Geneva, Switzerland: Author, from http://whqlibdoc.who.int/publications/2011/9799241564359_eng.pdf

Wrich, J. T. (1980). *The employee assistance program – A primer*. Troy, MI: Performance Resource Press, Inc.

Yamatani, H., Santangelo, L. K., Maue, C., & Heath, M. C. (1999). A comparative analysis and evaluation of a university employee assistance program. *Employee Assistance Quarterly, 15*(1), 107–118. doi:10.1300/J022v15n01_05.

Yin, P. (2011, October). *EAP in China: Not so foreign after all*. Presented at the Annual Conference of the Employee Assistance Professionals Association, Denver, CO..

Young, K. S. (2005). An empirical examination of client attitudes towards online counseling. *Cyberpsychology & Behavior, 8*(2), 172–177. doi:10.1089/cpb.2005.8.172.

Part V

Research, Evaluation, Diversity and Practice

Epidemiological Methods for Determining Potential Occupational Health and Illness Issues

22

J. Mark Melhorn, Charles N. Brooks
and Shirley Seaman

Introduction

Epidemiology requires a methodology for testing scientific hypotheses in groups of individuals. Indeed, with the understanding the fundamental strengths and limitations of the design, combined with the implementation of published studies, it is possible to evaluate the strength of the evidence derived from these studies, and even to make sense of conflicting results from different studies on the same issue. Thus, we present an overview of the basic terminology used in epidemiology and the characteristics, strengths, and limitations of analytic (hypothesis testing) study designs, with an emphasis on observational study designs. At the outset, it should be noted that the two most common types of epidemiologic studies are: descriptive epidemiology is the most common type and is used to monitor the health of a population, identifying health problems, and compiling information that can be used to develop causal hypotheses. Analytic epidemiology is designed to test specific a hypotheses.

Why Is Determining Causation Important?

In the occupational setting, causation analysis is most often used to determine legal and, hence, financial responsibility for the health condition. Causality assessment can also be used to develop prevention programs to: reduce the risk of disease or injury occurrence; establish eligibility for Social Security, welfare, or other entitlement programs; and to develop reasonable stay at work or return to work guides. To elaborate on the former, a causal determination in workers' compensation is typically based on physician opinion, and used to decide whether or not employers or their insurers are legally responsible for the costs of evaluation and treatment of the health condition in question, as well as any disability and/or impairment resulting therefrom. In the United States, workers' compensation is not a single system, but is a conglomerate of systems created by each State and Territory, in addition to

---

J.M. Melhorn, M.D. (✉) • S. Seaman, P.A.-C.
The Hand Center, 625 N Carriage Parkway Suite 125, Whichita, KS 67208, USA
e-mail: melhorn@onemain.com

C.N. Brooks, M.D.
Bellevue, WA, USA

federal statutes covering longshore and harbor workers, railroad employees, federal and postal workers, etc. The threshold for legal causation differs from one workers' compensation system to another, and from tort or liability cases, both of which may be quite different from the criteria for scientific-medical causation. This lack of uniformity injects additional complexities into occupational causation analysis, which has both a medical and legal component. A well-informed physician opinion on causality requires knowledge of the applicable medical literature on causation of the condition in question, legal criteria for causation in the applicable jurisdiction, and facts of the specific case.

Before workers' compensation statutes, suing the employer was the only legal means for a worker or the family to obtain compensation for an occupational injury or illness. Workers had to prove the employer's negligence to be compensated, a hurdle that often could not be overcome due to three common law defenses: contributory negligence; fellow servant rule; and assumption of risk. These defenses, which often resulted in denial of recovery to injured or ill workers by nineteenth century courts, became known as the "three wicked sisters." On the other hand, employers' potential liability was not limited to healthcare costs, wage loss, and permanent impairments, but also included compensatory damages (e.g., pain and suffering, and punitive). Additionally, both parties had to undergo a time consuming and costly trial to determine liability and damages. Consequently, legislators passed workers' compensation statutes as a compromise, ensuring that employees injured or made ill on the job received compensation in a timely manner, without need to prove negligence. Employers benefited via the preclusion of compensatory and punitive damages, thereby limiting their risk. Both parties and the courts were spared the temporal and financial costs of litigation.

Definitions

In order to provide a consistent approach to definitions and terms, this section has been provided with permission of the American Medical Association's Press *Guides to the Evaluation of Disease and Injury Causation* (Melhorn & Ackerman, 2008, Chapter 1: Introduction).[1]

Evidence-Based Literature

Evidence-based medicine has become the standard for determining appropriate medical care. The most common definition was provided by Dr. David Sackett: "Evidence-based medicine is the conscientious, explicit, and judicious use of current best evidence in making decisions about the care of individual patients… [which] means integrating individual clinical expertise with the best available external clinical evidence from systematic research" (Sackett, Rosenberg, Gray, Haynes, & Richardson, 1996). Unfortunately, randomized controlled clinical studies are difficult to perform in the workplace and, hence, are uncommon. Therefore, most of the information available is from epidemiologic studies which can disprove, but not prove, an association (Hadler, 1999).

Epidemiology

As noted earlier, epidemiology focuses on the distribution and determinants of disease in groups of individuals who happen to have some characteristics, exposures, or diseases in common. Viewed as the study of the distribution and societal determinants of the health status of populations, epidemiology

---

[1] Jmm 1—Permission to Use Granted by AMA.

is the basic science foundation of public health (Melhorn, 1999). The goal of epidemiologic studies is to identify factors associated (positively or negatively) with the development or recurrence of adverse medical conditions. A search strategy of bibliographic databases was used to identify epidemiologic literature that addresses causation of specific medical conditions as outlined in *Guides to the Evaluation of Disease and Injury Causation* (Melhorn & Hegmann, 2008, Chapter 4: Methodology). Although the referenced Chap. 4 is copyrighted, Drs. Melhorn and Hegmann have decided to offer the materials therein as "in the public domain and may be freely copied or reprinted" if appropriate acknowledgment of the reference source is used.

Specific Definitions

- Medical conditions are defined as: An injury or illness that meets the standard criteria for an ICD-10 diagnosis (Melhorn & Ackerman, 2008).
- Disability refers to an alteration of an individual's capacity to meet personal, social, or occupational demands or statutory or regulatory requirements because of impairment. Disability is a relational outcome, contingent on the environmental conditions in which activities are performed (AMA, 2001).
- Impairment refers to a loss, loss of use, or derangement of any body part, organ system, or organ function (AMA, 2001).
- Occupational exposures and physical factors at work are defined as: Identifiable occupational exposures to possible exacerbating or aggravating agents. For the musculoskeletal system, physical factors are often described in terms of Repetition, Force, Posture, Vibration, Temperature, Contact stress, and Unaccustomed activities (CtdMAP, 2006; Melhorn, 1998). For hearing, sound levels are measured in decibels. Radiation exposure is measured in millirads, and chemical exposure in milligram per cubic meter or parts per million.
- Nonoccupational exposures are defined as: Individual risk characteristics such as age, gender, hand preference, comorbid medical conditions such as diabetes, body mass index (BMI), depression, and hobbies.
- The work environment: Under paragraph 1904.5(b)(1), the Occupational Safety and Health Act (OSHA) defines the work environment as the establishment and other locations where one or more employees are working, or are present as a condition of their employment. The work environment includes not only physical locations but also the equipment or materials used by the employee during the course of his or her work (U.S. Department of Labor, 2006a).
- Aggravation refers to a preexisting injury or illness that has been significantly aggravated, for purposes of OSHA injury and illness recordkeeping, when an event or exposure in the work environment results in any of the following:
- Death, provided that the preexisting injury or illness would likely not have resulted in death but for the occupational event or exposure.
- Loss of consciousness, provided that the preexisting injury or illness would likely not have resulted in loss of consciousness but for the occupational event or exposure.
- One or more days away from work, or days of restricted work, or days of job transfer that otherwise would not have occurred but for the occupational event or exposure.
- Medical treatment in a case where no medical treatment was needed for the injury or illness before the workplace event or exposure, or a change in medical treatment was necessitated by the workplace event or exposure (U.S. Department of Labor, 2006a).
- The above are similar to aggravation as defined by the AMA *Guides to the Evaluation of Permanent Impairment*, 5th Edition: A factor(s) (e.g., physical, chemical, biological, or medical condition)

that adversely alters the course or progression of the medical impairment. Worsening of a preexisting medical condition or impairment (AMA, 2001).
- Exacerbation is defined as: A transient worsening of a prior condition by an injury or illness, with the expectation that the situation will eventually return to baseline or pre-worsening level (Talmage & Melhorn, 2005). Some take issue with this definition because the signs or symptoms of a preexisting injury or illness may be temporarily worsened by something (i.e., activity, exposure, weather, reinjury), but the "something" is not an injury or illness. For example, a set of tennis will temporarily worsen the symptoms of degenerative arthritis in the serving shoulder, but tennis is neither an injury nor illness. This concept is clarified by the following:
- Exacerbation is defined in the AMA *Guides to the Evaluation of Permanent Impairment*, 6th Edition as: *Temporary* worsening of a preexisting condition. Following a transient increase in symptoms, signs, disability, and/or impairment, the person recovers to his or her baseline status, or what it would have been had the exacerbation never occurred. Given a condition whose natural history is one of progressive worsening, following a prolonged but still temporary worsening, return to pre-exacerbation status would not be expected, despite the absence of permanent residuals from the new cause (p. 611 of reference) (Oakley, 2011).
- Recurrence is defined as: The reappearance of signs or symptoms of a prior injury or illness with minimal or no provocation and not necessarily related to work activities (Talmage & Melhorn, 2005).
- Apportionment is defined as: A distribution or allocation of causation among multiple factors that caused or significantly contributed to the injury or disease and resulting impairment. The factor could be a preexisting injury, illness, or impairment (AMA, 2001).
- For purposes of this present chapter, the words diagnosis, disorder, condition, injury, or illness are essentially considered the same.

What We Know and How We Know It

Epistemology (E·pis·te·mol·o·gy) [ih-pis-tuh-mol-uh-jee] is a branch of philosophy that investigates the origin, nature, methods, and limits of human knowledge. In other words "What We Know And How We Know It" or "What There Is to Know About Knowing" (Melhorn, 2008). Therefore, as is often the case, a decision on causation may be difficult because the determination is based on imperfect or inadequate information. This chapter is designed to address causation analysis while acknowledging these intrinsic limitations. Limiting causal conclusions to proven and established facts does not guarantee that future studies will not prove the current data wrong. Conversely, shunning everything unproven will result in rejection of many statements that are true but just not proven. The best illustration of this concept is in Fig. 22.1.

The Science

Healthcare providers are often asked whether a condition is work-related or not (i.e., if it is causally related to a specific occupational injury or exposure). It is incumbent upon the clinician to give an opinion based on a careful review and analysis of: the individual's clinical findings; his or her workplace exposures; the literature linking (or not) the injury or exposure of concern and the condition in question (Melhorn & Ackerman, 2008). In contrast to a witnessed occupational injury causing immediate symptoms and corroborated by objective physical and diagnostic test findings, a cause-and-effect relationship between the disease (nontraumatic injuries are classified by OSHA as illnesses) and

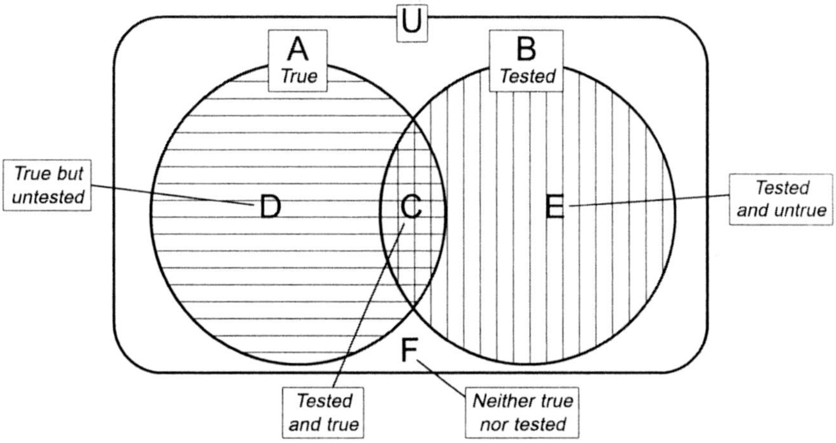

Fig. 22.1 Medical knowledge. A Venn diagram representing the universe (U) of medical knowledge. Area A represents all true statements and area B, all tested statements. Area C represents all validated (tested and true) statements, but it does not contain all truths: it is missing area D, which represents truths that have not been proved (true but untested). Area E represents invalidated knowledge, i.e., all tested and untrue statements. Area F is those statements that are neither true nor tested. A clinician using untested knowledge hopes to use statements that fall within area D but may in fact sample from area F. Permission to Used Granted. J. Bernstein. Evidence-based medicine. J Am Acad Orthop Surg 12 (2):80–88, 2004.

an agent or condition in the workplace, may be unclear. Occupational diseases may develop slowly, with months or years between exposure and onset of symptoms and/or signs. Disease manifestations may be confused with changes due to normal aging. Information on past work exposure is often unavailable, inadequate, or incomplete. In addition, not all individuals react or respond in the same way to similar exposures to disease-producing agents. In some cases, there is a clearly identifiable single cause for the condition, whether work-related or nonoccupational. More often, causation is multifactorial, with one or more nonoccupational cause(s) (e.g., age-related degeneration, smoking, or obesity), in addition to varying contribution from the workplace.

Causality determination may be difficult and result in contested claims. Honest differences of opinion are common when the facts are subject to different interpretations. Therefore, considerable judgment is necessary when data are lacking or incomplete. With occupational diseases, what appears obvious to some may nevertheless still be controversial, and it is important to: assemble a complete a database (history including occupational and nonoccupational exposures, physical and test findings, healthcare records, etc.); be familiar with the relevant medical literature; and then review and analyze the data in a logical and unbiased manner to ensure a correct and equitable decision on causation. In 1976, The National Institute for Occupational Safety and Health (NIOSH) created *A Guide To The Work-Relatedness of Disease* (1979, Publication No. 79-116) to assist clinicians and, therein, provided a six-step method to assist in this decision making process (Hegmann & Oostema, 2008). These six steps are listed in Table 22.1.

Consideration of Evidence

The first step in determining the probability of a cause-and-effect relationship between an exposure in the workplace and the subject illness is to establish that: a disease does in fact exist; and the disease and its manifestations appear to be the result of exposure to a specific harmful agent. Evidence elicited

Table 22.1 NIOSH causation decision making process

1. Consideration of evidence
2. Consideration of epidemiologic data
3. Consideration of evidence of exposure
4. Consideration of validity of testimony
5. Consideration of other relevant factors
6. Evaluation and conclusion

in the course of a medical evaluation should address these questions, and specifically include the following:
- Complete medical, personal, family, military, and occupational histories from the employee.
- A thorough physical examination and acquisition or review of appropriate radiographic, laboratory, or other diagnostic tests.
- Analysis and reporting of this clinical data.

The occupational history should include, but is not, limited to:
- Job titles
- Type of work performed (complete listing of actual duties)
- Duration of each type of activity
- Dates of employment and worker's age for each job activity
- Geographical and physical location of employment
- Product or service produced
- Condition of personal protective equipment used (if any), and frequency and duration of periods of use
- Nature of agents or substances to which worker is, or has been, exposed, if known (including frequency and average duration of each exposure situation)
- The resultant report should include a complete list of all diagnoses, with an opinion whenever possible at to which diagnoses are occupationally-related and which are not.

Consideration of Epidemiological Data

The essential approach of epidemiology is the investigation of relative and absolute measures of frequency, while comparing the characteristics of individuals with and without the condition. The most obvious measures of frequency are case counts and their variations, which are often referred to as *numerator data*. This number, the (numerator) describes the frequency of the disorder, without reference to the underlying population at risk (the *dominator* data). The United States Congress recognized that statistics on workplace injuries and diseases were essential to an effective national program of occupational disease prevention (Melhorn & Ackerman, 2008). Therefore, when the OSHA was passed in 1970, employers were required to maintain records on workplace injuries and illnesses (commonly labeled as OSHA 300 Logs). The Act delegated the responsibility for collecting statistics on these occupational injuries and illnesses to the Bureau of Labor Statistics (BLS). To comply with the OSHA, the BLS conducts an annual survey of the occupational injuries and illnesses in the United States (U.S. Department of Labor, 2006b). The survey compiles the OSHA 300 logs from over 200,000 establishments, grouped together by industry codes established by BLS as the North American Industry Classification System (NAICS) (http://www.bls.gov/bls/naics.htm). The frequency of the particular disorder can also be expressed as a proportionate ratio. The number of cases of the particular disorder, compared to cases of all disorders, in the study population. By itself, *numerator data* cannot provide useful information regarding the risk or probability of acquiring the disorder. The case frequency has to be related to the underlying population that could have potentially developed the disorder (the *denominator*). Without the denominator (the number of people at risk), it is not possible to estimate the risk of a specific condition in the population, or to test hypotheses regarding risk factors for a specific condition.

There are, though, known limitations of the BLS data. The survey estimates of occupational injuries and illnesses are based on a scientifically-selected probability sample, rather than a census of the entire population. Because the data are based on a sample survey, the injury and illness estimates probably differ from the figures that would be obtained from all units covered by the survey. Also, the survey measures the number of new work-related illness cases that are recognized, diagnosed, and reported during the year. Some conditions (e.g., long-term latent illnesses caused by exposure to carcinogens) often are difficult to relate to the workplace, and are not adequately recognized and reported. These long-term latent illnesses are believed to be understated in the survey's illness measures. In contrast, the overwhelming majority of the reported new illnesses are those that are easier to track (e.g., contact dermatitis or carpal tunnel syndrome) (Melhorn & Ackerman, 2008). Furthermore, employer bias in selecting which conditions to report may result in under-reporting. Additionally, the OSHA definition for work-relatedness is more inclusive than most. Injuries and illnesses that occur at work may not have a clear connection to an occupational activity or substance peculiar to the work environment. For example, an employee may trip for no apparent reason while walking across a level factory floor, be sexually assaulted by a coworker, or be injured accidentally as a result of an act of violence perpetrated by one coworker against a third party. For this reason, rates are often used when the objective is to assess the risk of the disorder or determinants of disorders or their outcomes.

Rates

Rates describe the frequency of a disorder (or disorder per unit size of the population per unit time of observation). The most common rates are *incidence* and *prevalence*. The incidence rate is based on new cases of a disorder, whereas the prevalence rate reflects existing cases. Because they are based on new versus existing cases, incidence and prevalence rates have different uses and limitations. Therefore, the incidence rate is a rate of change, often described as the frequency with which people change from healthy to injured, sick, or disabled. Thus, the appropriate denominator is the population at risk of acquiring the disorder (i.e., those who are free of the disorder at the start of the time interval). The incidence rate may be quantified in a number of ways when the population is stable and the number of new events is counted each year. This is often expressed as the number of new events per 1,000 persons per year. Alternatively, incidence rate may be quantified as the number of new events per 1,000 person-years, as is done in prospective studies where a fixed population is followed until the end of the study. In practice, although the best denominator for incidence rates is the number of people free of the disorder at the start of the time interval, surveillance incidence rates (and prevalence rates) that are based on case reports often use the total population derived from estimates or census data.

The prevalence rate is the number of existing cases of a disorder in a given population in a given time period, while *point prevalence* is the number of cases per unit population at one moment. For example, point prevalence would be the number of railroad employees receiving disability because of a medical condition on a specific day such as January 1, 2010. Therefore, the unit of time is not expressed. A *period prevalence* would be the number of cases existing at one time during a definable time interval such as 1-year. Lifetime prevalence (which is a form of period prevalence) is defined as the number of individuals in a population that, at some point in their life which could be several to more than 100 years, have the condition in question, compared to the total number of persons. Prevalence is sometimes not defined as a rate because, in practice, data are often derived from surveys that are difficult to assign to a specific time interval. A number of variables, other than the risk factor under study, may affect the incidence and prevalence rates. Examples include demographic characteristics of the underlying population. The most common variable is age distribution because aging is associated with the onset of most disorders. Gender and ethnicity distributions must also be taken into account. Other confounders that can distort the incidence rate include company policies, workers' compensation claims, and health care system influences that affect the likelihood of seeking medical attention, of being diagnosed with a given disorder, or of having the disorder reported. These variables must be considered when measures of disorder frequency are evaluated, particularly when changes are assessed over time or when different populations are compared. In order to eliminate the effects of differences in these variables, the rates may be adjusted or standardized algebraically. The adjusted rates express the risk of acquiring the disorder in the populations being compared as if they had the same age, sex, and ethnicity distributions. In other words, the "variables" have been accounted for. Sometimes, it is appropriate to not account for these variables (e.g., the morbidity rates within population strata defined by age, sex, and ethnicity). Remember, the number of existing cases of a disorder at any time is a function of both the rate of new cases (incidence) and the duration of that disorder. Accordingly, a change in prevalence may reflect changes in the incidence rate, duration, or both. Consequently, when a population is stable and the duration of a disorder is also stable, it is possible to estimate prevalence from incidence and vice versa, according to the following approximation:

$$\text{Prevalence} \approx \text{incidence} \times \text{duration}.$$

Therefore, rates become the first step in considering causality and lead to further epidemiological studies.

Epidemiological Study Design

Epidemiological studies are of two major types which can be subdivided. The first is the *descriptive epidemiology* study, which drives the need to explain variation and formulate causal hypotheses that draw on current available information. However, while it supports the development of causal hypotheses, descriptive epidemiology does not itself support conclusions about disorder causality or any hypotheses. In descriptive epidemiology, the frequency of a disorder in the population is characterized in terms of person (e.g., individual risk factors: age, gender, ethnicity-specific incidence rates, economic, behavioral, occupational, and other factors), place (country, rural, urban, type of industry, and job requirements), and time (day, week, month, year, and lifetime) as seen in Table 22.2.

Each epidemiologic study also has certain basic elements: occurrence relation, outcome, determinant(s), study population, and domain. Determinant(s) are defined as the risk factors related to the diagnosis. The study population must be well defined to allow the data obtained to be applied, or theoretically generalized, to a larger population called the domain. This requirement is often described as *external validity*.

Table 22.2 Descriptive epidemiology study design

Person
Place
Time
Condition or disorder

Specific hypotheses are developed by inductive reasoning to explain observed patterns of variation, and then evaluated using a study designed to test them. Studies that test specific hypotheses are *analytic epidemiologic* studies (the second major type of epidemiologic study). As the results of hypothesis testing (analytic) studies are accrued, and their data added to the basis for causal inference, depending on their strengths and generalizability, and hypotheses are supported, modified, or negated. Analytic (hypothesis testing) epidemiology relies on two types of study designs: Observational and experimental. In observational studies, exposure to the hypothesized causal factor and the subsequence development of the selected disorder in the population under study occur in the natural course of events; in other words, the investigator does not cause the exposure to the causal factor. The study is designed and implemented to maximize the extent to which it is a natural experiment. Extraneous sources of variation are eliminated, and only exposure to the alleged cause and the frequency of the selected disorder vary between populations being compared. Once substantial observational evidence has accrued, causality is often widely accepted. However, only prospective randomized interventional or experimental studies can prove causation; and these are unlikely to be performed in the workplace as it would require exposing individuals to known or suspected risk factors and, thereby, potential harm.

Literature Review Summaries

Epidemiological versus individual causal assessment requires determination that a "risk factor" is truly a disease determinant, rather than merely an associated factor (Hegmann & Oostema, 2008). If the risk factor is causal, then elimination of the risk factor must result in fewer cases of the particular disease. Literature review summaries require five steps, as listed in Table 22.3. To summarize, one must try to avoid omitting articles in the review of the literature. Of course, the purpose of a well-designed study is to provide insight into the "truth" regarding causation. The ability to determine the truth, or to infer from a limited sample to the whole, is compromised by a systematic or study design flaw in the form of bias and/or confounding. Alternatively, chance or random occurrence may influence whether the results of a study accurately reflect the truth. Etiologic epidemiology tests whether a hypothesized factor is a determinant or cause of disorder in previously healthy population whereas, in clinical epidemiology, one tests whether risk factors are determinants of the specific disease. The classic observational analytic study designs are the cohort study, the case–control study, and the cross-sectional study.

Figure 22.2 summarizes the various types of study designs, based on their strength.

Because it is not possible to study the entire universe of potentially eligible subjects (workers), epidemiologic studies are conducted on samples of the population of interest. Even a study of an entire city's work force constitutes a sample. The method of sampling should not introduce selection biases, but epidemiological studies are commonly affected by them. For example, no characteristics of the individuals should affect the likelihood of selection for the study; but a volunteer study is potentially susceptible to selection bias because the health behavior and health status of people who volunteer for research are known to be better than those who refuse.

Internal validity refers to both how well a scientific study was conducted, and how confidently one can conclude there is a cause-and-effect relationship. Research design, definitions used, what variables were and were not measured, how accurately they were measured, completeness of data collection, and other factors all influence validity. This applies to both descriptive and experimental studies. However, in experimental studies, one also wants to know how certain is it that the effect was caused by the independent variable rather than extraneous ones. For example, did the treatment really cause or contribute to the difference observed between subjects in the control and experimental groups? If there is inaccuracy (measurement error) in the information collected, the ability to detect the association

Table 22.3 Literature review. Table 3-1 page 35, Guides to the Evaluation of Disease and Injury Causation, editors J. Mark Melhorn and William E. Ackerman, Chapter 3 Causal Associations and Determination. Used with permission of Work-Relatedness (release done)

Table 3-1 Steps for concluding a causal association exists
1. Collect all epidemiologic literature on the disorder
2. Identify the design of each study

3. Assess the methods of each study
  (a) Exposure assessment methods and potential biases
  (b) Disease ascertainment methods and potential biases
  (c) Absence of significant uncontrolled confounders; consideration of residual confounding
  (d) Addressing of other potential biases
  (e) Adequacy of biostatistical methods and analytic techniques

4. Ascertain statistical significance and the degree to which chance may have produced the results

5. Assess the studies using the Updated Hill Criteria; apply the criteria to individual studies (especially 5a–5c) and to the studies as a whole (5a–5l)
  (a) Temporality
  (b) Strength of association
  (c) Dose–response relationship
  (d) Consistency
  (e) Coherence
  (f) Specificity
  (g) Plausibility
  (h) Reversibility
  (i) Prevention/elimination
  (j) Experiment
  (k) Analogy
  (l) Predictive performance

6. Conclusion about the degree to which a causal association is or is not present

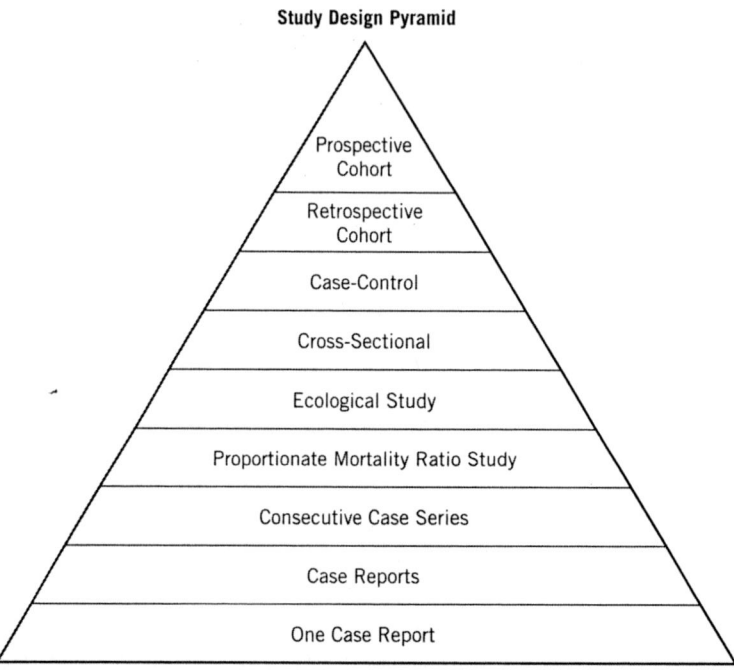

Fig. 22.2 Study Design Pyramid page 36, Guides to the Evaluation of Disease and Injury Causation, editors J. Mark Melhorn and William E. Ackerman, Chapter 3 Causal Associations and Determination of Work-Relatedness. Used with permission

Table 22.4 Common statistical tests.

Type of data	No. of groups	Independent	Paired
Continuous			
Normal	2	Student's t test	Paired t test
Non-normal	2	Mann–Whitney U test	Wilcoxon's signed rank test
Normal	>2	ANOVA test	Repeated measures ANOVA test
Non-normal	>2	Kruskal–Wallis test	Friedman's test
Proportions	2 (large number of observations)	Chi square test	
	2 (small number of observations)	Fisher's exact test	
Ordinal	2	Mann–Whitney U test	Wilcoxon's signed rank test
	>2	Kruskal–Wallis test	Friedman's test
Nominal	2	Fisher's exact test	McNemar's test
	>2	Pearson chi square test	Cochran's Q test
Survival	2/>2	Log-rank test	Conditional logistic regression

of interest is reduced. If the accuracy of information is worse for one exposure group than another, the effect on the study results may not be predictable. Hence, evaluation of the accuracy (or validity) of measurements is necessary for any study. Research reports should describe the validity of the sources of information. For example, questionnaires or reporting methods that have been validated in the study population, or in similar populations or circumstances, should be used.

Finally, the strength of evidence regarding etiology varies depending on the type of study. Prospective cohort studies are best, while retrospective cohort studies are of low-medium strength, and case–control and cross-sectional low strength. Frequently used analysis tools are listed in Table 22.4.

Cohort Study

Cohort studies can be *prospective* or *retrospective*. The direction of data inquiry can be seen in Fig. 22.3. When well designed and executed, a cohort study produces the soundest results for incidence rates, disorder etiology, and/or prognostic determinants of all the observational study designs. The hallmark of a cohort study is that a population is initially free of the disease of interest. Potential confounders and important covariates are identified and characterized with respect to the hypothesized risk factor. The population is observed for a period of time adequate for development of the disorder, and the new (incident) cases are recorded. Rates of disorder development are compared between those who are and are not exposed to the hypothesized risk factor. Loss to follow-up, though, is a potential problem. If a number of individuals are lost to follow-up, the observed relative risk underestimates the true relative risk. Selective survival or selective attrition bias can occur. Long latency periods increase the cost to continue these studies.

Case–Control Study

The essential feature of the case–control study that differentiates it from other observational study types is that individuals are selected for the study based on the presence of the disorder in question (cases) and compared with others who do not have the disorder (control subjects). The presence or absence of the hypothesized cause is then ascertained in both case and control subjects. Although this

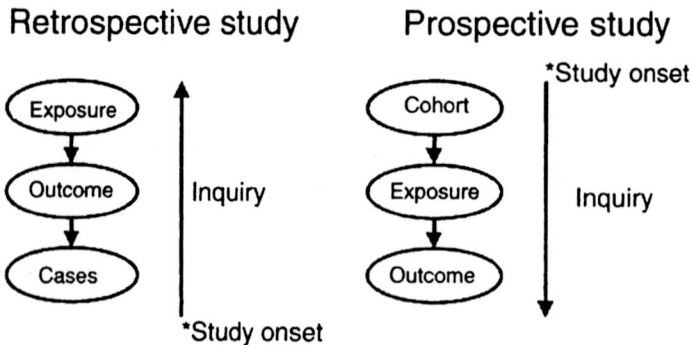

Fig. 22.3 Direction of inquiry. R.J. O'Keefe, G.R. Huffman, and S.V. Bukata. Orthopaedic Research: Clinical Epidemiology and Biostatistics. In: *Orthopaedic Knowledge Update*, edited by J.S. Fischgrund, Chicago, IL: American Academy of Orthopaedic Surgeons, 2008, p. 173-185.in JBJS 2004:86:607-620 direction of inquiry. Direction of inquiry (adapted with permission from Kocher MS, Zurakowki D: Clinical epidemiology and biostatistics: A primer for orthopaedic surgeons. J Bone Joint Surg Am 2004;86:607–620) Used with permission

appears to be a simple undertaking, case–control studies present a number of methodological challenges that must be solved for the study results to be valid. Case–control studies frequently suffer from information biases and unbiased recall failure.

Cross-Sectional Study

Cross-sectional studies simultaneously ascertain exposure to risk factors and the presence of the disorder in question in a population sampled without regard to the presence of either. This type of sampling is sometimes called naturalistic sampling. In contrast to a cohort study, which follows subjects over time and ascertains incidence, a cross-sectional study ascertains conditions present at the moment of study, that is, prevalence of the disorder. The estimates of relative risk derived from cross-sectional studies are therefore estimates of prevalence relative risk. Cross-sectional or survey studies are often undertaken because, unlike case–control studies, they require few a priori decisions regarding subject selection and, unlike cohort studies, it is not necessary to wait for the study outcome. These advantages are offset by their susceptibility to some of the problems of both cohort and case–control studies listed above, and resultant decreased strength of evidence.

Assess the Methods of Each Study

Strength and weakness of the data should be assessed. Another way of looking at this is to consider "threats to validity." There are three general reasons why the results of a study may not be valid: chance, bias, and confounding.
- Chance
  Chance is defined as the absence of any cause of events that can be predicted, understood, or controlled (Houghton Miffline Company, 2011). Measurements made during research are nearly always subject to random variation. Determining whether findings are due to chance is a key feature of statistical analysis. The best way to avoid error due to random variation is to ensure that sample size is adequate (O'Keefe, Huffman, & Bukata, 2008).

  The *confidence interval* is a plus-or-minus figure, and is often reported as the margin of error. For example, with a confidence interval of 5, if 40 % of a sample picks an answer, one can be reasonably certain that between 35 and 45 % (40±5) of the entire study population would have

selected the same answer if asked that question. The *confidence level* is the statistical likelihood that a variable lies within the confidence interval, expressed as a percentage, such as, 50, 95, or 99 %. It measures the reliability of a statistical result, and indicates the probability the result is correct. The 95 % confidence level is most commonly used. The sample size required depends on the confidence and confidence level (Creative Research Systems, 2011). For a given confidence level, the larger the sample size, the smaller your confidence interval, and the more certain one can be that the results truly reflect the entire population.

- Bias
  While chance is due to random variation, bias is caused by systematic variation. A systematic error in the selection of study subjects, disease or condition, outcome measures, or data analysis will lead to inaccurate results. The numerous types of bias can be broadly divided into three categories delineated below.
  - *Selection bias*. The selection of individuals for a sample or their allocation to groups may produce a sample not representative of the entire population. Random selection and allocation prevent this type of bias.
  - *Measurement bias*. Measurement of a condition or outcomes may be inaccurate due to inaccuracy in criteria for diagnosis of the disease or a measurement instrument, or bias in the expectations of study participants or researchers. The latter may be addressed by blinding both the subjects and investigators.
  - *Analysis bias*. The protection against bias afforded by randomization will be maintained only if subjects remain in the study group to which they were allocated and complete follow-up. Participants who change groups, withdraw from the study, or are lost to follow-up may be systematically different from those who complete the study. Analysis bias can be reduced by maximizing follow-up.

  There are also, other factors to be considered in determining the strength studies.

- Accuracy and precision
  Random variation (chance) leads to imprecise results, while systematic variation (bias) leads to inaccurate results. For example, a large observational study involving thousands of individuals may produce results that are precise (specific), but not accurate. A small, high quality randomized controlled trial may produce results that are accurate but not precise.

- Confounding
  This is similar to bias and is often confused. Bias involves error in the measurement of a variable, whereas confounding involves error in the interpretation of what may be an accurate measurement. A classic example of confounding is to interpret the finding that people who carry matches are more likely to develop lung cancer as a cause-and-effect relationship. Smoking is the confounder. Smokers are more likely to carry matches and also more likely to develop lung cancer. Confounding occurs when the study results can be explained by a factor unnecessary to the hypothesis being tested. A potential confounding factor must be associated with both the disorder in question and the hypothesized cause. That is to say, the study group with the disorder having the confounding exposure must be different from the study group without the disorder but also have the confounding exposure. Additionally, it is necessary that the study group of those with the hypothesized cause and confounding exposure are different from the group not exposed to the hypothesized cause but have the confounding factor. For example, a study finding an association between low job satisfaction and occupational carpal tunnel syndrome could be confounded by the physical requirements of work. Specifically, those individuals whose work involves repetitive high force activities in a cold environment are at greater risk of developing carpal tunnel syndrome, but this group also has a lower job satisfaction than individuals employed in less physically demanding occupations. So, which factor is actually responsible for the risk of occupational carpal tunnel syndrome?

Potential confounding factors can be eliminated in the design of the study by restricted or matched sampling or, in the data analysis phase, by stratified or multivariate analysis, for example. In the study just described, if statistical analyses controlled for the physical requirements of work, or if the researchers conducted an exploratory analysis and found no association between job satisfaction and the physical requirements of work, the confounding could be reduced or eliminated. In experimental studies, potential confounding should be eliminated by truly random assignment of individuals to the treatment and control groups. Comparability of the groups should be confirmed by presentation of the baseline characteristics of each group upon entry to the study. Thus, confounding invalidates a study as a test of the null hypothesis, and its results cannot be taken as evidence of causality. Lack of generalizability, unlike confounding, does not invalidate a study's results, but merely restricts inference to populations similar to those under study.

Because of its importance, we will summarize the concept of confounders.

- What is a confounder?
  A confounder is any factor that is prognostically linked to the disease of interest and unevenly distributed between the study groups. A factor is NOT a confounder if it lies on the causal pathway between the elements of interest. For example, the relationship between diet and coronary heart disease may be explained by serum cholesterol level. Elevated cholesterol is not a confounder because it may be the causal link between diet and coronary heart disease.
- Known confounders
  Dealing with confounding is relatively easy if the likely confounders are known. The data could be stratified. For example, in the study on diet and coronary heart disease, smokers and nonsmokers could be analyzed separately, or one could use statistical techniques to adjust for confounding.
- Unknown confounders
  Allocating for unknown confounders is much more difficult. There is always a risk that an apparent association between a risk factor and the disease is being mediated by an unknown confounder. This is particularly true of observational studies where selection is not randomized. Again, randomization suggests that both known and unknown confounders will be approximately evenly distributed between two study groups.

Ascertain Statistical Significance

Research is typically conducted on a sample of individuals (the study group) from a target population. Therefore, the results of such studies are estimates of the true means, proportions, relative risks, etc. of the populations from which the sample groups were selected. The precision of a study estimate of the population value is described by the *standard error of estimate*. The standard error (SE) is the square root of the ratio of the variance (s^2), or variability of the measurement in the sample, to the number of subjects (N) in the study, as expressed by the formula $SE_{mean} = \sqrt{(s^2/N)}$.

The statistical hypothesis test evaluates the null hypothesis: The study results observed occurred because of sampling error when there was no true association in the population from which the sample of study subjects was derived. If the observed association is large enough that this kind of error is improbable, the null hypothesis is rejected. The investigators then accept the alternative hypothesis, that the observed estimates of relative risk or association reflect the true situation in the sampled population. By convention, the cutoff for rejecting the null hypothesis is usually set at 0.05. Thus, if the probability (p value) that the observed results are due to sampling error is <0.05, the null hypothesis is rejected. The results are declared statistically significant because within an acceptable margin of error, they probably did not occur by chance. The larger the observed association, relative to the underlying variability of the outcome being measured, the more likely it will be statistically significant.

Table 22.5 Testing hypothesis

Study conclusions	Risk not different	Risk are different	
Risk not different	Correction conclusion	Type II error (probability = β)	Leads to PPV
Risk are different	Type I error (probability = α)	Correction conclusion	Leads to NPV
	Leads to sensitivity	Leads to specificity	

A *Type I error*, also known as a false positive, occurs when a statistical hypothesis test rejects the null hypothesis, even though it is true. For example, the null hypothesis states a new treatment is no better than an older, less expensive one. A Type I error would occur if researchers concluded the new treatment produced outcomes when in reality there was no difference. The rate of Type I errors is represented by the Greek letter alpha (α), and usually equals the significance level of a test. Relatedly, a Type II error, also known as a false negative, occurs when a statistical hypothesis test fails to reject a false null hypothesis. Continuing the prior example, a Type II error would occur if researchers concluded that there was no difference in outcomes between the new and old treatments when, in fact, the new treatment was more effective. False negative results are often due to too small sample sizes. The rate of Type II error is represented by the Greek letter beta (β).

The probability that a study will be able to correctly reject the null hypothesis when it is false, i.e., correctly detect an association when there is one in the population, is called *Statistical Power* $(1 - \beta)$. Table 22.5, illustrates the different conditions and possible results of a statistical hypothesis test.

In the planning phase of research, investigators should determine how strong an association (how large an estimated relative risk or how big a difference between treatments) would be statistically significant. Because a valid study requires that it be a true test of the research hypothesis, it is important to design it so the study has sufficient statistically power to detect a statistically significant association. The larger the sample size, the more power the statistical test has to detect associations. In other words, as expected differences or relative risks get smaller, the number of subjects studied must increase to have adequate statistically power to test the hypothesis. With very large sample sizes, it is possible to declare trivial associations statistically significant. When studies with small sample sizes report results that are not statistically significant, they should also report how large an association would have been required to detect it. One should also evaluate whether the observed difference and its upper confidence limit, although not statistically significant, are clinically significant. Conversely, when studies with large numbers of subjects report statistically significant results, then one needs to determine if the differences are clinically significant or not.

Other Important Terms

An *independent variable* is one whose value determines that of other variables. A *dependent variable* is that which is observed in a study, and whose changes are determined by the presence and extent of one or more independent variables. A *continuous variable* describes numerical information that can be any value within a range. Continuous data may be *parametric* or *nonparametric*. Parametric data may be represented in a distribution explained by a single mathematical equation. Nonparametric data are not represented by a single mathematical equation, and does not belong to any particular distribution. *Relative risk* (RR) estimates the magnitude of the association between the exposure and disease of interest. RR equals the incidence of disease in exposed subjects divided by that in unexposed individuals. A RR of 1.0 means the disease incidence rates are identical in the exposed and unexposed study groups. A RR >1.0 suggests a positive association (increased incidence in exposed group), while a RR of <1.0 suggests a negative or inverse association (decreased incidence in the exposed study group). Finally an *odds ratio* (OR) is used in retrospective case–control studies where incidence cannot be determined. OR equals the probability (odds) of being exposed in the group with the disease divided by the probability of exposure those without the disease.

Statistical tests of inference require assumptions about the data type and distribution. Examples of statistical tests were previously listed in Table 22.4.

It should also be noted that disease detection and correct diagnosis depend on the sensitivity and specificity of tests. A test that yields a positive result when the disease is present is called a *true positive*. A positive test result when the disease is not present is a *false positive*. A negative result when the disease is not present is a *true negative*, whereas a negative result when the disease is present is a *false negative*. The positive predictive value (PPV) of a test is the probability the patient has the disease when the test result is positive, specifically the number of true positives (TP) divided by the sum of true positives and false positives (FP). So, PPV=TP/(TP+FP). It can also be described as PPV = [(prevalence)(sensitivity)]/[(prevalence)(sensitivity) + (1 − prevalence)(1 − specificity)]. *Negative predictive value* (NPV) of a test is the probability the patient does not have the disease when the test result is negative, specifically the number of true negatives (TN) divided by the sum of true negatives and false negatives (FN). NPV = TN/(TN + FN). It can also be calculated as NPV = [(specificity)(1 − prevalence)]/[(specificity)(1 − prevalence) + (1 − sensitivity)(prevalence)]. Disease prevalence affects the PPV. Also note that PPV is not intrinsic to the test. Figure 22.4 summarizes some of the above review.

Conclusions About the Degree of Causal Association

Strength of evidence of causation in epidemiological studies can be combined using a point value to suggest an association between a risk factor and a disease or condition as very strong evidence, strong evidence, some evidence, or insufficient evidence (Melhorn & Hegmann, 2008). Additional details on this methodology are available in *Guides to the Evaluation of Disease and Injury Causation* (Editors

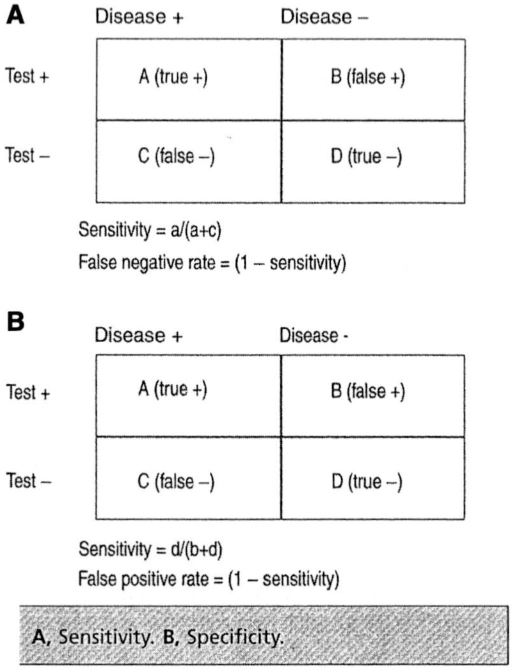

Fig. 22.4 Sensitivity and specificity. —R.J. O'Keefe, G.R. Huffman, and S.V. Bukata. Orthopaedic Research: Clinical Epidemiology and Biostatistics. In: Orthopaedic Knowledge Update, edited by J. S. Fischgrund, Chicago, IL: American Academy of Orthopaedic Surgeons, 2008, p. 173–185. Used with permission..

A

	Disease +	Disease −
Test +	A (true +)	B (false +)
Test −	C (false −)	D (true −)

Sensitivity = a/(a+c)
False negative rate = (1 − sensitivity)

B

	Disease +	Disease −
Test +	A (true +)	B (false +)
Test −	C (false −)	D (true −)

Sensitivity = d/(b+d)
False positive rate = (1 − sensitivity)

A, Sensitivity. B, Specificity.

Melhorn & Ackerman), Chapter 4 Methodology or can be downloaded from www.ctdmap.com/downloadsinfo/29101.aspx. This method is in the public domain and may be copied and used if appropriate acknowledgment is used.

Additional reading:

Users' Guide to Medical Literature by Gordon Guyatt and Drummond Rennie (editors) AMA Publication ISBN 1-57947-191-9.

Guides to the Evaluation of Disease and Injury Causation J. Mark Melhorn and William E. Ackerman (editors) AMA Press ISBN 978-1-57947-945-9.

Consideration of Evidence of Exposure

How does the evaluator take the general epidemiological data and apply this information to the specifics of the individual in question regarding causation? Occasionally, occupational data will be presented for each relevant job or duty. The following information would be helpful: the identification of risk factor(s); and data from industrial hygiene studies, especially any that indicates the magnitude of worker exposure. With regard to occupational disease, there is no generally accepted medical definition of *aggravation*. However, for workers' compensation, aggravation of a disease or impairment may be defined as any occupational occurrence, act, or exposure that permanently worsens, intensifies, or increases the severity of any preexisting physical or mental problem. The existence of a condition before exposure does not necessarily mean before employment. Furthermore, an individual may experience multiple exposures, while working for different employers having different workers' compensation insurance carriers. An example may be helpful.

A 35 year old man has worked as a chain saw logger for the past 15 years, and complains of a 10 year history of numbness in both hands and digits. History, physical examination, and nerve conduction study by a physician reveal bilateral carpal tunnel syndrome. A judge decided his condition was compensable under the current state's workers' compensation system and asked for an apportionment of the medical condition. During his 15 years of employment, he has worked for three different companies. The last employer changed insurance carriers 1 month before he filed the workers' compensation claim.

Apportionment

Workers' compensation boards in all jurisdictions are faced with an expanding challenge in the management of occupational disease claims. In some cases, there are multiple risk factors, with multifactorial causation, and the resultant need to clarify the contribution of each risk factor to the condition in question in order to apportion liability and financial costs. The process of adjudicating workers' compensation claims depends on the applicable statue, but may involve differentiation between occupational and nonoccupational causes of disease and injury. Although, in practice, this can be exceedingly difficult and, in some cases, impossible, establishing causation and *apportionment* are integral parts of the philosophy of workers' compensation. Apportionment by cause is the estimation in an individual case of the relative contribution of several risk factors or potential causal exposures to the disease. In the tort system, the equivalent concept is apportionment of harm (meaning responsibility for causing harm). However, because workers' compensation is a no-fault insurance system, assignment of blame or responsibility is generally irrelevant.

Apportionment by cause must be performed on the individual case, which may vary from the population as a whole. However, often apportionment cannot be determined with certainty, and epidemiologic data may then be used to derive an estimate of the relative contribution of risk factors in an individual claim. The estimate for apportionment of causation derived should not to be confused with the apportionment of its social derivative, disability. The benefits of fair and accurate apportionment, when it can be done, are obvious. Adjudication may be simpler, quicker, cheaper, and fairer to injured workers, employers, and insurers. Workers might be encouraged to take responsibility for their own health. The financial resources conserved could be used to increase benefits and/or decrease premium costs. Fiscal exposure for healthcare, disability, and impairment would be more fairly divided among payers, such as provincial or private healthcare plans, Social Security, or workers' compensation.

Although apportionment is an attractive option for adjudication in workers' compensation, it has many drawbacks and uncertainties (Melhorn, Andersson, & Mandell, 2001). The single greatest obstacle to apportionment is the availability of data and limitations on the methodology of assessment of relative contribution to the disease. Therefore, apportionment is often consensus- or expert-derived. Workers' compensation carriers are generally required to accept medical claims in their totality if a component of the disease is work-related. However, there is a wide variation between jurisdictions regarding how big the occupational component must be before the condition is accepted as work-related. A minimal contribution from work, even one iota, is sufficient to render a disease compensable in some states, whereas others require that work have been the substantial factor, the major contributing cause, or a significant contributor. Furthermore, defining what constitutes a substantial, significant, or even minimal component is often difficult. Apportionment is more often applied to the permanent impairment rating which is often used to determine a financial settlement in workers' compensation claims.

A special case of apportionment is *presumption*, of which there are two types. A *rebuttable presumption* shifts the burden of proof to the part against which the presumption applies (Melhorn, Ackerman, Glass, & Deitz, 2008). In law, it is an assumption by a court that is considered true until a preponderance of evidence disproves (rebuts) the presumption. For example, in criminal law a defendant is presumed innocent until proven guilty. On the other hand, an *irrebuttable presumption* establishes a legal conclusion which may be based, not on scientific or other evidence, but the desire for social justice and fair play (Melhorn et al., 2008). Judges and legislatures have the power to substitute convenience for science. For example, an irrebuttable presumption may be made based on information (not necessarily facts) that, because most cases of a disease in persons with a given job can be attributed to an occupational risk factor, any such case for which a claim is filed will be accepted as work-related. Many presumptions are written into law, often without good evidence, such as the presumption in California that heart disease among firefighters and police officers is work-related (Brooks & Melhorn, 2008). Others are "scheduled," or designated on lists. Presumption logically requires both strong evidence of an association and a risk that is at least doubled. A simple association can be accepted at a >50 % level of certainty for the occupational group overall at whatever degree of association, but a simple association is not the same as presumption. A presumption involves the same degree of certainty, but an actual proportion of the disease (attributable fraction) compatible with at least 50 % in the occupation or population overall. At such a high frequency, it is statistically likely that, for any one individual drawn from that population (and submitting a claim) who presents with the disease or outcome in question, the occupational cause would be the risk factor. For example, firefighters have a much higher risk of kidney cancer than the general population, but their risk of lung cancer is only elevated by about 50 % (Guidotti, 2006). One can justify a presumption for kidney cancer, but not for lung cancer. Any firefighter with kidney cancer probably would not have been at risk if he or she were not in that occupation.

Presumptions can also be legislated in the opposite fashion. For example, in 1996, the Virginia Supreme Court said that carpal tunnel syndrome does not make a person eligible for workers' compensation benefits even if a doctor insists the problem is work-related (Carrico, 1996). The effects of increasing requests for apportionment are reflected in the definition use in the AMA *Guides to the*

Evaluation of Permanent Impairment. The 4th edition, published in 1995, states apportionment is an estimate of the degree to which each of various occupational or nonoccupational factors may have caused or contributed to a particular impairment. For each alleged factor, two criteria must be met: the alleged factor could have caused or contributed to the impairment, which is a medical determination; and in the case in question, the factor did cause or contribute to the impairment, which usually is a nonmedical determination. The physician's analysis and explanation of causation is significant. The 5th edition, published in 2001, defines apportionment as the distribution or allocation of causation among multiple factors that caused or significantly contributed to the injury or disease and existing impairment. The 6th edition, published in 2008, states apportionment is the extent to which each of two or more probable causes are found responsible for an effect (injury, disease, impairment, etc.). Only probable causes (at least more probable than not) are included. Hence, the first step in apportionment is scientifically-based causation analysis. Second, one must allocate responsibility among the probable causes and select apportionment percentages consistent with the medical literature and facts of the case in question. Arbitrary, merely opinion-based unscientific apportionment estimates which are nothing more than speculations, must be avoided. When appropriate, the current impairment can also be apportioned to more than one cause.

The Changing Threshold for Workers' Compensation Compensability

Kansas House Bill No. 2134, An Act Concerning Workers Compensation, passed May 15 2011 as Law 04-18-2011 (Kansas House, 2011) defines "Prevailing Factor Test" which, under this test, the employee's work must be the "prevailing factor" for the injury to be considered work-compensable. If it is not the "prevailing factor," the injury is not compensable. It is believed that, under this standard, employers will have a defense against preexisting degenerative conditions not "caused" by work. In other words, employees will no longer have a compensable claim for an aggravation, acceleration, or intensification of a preexisting condition. Unfortunately, the legislature did not define "prevailing factor" and did not reference the Missouri law which could then have been used as "case law" to assist in the definition. Consensus opinion is that the need to define "prevailing factor" will increase ligation and the associated costs.

The Missouri Workers' Compensation Law was passed and is in Chapter 287 of the Revised Statutes of Missouri (www.moga.mo.gov/statutes/statutes.htm). The workers' compensation statute is the law that controls the rights and obligations of employees and employers when employees are injured at work. It outlines that the work injury must be the "prevailing factor" in causing the level of disability and medical condition for it to be compensable. Medical causation is needed in cases where a traumatic incident occurred or where an employee is injured by an occupational exposure or repetitive motion that is part of their employment. The prevailing factor is the primary factor in comparison to any other possible factor resulting in the employee's injury.

Oklahoma SB878 (Oklahoma, 2011), passed May 2011, now requires "major cause provision" (which has yet to be defined by case law but will probably be "contributes more than half"), and the requirement that objective medical evidence be determined by the Daubert criteria (Fed Rule of Evidence 702) for the opinion of "major cause."

Consideration of Validity of Testimony

Nonprofessional persons cannot be expected to collect and evaluate all the information needed in causation analysis. In most cases, physicians will provide testimony on test results, medical conditions, and causation using information from industrial hygienists regarding exposure and epidemiologists regarding epidemiologic data. These professionals must consider all pertinent facts and literature in their area of expertise to present an accurate and meaningful evaluation of the available data. The judicial entity requesting the information or determination may have additional expert witness criteria, such as the *Daubert Standard*, to be discussed next. The law of evidence governs whether testimony (e.g., oral or written statements, such as an affidavit), exhibits (e.g., physical objects), and other documentary material are admissible (i.e., allowed to be considered by the trier of fact, whether a judge or jury) in a judicial or administrative proceeding (e.g., a court of law) and how they are used (Wikipedia, 2011). In 1993, the United States Supreme Court established the current standards for the admissibility of scientific evidence in Daubert v. Merrell Dow Pharmaceuticals, Inc. This decision abolished the old "general acceptance" test and set forth a new standard which focuses on the reliability and relevance of scientific testimony. In evaluating scientific testimony, trial courts will consider the following factors: whether the research was conducted prior to the litigation; whether it has been tested; whether it had been subjected to peer review and publication; whether there is a known or potential rate of error; whether the research was conducted according to fixed standards; and whether the technique is generally accepted in the scientific community (Klimek, 2001).

The Daubert Standard is a rule of evidence regarding the admissibility of expert witness testimony during United States federal legal proceedings (Wikipedia, 2011). Pursuant to this standard, a party may raise a Daubert motion, which is a special case of motion in limine raised before or during trial to exclude the presentation of unqualified evidence to the jury. A motion in limine (Latin: "at the threshold") is one made before the start of a trial requesting that the judge rule that certain evidence may, or may not, be introduced at trial. This is done in judge's chambers, or in open court with the jury absent. Usually, it is used to shield the jury from evidence that may be inadmissible and/or unfairly prejudicial. Nonexpert witnesses are permitted to testify only about facts they observed and not their opinions about these facts. An expert (professional) witness is one who, by virtue of education, training, skill, or experience, has knowledge and expertise in a scientific, technical, or other subject beyond that of a layperson, sufficient that others may rely upon his or her opinion on evidence and facts within the expert's area of expertise, even though he or she was not present at the time of the injury, exposure, or other event. In law and religion, testimony is a solemn attestation as to the truth of a matter, and the expert opinion is intended to educate the judge and/or jury on a specialized subject matter, thereby assisting the trier of fact.

Consideration of Other Relevant Factors

Medical causation is drawn from science, while in-law causation is the connection between a wrongful act and harm (Melhorn et al., 2008). Work-relatedness, in the context of occupational injury or illness, involves concepts of both medical and legal causation. The two may be mutually exclusive. Definitions of medical causation and legal causation arise from different sources—one from science and the other from desire for social justice (with origins in religion). This has been described by Melhorn as "the difference between why things are as they are, and how things ought to be" (Melhorn, 2008). For physicians treating injured or ill workers, understanding the differences between the two concepts is essential. Legal causation requires two components: cause in fact, and proximate (or "legal") cause (Melhorn et al., 2008). Both must be present. If the occurrence of one event brings about another, the former can be considered the cause in fact of the latter. This is true regardless of the number of events involved. Causal fallacies exist, and at least one of them requires attention here. The *"post hoc ergo propter hoc"* fallacy occurs when "after this, therefore because of this" reasoning leads to the assertion of a causal relationship. It is a fallacy to conclude that the occurrence of one event followed by a second necessarily demonstrates a causal relationship between the two. The second part of the legal analysis of causation seeks to determine whether two events that are linked in fact should also be linked in law. This second test, proximate or legal cause, is whether the two events are so closely linked that liability should be attached or assigned to the first event that produced the harm, the second event. The most common legal threshold is "that the injury arises, in whole or in significant part, out of or in the course and scope of employment" (Melhorn, 2000). The most common level of legal certainty needed to establish medical causation in the legal system is "more likely than not" or "more probable than not" (Melhorn, 2007).

Evaluation and Conclusions

What is cause? What is risk? Precisely which factors predominate in the etiology of work-related medical conditions? Answering the following seven questions will allow the examiner to answer the question of causation based on the best available science.
1. Has a disease condition been clearly established?
2. Has it been shown that the disease can result from the suspected agent(s)?
3. Has exposure to the agent been demonstrated (by work history, sampling data, expert opinion)?
4. Has exposure to the agent been shown to be of sufficient degree and/or duration to result in the disease condition (by scientific literature, epidemiologic studies, special sampling, and replication of work conditions)?
5. Has nonoccupational exposure to the agent been ruled out as a causative factor (or a contributory factor—suggesting apportionment)?
6. Have all special circumstances been considered?
7. Has the burden of proof been met—did the evidence prove that the disease resulted from, or was aggravated by, conditions at work?

Summary and Conclusions

What is cause?: An event, condition, or characteristic that plays an essential role in producing an occurrence of a disease.
What is causation?: The act of causing.
  What is causality?: The relationship of cause to effect.
  What is risk?: Risk is the probability that an event will occur if exposed to the risk factor.
  What is a causal relationship?: Inferring a causal relationship requires an understanding of epidemiology. Epidemiology is a science and, as such, adopts the scientific standard of proof, generally greater than or equal to 95 % probability. However, civil litigation and adjudication hold to a different standard. How does one apply epidemiology when the standard is "more likely than not?" In general, this requires a relative risk odds ratio of greater than 2.0. Unfortunately, there is often insufficient data to establish a relative risk. Furthermore, conventional statistics for risk derived from epidemiologic research are generalized and may be difficult to apply to an individual case since the individual's experience in the future may not be similar to the group studied.
  Health and medical knowledge are essential to the resolution of disputes in legal and administrative applications (such as workers' compensation) and provide essential input into public policy decisions. There are no socially agreed-upon rules for the application of this knowledge except in the law. On a practical level, the legal system lacks the capacity to evaluate the validity of knowledge as evidence and therefore relies heavily on expert opinion.

The determination of causation may be extremely difficult in contested claims. Honest differences of opinion are common when the "facts" may be subject to different interpretations. The practitioner faced with the above questions should know the legal definitions that determine whether the condition is considered work-related. Although the condition may not meet the medical criteria of causation, the condition may meet the legal threshold and therefore be considered work-compensable. Considerable judgment is necessary when data are lacking or incomplete. It is important to assemble complete information in a logical and orderly sequence wherever possible to ensure a correct and an equitable decision regarding causation.

Future Directions

Epidemiology will play a major role in future research into the ever broadening field of health care and public health concerns. This is evidenced by the exponential growth of research studies claiming to be "evidence-based." This growth will not occur without challenges and opportunities, examples are listed below.

The challenges include:
1. The growing threats to data access. Unfortunately, many recent attempts to place limits on the collection and storage of personal health data have completely ignored the potential impact of the proposed legislation on epidemiological medical research. This has been less of a problem for Europe which has "universal health care" and government data available for research. For perspective, remember, this limitation of health care data access is occurring at a time when "social data" is commonly share by individuals on the internet on multiple Web sites.
2. The challenge of communicating epidemiologic data to the public. Often the science is not intuitive and therefore can be difficult to accept.
3. The intensifying interface between epidemiologic data and the legal and legislative system.

The opportunities include:
1. Scientific answers or insight to specific questions.
2. The ability to convert global data to the individual and thereby reduce individual risk factors.
3. The potential to maintain and improve the public and thereby reduce impairment and disability while improving the quality of life for the individual.

Acknowledgment Funding was provided by The Hand Center, Wichita, KS. As part of the grant/funding, the information contained becomes public domain after 3 years from the date of publication and the authors retain the right to use these materials in continuing education programs and future works without additional written approval as long as appropriate acknowledgement of the source is provided.

References

Houghton Miffline Company. (2011). *The American Heritage Dictionary of the English Language, Fifth Edition* published by Houghton Miffline Company.

Melhorn, J. M., & Ackerman, W. E. (2008). Introduction. In J. M. Melhorn & W. E. Ackerman (Eds.), *Guides to the evaluation of disease and injury causation* (pp. 1–12). Chicago, IL: AMA.

Sackett, D. L., Rosenberg, W. M., Gray, J. A., Haynes, R. B., & Richardson, W. S. (1996). Evidence based medicine: What it is and what it isn't. *BMJ, 312*, 71–72.

Hadler, N. M. (1999). *Occupational musculoskeletal disorders* (2nd ed.). Philadelphia, PA: Lippincott Williams & Wilkins.

Melhorn, J. M., & Melhorn, J. M. (1999). Epidemiology of musculoskeletal disorders and workplace factors. In T. G. Mayer, R. J. Gatchel, P. B. Polatin, T. G. Mayer, R. J. Gatchel, & P. B. Polatin (Eds.), *Occupational musculoskeletal disorders function, outcomes, and evidence* (pp. 225–266). Philadelphia, PA: Lippincott, Williams & Wilkins.

Melhorn, J. M., & Hegmann, K. T. (2008). Methodology. In J. M. Melhorn & W. E. Ackerman (Eds.), *Guides to the evaluation of disease and injury causation* (pp. 47–60). Chicago, IL: AMA.

AMA. (2001). *Guides to the evaluation of permanent impairment* (5th ed.). Chicago, IL: American Medical Association.

Melhorn, J. M. (1998). Upper-extremity cumulative trauma disorders on workers in aircraft manufacturing [Letter, Response] Upper extremities cumulative trauma disorders. *Journal of Occupational and Environmental Medicine, 40*, 12–15.

CtdMAP. (2006). *Workplace activity risk factors. CtdMAP occupational health intervention technologies*. Wichita, KS: MAP Managers.

U.S. Department of Labor. (2006a). *OSHA occupational safety and health administration home page*. Washington, DC: U.S. Department of Labor.

Talmage, J. B., & Melhorn, J. M. (2005). *A physician's guide to return to work*. Chicago, IL: AMA.

Oakley C. (2011). Sunny side up. *Parade Jul 30, 2011 issue*.

Melhorn, J. M. (2008). *Causation of occupational injuries: Fact & fiction*. Fairmount, MA: SEAK, Inc.

U.S. Department of Health, Education, and Welfare. (1979). *A guide to the work relatedness of disease (Revised). DHEW (NIOSH) Publication No. 79-116 ed.*. Washington, DC: U.S. Department of Health, Education, and Welfare.

Hegmann, K. T., & Oostema, S. J. (2008). Causal associations and determination of work-relatedness. In J. M. Melhorn & W. E. Ackerman (Eds.), *Guides to the evaluation of disease and injury causation* (pp. 33–46). Chicago, IL: AMA.

U.S. Department of Labor. (2006b). *Workplace injuries and illnesses in 2005*. Washington, DC: Bureau of Labor Statistics.

O'Keefe, R. J., Huffman, G. R., & Bukata, S. V. (2008). Orthopaedic research: Clinical epidemiology and biostatistics. In J. S. Fischgrund (Ed.), *Orthopaedic knowledge update* (9th ed., pp. 173–185). Chicago, IL: American Academy of Orthopaedic Surgeons.

Creative research systems (2011) Sample Size Calculator by Creative Research Systems accessed at http://www.survey-system.com on August 2011.

Melhorn, J. M., Andersson, G. B. J., & Mandell, P. J. (2001). Determining impairment and disability. In J. M. Melhorn (Ed.), *The fundamentals of workers' compensation* (pp. 13–21). Rosemont, IL: American Academy of Orthopaedic Surgeons.

Melhorn, J. M., Ackerman, W. E., Glass, L. S., & Deitz, D. C. (2008). Understanding work-relatedness. In J. M. Melhorn & W. E. Ackerman (Eds.), *Guides to the evaluation of disease and injury causation* (pp. 13–32). Chicago, IL: AMA.

Brooks, C. N., & Melhorn, J. M. (2008). Apportionment. In J. M. Melhorn & W. E. Ackerman (Eds.), *Guides to the evaluation of disease and injury causation* (pp. 61–72). Chicago, IL: AMA.

Guidotti, T. L. (2006). Evidence-based medical dispute resolution. In S. L. Demeter & G. B. J. Andersson (Eds.), *Disability evaluation* (2nd ed., pp. 86–94). St. Louis, MO: Mosby.

Carrico, H. L. (1996). Virginia declares carpal tunnel not a job injury. *Occupational Health Management*, 79–80 Vol 60, issue july.

Kansas House. (2011). *Kansas House Bill No. 2134 an act concerning workers compensation*. Topeka, KS: Kansas State Legislature.

Oklahoma. (2011). *Oklahoma SB878 enrolled May 2011 Workers Compensation*.

Wikipedia (2011). *Wikipedia the free encyclopedia*.

Klimek, E. H. (2001). *or4936 Klimek References*.

Melhorn, J. M. (2000). Identifying risk in the workplace and management of musculoskeletal disorders. *Tenth annual national workers' compensation and occupational medicine seminar*. Falmouth, MA: SEAK, Inc., pp. 11–30.

Melhorn, J. M. (2007, November/December). Understanding causation: An example using carpal tunnel syndrome. *AMA Guides Newsletter*, 5–9.

Program Evaluation of Prevention and Intervention Methods

23

Richard C. Robinson, John P. Garofalo, and Pamela Behnk

Overview

As Americans continue to grow ever sicker from chronic illnesses, such as heart disease, cancer, and stroke, the need for comprehensive interventions has also grown (Kung, Hoyert, Xu, & Murphy, 2008). An estimated 70% of deaths each year are attributable to chronic illness, with heart disease, cancer, and stroke accounting for 50% of those deaths (Kung et al., 2008). Americans spend a large majority of their time in the workplace and, as can be seen in other chapters of this Handbook, that fact has made occupational settings an ideal place for prevention and health intervention programs for many years (Haskell & Blair, 1980). However, the effectiveness of these programs has to be measured and evaluated if they are to survive. The importance of *program evaluation*, therefore, cannot be underestimated. The purview of *program evaluation* exists within the social sciences, but also within the private business sector and governmental programs. In fact, The Health Communication Unit at the University of Toronto (2007) goes as far as to define a program as follows: "…any group of related complementary activities intended to achieve specific outcomes or results. For example, community gardens, shopping skill classes and health cooking demonstrations…" (p. 5). Furthermore, they define

---

R.C. Robinson, Ph.D. (✉)
The University of Texas Southwestern Medical Center at Dallas,
5323 Harry Hines Blvd, Dallas, Texas 75390, USA
e-mail: richard.robinson11@gmail.com

John P. Garofalo, PhD
Associate Chair and Associate Professor
Washington State University
14204 NE Salmon Creek Ave
VCLS208
Vancouver, WA 98686

Pamela Behnk, MPH
University of Kansas School of Medicine
1010 North Kansas
Witchita, KS 67214

Table 23.1 Importance of evaluating health promotion programs (Valente, 2002)

- Improves chance of developing an effective program
- Allows researchers and organizations to understand the effect of intervention
- Evaluation plan encourages planners to establish clear goals
- Allows researchers and organizations to understand how a program worked
- Information from evaluation can be used for future planning
- Provides an opportunity for research on human behavior

a program evaluation as, "…the systematic gathering, analysis and reporting of data about a program to assist decision making" (p. 6).

Program evaluation consists of a trajectory of methods for collecting, assessing, and evaluating outcomes of interventions; in this case, applied in the workplace to improve health and wellness (Valente, 2002). *Program evaluation* allows interventions that prove ineffectual, or deliver results through unsustainable costs, to be modified or eliminated. In essence, *program evaluation* makes good programs stronger and bad programs crumble. Table 23.1 provides a summary of the benefits of *program evaluation*.

Research Methods/Concepts

Federal agencies played an instrumental role in developing the concept of program evaluation by applying the scientific method to evaluate the outcomes of educational and public health initiatives (Rossi & Freeman, 1993). Shadish, Cook, and Leviton (1991) described the three stages that program evaluation has undergone since World War II. The *first stage* emphasized a stringent application of the scientific method to program evaluation. The *second stage* focused on the inherent barriers and limitations to program evaluation, using a traditional scientific approach and emphasized the development of other methodologies. An emphasis was placed on more observational and informal methods of assessment, but these methods were not without structure. The final, and current, *third stage* attempted to synthesize the first two stages by employing multiple theories and techniques, as well as considering the context of the program (Shadish et al., 1991). For instance, empirically-sound research designs and valid outcome measures remain useful in this third stage, but an appreciation for stakeholder feedback has been seen as crucial for the successful implementation of health promotion programs.

Valente (2002) cogently describes the difficulty with research design in program evaluation: "The central challenge to designing studies is that they must be rigorous enough to make conclusions about program impact, yet face constraints of time, resources, program staff, and the willingness and protection of human subjects" (p. 88). For a program to be effective, a change in perception, attitude, knowledge, behavior, or health outcome must occur. Research designs are intended to provide evidence for "causality" (Henry, 2010). In the area of occupational health psychology, an evaluator wants to demonstrate that a program caused, or contributed to, a positive health-related change (Valente, 2002).

As mentioned, historically, rigorous quantitative research methods were employed for program evaluation. *Quantitative* research involves the systematic examination of an independent variable upon a dependent variable or variables (Creswell, 2003). For instance, when attempting to decrease heart disease, a health intervention may randomize individuals into health and unhealthy diets (independent variable) and a measure of heart disease would be the dependent variable. It is understandable how practical limitations of a purely quantitative approach led to the development and use of qualitative methodology in program evaluation. *Qualitative* methods are frequently used in the social sciences, but are often poorly understood by business organizations (Denzin & Lincoln, 2000). A qualitative approach relies upon more naturalistic and less structured data-gathering techniques, but does not lack systematic observation and coding (Creswell, 2003). Involvement of the stakeholders through the widely-used qualitative methods of interviews or focus groups at the initial, middle, and end-phases of program evaluation increases the likelihood of acceptance and positive results (Bryson & Patton, 2010). Unfortunately, focus groups and interviews, if haphazardly applied, face the risk of collecting information in an unsystematic way, and the results will offer limited value (Holliday, 2007).

Differences exist between program evaluation and other traditional forms of research in the social sciences. In addition to understanding differences between qualitative and quantitative research, an understanding of research methods in general is necessary to understand the complexities of program evaluation. First, a distinction must be made between *efficacy* and *effectiveness* studies. An intervention is said to be "efficacious" if it produces desired results within the context of a controlled environment in which error variance is minimized. The term "effectiveness" refers to the implementation of an intervention in a real-world environment. However, systematic controls are in place within an effectiveness trial, but the ability to control extraneous variables is minimal when compared to an efficacy trial. As can be seen, program evaluation is more accurately viewed as an effectiveness trial rather than a process that leads to the determination of efficacy (Hallfors et al., 2006). In other words, the general evaluation of the efficacy and effectiveness of interventions in the workplace relies on systematic observation and quantitative, as well as qualitative, research, and analytic methods.

Study validity is defined as the accuracy of the evaluation of the program's impact. A further distinction can be made between external and internal validity. *External validity* is closely tied to the concept of "generalizability." A study is determined to be externally valid and generalizable if it can be applied to a larger population. Generalizability is determined by the context of the intervention and the sample drawn upon for the evaluation (Valente, 2002). For instance, a program to improve sleep hygiene among a large, culturally diverse sample of United States (US) based factory employees would likely be generalizable to other factory shift workers in the United States. An intervention that targets Laotian immigrants, while important, would not be considered as generalizable and would have lower external validity. A study's *internal validity* refers to a researcher's confidence that the study evaluates what it intended to evaluate, and that the results are accurate in that the manipulation of one variable resulted in the change of another. Numerous threats to internal validity exist. First, uncontrollable events or factors can threaten internal validity (Valente, 2002). By definition, these factors cannot be controlled, only monitored and statistically controlled for at a later date. For instance, a program designed to change attitudes regarding stress management may be impacted by the sudden departure of a manager. Maturation or development of a subject over time is another potential threat to internal validity, but is typically of minimal concern for health promotion interventions, which are usually limited in time (Valente, 2002).

Internal threats to validity that can be controlled include *testing*, *instrumentation*, and *sensitization*. With regard to *testing*, certain practice effects can impact the true meaning of test results when testing is given in a repeated manner. Alternative forms of a test or use of a control groups diminish this threat to validity. *Instrumentation* or the impact that observation has on outcomes should be considered (Valente, 2002). Asking employees to simply record the number of vegetables they eat daily may be overly burdensome and unreliable and can impact the results. Finally, *sensitization* is the impact that the knowledge of the intervention will have on the baseline findings (Valente, 2002). For example, if a company announces a program to increase exercise, an employee may begin to exercise prior to the program.

Statistics Used in Program Evaluation

The application and correct use of statistics can appear to be a daunting task for many organizations. However, the understanding of basic statistical concepts can strengthen the validity of the program evaluation. Furthermore, a facile understanding of methodology and research design will allow program evaluators to more effectively communicate and generate support from stakeholders and managers as to the importance of certain program elements necessary for program evaluation. Therefore, a brief review of basic statistical concepts is warranted. Consideration of the data generated by the program evaluation influences the choice of statistics required. Data can be classified into two broad groups—categorical or continuous. Categorical variables have a limited number of response values, while continuous variables have a potentially infinite number of values and equal intervals between values. Further classification of data results in three broad categories of levels of measurement: nominal, ordinal, and interval-ratio. Nominal data are categorical and values are unordered or equivalent, such as gender or race. Ordinal data are also categorical, but values exist in relationship with one another in a ranked fashion (Stevens, 1946). For instance, an ordinal scale may ask employees how often they exercise with choices as *never, rarely, sometimes,* and *often*. Demographic data may also be ordinal, such as socioeconomic status, which does not reflect a greater inherent value, but a rank-order value within the dataset. Finally, interval-ratio data are continuous, ranked, and equidistant between values. Although there is a distinction between interval and ratio data, (i.e., ratio data have a true-zero and interval data do not), statistically they are treated essentially the same (Valente, 2002).

Choice of independent and dependent variables also influence the selection of statistics to be utilized. As mentioned, independent variables are considered to influence the dependent variable and be uninfluenced by other variables (Given, 2008). Program evaluators *hypothesize* that a program (the independent variable) will result in a change in an attitude, knowledge, or behavior in a health outcome (the dependent variable). More sophisticated hypotheses regarding behavior change also take into consideration moderating and mediating variables. *Moderating variables* weaken/strengthen the relationship between independent and dependent variables (Baron & Kenny, 1986). Gym membership (moderating variable) may strengthen the relationship between a work program to increase exercise (independent variable) and number of hours exercising a week (dependent variable.) *Mediating variables* play a more direct role in the relationship between the independent and dependent variables, and typically occur between the independent and dependent variable (Baron & Kenny, 1986). In our last example, gym membership existed prior to the independent variable. An onsite gym added to our fictitious organization, as part of a campaign to increase exercise, would be considered a mediating variable. The measures used to assess outcomes (dependent variables) must also be psychometrically-sound in order to begin to establish causality and impact. A measure is *reliable* if it consistently measures what it intends to measure. Although related to accuracy, reliability is synonymous with consistency. Validity refers to the extent that a measure assesses what it purports to assess. Validity is impacted by a measures reliability, or consistency, but is best understood as being synonymous with accuracy (Lambert et al., 1996).

In addition to reliability and validity, the concepts of *sensitivity* and *specificity* should also be considered. A measure is *sensitive* if it accurately measures the proportion of people who are positive for a state or trait. For instance, a measure of anxiety correctly identifies all those who are anxious. *Specificity* refers to the percentage of negatives that are accurately identified and, in our example, a measure with high specificity would have a low number of individuals who would score in the anxious range when not anxious. As can be seen, there is a balance between sensitivity and specific for most measures (Altman & Bland, 1994).

Types of Program Evaluation

Prior to implementation of an occupational health intervention, an assessment period is needed to increase the likelihood that an impactful and cost-effective intervention can be implemented. Rossi, Lipsey, and Freeman (2004) highlight the different types of assessment that can be offered at different stages of the

Fig. 23.1 Types of program evaluation

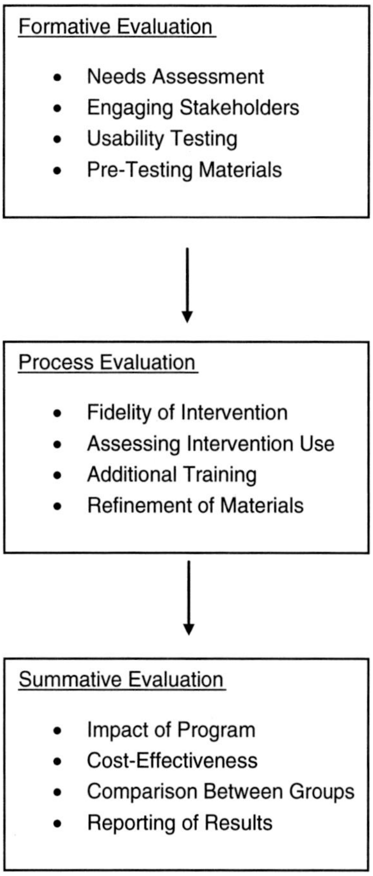

Formative Evaluation
- Needs Assessment
- Engaging Stakeholders
- Usability Testing
- Pre-Testing Materials

Process Evaluation
- Fidelity of Intervention
- Assessing Intervention Use
- Additional Training
- Refinement of Materials

Summative Evaluation
- Impact of Program
- Cost-Effectiveness
- Comparison Between Groups
- Reporting of Results

process. These assessments include the following: (1) evaluating the program's cost and efficiency; (2) evaluating the program's outcome; (3) examining the fidelity of program implementation; (4) assessment of program design and theory; and (5) assessment of the need for the program. Jacobs (2003) developed a similar *Five-Tiered Approach* to program evaluation. The five tiers are described as incremental in this approach, and include the following: (1) needs assessment; (2) monitoring and accountability; (3) quality review and program clarification; (4) achieving outcomes; and (5) establishing impact.

Potter (2006) also describes three paradigms regarding program evaluation, which the author refers to as the *positivist, interpretive,* and *critical-emancipatory* approaches. The *positivist approach* appears to be the most common, and relies on objective results derived primarily from quantitative data. Unfortunately, while ideal in the mind of many social scientists, the reality of the workplace and its naturally occurring obstacles may limit the effective implementation of a positivist design. The *interpretive approach* relies heavily on the perspectives and expectation of the stakeholders involved in the intervention. Emphasis is placed on more observation and information derived from qualitative methods, such as focus groups. The *critical-emancipatory approach* is a more ideologically-driven approach to program evaluation, and it is heavily influenced by social activism (Potter, 2006). The positivist and interpretive approaches appear most suited for program evaluation in occupational health promotion programs.

Program evaluation, within both the social sciences and business consulting literatures, are replete with steps and guidelines for its development. Traditionally, program evaluation can be separated into formative evaluations, process evaluations, and summative evaluations (Valente, 2002; see Fig. 23.1). Many organizations equate the summative evaluation with program evaluation, or evaluating the impact of a program once it has been completed. As will be seen, program evaluation is critical in all stages of the planning, implementation, and summation of a program.

Formative Evaluation

Formative evaluation refers to the evaluation of steps needed to undertake an effective program. Information is needed regarding the population, work-environment, and culture in which a program will be enacted. A review of the literature on the topic of interest, and a careful consideration of the theoretical basis for the intervention, are also required. Furthermore, area experts and potential stakeholders should be convened to further assess the problem area to be addressed in order to ensure that the problem is significant (Bartholomew, Parcel, Kok, & Gottlieb, 2001). Often, a needs assessment is undertaken, as well as pretesting of materials, tests, or technologies to be employed (Itschuld & Kumar, 2010). Programs fail for many reasons, but beginning with the end in mind, and understanding that program evaluation is needed from start to finish, increases the chance of program success. In other words, an appreciation for the trajectory of program evaluation and the questions that are being asked from this process are paramount.

Planning and implementation of health interventions in the workplace should include program evaluation at the outset. Decisions about the need for a program, scope of a problem, and ways in which a problem will be addressed should include consideration of evaluation along each step of the way. An exciting idea to improve health, but lacking a systematic way to assess the outcomes, is doomed to a relatively brief life-span. Furthermore, adding outcomes after an intervention has been planned or implemented will either interfere with the potential effectiveness of the program or provide uninterpretable outcomes.

Formative evaluations often rely heavily on qualitative, rather than quantitative, methods and techniques (Huhta, 2010). As discussed, qualitative data are gathered in a more observational, naturalistic, and unstructured way compared to quantitative data. As one would imagine, understanding the needs and wishes of the employees is critical to designing an effective program, and can often be more effectively gathered through qualitative techniques such as in-depth interviews and focus groups (Armenakis, Harris, & Mossholder, 1993). Although less structured than quantitative research, qualitative research requires a systematic approach. Miles and Huberman (1994) argue for the following criteria of strong qualitative research:

- *Systematic*. The same processes and procedures are delineated and applied to multiple settings.
- *Iterative*. Data collection is ongoing and builds upon previous findings.
- *Flexible*. Adaptations are made as more information is collected.
- *Triangulate*. Use of multiple (at least three) methods of measurement.

As part of a formative evaluation, the overall impact of the assessment needs to be addressed and entails answering the question, "What impact will have intervention have on the population of interest?" For instance, improving sleep and decreasing fatigue among emergency responders has the potential of having a significant overall impact. However, decreasing the risk of skin cancer among shift workers, while an important health outcome, would be judged to have a relatively low overall impact.

Although many observational and interview formats are considered qualitative research, *focus groups* provide a unique opportunity to efficiently collect reliable, valid, qualitative data. In a classic work, Merton and colleagues (1956) developed the basic principles of focus-group testing that still guides researchers today. An ideal focus group should be comprised of 8–10 similar participants, and potential attrition (cancelation by participants) requires recruiting more subjects than needed (Krueger, 1994). A trained moderator asks scripted, but open-ended, questions in a manner that allows for the open exchange of ideas, values, and preferences for the potential program. The results of the focus

Table 23.2 Common theoretical models for behavior change in program evaluation

- Diffusion of innovations (Ryan & Gross 1943)
- Hierarchy of effects and steps to behavior change (McGuire, 1989)
- Stages of change and the transtheoretical model (Prochaska, Diclemente, & Norcross 1992)
- Theory of reasoned action (Fishbein & Ajzen 1975)
- Social learning theory and self-efficacy (Bandura, 1986)
- Health belief model (Rosenstock, 1974)

group discussion can be recorded, transcribed, and coded through various techniques (e.g., word-clouds or concept mapping). Valente (2002), though, describes three ways in which focus groups may produce misleading information. First, the group discussion may be overly influenced by a subset of individuals. Second, individuals may be reluctant to diverge from what is considered normal. Finally, the topic may lack interest to the participants and, thus, limited information is gathered (Valente, 2002).

Over the last two decades, interactive, internet-based interventions have been developed to improve health in occupational settings (Chumley-Jones, Dobbie, & Alfor, 2002). Multiple platforms have evolved through the last two decades, from CD-ROMS, to Web-based to applications for smart phones. However, with technologically advanced health promotion delivery systems, come additional opportunities for formative evaluations. Specifically, *usability testing* has developed as a qualitative technique to evaluate the design, ease-of-use, and acceptability of internet-based interventions, as well as other computer interfaces and devices with potential end-users (Nielsen, 1994). Usability testing is atheoretical and, thus, a *black box* evaluation that focuses upon efficiency, accuracy, recall, and emotional response (Nielsen, 1994). Virzi (1992) established that a sample size of 5 users was sufficient to identify potential problems with usability during initial stages of testing.

The theoretical basis of the intervention is needed to assess whether the intervention is achieving results in the manner expected. For example, simple educational methods to improve health and wellness have underperformed compared to other models, such as the *Health Belief Model* (Nutbeam, 2000). The theoretical model also guides the determination of outcomes to be chosen to examine. However, certain health outcomes occur distally and are affected by a variety of factors. A clear, sound theoretical model allows for the assessment of shorter-term moderating and mediator variables. For instance, exercise has been shown to decrease risk of heart disease. Prospectively following an intervention over a long period of time in order to determine which employees have a lower incidence of heart disease is impractical, but assessing degree of knowledge and increased exercise are noteworthy outcomes.

In the past, interventionists would design a program and independent researchers would evaluate its impact and effectiveness (Valente, 2002). This process helped to promote evaluator objectivity, and is referred to as *black box evaluation* (Chen & Rossi, 1983). This approach appears to have been largely abandoned and replaced by *theory-based evaluations* (Valente, 2002). Valente (2002) goes so far as to argue that theory influences all aspects of program evaluation. Table 23.2 provides a list of major theories commonly used in program evaluation today.

Finally, ethical, legal, and regulatory constraints are considered during formative evaluations. In the workplace, the right to privacy requires significant consideration, and difficulties with mental illness, substance abuse, and sexually transmitted diseases are protected information for most employees. For instance, evaluating a work-based program to decrease heavy drinking among employees not directly involved in public safety presents many challenges. Not only may employees be reluctant to report problems or changes in drinking, but such programs, if poorly designed, may violate an employee's rights.

Within formative evaluations, the impact of the evaluation is not being directly studied, but the study validity is increased if input from potential end-user is sought and the methods of program deployment are examined. Without this input, interventions may be less than engaging, poorly focused, or potentially offensive. Usability testing decreases the chances of user frustration and poor adherence with overly complex or flawed technologically-based interventions.

Process Evaluation

Process evaluation focuses upon programs that are already proceeding, and examines the activities needed to run the program. Furthermore, process evaluation tracks those who are being served and the manner in which they are being served. The theoretical basis of the intervention is needed to assess whether the intervention is achieving results in the manner expected. Valente (2002) argues that programs should engage in process evaluations, but disproportionately focus on whether a program demonstrates success, rather than *why* it may be successful. Therefore, process evaluation increases internal study validity, and ensures that changes in outcome measures can be attributed to the success or failure of the program.

Adherence to the original intent and implementation of the program is referred to as *fidelity* (Valente, 2002). During the process evaluation phase, assessment as to whether the critical components of the intervention are being administered effectively and uniformly is necessary (Saksvik, Nytro, Dahl-Jorgensen, & Mikkelsen, 2002). Furthermore, technical issues related to interventions using Web-based or other technologically-laden platforms are assessed. Although usability of the platform should have occurred previously, additional changes may be required to ensure effective implementation. Additional training may be required for the individuals implementing the program. As noted, health promotion programs involve the development of protocols for implementation and, over time, a drift from the original protocol can be detected and corrected with process evaluation. Changes in the staff implementing a specific protocol and the passage of time can both threaten the fidelity of a program. Finally, a second variable relevant to process evaluation is *dose*. Dose refers to the amount of exposure an employee has to a program, as well as to the intensity (Valente, 2002). For example, a Web-based intervention can be evaluated by frequency of visits by end-users.

Challenges to Process Evaluation

Saksvik and colleagues (2002) performed one of the few studies to evaluate the implementation process of a health promotion program. Griffiths (1999) argues that the reason for the sparse body of literature addressing process evaluation is that most of the studies suffer from poor research design and other methodological limitations. Lipsey and Cordray (2000) also state, from a review of the literature, that intervention programs are inherently difficult to implement. Unfortunately, there is also often a lack of attention to implementing process evaluations in different environments (i.e., inattention to generalizability). Further hampering effective evaluations are differences among researchers, bot theoretically and methodologically (Burke, 1993; Colarelli, 1998; Handy, 1988). Social and political realities may also hamper process evaluations, and a growing emphasis has been on *contextualization*, which emphasizes the importance of understanding the uniqueness of the political and social realities within organizations. Lastly, a lack of detailed description of the intervention program can often hamper implementation efforts (Lipsey & Cordray, 2000). Given these barriers to process evaluation, a more "nuanced" definition is required. Nytrø, Saksvik, Mikkelsen, Bohle, and Quinlan (2000) define process as, "…individual, collective or management perceptions and actions in implementing any intervention and their influence of the overall result of the intervention." (p. 214). This definition takes into account the contextual challenges and differences within and among organizations than more traditional definitions of process evaluation. Finally, Sechrest and Figueredo (1993) indicated that organizations have focused on formative over process evaluations. As previously discussed, formative evaluations have often been atheoretical *block box* evaluations, rather than evaluation of programs with a strong theoretical basis. As a result, the lack of theoretical basis during formative evaluations has hampered subsequent process and summative evaluations (Saksvik et al., 2002).

Despite their systematic nature, theory-driven approaches have been stressed in this present Chapter. Colarelli (1998) describes an evolutionary perspective on process evaluation that merits consideration. The evolutionary perspective accurately brings attention to the fact that, within organizations, change processes are often founded on simple heuristics, ecological adaptations, and tacit knowledge rather than on empirical analyses or clear, reasoned rationales (Colarelli, 1998). Although these factors are important to remember, the methodological considerations to successfully employ a process evaluation from an evolutionary perspective remain elusive (Saksvik et al., 2002). However, Saksvik and colleagues (2002) approached their study on process evaluation from a systematic, theory driven approach while remaining mindful of evolutionary perspective factors by evaluating, "…not only at the shop floor level, but also in a larger context including external constraints from, for example, company top managers or working life partners." (p. 39).

Several researchers have outlined and recommended ways to investigate *formal* process factors. Below, Goldenhar, Lamontagne, Katz, Heaney, and Landsbergis (2001) provide a summary of five important approaches:

"1. Gathering background information about former experiences with similar interventions in the organization and finding out what is known about the selected intervention (e.g., application, efficacy, effectiveness and quality of existing data).
2. Securing stakeholder involvement and multidisciplinary teams in the evaluation.
3. Choosing methods and designs that are related to scientific quality, but also address the practical limitations.
4. Identifying implementation barriers, (e.g. changes in participation and factors that confound the measurement).
5. Communicating findings to both participants and non-participants who are capable of taking action based on the results." (Saksvik et al., 2002; p. 40)

Evaluating formal process factors is a necessary step that is enhanced by gathering information about informal process factors. Informal factors, related to the culture and politics of an organization, while difficult to glean, represent variables that can doom a program, or program evaluation, as well as offer the opportunity for enhanced success. Below, are Nytrø and colleagues' (2000) suggestions of *informal* processes to be considered when developing a process evaluation.

"1) The establishment of social climate of learning from failure. This means that one has to move beyond merely building on experience if there appear to be strong cultural, social and psychological prohibitions against learning from failure.
2) Providing opportunities for multi-level participation and negotiation in the design of interventions. The pitfall here is often that the managers and employees may agree on the objective of the intervention (e.g. lower absenteeism), but have different ideas about what may constitute important methods for achieving this objective. Possible differences in organizational perceptions have to be uncovered early in the project.
3) Facilitating cultural maturity. If an organization is immature in its competence to manage change processes, it may be appropriate to pursue greater empowerment of employees. It may be hard to gain insight into such a lack of cultural maturity, and an acceptance that this trait characterizes the organization in question is not always easily archived.
4) Reaching awareness of tacit and informal organizational behavior that undermines the objectives of interventions. Both managers and workers can invent their own idiosyncratic justifications for change from their own locally-bound perspectives. Novel insights may create frustrations, suspicions, and norms that, unintentionally, support dysfunctional behavior.
5) Monitoring readiness to change. It is wise to monitor employee attitudes towards the interventions introduced in order to asses to what degree these interventions are appreciated as appropriate means towards alleviating the current state of affairs. The most fit and healthy employees may find the intervention attractive, while those who really need to change health behaviors may find it stigmatizing and unattractive.
6) Defining roles and responsibilities before and during the intervention period. Different projects of change require different roles from both employers' and employees' representatives and different roles require dif-

ferent skills. One person (the manager) cannot (and should not) hold all roles at the same time. In practice, however, this is often the case." (Saksvik et al., 2002; p. 40–41)

Finally, Saksvik and colleagues (2002) blended formal and informal process factors and identified the following key process factors:

"1) The ability to learn from failure and to motivate participants.
2) Multi-level participation and negotiation, and differences in organizational perception.
3) Insight into tacit informational organizational behavior.
4) Clarification of roles and responsibilities, especially the role of middle management.
5) Competing projects and reorganization." (Saksvik et al., 2002; p. 41)

Summative Evaluation

Summative evaluation can be used to assess programs that are underway, but typically focus on programs that have been completed in order to assess their impact. The summative evaluation, sometimes referred to as impact evaluations, examines whether the stated goals and objectives of the program were met (Henry, 2010). Determining the impact of the intervention is one of the more challenging aspects of effective program evaluation. Without a sound program evaluation design, it will be impossible to determine if the intervention does generate positive outcomes and what factors in concert with the intervention contribute to these positive outcomes. Although several study designs exist that are commonly used for summative evaluations, comparison groups, and randomized control trials are two of the more rigorous designs. A randomized control trial, the "gold standard" of research, is considered the most robust and empirically-sound study design to establish *causality* (the key factor in summative evaluations). Randomization is the best manner in which to ensure that the makeup of the control and experimental groups are essentially the same, and therefore minimize the risk of *selection bias*, where selection into a group influences the outcomes (Torgerson, Torgerson, & Taylor, 2010). A common constraint among program evaluations involves voluntary participation in a program. It may be that individuals who voluntarily participate in a weight loss program are more interested in their health than those who do not. A comparison between those groups is likely to result in confounded results, which will greatly limit the interpretation of the findings. Moreover, failure to control for potential confounds will limit the generalizability of the results.

Although the randomized clinical trial represents the most rigorous design, there are several inherent threats to randomization, as well as practical limitations within the workplace setting. *Contamination* occurs when control participants are exposed to, or contaminated by, the interventions intended for the treatment condition. It is often difficult to blind all research staff to an individual's group assignment; thus, researchers can inadvertently bias the outcomes. Furthermore, control condition employees may be exposed to educational or interventions designed for the treatment condition (Torgerson et al., 2010). For example, Kwak and colleagues (2006) developed a weight prevention program and used prompts at elevators at worksites to promote taking the stairs. As can be seen, it would be impossible to randomize in this example. Finally, *attrition* (i.e., loss of participants prior to conclusion of the program evaluation) and participants' preference for a specific group allocation, also threaten randomized control trials (Torgerson et al., 2010). Even though they are less rigorous than randomized control trials, comparison groups offer practical benefits, and will likely fit more easily into the demands of an operational organization. Furthermore, several comparison designs exist that may minimize, but not eliminate, selection bias (Henry, 2010). The *naïve design* is the simplest of the comparison designs, and it compares those who participated, or could have participated, in a program to those who did not. A *basic value-added design* relies on pre-intervention outcome measures and employs a regression analysis, thus statistically controlling for pre-intervention differences in outcome measures. Similarly, a *regression-adjusted covariate design* also utilizes a regression analysis and controls for multiple known variables that may bias group membership and, ultimately, outcomes (Henry, 2010). There is significant evidence that this approach reduces, but does not eliminate, bias (Glazerman, Levy, & Meyers, 2003). Finally, *matched designs* involve matching members in each group on several variables, such as age, race, marital status, that are known, or suspected, to impact the outcome. Unfortunately, matching becomes challenging without a large sample size, and unforeseen relevant participant characteristics may bias the outcomes in unpredicted ways (Henry, 2010).

The number of participants needed to provide meaningful results can be determined by one of several methods, including the tabulation method, the proportion method, the differences method, and power analysis. The simplest, *tabulation method*, requires at least 50 participants for each level of an independent variable. However, this method is likely best suited for very initial assessments of sample size. The most rigorous and most common manner to determine sample size is a power analysis. Cohen (1977) defines power analysis as: "The power of a statistical test of a null hypothesis is the probability that it will lead to the rejection of the null hypothesis, i.e., the probability that it will result in the conclusion that the phenomenon exists." (p. 4). Three elements are needed to calculate sample size using a power analysis: (a) effect size; (b) significance level; and (c) power (an estimate of confidence in results).

Cost-Effectiveness

Cost-effectiveness analysis (CEA) and cost-benefit analysis (CBA) are important elements of program evaluation that can occur during formative, process, or summative evaluations. Cellini and Kee (2010) define cost-effectiveness analysis as, "…a technique that relates the costs of a program to its key outcomes or benefits." (p. 536). Cost-benefit analysis, in comparison, takes into account the ratio of costs compared to all of the program's benefits. The formula for calculating a cost-effective ratio is as follows:

$$\text{Cost - Effectiveness Ratio} = \frac{\text{Total Costs}}{\text{Units of Effectiveness}}$$

The units of effectiveness are typically a clear outcome of the program (e.g., number of hours at the gym or percentage of weight decrease). In program evaluations to promote health change, distal health outcomes, such as decreases in the number of employees with heart disease, would likely be outside the scope of a cost-effective analysis. However, assessment of mediating variables, such as hours a week engaged in physical activity, would be extremely relevant (Cellini & Kee, 2010).

With cost-benefit analysis, researchers weigh costs against the estimated value of the program benefits. Costs are subtracted from benefits in this analysis in order to obtain the *net benefits*. A further distinction can be made between financial cost analyses and social cost analyses. Within social cost analyses, both financial and nonfinancial costs and benefits are taken into account. A social cost analysis considers negative outcomes of a program a budgetary cost, and positive impacts as budgetary benefits (Cellini & Kee, 2010). The formula for cost-benefit analysis is presented below:

$$\text{Net Benefits} = \text{Total Benefits} - \text{Total Costs}$$

Despite the apparent simplicity for the formulas to determine cost-effectiveness and cost-benefit, these analyses require multiple assumptions and estimations. However, Cellini and Kee

(2010) adapted a ten step process from Boardman, Greenberg, Vining, and Weimer (2006) that take program evaluators through the needed components of a cost-effective or cost-benefit analysis. The outline of the steps that can be use in both cost-effectiveness and cost-benefit analysis are presented below:

> "1. Set the framework for the analysis.
> 2. Decide whose costs and benefits should be recognized.
> 3. Identify and categorize costs and benefits.
> 4. Project costs and benefits of the life of the program, if applicable.
> 5. Monetize costs.
> 6. Quantify benefits in terms of units of effectiveness (for CEA), or monetize benefits (for CBA).
> 7. Discount costs and benefits to obtain present values.
> 8. Compute a cost-effectiveness ratio or net present value.
> 9. Perform sensitivity analysis.
> 10. Make recommendation when appropriate." (p. 537–538)

Additional Barriers to Program Evaluation

Frequent, real-world limitations to program evaluation include money and time constraints, as well as the methodological and ethical limitations imposed when evaluating outcomes in workplace settings (Bamberger, Rugh, Church, & Fort, 2004). In fact, most programs do not allocate a budget for program evaluation at the outset (Bamberger et al., 2004). Therefore, flexibility and relying on both qualitative and quantitative methods, as well as statistically controlling for internal and external threats to study validity, are often the norm for program evaluation. This, though, should not deter researchers from evaluating the impact of the program. Jacobs (Jacobs, 2003) developed the *Five-Tiered Approach* of program evaluation to manage monetary, data, and time constraints by condensing and simplifying key elements of formative, process, and summative evaluations. It assumes that many program evaluations will not be fully considered or budgeted by the parties interested in developing a program. Therefore, it takes an incremental and iterative approach where program evaluators can build upon previous tiers if possible. The approach could be accurately described as a blend between qualitative and quantitative methods, and techniques that emphasize the unique aspects of an organization and population. The five tiers include the following:

- *Needs Assessment.* The needs assessment is conducted in a contextual manner and gathers information about the problem to be addressed, in the organization to be addressed, and about previous success with similar interventions.
- *Monitoring and Accountability.* At this tier, emphasis is placed on accurate description of clients, services, personnel, and costs.
- *Quality Review and Program Clarification.* Three standards are assessed at this tier, including model standards (or how a program is intended to operate), program-generated standards (process evaluation based on goals set by the program rather than external source), and participant-generated standards (the preferences of the participants).
- *Achieving Outcomes.* Emphasis at this tier is typically on short-term objectives, using systematic, but less than rigorous, designs to provide useful and interesting results to interested parties.
- *Establishing Impact.* This tier is reserved for large, well-funded summative research with rigorous research designs.

Although the above *Five-Tiered Approach* may appear less than ideal from a methodological perspective, it provides a path to develop useful data under common time, data, and budget constraints.

Intervention Mapping

Kwak et al., 2006 described an exceptional example of program evaluation that implemented a theory-driven and systematic approach to a health intervention regarding the prevention of weight gain. Prior to program development and design, the researchers conducted a needs assessment (i.e., identified physical and behavioral factors related to weight gain via a thorough review of the literature). Based on the needs assessment, the following clear objective was defined: "...to decrease overall dietary energy intake and/or increase daily routine physical activity in order to prevent weight gain in young adults aged 25–40 years." (p. 349). The investigator applied a five step *Intervention Mapping* protocol that relies on theoretical, empirical, and practical factors to develop a health promotion program (Bartholomew et al., 2001). This study's use of *Intervention Mapping* provides an excellent example and roadmap for how program evaluation can be incorporated at each stage of program development, implementation, and summation.

Step 1. Defining Proximal Program Objectives. Based upon the needs assessment, researchers translate risk behaviors into behaviors demonstrated to impact the outcome. In the example of the Kwak and colleagues (2006) study, specific behaviors were identified as targets to increase energy expenditure (walking and biking to work and increase physical activity at work), as well as decreasing calories (decreasing portion size, replacing high-fat foods with low-calorie food, increase fiber, and replacement of saturated fats by unsaturated fats). Furthermore, these goals were further broken down into performance objectives, such as increased knowledge of fiber-rich food, self-assessment of fiber intake, etc. Lastly, in Step 1, relevant, alterable personal, and environmental determinants are selected. In the Kwak et al. (2006) study, knowledge, awareness, preferences, attitude, self-efficacy, and habit were identified as personal determinants. Environmental determinants included availability of health food, management commitment and support, social support, company rules, and cost of healthier food.

Step 2. Selecting Theory-based Intervention Methods and Practical Strategies. From an intervention mapping perspective, after personal and environmental determinants are selected, an appropriate theoretical model of behavior change is selected. For this program, multiple theories were applied, including self-monitoring, tailoring, and skills training. Next, practical strategies based on the above steps and sub-steps were developed, such as launching a Web site for information and interactive features for tailoring, placing cues at elevators to increase use of stairs, and making healthier food choices available in vending machines.

Step 3. Producing and Integrating the Intervention Program. This step refers to the development of the intervention protocol, materials, and measurements. The program developed consisted of two components: an individual and worksite component. With regard to the individual component, materials produced included: information on an individual's body mass index, fat percentage, and waist size; a kit which contained a pedometer, waist circumference tape, and calorie guide; and a Web site and CD-ROM. The main environmental components were developed into a handbook with clear guidelines for employers.

Step 4. Adoption and Implementation Plan. In this stage, it is often useful to develop a plan that facilitates interactions among the program developers and end users. In this study, working groups were formed that contained employees who could influence the stated objectives, such as cafeteria workers and managers, and members of the research team. Also, materials were pretested to assess usability and acceptability, thus increasing the chances for success.

Step 5. Monitoring and Evaluation Plan. Within *Intervention Mapping*, process evaluation and summative evaluation are the last steps of the Map. The previous four steps could accurately be described as a formative evaluation. It is important to note that all five steps are developed prior to the initiation of the actual program. For the process evaluation, the researchers selected Roger's *Diffusion of Innovations Model* and examined intervention delivery, participation, comprehension, satisfaction, level of use, fidelity, and institutionalization. Furthermore, measures of success for the process evaluation were divided into indirect, immediate, and outcome categories. For the summative evaluation, 12 worksites with over 500 participants were utilized, and the researchers employed a nonrandomized pretest multiple posttest control group design. The primary outcome was weight loss, and was collected after the year-long intervention and then another year later. However, other physiological measures, such as waist circumference, were also examined. Thoughts, intentions, and physical activity were evaluated with paper and pencil measures, but 10% of the sample underwent more expensive, but valid, physical performance assessments, such as VO2-max test (Kwak et al., 2006).

As can be seen, this *Intervention Mapping* approach provides a clear, structured method for program evaluation that takes into consideration all of the factors discussed throughout this Chapter. Although this approach is not always be practical or possible, it represents an ideal that could be applied to many health promotion programs in occupational settings.

Summary and Future Directions

As noted throughout this present Handbook, the need for effective interventions in the workplace is growing (Kung et al., 2008). Program evaluation has undergone several transitions after beginning in the period following World War II. A rigorous method of evaluation of these programs had once been the "gold-standard" for evaluating the impact of interventions. Unfortunately, many rigorous methodologies were impractical, or impossible, to implement in work settings. Worker safety and confidentiality posed barriers for strict intervention protocols, as well as the practical limitations of providing an intervention in an operational worksite. It had been seen as ideal to exclude evaluators from the program design in order to increase evaluator objectiveness. As a result, qualitative methods that allowed the gathering of stakeholder input began to be more widely used in favor of stricter quantitative methods. In most workplace settings, a combination of both quantitative and qualitative methods is required to ensure effective program evaluation while operating within the constraints of a functioning workplace. For instance, in order to evaluate the effectiveness of a weight loss program in the workplace from a quantitative perspective: the sample size of willing participants would need to be large; all participants would be required to participate and randomly assigned to control or experimental condition; and the dependent variable would consist of weight lost. Although ideal from an empirical perspective, this approach cannot realistically be implemented in most work settings.

With regard to program evaluation of workplace interventions, a blended approach is required that utilizes the structure of empirical techniques and is informed by more qualitative methods. As discussed in this Chapter, randomized control trials provide the most rigorous assessment, but comparison designs with statistical control provide a more realistic avenue for inquiry. In addition to the theme of a blended methodological approach being the most value in program evaluation, a second theme was emphasized in this Chapter—namely, that program evaluation is needed from the outset, including during initial planning stages (formative evaluation), during the implementation of the program (process evaluation), and at the conclusion (summative evaluation). As seen in the study by Kwak and colleagues (2006), effective interventions are integrated throughout all stages of program development.

Thus, the goals for program evaluation are complex. The integration of intervention programs in the work setting continues. However, accompanying an evaluation process, it will need to be seamless and organic to the industry being targeted. The aforementioned budgetary woes and the fiscal climate represent major hurdles in utilizing the worksite in implementing potentially health-enhancing prevention programs. The appreciation for the work environment to implement health-behavior interventions is not novel—the solution to overcome the barriers to the implementation and its evaluation require will require the development of novel research/methodological techniques in the future. It should also be noted that, with the staggering and growing healthcare cost in the USA, the federal government is moving towards funding the best ways to design guidelines for treatment that are both beneficial and cost-effective (Lauer & Collins, 2010). This has stimulated the need for more Comparative effectiveness research (CER; Manchikanti, Falco, Boswell, & Hirsch, 2010; Sox, 2010). One vital aspect of CER is the use of cost-effectiveness analysis in order to help objectively document the most cost-effective intervention methods. Thus, approaches such as CEA and CBA (discussed earlier in this Chapter) will be at the forefront of needs for future program evaluation of prevention and intervention methods in the workplace.

References

Altman, D. G., & Bland, J. M. (1994). Diagnostic tests. 1: Sensitivity and specificity. *BMJ: Brittish Medical Journal, 308*(6943), 1552.

Armenakis, A., Harris, S. G., & Mossholder, K. W. (1993). Creating readiness for organizational change. *Human Relations, 46*, 681–703.

Bamberger, M., Rugh, J., Church, M., & Fort, L. (2004). Shoestring evaluation: Designing evaluations under budge, time and data constraints. *American Journal of Evaluation, 25*(1).

Bandura, A. (1986). *Social foundations of thought and action: A social cognitive theory.* Englewood Cliffs, NJ: Prentice-Hall.

Baron, R. M., & Kenny, D. A. (1986). The moderator-mediator variable distinction in social psychology research: Conceptual, strategic, and statistical considerations. *Journal of Personality and Social Psychology, 51*(6), 1173–1182.

Bartholomew, L. K., Parcel, G. S., Kok, G., & Gottlieb, N. H. (2001). *Intervention mapping: Designing theory-evidence-based health promotion programs.* New York: McGraw-Hill.

Boardman, A. A., Greenberg, D. H., Vining, A. R., & Weimer, D. L. (2006). *Cost-benefit analysis: Concepts and practice.* Upper Saddle River, NJ: Prentice Hall.

Bryson, J. M., & Patton, M. Q. (2010). Analyzing and engaging stakeholders. In J. S. Wholey, H. P. Hatry, & K. E. Newcomer (Eds.), *Handbook of practical program evaluation* (3rd ed.). San Francisco, CA: Jossey-Bass.

Burke, R. J. (1993). Organizational-level interventions to reduce occupational stressors. *Work and Stress, 7*, 77–87.

Cellini, S. R., & Kee, J. E. (2010). Cost-effectiveness and cost-benefit-analysis. In J. S. Wholey, H. P. Hatry, & K. E. Newcomer (Eds.), *Handbook of practical program evaluation* (3rd ed.). San Franciscol, CA: Jossey-Bass.

Chen, H. T., & Rossi, P. H. (1983). Evaluation with sense: The theory-driven approach. *Evaluation Review, 7*(3), 283–302.

Chumley-Jones, H. S., Dobbie, A., & Alfor, C. L. (2002). Web-based learning: Sound educational method or hype? A review of the evaluation literature. *Academic Medicine, 77*(10), S86–S93.

Cohen, J. (1977). *Statistical power analysis for the behavioral sciences (Rev ed.).* New York: Academic.

Colarelli, S. M. (1998). Psychological interventions in organizations. An evolutionary perspective. *The American Psychologist, 53*, 1044–1056.

Creswell, J. W. (2003). *Research design: Qualitative, quantitative and mixed method approaches.* Thousand Oaks, CA: Sage.

Denzin, N. K., & Lincoln, Y. S. (2000). *Handbook of qualitative research.* Thousand Oaks, CA: Sage.

Fishbein, M., & Ajzen, I. (1975). *Belief, attitude, intention and behavior: An introduction to theory and research.* Boston: Addison-Wesley.

Given, L. M. (2008). *The Sage encyclopedia of qualitative research methods.* Los Angeles, CA: Sage.

Glazerman, S., Levy, D. M., & Meyers, D. (2003). Nonexperimental versus experimental estimates of earnings impacts. *The Annals of the American Academy of Political and Social Science, 589*, 63–93.

Goldenhar, L. M., Lamontagne, A., Katz, T., Heaney, C., & Landsbergis, P. (2001). The intervention research process in occupational safety and health: An overview from the national occupational research agenda intervention effectiveness team. *Journal of Occupational and Environmental Medicine, 43*, 616–622.

Griffiths, A. (1999). Organizational interventions. Facing the limits of the natural science paradigm. *Scandinavian Journal of Work, Environment and Health, 25*, 589–596.

Hallfors, D., Hyunsan, C., Sanchez, V., Khatapoush, S., Kim, H. M., & Bauer, D. (2006). Efficacy vs defectiveness trial results of an indicated "model" substance abuse program: Implications for public health. *American Journal of Public Health, 96*(12), 2254–2259.

Handy, J. A. (1988). Theoretical and methodological problems within occupational stress and burnout research. *Work and Stress, 41*, 351–369.

Haskell, W. L., & Blair, S. N. (1980). The physical activity component of health promotion in occupational settings. *Public Health Reports, 95*(2).

Henry, G. T. (2010). Comparison group designs. In J. S. Wholey, H. P. Hatry, & K. E. Newcomer (Eds.), *Handbook of practical program evaluation* (3rd ed.). San Francisco, CA: Jossey-Bass.

Holliday, A. R. (2007). *Doing and writing qualitative research* (2nd ed.). London: Sage.

Huhta, A. (2010). Diagnostic and formative assessment. In B. Spolsky & F. M. Hult (Eds.), *The handbook of educational linguistics* (pp. 469–482). Oxford, UK: Blackwell.

Itschuld, J. W., & Kumar, D. D. (2010). *Needs assessment: An overview*. Thousand Oaks, CA: Sage.

Jacobs, F. H. (2003). Child and family program evaluation: Learning to enjoy complexity. *Applied Developmental Science, 7*(2), 62–75.

Krueger, R. A. (1994). *Focus groups: A practical guide for applied research*. Newbury Park, CA: Sage.

Kung, H. C., Hoyert, D. L., Xu, J. Q., & Murphy, S. L. (2008). Deaths: Final data for 2005. *National Vital Statistics Reports, 56*(10).

Kwak, L., Kremers, S. P. J., Werman, A., Visscher, T. L. S., van Baak, M. A., & Burg, J. (2006). The NHF-NRG IN Balance-project: the application of Intervention Mapping in the development, implementation and evaluation of weight gain prevent at worksite. *Obesity Reviews, 8*, 347–361.

Lambert, M. J., Burlingame, G. M., Umphress, V., Hansen, N. B., Vermeersch, D. A., Clouse, G. C., et al. (1996). The reliability and validity of the outcome questionnaire. *Clinical Psychology & Psychotherapy, 3*(4), 249–258.

Lauer, M. S., & Collins, F. S. (2010). Using science to improve the nation's health system. *JAMA: The Journal of the American Medical Association, 303*(21), 2182–2183. doi:10.1001/jama.2010.726.

Lipsey, M. V., & Cordray, D. S. (2000). Evaluation methods for social intervention. *Annual Review of Psychology, 51*, 345–375.

Manchikanti, L., Falco, F. J., Boswell, M. V., & Hirsch, J. A. (2010). Facts, fallacies, and politics of comparative effectiveness research: Part I. Basic considerations. *Pain Physician, 13*(1), E23–E54.

McGuire, W. J. (1989). Theoretical foundations of campaigns. In R. E. Rice & C. K. Atkins (Eds.), *Public communications campaigns* (3rd ed.). Thousand Oaks, CA: Sage.

Merton, R. K., Fiske, M., & Kendall, P. (1956). *The focused interview: A manual of problems & procedures*. Glencoe, IL: Free Press.

Miles, M. B., & Huberman, A. M. (1994). *Qualitative data analysis: An expanded sourcebook*. Newbury Park, CA: Sage.

Nielsen, J. (1994). Heuristic evaluation. In J. Nielsen & R. L. Mack (Eds.), *Usability inspection methods*. New York, NY: John Wiley & Sons.

Nutbeam, D. (2000). Health literacy as a public health goal: A challenge for contemporary health education and communication strategies into the 21st century. *Health Promotion International, 15*(3), 259–267.

Nytrø, K., Saksvik, P. O., Mikkelsen, A., Bohle, P., & Quinlan, M. (2000). An appraisal of key factors in the implementation of occupational stress interventions. *Work and Stress, 14*, 213–225.

Potter, C. (2006). Program evaluation. In K. Durrheim, D. Painter, & M. Terre Blanche (Eds.), *Research in practice: Applied methods for the social sciences* (2nd ed.). Cape Town: UCT Press.

Prochaska, J. O., Diclemente, C. C., & Norcross, J. C. (1992). In search of how people change: Applications to addictive behaviors. *The American Psychologist, 47*, 1102–1114.

Rosenstock, I. M. (1974). Historical origins of the health belief model. *Health Education Monographs, 2*, 328–335.

Rossi, P. H., & Freeman, H. E. (1993). *Evaluation: A systematic approach* (5th ed.). Newbury Park, CA: Sage.

Rossi, P., Lipsey, M. W., & Freeman, H. E. (2004). *Evaluation: A systematic approach* (7th ed.). Thousand Oaks, CA: Sage.

Ryan, R., & Gross, N. (1943). The diffusion of hybrid seed corn in two Iowa communities. *Rural Sociology, 8*, 15–24.

Saksvik, P. O., Nytro, K., Dahl-Jorgensen, C., & Mikkelsen, A. (2002). A process evaluation of individual and organizational occupational stress and health interventions. *Work and Stress, 16*(1), 37–57.

Sechrest, L., & Figueredo, A. J. (1993). Program evaluation. *Annual Review of Psychology, 44*, 645–674.

Shadish, W. R., Cook, T. D., & Leviton, L. C. (1991). *Foundations of program evaluation; Theories of practice*. Newbury Park, CA: Sage.

Sox, H. C. (2010). Comparative effectiveness research: A progress report. *Annals of Internal Medicine, 153*, 469–472.

Stevens, S. S. (1946). On the theory of scales of measurement. *Science, 103*(2684), 677–680.

Torgerson, C. J., Torgerson, D. J., & Taylor, C. A. (2010). Randomized controlled trials and nonrandomized designs. In J. S. Wholey, H. P. Hatry, & K. E. Newcomer (Eds.), *Handbook of practical program evaluation* (3rd ed.). San Francisco, CA: Jossey-Bass.

The Health Communication Unit at the Centre for Health Promotion University of Toronto title: Evaluating Heatlh Promotion Programs Year: 2007

Valente, T. (2002). *Evaluating health promotion programs*. New York: Oxford University Press.

Virzi, R. A. (1992). Refining the test phase of usability evaluation: How many subjects is enough? *Human Factors, 34*(4), 457–468.

Gender and Cultural Considerations in the Workplace

24

Nicolette Lopez, Hollie Pellosmaa, and Pablo Mora

"The challenge posed by the increasing cultural diversity of the U.S. workforce is perhaps the most pressing challenge of our times" (Fine, 1996, p. 499).

The Changing Workplace: An Overview

Rapid and continual changes in technology, and an aggressive and competitive business climate, are often noted as some of the more decisive forces that have directly impacted the modern workplace. Globalization, the "economic interdependence among countries that develops through cross-national flows of goods and services, capital, know-how, and people" (Gelfand, Erez, & Aycan, 2007, p. 481), is another powerful event that has irrevocably altered business and industry. The growing global connection among businesses has had a substantial impact on the people who work in organizations, as many workers are now venturing out on short- and long-term international assignments. Yet, it is important to note that both cross-national and *intra*-national events have influenced today's business environment. For example, while globalization has resulted in more and more international workers joining US organizations, US minority populations in the past decade have significantly increased. According to the 2010 US Census, both the Asian and Latino populations grew a dramatic 43% each since 2000. Moreover, the Department of Labor reports that today's minority labor force (which includes both the employed and unemployed) is made up of 47% women, 15% Latino, 12% African–American, 5% Asian–American, and 15.8% foreign-born workers. Employment projections reported by the Bureau of Labor Statistics (2009) note that, by 2018, the minority labor force will increase considerably (Latinos by 33%, Asian-American by 30%, African-American by 14%, women by 9%), compared to White workers (5.5%). These numbers, along with increases in minority populations, indicate that this cultural shift in the work environment is not simply a temporary situation but rather a progressive pattern that will continue to have an effect on organizations and employees. People who

---

N. Lopez, Ph.D. (✉) • H. Pellosmaa, M.Hu.Serv. • P. Mora, Ph.D.
Department of Psychology, University of Texas at Arlington,
501 S. Nedderman Dr, Box 19528, Arlington, TX 76019, USA
e-mail: nlopez@uta.edu; hollie.pellosmaa@mavs.uta.edu; pmora@uta.edu

R.J. Gatchel and I.Z. Schultz (eds.), *Handbook of Occupational Health and Wellness*,
Handbooks in Health, Work, and Disability, DOI 10.1007/978-1-4614-4839-6_24,
© Springer Science+Business Media New York 2012

represent various countries, ethnicities, and cultures are now, and will continue to be, closely interacting with one another at work.

Many researchers proclaim the enhanced organizational benefits that result from a having diverse workforce, such as increased competitiveness, innovation, and creativity (Chavez & Weisinger, 2008; Fine, 1996; Hobman, Bordia, & Gallois, 2004; Meares, Oetzel, Torres, Derkacs, & Ginossar, 2004). These claims have been received with caution by researchers who warn that simply hiring individuals from diverse backgrounds will not necessarily guarantee that organizations will reap the benefits associated with a diverse workforce (Jayne & Dipboye, 2004; Roberson, 2006). It is the organization's mindset (i.e., its general philosophy that guides specific practices, policies, and procedures) that will be the best indicator of how companies approach this changing work environment (Findler, Wind, & Mor-Barak, 2007; Meares et al., 2004; Mor-Barak & Levin, 2002), and the impact that these changes will have on individual workers. Is workplace diversity a "problem" that organizations must "deal with?" Or, is workplace diversity an opportunity that will give organizations an advantage in an increasingly competitive global market? To answer these questions, organizations must first assess their objectives for establishing diversity[1]. If the decision to increase diversity is based only on legal obligations, the resulting organizational environment will be much different than if the decision is based on the desire to accumulate unique perspectives. In order to fully capitalize on the potential benefits of a diverse workforce, organizations need to shift from a mindset of tolerating differences to one of inclusion where diversity is perceived as a valuable component to organizational effectiveness (Erez, 2011). Altering the organization's mindset in this manner lays the foundation for building a multicultural organization which, in turn, will lead to a healthy work environment.

As organizations continue to employ people from a variety of culturally diverse backgrounds, the effects on behavior at work, including the way in which individuals are treated and the subsequent physical, psychosocial, and emotional effects of that treatment, are likely to be significant. Thus, it is the purpose of this chapter to address the workplace consequences of this demographically shifting US population. What are the organizational objectives in terms of increasing diversity in the workplace? If a diverse workforce contributes to an organization's competitive advantage, why do many organizations struggle to achieve the promised results? This chapter addresses these and other questions in detail and presents a framework that conceptualizes a variety of organizational environments derived from the combination of specific organizational elements. The framework also describes the associated health-related consequences that may potentially result from these various organizational environments. Finally, the chapter ends with a discussion about how organizations can create and promote a healthy, inclusive work environment. The key for organizations will be to develop a shared organizational identity, while simultaneously allowing for individuals to retain their own cultural characteristics. In this sense, true multiculturalism is achieved along with total organizational health.

A Focus on Diversity and Health

One of the recent challenges of occupational health psychology, as noted by Tetrick and Quick (2011), is related to the demographical shifts occurring in the workplace. To the extent that occupational health psychology is still an emerging field (Barling & Griffiths, 2011; Peiró & Tetrick, 2011), issues

---

[1] For purposes of this discussion, we focus on gender, cultural, and ethnic diversity. The authors acknowledge that diversity can be defined using "the entire spectrum of human differences" (Jayne & Dipboye, p. 410) including age, sexual orientation, level of education, physical and/or mental disability, physical appearance, political affiliation, marital status, organizational tenure, job class, personality, socioeconomic status, religious beliefs, or any other characteristic or attribute that differentiates one individual or group from another.

related to organizational demographics can be considered recent challenges; however, organizational problems associated with culture and diversity are certainly not new. Historically, in the USA, women, minorities, and migrant workers have experienced pervasive, flagrant, and even state-sponsored workplace discrimination. The psychosocial, physical, and institutional effects of discrimination are well-documented (Clark, Anderson, Clark, & Williams, 1999; D'Anna, Ponce, & Siegel, 2010; Thompson, 1996; Williams, Yu, Jackson, & Anderson, 1997). In general, perceived discrimination has been shown to impact blood pressure (e.g., Armstead, Lawler, Gorden, Cross, & Gibbons, 1989), perceived stress, anxiety, and depression (e.g., Landrine & Klonoff, 1996; Pascoe & Richman, 2009), psychosocial distress and well-being (Kessler, Michelson, & Williams, 1999), quality of, and access to, health care (Briggance & Burke, 2002), illness and workplace accidents (Gany et al., 2011) and injuries and disease rates on the job (Murray, 2003). Specifically in the workplace, perceived discrimination affects job satisfaction and increases the likelihood of job burnout, job stress, and poor mental health (Roberts, Swanson, & Murphy, 2004). Clearly, the current focus of attention on workplace health and diversity is both urgent and welcomed.

Defining the Constructs

Organizations that implement diversity initiatives, such as training and development programs and hiring strategies, yet struggle to achieve the desired outcomes, may focus on such factors as culture, ethnicity, race, and/or gender to describe or identify potential causes. Rarely, however, are these terms properly distinguished or defined in specific and concrete ways (e.g., practices, behaviors, or beliefs) so that they can more easily be assessed and modified (Betancourt & Lopez, 1993). To provide a clearer and more detailed account of the relationship among occupational health, culture, and gender, it is necessary to clearly define the constructs used in practice that pertain to diversity in order for organizations to better address the health problems that are implicated in the specific aspects of these constructs. For example, as noted in Table 24.1, culture can be conceptualized as systems of meaning that are learned and shared by a people or a segment (or segments) of a population (Rohner, 1984). Subjective aspects, such as shared social norms, roles, beliefs, values, and practices are elements of culture (Triandis & Brislin, 1984). Subjective culture can be further specified in terms of gender roles, familial roles, communication patterns, affective styles, values regarding personal control, individualism, collectivism, spirituality, and religiosity. Ethnicity has been used interchangeably with culture; however, ethnicity refers to groups of people characterized in terms of a common nationality, culture, and/or language (Gelfand et al. 2007). Specifically, ethnicity refers to the national or tribal affiliation of a group. Both ethnicity and culture are closely related and sometimes are hard to differentiate; cultural backgrounds can shape people's ethnic identity or affiliation, and being part of an ethnic group or groups can shape cultural patterns. Finally, ethnicity and race have also been hard to differentiate due, in part, to both being utilized interchangeably with culture and nationality by a variety of disciplines including psychology, law, government, and business. Historically, racial categories have been used to classify people in terms of observable physical characteristics with the purpose of creating hierarchies among human beings (Corcos, 1997; Smedley & Smedley, 2005). However, evidence has shown that there is no scientific support for the idea that races exist (Olson, 2005). Data have demonstrated that genetic variability is greater within than between "racial" groups (Bamshad, Wooding, Salisbury, & Stephens, 2004).

The meanings that people attribute to these constructs compound the problems that organizations experience. Often, these terms are used synonymously, and people behave and make decisions based on their view that race, ethnicity, and culture are not distinguishable. For example, out-group categorization and discrimination against minority coworkers may occur due to the color of an individual's

Table 24.1 Summarizing the constructs

Construct	Definition	EEOC definition	Discrimination defined by EEOC
Culture	Learned beliefs, norms, and values shared by a group	No definition for culture	Used interchangeably with ethnicity and race
Ethnicity	Common nationality, culture, and/or language	The place of origin of an individual or his or her ancestors, or because an individual has the physical, cultural, or linguistic characteristics of a national origin group	Employment discrimination against a national origin group includes discrimination based on ethnicity, physical, linguistic, or cultural traits
Race	Socially constructed term that refers to observable physical characteristics	No definition for race	Race discrimination encompasses ancestry, physical characteristics, culture, and "reverse" discrimination
Sex	Biological/physiological differences between men and women	No definition for sex	Sex discrimination involves treating someone (an applicant or employee) unfavorably because of that person's sex
Gender	Behaviors that society deem appropriate for men and women	No definition for gender	Used interchangeably with sex

skin. Furthermore, people may make attributions about a coworker's beliefs and behaviors based solely on this type of superficial characteristic. Current classification systems used by the US federal government facilitate and reinforce the idea that racial categories exist, which further contributes to the ongoing confusion regarding ethnicity and race. The Equal Employment Opportunity Commission (EEOC) continues to use race as a descriptor that often overlaps with ethnicity. As noted on Table 24.1, the EEOC's definition of ethnicity (i.e., national origin) uses physical characteristics as an indicator equivalent to language and culture. As further evidence of the blur between the constructs, Table 24.1 also summarizes how the EEOC defines discrimination. Despite the evidence against the concept of race or the idea that physical characteristics can be used as markers of ethnicity and culture, this classification system is widely used by researchers and practitioners. We distinguish between ethnicity and culture (although we acknowledge their relatedness), specifying ethnicity in terms of group affiliation and culture as a system of shared beliefs, norms, and values of a (ethnic) group. We further argue that race is a socially constructed term that may impede the understanding of the relationship between culture and health, and may contribute to discrimination in the workplace. A similar problem occurs between the definitions of sex and gender, as both tend to be used interchangeably which hinders the understanding of the processes that link organizational diversity initiatives and health (see Table 24.1). Sex refers to the biological and physiological differences between men and women. Behaviors and activities directly related to biological differences are defined as sex roles (e.g., pregnancy or breastfeeding). Gender, on the other hand, refers to behaviors or patterns of activities that society or culture deem appropriate for men and women. Gender roles are the expectations for behaviors and attitudes that a particular culture defines as appropriate for men and women (e.g., expectation that women stay at home to rear children, or the assumption that women do not need competitive salaries because their male partners are the main breadwinners). Because these distinctions between sex and gender are often blurred, the potential to attribute and conflate gender differences to inherent biological differences increases. This, in turn, may lead to the belief that the causes of behaviors, and the behaviors themselves, are hard or even impossible to change (e.g., women cannot be good leaders because they are "too emotional").

Cultural Differences in Values and Behavior

Cultural values are associated with differences in beliefs, attitudes, and behaviors, and these differences can shape the structure of organizations as well as the relationships within. Therefore, a helpful way to understand the impact of culture and gender on organizations is by examining how cultural values may facilitate and/or hinder some behaviors (e.g., discrimination, acceptance, harassment). Cultural values reflect the learned beliefs and behaviors that are shared by specific groups of individuals which distinguish them from other groups of individuals, and are shaped by culturally guided norms, emotions, and patterns in thinking (Plaut, Markus, & Lackman, 2002). In his seminal work, Hofstede (1994) identified four major dimensions of cultural values: collectivism–individualism, power distance, masculinity–femininity, and uncertainty avoidance. These dimensions have been extensively used to explain and predict cross-national differences in values and behaviors (Spector et al., 2004). The collectivism–individualism dimension relates to the degree to which a culture is more or less group oriented. Cultures that are high in individualism emphasize an independent, self-focused orientation, while cultures that are high in collectivism emphasize an interdependent, group-focused orientation. Power distance refers to the extent to which cultures encourage or maintain differences in power and status in interpersonal relationships. High power distance cultures favor centralized and authoritarian decision-making. The masculinity–femininity dimension relates to the degree to which cultures maintain stereotypical differences between men and women. For example, in a feminine society, men and women would be similar in feminine-type traits such as caring and modesty, whereas, in a masculine society, men would be more assertive and competitive compared to women. Uncertainty avoidance refers to a culture's degree of comfort or discomfort in ambiguous or unstructured environments. Cultures that are low on uncertainty avoidance would be more comfortable with, and tolerant of, vague situations.

Organizations that are composed of individuals from different cultures naturally will experience a wider range of diversity in employees' attitudes and behaviors. For example, research notes that, in certain collectivistic cultures, maintaining indirect eye contact while conversing is considered a sign of respect (Chang & Spector, 2011). However, in other cultures, this act may infer that one group is more dominant over another. Hofstede's (1994) dimensions have also been used to demonstrate cross-cultural differences and similarities in how conflict is expressed and resolved. For example, in low power cultures, such as the USA, workers may be more likely to cooperate and use open communication instead of avoidance or conformity when resolving conflicts with coworkers (Tinsley, 2001). Similarly, in high femininity cultures, conflict is more likely to be resolved by engaging in problem-solving (Van Oudenhoven, Mechelse, & de Dreu, 1998). These types of conflict resolution methods can result in lower levels of physical problems. Additionally, in terms of resolving conflict, research has shown that individualistic cultures prefer a direct, competitive style where one person's goals are achieved at the expense of another's and winning is key, whereas in collectivistic cultures, compromise is key and individuals prefer to resolve conflict indirectly using avoidance (Gelfand et al., 2007; Liu, Spector, & Shi, 2007). Avoidance is not invoked in order to ignore issues, but rather to protect relationships and maintain harmony.

Other research highlights the negative outcomes associated with culture and interpersonal relations at work. Of special concern is verbal abuse and bullying. For instance, research has shown that high power distance, individualistic, and masculine organizations may facilitate organizational bullying (e.g., Einarsen, Raknes, & Matthiesen, 1994; Vartia, 1996). Bullying in an organizational context has been related to low job satisfaction (Loh, Restubog, & Zagenczyk, 2010) and increased anxiety (Mikkelsen & Einarsen, 2001). It must be noted that bullied individuals may be more likely to be perceived as being part of the "out-group" and as having lower status (Loh et al., 2010). These perceptions may result in increased victimization of those individuals who hold lower-level jobs, such as minorities and women, and result in worse health outcomes for those who suffer from bullying. When the values of an organization (i.e., an organization's mindset) are not consistent with the values of the larger culture, individuals may interpret and react to conflict and bullying in a way that may be more detrimental to their health. For example, women from a low power distance country, such as the USA, but who work in a high-power distance organization, may experience more health problems and lower job satisfaction than women from a culture where high power differences between supervisor and supervisee are more accepted (Mikkelsen & Einarsen, 2001). Differences in cultural values have also have been shown to affect the workplace in terms of job satisfaction and perceptions of justice which, in turn, can affect individuals' mental and physical health (Robbins, Ford, & Tetrick, 2012). For instance, low levels of perceived justice within the organization have been associated with more sleeping problems, sickness absences, and mental health (Elovainio, Kivimaki, & Vahtera, 2002; Tepper, 2001). These differences can exacerbate work and perceived organization conflict. Research has shown that conflict with supervisors is indirectly associated with mental and physical health via job satisfaction (Faragher, Cass, & Cooper, 2005); whereas conflict with coworkers has a direct impact on mental and physical health (Frone, 2000).

Cultural values can also affect workers' health by favoring males or females at work and/or by influencing where work is performed, the types of jobs available, and the number of hours worked. For example, in some high masculine societies, men tend to choose more hazardous jobs than women (e.g., construction and manual labor), which can have a negative cumulative effect on their physical health. These types of jobs may result in early disability and physical dysfunction which, in turn, may lead to early retirement. Health risks associated with job choice have been related to the shortened life expectancy for men, although this accounts for a small percentage of the difference (Donkin, Goldblatt, & Lynch, 2002). Job choice can also negatively affect women's health. Traditionally feminine jobs, such as some health professions (e.g., nurse or midwifery) or care-giving occupations (e.g., teacher), may increase health risks such as infectious diseases and/or burnout for women who tend to be overrepresented in these lines of work. Preoccupation with one's job may also have differential effects on health outcomes. In societies where females are expected to raise children at home, and males are expected to be the main source of household income, men invest more time at work than women and are at higher risk for workaholism (Snir & Harpaz, 2009). Workaholics have been found to report higher levels of physical problems and poorer emotional health (Burke, 2000; Andreassen, Ursin, & Eriksen, 2007). Women, on the other hand, are more likely to show presenteeism (i.e., the tendency to attend or stay at work despite being ill). Presenteeism can negatively affect the health of women who are in highly demanding jobs, such as nursing, midwifery, and teaching, by exacerbating the effects of the illness conditions (Aronsson, Gustafsson, & Dallner, 2000; Martinez & Ferreira, 2011). In collectivist communities, where men's and women's social roles are similar (for both work and household contributions), gender differences in health tend to disappear (Anson, Levenson, & Bonneh, 1990), and the male–female mortality gap is smaller (Leviatan & Cohen, 1985).

Differences in cultural values not only exist and affect behavior at the cross-national level but also at the regional or intra-national level. In fact, Plaut et al. (2002) state that "...regional culture should not be ignored as an important shaper of psychological functioning" (p. 166). Plaut and colleagues assessed indicators of well-being in the USA, finding both agreement and variability across five US regions. Consistent with American ideology, one indicator of well-being that did not vary across the USA was control (i.e., feeling that one can accomplish anything if one wanted). However, between-region variability was found for many of the indicators. For example, compared to areas in New England, people in southeastern regions of the USA were less likely to view autonomy as an indicator of well-being. Also, compared to north-central regions, people in certain southwestern regions were more likely to describe themselves as lively and outgoing.

Summary

In a diverse organizational environment, interactions among people are complex and are further complicated by the beliefs and social norms held by different groups. Strong evidence points to a connection in how differences in culture, cultural values, and gender shape and affect individuals and relationships at work. The above examples demonstrate that differences in values and cultural characteristics can exist anywhere. Individuals who engage in behaviors that are consistent with their cultural-specific or gender-specific norms, yet perform outside of a certain accepted model, may be viewed as atypical and thus may be a target for discrimination and exclusion. It is this dynamic which can lead to psychosocial and physical health-related problems.

Discrimination and Exclusion

That women and minorities in the workplace have experienced, and continue to experience, more discrimination compared to their White male counterparts, including mistreatment (Meares et al., 2004), alienation (Findler et al., 2007; Mor-Barak & Levin, 2002), and bias and harassment (Morris, 1996), points to how organizations have traditionally approached diverse cultural viewpoints. The recent influx of international workers into the USA adds another layer of complexity to what has already been an existing challenge associated with workplace diversity. Discrimination at work is of great concern because perceived discrimination has been associated with poorer mental and physical health, and increased stress in a variety of settings (Pascoe & Richman, 2009). Similarly, research in organizational settings has revealed that individuals who report high levels of racial discrimination are more likely to report worse physical health (De Castro, Gee, & Takeuchi, 2008), and greater levels of perceived stress (Wadsworth et al., 2007), than their colleagues who report low levels of discrimination. At the forefront of this challenge is an organizational mindset which has traditionally excluded women and minorities from the mainstream culture (Cox & Nkomo, 1990; Mor-Barak & Levin, 2002). Power, in terms of decision making, access to information, and other organizational processes, is typically held by the mainstream culture, and this majority culture is the basis for comparison and judgment of the values and workplace behavior of every other culture (Fine, 1996; Meares et al. 2004). Karasek and collaborators have shown that lack of access to decision-making can result in negative health outcomes for workers (e.g., Karasek, 1990), such as increased depression and anxiety (Egan et al., 2007). For women, low decision control on the job can negatively affect physical and mental health, especially if coupled with high job demands. For example, in a large study with over 30,000 women, Amick et al. (1998) found that women in high demand jobs who have low levels of control reported increased physical and mental strains when compared to women with high demands/high control jobs. By virtue of their dissimilar characteristics compared to the majority culture, women and minorities may continue to experience lack of decision control and exclusion from the core functioning of the organization. Findler et al. (2007) stated that diversity characteristics are related to the way employees are treated. Therefore, those who have dissimilar characteristics are more likely to perceive detachment from the mainstream group. Over time, the concerns of the mainstream become the only concerns and, it is the responsibility of groups outside of the mainstream to conform to these established norms.

Fine (1996) indicates that, historically, African-Americans and women are often judged using White males as the norm. She also notes the psychological and physical damage associated with individuals who feel compelled to assimilate into the dominant culture. Assimilation requires a great deal of energy to keep the genuine, true self repressed in order to "fit" with the mainstream, but assimilation does not necessarily equate to lack of discrimination. On the contrary, it merely highlights the division between the majority and the minority. Eventually, the effort expended on assimilation takes its toll in the form of anger and stress. The phenomenon of working hard at the expense of one's health has been termed "John Henryism," and refers to an individual's predisposition to display unrelenting attempts to cope with stressors even in the face of significant barriers (James, 1994). John Henryism has been associated with an increased risk of hypertension among African-Americans of lower socioeconomic status (Taylor, 2006). Given an organizational environment where clear boundaries exist between the majority and the minority, fit by assimilation will never be achieved and those individuals who continue to work hard despite the unachievable will be at a higher risk of developing more adverse physical and psychosocial conditions. Moreover, people who expend energy on coping and assimilating will have less energy to perform their jobs well. Thus, the consequences to the organization are also negative (Fine, 1996).

An additional line of research has investigated the role of gender stereotyping and discrimination against women in the workplace. Because women make up a minority portion of managerial positions, confusion exists regarding how women should act in management roles to be perceived as effective leaders. If a female leader acts in a caring manner, her behavior may be perceived as a sign of weakness yet, if she acts using stereotypical male characteristics (e.g., assertiveness, competitiveness), her behavior can be perceived as going against typical gender roles. This ambivalent approach can lead to fewer women succeeding in top positions. However, women that do succeed in incongruent job positions (i.e., careers considered typically male) may be more likely to experience negative health outcomes, such as increased levels of stress (Jacobs, Tytherleigh, Webb, & Cooper, 2010).

Lyness and Thompson (2000) identified several barriers to women's advancement in managerial positions, including lack of fit with male-dominated cultures, stereotyping about women's abilities, and exclusion from informal networks with males peers. Women, regardless of their job positions, are also more vulnerable to hostile behaviors such as sexual harassment. Approximately one-quarter of women in the workforce report having experienced sexual harassment (Ilies, Hauserman, Schwochau, & Stibal, 2003; Krieger et al., 2006). High levels of harassment are associated with lower job satisfaction, poorer mental health, less satisfaction with life (Schneider, Swan, & Fitzgerald, 1997) and increased blood pressure levels (Krieger et al., 2008).

Summary

The harmful physical and psychosocial effects of workplace discrimination are clear. Workers who are subjected to an adverse or hostile organizational environment will not be in a position to add value to the organization. Moreover, it is likely that workers will not want to contribute to organizational functioning if they are not feeling valued. This places organizations at risk of not successfully achieving their goals, as organizations that continue to repress individuals lose out on the opportunity to explore diverse points of view. Not tapping into the knowledge and experiences of every employee limits organizational learning, and the promised benefits of a diverse workforce will not be achieved.

The Importance of Context

Erez (2011) notes that culture is a construct that can be represented at multiple levels (cross-national, intra-national, organizational, group, etc.) which suggests that, depending on the context, (e.g., organizational philosophy, structure, values), cultural characteristics can range from very similar to very dissimilar. Mor-Barak (2000) indicates that the definition of diversity is context-dependent. Therefore, context should not be overlooked when evaluating what is considered typical. As an example of this, suppose a Muslim woman employed at an American Halal food processing company dresses in traditional Islamic clothing, including a hijab or headscarf. In this context, she may not be perceived as atypical. However, within a different context, such as in an American retail clothing store, she is likely to have more trouble fitting in (e.g., see *EEOC v. Abercrombie & Fitch Stores*). In the context of a majority/minority organizational environment, control and the retention of power and privilege of the majority are main characteristics that separate the mainstream group from all other groups. Although Meares et al. (2004) found that cultural groups who are silenced at work can resist (e.g., muted group theory), oftentimes those who are considered in the minority group will be excluded from organizational events. Findler et al. (2007) describe exclusion in terms of an inclusion exclusion continuum, where individual characteristics dictate where a person falls. Salient characteristics, such as skin color, sex, accent, and language, are likely to be the primary means to identify mainstream versus minority group membership. Research has shown significant mean differences between groups where Whites felt more included than African-Americans and Native Americans, and males felt more included than females (Mor-Barak & Levin, 2002). Yet, characteristics that are capable of excluding individuals are not limited to physical characteristics. Differences in cultural values, beliefs, attitudes, and behaviors can affect how people approach work (Fine, 1996; Meares et al., 2004) which, in turn, can affect how people are treated in the workplace, particularly when different from expectations of the mainstream (Thomas & Inkson, 2004).

It is important to note that, although women and minorities have historically been the targets of workplace exclusion (Mor-Barak & Levin, 2002), the agents of the exclusionary acts are not necessarily

White and male. Rather, the source of an exclusionary environment lies with the organization's culture (i.e., mindset) where the organizational norms and expectations are cultivated. Culture, in this sense, refers to the shared and deeply embedded belief system that usually stems from, and is filtered through, the organization's founders and leaders (Schein, 1990). It is safe to say that a majority of US organizations have been established by White males, which may be reason enough to explain why the shared values common to that particular demographic have, in general, dictated the beliefs, traditions, norms, and behavior of most US organizations. Statistics show that White males continue to occupy a majority (70%) of *Fortune 100* board of director seats (Alliance for Board Diversity Census, 2010). However, if culture can be portrayed as context-dependent and multilevel, "mainstream" is likely to change from context to context depending on the dominant set of practices and ideas in a given environment (Mor-Barak, 2000). The mainstream is not designated to one particular culture or set of ideals exclusive of all others in every circumstance or environment. A non-Spanish speaking White employee working in a company that values bilingualism may be just as likely to face exclusion and discrimination as a non-English speaking Latino employee working in a company that holds traditional Anglo values. In fact, in a study conducted using New York City police officers, Morris (1996) found that, compared to women and minority officers, White male officers who worked within an ethnically diverse department and who served an ethnically diverse population perceived less positive social interactions with supervisors and felt more alienation. Thus, the mainstream adjusts based on contextual factors. In this sense, *any* group or individual is a potential target of discrimination and exclusion.

Research and theory from social psychology have demonstrated the complex dynamics of exclusion in terms of the impact on it has relationships between people. In essence, exclusion occurs because individuals deviate from a prototype envisioned by the majority group. Abrams, Hogg, and Marques (2005) assert that "the effects of exclusion are almost wholly negative" (p.14). Exclusion threatens the self-concept and an individual's need to belong, and results in a variety of adverse physical and psychosocial conditions. Empirical investigations have shown that exclusion lowers an individual's sense of well-being (Mor-Barak & Levin, 2002), and leads to more aggression and procrastination, and less cooperation and intelligent thought (Twenge & Baumeister, 2005). In the workplace where group coordination and interaction are vital to many organizational processes, exclusion will have a powerful impact on organizational productivity and effectiveness. Rather than providing an environment where all employees participate fully, often individuals from diverse backgrounds are marginalized which, in turn, prohibits organizations from gaining the competitive advantage that a diverse workforce is supposed to provide (Mor-Barak, 2000). Although little research on the effects of exclusion on health has been conducted in the workplace, this evidence suggests that perceived exclusion or rejection is associated with poor psychosocial health (Hitlan, Cliffton, & DeSoto, 2006), specifically increased levels of depression (Penhaligon, Louis, & Restubog, 2009).

Whether individuals perceive themselves to be included or excluded will be based on a comparative evaluation relative to others (Mor-Barak & Cherin, 1998; Roberson, 2006), and this comparison will affect an individual's interpretation of where he or she stands in the social environment. Mor-Barak and Cherin (1998) note that "…inclusion and exclusion are at the root of psychosocial well-being" (p. 49). Indeed, other research (Mor-Barak & Levin, 2002) has demonstrated a strong relationship between inclusion and both job satisfaction and employee general well-being (absence of depression and strain). Often, however, these "soft" outcomes are given minimal attention by organizations in favor of more financially based indicators of effectiveness such as organizational productivity. Thus, given the conventional wisdom that proclaims a diverse workforce leads to improved organizational performance, bottom-line productivity may be an organization's main or sole motivation in establishing a diverse workforce, while employee well-being is overlooked or dismissed altogether. In some instances, organizations may welcome diversity, but employee inclusion may be assumed rather than proactively managed. In other instances, the organization's culture may be far from

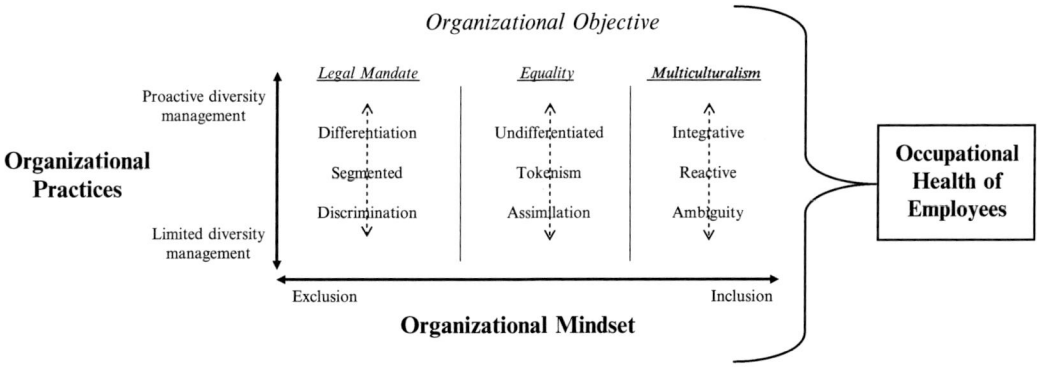

Fig. 24.1 A framework for conceptualizing diversity environments

embracing diverse viewpoints, choosing instead to dismiss or ignore those who deviate from the mainstream. A truly healthy organizational environment is one that considers not only the organizational financial bottom line but also the well-being of all employees within (Grawitch, Gottschalk, & Munz, 2006), as ultimately the success of any organization rests with its employees. Therefore, organizations that wish to promote total health and success will need to first assess the factors that influence the existing organizational environment.

A Framework for Conceptualizing Diversity Environments

Research reveals the reciprocal influence of the organization's embedded philosophy or values (i.e., the organization's mindset) and the organization's observable practices, policies, and procedures. That is to say, the organization's values guide the practices that employees engage in, and implementing new organizational practices and policies can influence existing values (Schneider, Brief, & Guzzo, 1996; Schneider, Ehrhart, & Macey, 2010). The development and implementation of the organization's overall strategic objectives are also influenced by the values and practices of the organization. This interplay among organizational values, practices, and objectives is a key factor in determining the organizational environment. The resulting organizational environment, in turn, could have a critical impact on workers' health. Figure 24.1 provides a framework that combines these organizational elements to produce an organizational environment wherein employees' attitudes and behaviors are cultivated. Drawing on, and integrating, a variety of research and conceptualizations, this framework is designed to show how the organizational environment develops through the relationship between the mindset of the organization and the actual practices that organizations engage in. The organizational mindset is depicted through an exclusion–inclusion continuum as discussed previously. Organizational practices are represented by degree of management activity and effort expended toward creating and managing diversity initiatives, such as hiring strategies, and training and development programs. Both researchers and practitioners stress the critical influence of management involvement on organizational practices because managers are the key representatives who develop and enforce these practices. In addition, actions by management provide cues regarding appropriate attitudes and behaviors of employees (Cox, 1991; Peiró & Tetrick, 2011).

***The framework also provides de facto organizational objectives to show how this particular organizational element may be at odds with what the organization claims or thinks are its objectives. The misalignment between objectives and the environment could be the critical factor that hinders organizations from capitalizing on the full potential of a diverse workforce. Including organizational objectives on the framework will help those organizations to better understand why diversity initiatives may not be contributing to the success of the organization so action can be taken to ameliorate the environment. Finally, the framework conceptualizes the influence that all of these organizational factors have on workplace health. As noted throughout this chapter, research has verified that an environment of intentional discrimination increases stress levels and mental health problems. A similarly stressful yet different atmosphere is an ambiguous environment where the organization's espoused objectives are at odds with the actual practices of management (Podsakoff, LePine, & LePine, 2007). In fact, the alignment between what the organization values and its practices has been recognized as being critical to workplace health (Grawitch et al., 2006). Ultimately, the framework will allow an organization to reflect upon what it wants to achieve (objectives), what it is actually able to achieve (mindset and practices), what might be expected as a result (environment), and the consequences of these on employee occupational health. The following section describes a variety of organizational environments produced from the combination of practices and mindset, and the resulting health outcomes from those environments. It should be noted that the organizational environments are arranged vertically and quasi-hierarchically on the framework, under the three main columns of organizational objectives. Until future studies verify the placement of each environmental construct, it is impossible to pinpoint the exact location of organizational environments in relation to the other constructs represented on the framework (i.e., organizational practices, organizational mindset). Each environmental construct may (or may not) overlap with another and to an unknown degree. This contingency is noted by the dotted lines within the framework.

Legal Mandate

In the least inclusive sense, the organization's de facto objective behind diversity hiring may be only to comply with EEOC requirements. In this organization, the majority culture dictates the policies and procedures, and diverse viewpoints are of little importance. Thus, there is little need to proactively manage diversity initiatives beyond monitoring EEOC compliance requirements. This type of organization might be compared to Cox's (1991) monolithic organization, where the organizational environment is composed of high levels of segregation and cultural bias, both of which produce prejudice and *discrimination*. Although the civil rights movement significantly reduced the overt monolithic organization in its truest sense, the fact that thousands of reasonable cause discrimination charges are filed with the EEOC annually (nearly 5,000 in 2010) is a demonstration that discrimination continues to plague organizations. Beyond satisfying hiring quotas, diversity initiatives meant to benefit the organization will likely fail, and the discriminatory environment will continue to produce negative health-related outcomes for workers (e.g., Wadsworth et al., 2007).

Organizations that maintain an exclusionary mindset yet provide a moderate amount of active management might perpetuate an environment of *segmentation*, both across and within jobs where (a) lower status jobs are overly represented by women and minorities and (b) higher status jobs keep women and minorities isolated and underutilized. These organizations may engage in particular job placement strategies, for example, relegating lower status jobs to individuals based on certain ethnic or gender characteristics. Physical demands of these lower status jobs may result in increased health problems for ethnic minorities and women (Lundberg, 1999). For those individuals who do rise to management positions, participation in organizational processes and decision making is limited or nonexistent. This incongruence between what individuals expect to do on the job compared to what the organization allows them to do can produce physical and/or psychosocial distress. Research has demonstrated the negative effects that perceived racial segmentation has on the psychosocial well-being of African-Americans, particularly in jobs of higher status (Forman, 2003).

Even when a proactive management approach is taken, the emphasis of diversity initiatives will be on differences rather than on the potential for a collective organizational identity because the mindset continues to be exclusionary. For example, research has documented that the failure of diversity training programs is due in part to the training's focus on differences that serve to perpetuate stereotyping and promote a "we-they" perception (Chavez & Weisinger, 2008). *Differentiation* is underscored in Thomas and Ely's (1996) access-and-legitimacy organizational paradigm, which notes that this type of environment "pigeonholes" workers into positions where their physical attributes (i.e., perceived race), gender, or ethnicity is highlighted and aligned with demographically similar customers. Diverse viewpoints are not integrated into the organization's mainstream culture but are considered only to the extent that they correspond to demographically similar customer markets. "Exploited" and "devalued" are terms that workers have used when describing how they feel within this type of environment (Thomas & Ely). Overall, if the driving organizational strategy behind diversity hiring is a legal obligation, both individual health and well-being, and total organizational health, suffer.

Equality

Midway between the inclusion and exclusion continuum lays the organizational objective of equality. Similar to the access-and-legitimacy paradigm, hiring quotas and compliance still strongly influence diversity initiatives. However, unlike the emphasis on differences of the access-and-legitimacy paradigm, here the emphasis is on sameness. Additionally, unlike the monolithic typology of total exclusion, this organization's mindset can be described as fair and respectful. Thus, the organization is more comparable to Thomas and Ely's (1996) discrimination-fairness paradigm where fairness is enforced. Within this environment, women and minorities are respected and overt discrimination is significantly reduced. However, the organization does not go so far as to allow the contribution of differing viewpoints. This sameness-fairness organizational mindset can produce a variety of organizational environments depending on the level of active diversity management. For example, combined with limited management, an environment of *assimilation* might evolve where minorities are expected to adopt the norms of the majority culture at the expense of losing their own cultural identity. An assimilation environment might also exist even in organizations where a moderate amount of active diversity management occurs. This type of organization might be compared to Cox's (1991) pluralistic organizational. Cox noted that this organizational typology falls short of full cultural integration much like the discrimination-fairness organizational paradigm where minority workers must resign their cultural norms in order to fit in with the majority culture. Forcing people to assimilate, rather than allowing them to express their cultural individuality, affects self-esteem and perpetuates feelings of social isolation. The health-related problems of assimilation were discussed previously and were noted as being particularly detrimental to both the individual and the organization (Fine, 1996).

Cox's (1991) pluralistic organization is also characterized by a skewed minority worker population so, along with an environment of assimilation, this organization may also produce an environment of *tokenism*. A moderate amount of diversity management under the discrimination-fairness paradigm may equate to ensuring the minimum percentage of women and minorities are represented in the hiring process. In turn, an even smaller percentage of minorities are actually hired. In this sense, diversity hiring is seen as symbolic, which serves to draw attention to those "token" employees who are hired. Although the organization enforces color blindness and gender blindness, the fact that women and minorities represent a significantly smaller percentage of the organization's workforce tends to make them stand out (in addition to the obvious physical differences). This type of visible notoriety can result in increased pressures to perform. Researchers have noted that tokenism is complex, involving more than just minority representation and percentages in the workplace (Stichman, Hassell, &

Archbold, 2010), but also includes psychosocial factors such as feelings of inadequacy which leads individuals to question their own competence. Some consequences of tokenism include increased depression, anxiety, lower levels of self-esteem, and stress on the job (Jackson, Thoits, & Taylor, 1995; Krimmel & Gormley, 2003).

An organization that practices a proactive management style within the objective of equality may take fairness to the extreme because fairness is not part of the cultural integration process, it is the end itself. The zeal to better integrate minorities and women into the organization may even lead to reverse discrimination and preferential hiring. Mostly, however, the organization devotes a great deal of effort to ensure that hiring quotas are met and everyone is treated equally. Differences among employees are not acknowledged, thus the environment might be characterized as *undifferentiated*. Sameness and conformity are emphasized in an attempt to maintain harmony, yet the organization continues to operate within a majority/minority mindset. The combination of a suppressed minority workforce and a persisting mainstream culture causes tension among employees and leads to resentment and distrust of management. Individuals' unique contributions are not supported. Thus, women and minorities will continue to be marginalized resulting in a higher risk for health problems (Hitlan et al. 2006).

Multiculturalism

Cox (1991) notes that the multicultural organization is characterized by (a) full organizational integration of minority cultures, (b) the elimination of cultural bias, and (c) the elimination of the majority/minority gap. This type of organization can be compared to Ely and Thomas's (2001) integration-and-learning paradigm. Keys to this organizational typology are the emphasis placed on the inclusion of diverse perspectives and the integration of these perspectives into the organization's core functioning. A true multicultural organization is composed of individuals from diverse backgrounds whose ideas are valued, supported, and incorporated into the organization's overall operation (Cox, 1991; Nahavandi & Malekzadeh, 1988; Thomas & Ely, 1996). Improved productivity and organizational effectiveness are much more likely within a multicultural organization, but are highly dependent upon top management's commitment toward true multiculturalism. As noted on the framework, inclusion is maximized in the multicultural organization, meaning that this organization will have a mindset that focuses on valuing human relationships. Therefore, the critical factor for this organization in achieving the full benefits of a diverse workforce will rest mainly on the organizational practices and the proactive management of diversity initiatives.

The multiple perspectives inherent within a multicultural organization produce a variety beliefs and attitudes. Thus, effort is required by leaders to implement and direct the policies that will guide appropriate employee behavior. Organizations that acquire an inclusionary mindset, but do not actively manage diversity issues, may produce an environment of *ambiguity*. The organization may have good intentions in terms of welcoming diversity, but may fall short of achieving the full benefits of a diverse workforce because diversity management is assumed rather than being proactively attended to. Inclusion is a necessary but not a sufficient element of true multiculturalism. Meares et al. (2004) noted how ambiguous policies kept employees from clearly understanding the organization's expectations. This resulted in the continuation of mistreatment of minorities, as well as the continuation of a majority/minority gap. Furthermore, when this ambiguity is reflected in poorly defined roles (i.e., role ambiguity), workers' motivation, performance, commitment and, more importantly, mental and physical health are negatively affected (Örtqvist & Wincent, 2006). Limited management of diversity initiatives might also lead to a *reactive* environment where organizations spend a great deal of time problem solving and developing solutions that occur after the fact, but fail to actually resolve the central issue. For example, organizations may develop diversity training that informs employees about respecting diversity, yet never assess the alignment between the training and the goals of diversity programs. If the goal is to fully integrate the workforce, training that teaches respect and awareness may not be enough. Research has noted how diversity training initiatives typically fail due to conventional attitudes towards diversity issues (Chavez & Weisinger, 2008). Although an important element in ensuring a fully integrated environment is the effort made to align and manage diversity initiatives, such as employee training and selection, this effort should not be confined to diversity initiatives only, but something that should be instilled within the organization's core functions.

A true multicultural organization is characterized by the full integration of cultural differences. Individuals' various points of view are valued and, even more importantly, are considered vital resources that aid in the organization's learning and overall functioning (Ely & Thomas, 2001). To be successful in achieving a multicultural organization, management must be committed to ensuring that, to greatest extent possible, all employees who want to be involved in organizational events, such as decision making and information and knowledge sharing, are encouraged to do so (McMahan, Bell, & Virick, 1998; Wood & Wall, 2007). Grawitch and colleagues (Grawitch, Trares, & Kohler, 2007; Grawitch, Ledford, Ballard, and Barber, 2009) note that employee involvement influences various indicators of employee physical and psychosocial well-being, and organizational commitment. Given that inclusion has been shown to promote well-being, whereas exclusion has been shown to lower well-being (Mor-Barak & Levin, 2002), it might be argued that proactively promoting and encouraging diversity may be considered a healthy organizational practice. In the *integrative* environment, the goals for management will extend beyond implementing traditional diversity initiatives towards creating a shared organizational identity. Nahavandi and Malekzadeh (1988) note that a shared organizational identity is where everyone belongs to the same social group (i.e., the organization) while, at the same time, each individual is allowed to retain his/her own cultural identity. Rather than suppressing individuality which leads to increased stress levels, unique perspectives are encouraged because the more ideas generated, the greater the likelihood of more creative solutions (Lauring, 2009).

Toward a Healthy Organizational Environment

Tetrick and Quick (2011) provide insight into how organizations might move toward true multiculturalism. For example, changing the organization's culture might be considered a primary intervention (i.e., prevention before people are at risk). Quite often, organizations implement change programs out of a desire to keep up with current trends yet, over time, these initiatives will lose momentum because the crux of the issue has not been addressed. If multiculturalism in its truest sense is desired and possible in an organization, successful culture change will start with top management and an assessment of the potential barriers to successful diversity integration (e.g., embedded beliefs and values). Rather than an organizational culture being defined by the physical or cultural characteristics of the leaders and founders, organizations can change the culture so that it is driven by the organization's mission and goals. The main focus of any organization should be on achieving its goals. An integrated, multicultural organization should be guided by the goals that reflect the objectives, mission, and strategies. This, in turn, will help to reduce and even eliminate the majority/minority gap and move employees toward a shared organizational identity. However, the major shift in organizational thinking is not without its challenges. The strength of the multicultural organization is in its ability to draw upon diverse perspectives. If not managed effectively, the organization's ability to capitalize on that strength may be threatened. Leaders will have to manage employee involvement and participation by not allowing one group to dominate over another. At the same time, leaders will need to ensure that employees are allowed to retain their individual cultural identity. People who feel they must hide their own cultural uniqueness will be less willing to share information, whereas those who feel valued and respected for their competence will be more willing to contribute (Ely & Thomas, 2001). Full contribution and participation by employees is what differentiates the multicultural organization from all others. Therefore, one challenge for the multicultural organization will be the balancing act between uniting people to the goals of the organization, while at the same time respecting the differences among individual cultures.

Inherent to this atmosphere of open dialogue, another challenge will be for leaders to manage the inevitable conflict that naturally occurs when different perspectives are allowed to emerge. Tense discussions are likely, but will be expressed by disagreements based on differences of opinion and not based on the characteristics of the individual. The multicultural organization encourages this type of open communication because it serves to expand the organization's overall learning. In this regard, training initiatives on specific topics, such as effective communication and managing conflict, are likely to be more successful because the training's purpose and the goals of the organization are aligned. Moreover, learning will not stop once training is over, but will continue outside of the training room because the behaviors and attitudes will be expressed consistently throughout the organization. For organizations that wish to adopt a multicultural perspective, a final challenge will be a potential change to the existing organizational culture. Due to the deeply held, embedded beliefs and values, changing an organization's culture is difficult, yet not impossible. The reciprocal influence between an organization's culture and its policies and practices as noted previously represents a starting point for organizations. Redefining what is considered acceptable behaviors and attitudes on the job can be achieved through enacting new policies. By frequently communicating these new policies, and having management at all levels of the organization consistently model desired practices and behaviors, over time culture change can occur.

Conclusions

Issues associated with organizational diversity have existed long before the recent appeal was made by occupational health psychologists to focus on total organizational health. Moreover, in recent times, the literature has clearly articulated the potential benefits of a culturally diverse workforce. If organizations wish to capitalize on these benefits, the framework presented here can be used as a starting point for organizations to assess the alignment among objectives, mindset, and practices. Merely acquiring individuals from diverse backgrounds, without providing a foundation that supports their success, will not produce the desired results. Even for those organizations with the best intentions, this strategy will eventually prove detrimental to the health and well-being of both the workers and the organization.

In 1996, the call for valuing differences in the workplace was made by Fine, who described how the organizational mindset at that time was starting to shift from suppression of women and minorities to awareness. A decade and a half later, it would seem another shift is in order: from awareness of differences to the active promotion and integration of diversity into the organization's core functioning. The organization that proactively embraces this shift will certainly be in a better position to realize the full benefits that have been promised from implementing a diverse workforce. The heart of the matter lies with the overall values of the organizational that perpetuates established behaviors. Thus, whether organizations support or block the establishment of healthy workplace practices, such as integrating diversity, will be based on its underlying mindset, as this will be the ultimate determinant of success and sustainment over the long term.

Future Research Directions

As organizations become more diverse, interest in the relationships among culture, gender, and occupational health will continue to grow. To meet the future demands from both practitioners and academics, researchers will have to develop and test more integrative, mechanistic models that can account for these relationships. Currently, support for the associations is indirect; there is strong evidence that culture influences organizational behavior, such as conflict at work and perceptions of fairness, and that these psychosocial factors, in turn, influence workers' physical and mental health. However, the complete models and the specific pathways have not been fully examined. Future research is required to determine how the organization's mindset and practices combine to produce the various environments, and result in organizational changes that affect individuals' health. The knowledge resulting from this type of research will be critical for the identification of specific organizational practices that can be the target for modification.

This work will require further specification and clarification of the terms used and constructs examined. As indicated above, there is still great confusion about the meaning and in the usage of key concepts such as culture, ethnicity, race, gender, and sex. A strong and useful theoretical body requires specific explanations which can only be achieved by increasing the rigor in the use and measurement of these terms. For instance, using race as a proxy for ethnicity or culture will most likely hinder the understanding of a phenomenon, as skin color does not tell us anything about the specific aspects of culture that may influence organizational behaviors and occupational health. However, if one is attempting to understand how individuals' perceptions of coworkers may affect conflict at work, this may require the use of race as a descriptor of the ways in which individuals categorize coworkers. Something similar is required when sex and gender are the focus of studies. Women or men may experience differential health outcomes because of culturally prescribed roles (e.g., type of job one chooses) or because of sex-based discrimination.

These recommendations also require that greater attention is paid to the quality of measurement. Specifically, it is critical that researchers test the assumption that the instruments are measuring the same construct, and in the same way (i.e., measurement invariance) for all groups (e.g., countries, ethnicity, or sex). Group comparisons or the examination of group differences in psychosocial processes across groups will result in biased results in the absence of measurement invariance. Psychometric research needs to be more closely integrated into the work conducted by researchers and practitioners to ensure the validity of inferences.

The road ahead is challenging but has the potential to be extremely rewarding for both researchers and practitioners. This will be especially true if investigators can produce knowledge about organizational processes that can be used by managers to enact changes to improve their organizations.

References

Abrams, D., Hogg, M. A., & Marques, J. M. (2005). A social psychological framework for understanding social inclusion and exclusion. In D. Abrams, M. A. Hogg, & J. M. Marques (Eds.), *The social psychology of inclusion and exclusion* (pp. 1–23). New York: Psychology Press.

Alliance for Board Diversity Census. (2010). Retrieved on August 8, 2011 from http://theabd.org/ABD_report.pdf.

Amick, B., Kawachi, I., Coakley, E., Lerner, D., Levine, S., & Colditz, G. (1998). Relationship of job strain and isostrain to health status in a cohort of women in the United States. *Scandinavian Journal of Work, Environment and Health, 24*(1), 54–61.

Andreassen, C., Ursin, H., & Eriksen, H. (2007). The relationship between strong motivation to work, "workaholism", and health. *Psychology and Health, 22*(5), 615–629.

Anson, O., Levenson, A., & Bonneh, D. (1990). Gender and health on the kibbutz. *Sex Roles, 22*(3), 213–236.

Armstead, C. A., Lawler, K. A., Gorden, G., Cross, J., & Gibbons, J. (1989). Relationship of racial stressors to blood pressure responses and anger expression in Black college students. *Health Psychology, 8*(5), 541–556.

Aronsson, G., Gustafsson, K., & Dallner, M. (2000). Sick but yet at work: An empirical study of sickness presenteeism. *Journal of Epidemiology and Community Health, 54*, 502–509.

Barling, J., & Griffiths, A. (2011). A history of occupational health psychology. In J. C. Quick & L. E. Tetrick (Eds.), *Handbook of occupational health psychology* (pp. 21–34). Washington, DC: American Psychological Association.

Bamshad, M., Wooding, S., Salisbury, B. A., & Stephens, J. C. (2004). Deconstructing the relationship between genetics and race. *Nature Reviews Genetics, 5*(8), 598–609.

Betancourt, H., & Lopez, S. R. (1993). The study of culture, ethnicity, and race in American psychology. *American Psychologist, 48*(6), 629–637. doi:10.1037/0003-066X.48.6.629. http://dx.doi.org/.

Briggance, B. B., & Burke, N. (2002). Shaping America's health care professions: The dramatic rise of multiculturalism. *The Western Journal of Medicine, 176*(1), 62–66.

Bureau of Labor Statistics. (2009). Retrieved on August 19, 2011 from http://www.bls.gov/news.release/archives/ecopro_12102009.pdf on.

Burke, R. (2000). Workaholism in organizations: Psychological and physical well-being consequences. *Stress Medicine, 16*, 11–16.

Chang, C. H., & Spector, P. E. (2011). Cross-cultural organizational health psychology. In J. C. Quick & L. E. Tetrick (Eds.), *Handbook of occupational health psychology* (pp. 119–137). Washington, DC: American Psychological Association.

Chavez, C. I., & Weisinger, J. Y. (2008). Beyond diversity training: A social infusion for cultural inclusion. *Human Resource Management, 47*(2), 331–350.

Clark, R., Anderson, N. B., Clark, V. R., & Williams, D. R. (1999). Racism as a stressor for African Americans: A biopsychosocial model. *American Psychologist, 54*(10), 805–816.

Corcos, A. F. (1997). *The myth of human races*. East Lansing: Michigan State University Press.

Cox, T., Jr. (1991). The multicultural organization. *The Academy of Management Executive, 5*(2), 34–47.

Cox, T., Jr., & Nkomo, S. M. (1990). Invisible men and women: A status report on race as a variable in organizational behavior research. *Journal of Organizational Behavior, 11*, 419–431.

D'Anna, L. H., Ponce, N. A., & Siegel, J. M. (2010). Racial and ethnic health disparities: Evidence of discrimination's effects across the SEP spectrum. *Ethnicity and Health, 15*(2), 121–143.

De Castro, A., Gee, G., & Takeuchi, D. (2008). Workplace discrimination and health among Filipinos in the United States. *American Journal of Public Health, 98*(3), 520–526.

Department of Labor. (2011). Retrieved on August 19, 2011 from http://www.dol.gov/_sec/media/reports/asianlaborforce/.

Donkin, A., Goldblatt, P., & Lynch, K. (2002). Inequalities in life expectancy by social class, 1972–1999. *Health Statistics Quarterly, 15*, 5–15.

Egan, M., Bambra, C., Thomas, S., Petticrew, M., Whitehead, M., & Thomson, H. (2007). The psychosocial and health effects of workplace reorganization: A systematic review of organizational-level interventions that aim to increase employee control. *Journal of Epidemiology and Community Health, 61*(11), 945–954.

Einarsen, S., Raknes, B., & Matthiesen, S. (1994). Bullying and harassment at work and their relationships to work environment quality: An exploratory study. *The European Work and Organizational Psychologist, 4*(4), 381–401.

Elovainio, M., Kivimaki, M., & Vahtera, J. (2002). Organizational justice: Evidence of a new psychosocial predictor of health. *American Journal of Public Health, 92*(1), 105–108.

Ely, R. J., & Thomas, D. A. (2001). Cultural diversity at work: The effects of diversity perspectives on work group processes and outcomes. *Administrative Science Quarterly, 46*, 229–273.

EEOC v. Abercrombie & Fitch Stores, Inc. Case No. 09-CV-602-GKF-FHM. Retrieved August 15, 2011 from http://www.hecouncil.org/files/2011/20110802_6.pdf.

Equal Employment Opportunity Commission. (2011). Retrieved on December 13, 2011. from http://www.eeoc.gov/.

Erez, M. (2011). Cross-cultural and global issues in organizational psychology. In S. Zedeck (Ed.), *APA handbook of industrial and organizational psychology* (Vol. 3, pp. 807–854). Washington, DC: American Psychological Association.

Faragher, E., Cass, M., & Cooper, C. (2005). The relationship between job satisfaction and health: A meta-analysis. *Occupational and Environmental Medicine, 62*, 105–112.

Findler, L., Wind, L. H., & Mor-Barak, M. E. (2007). The challenge of workforce management in a global society: Modeling the relationship between diversity, inclusion, organizational culture, and employee well-being, job satisfaction and organizational commitment. *Administration in Social Work, 31*(3), 63–94.

Fine, M. G. (1996). Cultural diversity in the workplace: The state of the field. *Journal of Business Communication, 33*(4), 485–502.

Forman, T. A. (2003). The social psychological costs of racial segmentation in the workplace: A study of African Americans' well-being. *Journal of Health and Social Behavior, 44*(3), 332–352.

Frone, E. (2000). Work-family conflict and employee psychiatric disorders: The national comorbidity study health: A meta-analytic integration. *The Journal of Applied Psychology, 85*(6), 888–895.

Gany, F., Dobslaw, R., Ramirez, J., Tonda, J., Lobach, I., & Leng, J. (2011). Mexican urban occupational health in the U.S.: A population at risk. *Journal of Community Health, 36*, 175–179.

Gelfand, M. J., Erez, M., & Aycan, Z. (2007). Cross-cultural organizational behavior. *Annual Review of Psychology, 58*, 479–514.

Grawitch, M. J., Gottschalk, M., & Munz, D. C. (2006). The path to a healthy workplace: A critical review linking healthy workplace practices, employee well-being, and organizational improvements. *Consulting Psychology Journal: Practice and Research, 58*(3), 129–147.

Grawitch, M. J., Trares, S., & Kohler, J. M. (2007). Healthy workplace practices and employee outcomes. *International Journal of Stress Management, 14*(3), 275–293.

Grawitch, M. J., Ledford, G. E., Jr., Ballard, D. W., & Barber, L. K. (2009). Leading the healthy workforce: The integral role of employee involvement. *Consulting Psychology Journal: Practice and Research, 61*(2), 122–135.

Hitlan, R., Cliffton, R., & DeSoto, M. (2006). Perceived exclusion in the workplace: The moderating effects of gender on work-related attitudes and psychological health. *North American Journal of Psychology, 8*(2), 217–236.

Hobman, E. V., Bordia, P., & Gallois, C. (2004). Perceived dissimilarity and work group involvement: The moderating effects of group openness to diversity. *Group and Organization Management, 29*(5), 560–587.

Hofstede, G. (1994). The business of international business is culture. *International Business Review, 3*(1), 1–14.

Ilies, R., Hauserman, N., Schwochau, S., & Stibal, J. (2003). Reported incidence rates of work-related sexual harassment in the United States: Using meta-analysis to explain reported rate disparities. *Personnel Psychology, 56*(3), 607–631.

Jackson, P., Thoits, P., & Taylor, H. (1995). Composition of the workplace and psychological well-being: The effects of tokenism on America's black elite. *Social Forces, 74*(2), 543–557.

Jacobs, P., Tytherleigh, M., Webb, C., & Cooper, C. (2010). Breaking the mold: The impact of working in a gender-congruent versus gender-incongruent role on self-reported sources of stress, organizational commitment, and health in U.K. universities. *International Journal of Stress Management, 17*(1), 21–37.

James, K. (1994). Social identity, work stress, and minority workers' health. In G. P. Keita & J. J. Hurrell Jr. (Eds.), *Job stress in a changing workforce: Investigating gender, diversity, and family issues* (pp. 127–146). Washington, DC: American Psychological Association.

Jayne, M. E. A., & Dipboye, R. L. (2004). Leveraging diversity to improve business performance: Research findings and recommendations for organizations. *Human Resource Management, 43*(4), 409–424.

Karasek, R. (1990). Lower health risk with increased job control among white collar workers. *Journal of Organizational Behaviour, 11*, 171–185.

Kessler, R. C., Michelson, K. D., & Williams, D. R. (1999). The prevalence, distribution, and mental health correlates of perceived discrimination in the United States. *Journal of Health and Social Behavior, 40*(3), 208–230.

Krieger, N., Chen, J., Waterman, P., Hartman, C., Stoddard, A., Quinn, M., Sorensen, G., & Barbeau, E. (2008). The inverse hazard law: Blood pressure, sexual harassment, racial discrimination, workplace abuse and occupational exposures in US low-income black, white and Latino workers. *Social Science and Medicine, 67*(12), 1970–1981.

Krieger, N., Waterman, P., Hartman, C., Bates, L., Stoddard, A., Quinn, M., Sorensen, G., & Barbeau, E. (2006). Social hazards on the job: Workplace abuse, sexual harassment, and racial discrimination—A study of black, Latino, and white low-income women and men workers in the United States. *International Journal of Health Services, 36*(1), 51–85.

Krimmel, J. T., & Gormley, P. E. (2003). Tokenism and job satisfaction for policewomen. *American Journal of Criminal Justice, 28*(1), 73–88.

Landrine, H., & Klonoff, E. A. (1996). The schedule of racist events: A measure of racial discrimination and a study of its negative physical and mental health consequences. *Journal of Black Psychology, 22*(2), 144–168.

Lauring, J. (2009). Managing cultural diversity and the process of knowledge sharing: A case from Denmark. *Scandinavian Journal of Management, 25*, 385–394.

Leviatan, U., & Cohen, J. (1985). Gender differences in life expectancy among Kibbutz members. *Social Science and Medicine, 21*(5), 545–551.

Liu, C., Spector, P. E., & Shi, L. (2007). Cross-national job stress: A quantitative and qualitative study. *Journal of Organizational Behavior, 28*, 209–239.

Loh, J., Restubog, S., & Zagenczyk, T. (2010). Consequences of workplace bullying on employee identification and satisfaction among Australians and Singaporeans. *Journal of Cross-Cultural Psychology, 41*(2), 236–252.

Lundberg, U. (1999). Stress responses in low-status jobs and their relationship to health risks: Musculoskeletal disorders. *Annals of the New York Academy of Sciences, 896*, 162–172. doi:10.1111/j.1749-6632.1999.tb08113.x.

Lyness, K., & Thompson, D. (2000). Climbing the corporate ladder: Do female and male executives follow the same route? *The Journal of Applied Psychology, 85*(1), 86–101.

Martinez, L. F., & Ferreira, A. I. (2011). Sick at work: Presenteeism among nurses in a Portuguese public hospital. *Stress and Health*. doi:10.1002/smi.1432.

McMahan, G. C., Bell, M. P., & Virick, M. (1998). Strategic human resource management: Employee involvement, diversity, and international issues. *Human Resource Management Review, 8*(3), 193–214.

Meares, M. M., Oetzel, J. G., Torres, A., Derkacs, D., & Ginossar, T. (2004). Employees mistreatment and muted voices in the culturally diverse workplace. *Journal of Applied Communication Research, 32*(1), 4–27.

Mikkelsen, E., & Einarsen, S. (2001). Bullying in Danish work-life: Prevalence and health correlates. *European Journal of Work and Organizational Psychology, 10*(4), 393–413.

Mor-Barak, M. E. (2000). Beyond affirmative action: Toward a model of diversity and organizational inclusion. *Administration in Social Work, 23*(3), 47–68.

Mor-Barak, M. E., & Cherin, D. A. (1998). A tool to expand organizational understanding of workforce diversity: Exploring a measure of inclusion-exclusion. *Administration in Social Work, 22*(1), 47–64.

Mor-Barak, M. E., & Levin, A. (2002). Outside of the corporate mainstream and excluded from the work community: A study of diversity, job satisfaction and well-being. *Community, Work and Family, 5*(2), 133–157.

Morris, A. (1996). Gender and ethnic differences in social constraints among a sample of New York City police officers. *Journal of Occupational Health Psychology, 1*(2), 224–235.

Murray, L. R. (2003). Sick and tired of being sick and tired: Scientific evidence, methods, and research, implications for racial and ethnic disparities in occupational health. *American Journal of Public Health, 93*(2), 221–226.

Nahavandi, A., & Malekzadeh, A. R. (1988). Acculturation in mergers and acquisitions. *Academy of Management Review, 13*(1), 79–90.

Olson, S. (2005). The use of racial, ethnic, and ancestral categories in human genetics research. *American Journal of Human Genetics, 77*(4), 519–532.

Örtqvist, D., & Wincent, J. (2006). Prominent consequences of role stress: A meta-analytic review. *International Journal of Stress Management, 13*(4), 399–422.

Pascoe, E., & Richman, L. (2009). Perceived discrimination and health: A meta-analytic review. *Psychological Bulletin, 135*(4), 53–554.

Peiró, J. M. & Tetrick, L. (2011). Occupational health psychology. In P. R. Martin, F. M. Cheung, M. C. Knowles, M. Kyrios, L. Littlefield, B. J. Overmier, & J. M. Prieto (Eds). *IAAP Handbook of Applied Psychology* (pp. 292–315). West Sussex, UK: Wiley-Blackwell.

Penhaligon, N., Louis, W., & Restubog, S. (2009). Emotional anguish at work: The mediating role of perceived rejection on workgroup mistreatment and affective outcomes. *Journal of Occupational Health Psychology, 14*(1), 34–45.

Plaut, V. C., Markus, H. R., & Lackman, M. E. (2002). Place matters: Consensual features and regional variation in American well-being and self. *Journal of Personality and Social Psychology, 83*(1), 160–184.

Podsakoff, N. P., LePine, J. A., & LePine, M. A. (2007). Differential challenge stressor-hindrance stressor relationships with job attitudes, turnover intentions, turnover, and withdrawal behavior: A meta-analysis. *The Journal of Applied Psychology, 92*(2), 438–454.

Robbins, J. M., Ford, M. T., & Tetrick, L. E. (2012). Perceived unfairness and employee health: A meta-analytic integration. *The Journal of Applied Psychology, 97*(2), 235–272. doi:10.1037/a0025408.

Roberson, Q. M. (2006). Disentangling the meanings of diversity and inclusion in organizations. *Group and Organization Management, 31*(2), 212–236.

Roberts, R. K., Swanson, N. G., & Murphy, L. R. (2004). Discrimination and occupational mental health. *Journal of Mental Health, 13*(2), 129–142.

Rohner, R. P. (1984). Toward a conception of culture for cross-cultural psychology. *Journal of Cross-Cultural Psychology, 15*(2), 111–138. doi:10.1177/0022002184015002002.

Schein, E. H. (1990). Organizational culture. *American Psychologist, 45*(2), 109–119.

Schneider, B., Brief, A. P., & Guzzo, R. A. (1996). Creating a climate and culture for sustainable organizational change. *Organizational Dynamics, 24*(4), 7–19.

Schneider, B., Ehrhart, M. G., & Macey, W. H. (2010). Perspectives on organizational climate and culture. In S. Zedeck (Ed.), *APA handbook of industrial and organizational psychology* (Vol. 1, pp. 373–414). Washington, DC: American Psychological Association.

Schneider, K., Swan, S., & Fitzgerald, L. (1997). Job-related and psychological effects of sexual harassment in the workplace: Empirical evidence from two organizations. *The Journal of Applied Psychology, 82*(3), 401–415.

Smedley, A., & Smedley, B. D. (2005). Race as biology is fiction, racism as a social problem is real: Anthropological and historical perspectives on the social construction of race. *American Psychologist, 60*(1), 16–26.

Snir, R., & Harpaz, I. (2009). Workaholism from a cross-cultural perspective. *Journal of Cross-Cultural Research, 43*(4), 303–308.

Spector, P. E., Cooper, C. L., Poelmans, S., Allen, T. D., O'Driscoll, M., Sanchez, J. I., et al. (2004). A cross-national comparative study of work-family stressors, working hours, and well-being: China and Latin America versus the Anglo world. *Personnel Psychology, 57*(1), 119–142.

Stichman, A. J., Hassell, K. D., & Archbold, C. A. (2010). Strength in numbers? A test of Kanter's theory of tokenism. *Journal of Criminal Justice, 38*(4), 633–639.

Taylor, S. E. (2006). *Health psychology*. New York: McGraw Hill.

Tepper, B. (2001). Health consequences of organizational injustice: Test of main and interactive effects. *Organizational Behavior and Human Decision Processes, 86*(2), 197–215.

Tetrick, L. E., & Quick, J. C. (2011). Overview of occupational health psychology: Public health in occupational settings. In J. C. Quick & L. E. Tetrick (Eds.), *Handbook of occupational health psychology* (pp. 3–20). Washington, DC: American Psychological Association.

Thomas, D. A., & Ely, R. J. (1996). Making differences matter: A new paradigm for managing diversity. *Harvard Business Review, 74*(5), 79–90.

Thomas, D. C., & Inkson, K. (2004). *Cultural intelligence.* San Francisco: Berrett-Koehler.

Thompson, V. L. S. (1996). Perceived experiences of racism as stressful life events. *Community Mental Health Journal, 32*(3), 223–233.

Tinsley, C. H. (2001). How negotiators get to yes: Predicting the constellation of strategies used across cultures to negotiate conflict. *The Journal of Applied Psychology, 86*(4), 583–593. doi:10.1037/0021-9010.86.4.583.

Triandis, H. C., & Brislin, R. W. (1984). Cross-cultural psychology. *American Psychologist, 39*(9), 1006–1016. doi:10.1037/0003-066X.39.9.1006. http://dx.doi.org/.

Twenge, J. M., & Baumeister, R. F. (2005). Social exclusion increases aggression and self-defeating behavior while reducing intelligent thought and prosocial behavior. In D. Abrams, M. A. Hogg, & J. M. Marques (Eds.), *The social psychology of inclusion and exclusion* (pp. 27–46). New York: Psychology Press.

United States Census. (2010). Retrieved on May 28, 2011 from http://2010.census.gov/2010census/

Van Oudenhoven, J., Mechelse, L., & de Dreu, C. (1998). Managerial conflict management in five European countries: The importance of power, distance, uncertainty avoidance, and masculinity. *Applied Psychology, 47*(3), 439–455.

Vartia, M. (1996). The sources of bullying: Psychological work environment and organizational climate. *European Journal of Work and Organisational Psychology, 5*(2), 203–214.

Wadsworth, E., Dhillon, K., Shaw, C., Bhui, K., Stansfeld, S., & Smith, A. (2007). Racial discrimination, ethnicity and work stress. *Occupational Medicine, 57,* 18–24.

Williams, D. R., Yu, Y., Jackson, J. S., & Anderson, N. B. (1997). Racial differences in psychical and mental health: Socio-economic status, stress, and discrimination. *Journal of Health Psychology, 2*(3), 335–351.

Wood, S. J., & Wall, T. D. (2007). Work enrichment and employee voice in human resource management-performance studies. *International Journal of Human Resource Management, 18*(7), 1335–1372.

Addressing Occupational Workplace Issues "In Action": An Ongoing Study of Nursing Academic Program Directors

25

Ronda Mintz-Binder

Overview

Higher education is a major financial industry in its own right. Indeed, in a report by New York State's Comptroller (entitled *The Economic Impact of Higher Education in New York State*), the following data were cited.
- In 2009, the State's colleges and universities employed 266,110 people and paid $13.2 billion in wages.
- Taking into account student spending (on housing, food, etc.), it generated $62.2 billion in economic activity in the State.
- Research conducted at these institutions also helped to generate new technologies, products, and services that also added to the economy (such as $380 million in licensing of technologies' agreements, as well as economic growth produced by 42 start-up companies that were developed to use the technology licensed from these institutions (www.osc.state.ny.us), March, 2012).

In spite of such statistics, higher education institutions are rarely considered when talking about occupational health and wellness issues. The present chapter is being written to fill this void.

At the outset, it should also be noted that many of the issues to be discussed in the present chapter will have been reviewed in greater detail in other chapters of this handbook because of its occupational theme. For example, the chapter by Dewe, O'Driscoll and Cooper explores the relationship between work-related strain and well-being, and these authors presented a *Job Demand-Control-Support,* which emphasized the importance of high job demands and a low degree of control in producing high job strain. In another chapter, Theorell further elucidated the physiological/health consequences of high- versus low-strain jobs on workers. In addition, McGeary's and McGeary's chapter on *Occupational Burnout* explored the role of job demands, weighed against perceived job resources, in explaining the complex relationship between job burnout and work engagement, regardless of the occupation being examined. As will be seen in this chapter, many of these same

R. Mintz-Binder, D.N.P., R.N., C.N.E. (✉)
Department of Nursing, College of Nursing, The University of Texas at Arlington,
701 S. Nedderman Dr., Box 19407, Arlington, TX 76019-0407, USA
e-mail: rondamb@uta.edu

dynamics can play out in one specific job that will be reviewed, that of a community college academic administrator.

There is a wide diversity of organizations, with unique models of management, hierarchical levels of responsibility and power, and styles of leadership. Colleges and universities are such unique organizations with their own structure, organization and levels of responsibility. Successful colleges and universities manage their budgets and fiscal resources by balancing the costs of education, subsidized support from the government or private sector, and the tuition costs paid for by students. State-funded colleges and universities are dependent on each state's annual budget and, as states have experienced, their own fiscal crises over the last 5 years. Higher education has also been struggling with the price of education in comparison to the efficiency of successfully educating the student of today.

A common thought and/or expectation is that college and university administrators are simply strong and long-standing faculty members who choose to move into the administrative sector of their institution. Although this style of promoting from within has been common in the past, it is no longer the most useful paradigm. One of the biggest differences between the faculty perspective and the administrator perspective is the job related focus (Foster, 2006). The faculty role is considered to be program focused with great emphasis on strengthening the course offerings, the faculty members, recruitment and graduation rates of students, and meeting yearly budgetary expectations. In contrast, an administrator's role is considered to be institutional focused with emphasis on managing departments collectively, advocating for the needs of their departments and incorporating both of these components into strategic planning efforts geared toward the yearly goals of the overall institution. To be successful at transitioning from a faculty role to an administrative role, one must move from a specialist to a generalist and place to the side a discipline-specific focus or bias, and take on a broader multidiscipline view (Plater, 2006). Understanding the distinctions in these two viewpoints is critical in considering: (a) why not all faculty can be administrators; (b) why a transition from faculty to administration is noted to be difficult; (c) why the workload dramatically increases when one moves into administration; and (d) why many new administrators choose to return to faculty positions quickly or have difficulty understanding and mastering these new skill sets.

When exploring an organization's strength and fiscal health, it is quite common to look at the length of tenure of the top-tier administrators; the world of higher education is no different. In most colleges and universities, the President is the top-level position, followed by Vice Presidents, Provosts, Deans, Assistant and/or Associate Deans, and then the Department Chairs. Each role has designated job descriptions varying in levels of responsibility, from Deans overseeing multiple clusters of departments, to Department Chairs managing and overseeing their own faculty, staff, and students. The Vice Presidents and President oversee varying levels of responsibility of the college and/or university. Participants and members of the American Association of Community Colleges (AACC) created a model of six primary competencies for current and future Community College Leaders (American Association of Community Colleges, 2005, p. 1). These six competencies are listed in Table 25.1.

The administrative roles investigated in the literature have ranged from the Presidents, the Vice Presidents, Deans, and Department Chairs, along with a variety of other similar titles. What appears clear is that strong and well-functioning institutions of higher education have continuity and consistency in their top leadership positions. However, increasing concern is mounting related to a severe shortage of community college leaders in the very near future. This trend appears to be due to a decrease in the number of advanced degrees now being awarded in community college leadership, complexities and increased workloads noted at the academic leadership level, and numerous barriers to advancement including the dissolution of preparatory administrative positions during state fiscal crises (Keim & Murray, 2008; McNair, Duree, & Ebbers, 2011). Reille and Kezar (2010) suggest that at least 1,500 top community college personnel (e.g., Presidents and Chief Academic Officers) either have or will be retiring by the end of 2012. However, vacancies are also becoming apparent at all

Table 25.1 American Association of Community Colleges competencies for leaders

Competencies	Description/focus
Organizational strategy	Educational quality; mission and trends; college wide decision making
Resource management	Equitable; physical and financial aspects
Communication	Honest, open dialogue amongst all stakeholders, students, employees
Collaboration	Cooperative, mutually beneficial relationships for the good of the college
Advocacy	Supports and promotes the mission and vision of the college within the community and at large
Professionalism	Establishes and maintains high standards and expectations for all; authentic leadership practices

Summarized from http://www.aacc.nche.edu/Resources/leadership/Pages/six_competencies.aspx

levels of academic administration, and as those in the lower ranks are promoted or hired for higher position, their vacated positions are not being readily filled. Steady turnover at these higher positions is not only costly, due to the price of recruitment, interviewing, and acclimating a new administrator into their new role, but also often creates a wave of other changes. Additional vacancies may occur, conflicts may arise, and a period of unsettling and unrest is not uncommon. Knowing that these sorts of responses are possible, administrators, and researchers have searched for ways to understand and ultimately increase longevity in these critical academic management positions.

Filan and Seagren (2003) delineated six-specific leadership characteristics that they found to be critical for success at the midlevel management level in higher education. The Academy of Leadership Training and Development was created in 1992 in Mesa, Arizona to offer internationally recognized leadership training for department chairs and assistant/associate deans to evolve within their new or current positions. The six critical focus areas for academic middle managers are (a) understanding one's self—strengths and limitations; (b) understanding transformational leadership—encouraging others to grow and develop; (c) establishing and maintaining relationships—effective and positive rapport with all levels; (d) leading teams—striving for high performance and balanced successful teamwork; (e) leading strategic planning and change—aids the focus, direction, and quality of the institution every year; and (f) connecting through community—bringing all players within the college or university to the community for mutual gain (Filan & Seagren, 2003).

Review of Major Organizational Management Concepts

A host of variables have been studied over the last 20 years with respect to varying administrative positions within colleges and/or universities. Job satisfaction, intention to leave, stress, workload concerns, and social support are but a few of the work-related variables examined. Inevitably, if these specific work-related concepts are not managed well, the process of job burnout can ensue. To explore how these concepts interrelate in an academic administrative setting, understanding the phenomena and evolution of job burnout is critical.

Job Burnout

The general area of occupational burnout has been more comprehensively reviewed in another chapter of this handbook, by McGeary and McGeary. The concept of burnout became part of

Table 25.2 Six worklife areas related to burnout: Maslach and Leiter model

Worklife area	Description
Workload	Emotional or cognitive work; amount in relation to energy available
Control	Resources or authority may be mismatched in relation to what is necessary for job performance
Reward	Lack of recognition (financial or personal) in relation to expectation
Community	Interpersonal relationships within the workplace; positive, happy or conflict ridden
Fairness	Level or respect, equality, pay, workload, etc.
Values	Inherent existing conflict between values and ethics or job expectations

Derived from Maslach and Leiter (1997)

psychosocial and human services research in the 1970s. Maslach (1976) is most noted for her dedication to researching the phenomenon of burnout in the workplace, and creating the *Maslach Burnout Inventory Tool* (Maslach & Jackson, 1981). What has evolved over the last 30 years is a concise portrait of burnout that involves three key aspects: (a) overwhelming exhaustion which is related to amount and severity of stress; (b) feelings of doubt, mistrust and/or detachment from their work position most representative of an interpersonal nature; and (c) a growing sense of ineffectiveness and not accomplishing or completing tasks related to a personal view of not achieving a set level of performance (Maslach, Schaufeli, & Leiter, 2001). As research into burnout has progressed, there appear to be individual factors unique to those who experience burnout, such as individual factors like age, marital status, and educational level. Personality characteristics, such as low hardiness (which will be addressed later in this chapter), lower level self-esteem and/or an avoidant means of coping with conflict appear to show greater signs of burnout in the work environment. Lastly, an individual's personal job attitudes or expectations may predict burnout levels. If personal expectations are extremely high or even unrealistic, burnout can ensure. Most recently, Maslach and Leiter (1997) began addressing the proper match between an employees' personality and qualities of their job position. Six concepts appear to be critical variables in understanding the relationship between an occupation or position, and whether a person finds work dimensions acceptable or not. These concepts are explored in Table 25.2.

Job Satisfaction

Another major area of research of renewed concern is job satisfaction measures of academic administrators as well as of faculty. One of the foremost early researchers on job satisfaction is Locke (1969) who defined job satisfaction as a "…pleasurable emotional state resulting from the appraisal of one's job as achieving or facilitating the achievement of one's job values" (p. 316). It stands to reason that if someone is happy in their job, they will remain and, if they are not, they will at some point leave that position. Because expanding and enhancing academic administrators' tenure in leadership positions is critical for continuity (for a highly positive and well-functioning administrative team and for the public view of a community college's importance to a community) it therefore becomes essential to try to enhance job satisfaction. Indeed, job satisfaction continues to be a critical variable in studies across administrators, department chairs, and faculty. All of these college employees may impact a student's collegial satisfaction which has fiscal and publicity-related implications.

Table 25.3 Overview of job responsibilities of Department Chairs

College level	Committee meetings with top administrators
	Decision making/college planning/retreats
Departmental level	Hire/Evaluate/Counsel Faculty and performance
	Create/revise departmental budget
	Arrange/confirm course offerings each semester
	Conflict resolution with faculty
Student level	Handle concerns with other students, grades, and/or faculty
	Assist with admission criteria within programs
	Assist with graduation processing and ceremonies

Other Concepts to Consider

Trends of decreasing length of times in these key academic administrative positions have been reported. Turnover at this level can be quite expensive, with cost estimates ranging from 5- to 25 times of an employee's monthly salary (Glick, 1992). It is also documented that efforts to offset turnover are underutilized. However, with fiscal crises affecting multiple state budgets, higher workloads are contributing to increased levels of stress at the Assistant and/or Associate Dean, Program Director and Department Chair levels. Stress can be caused by numerous factors that include role ambiguity and lack of social support. Understanding all aspects of the role one is undertaking is critical to job satisfaction and managing stress. Yet, as budget cuts occur, community colleges have been faced with trimming their administrative tier of positions, and then consolidating the positions that remained. Role ambiguity relates to a lack of complete confidence as to what the role is, as well as new levels of authority and amount of responsibility. When a job position is expanded or altered, this can have a negative effect on the administrator, as well as the staff and faculty involved. The ramifications of a job position change, including changes in stress level and workload, can be felt by subordinates. That administrator may no longer be as available for consultation, may not be as invested, and may not be able to engage in supportive exchanges with subordinates. Removing some of the "perks" from the prior position and replacing them with higher labor-intensive or cognitive expectations can diminish one's prior positive job satisfaction, as well as affect the satisfaction of those in the same department. As is noted in the chapter by McGeary and McGeary in this present handbook, this can be a precursor to the development of job burnout.

Summary of Job Responsibilities

Mid-level administrative positions are keys to a well-functioning institution. This group of administrators interfaces at the college level, the departmental level and with students alike. This particular group of administrators hire and evaluate faculty performances, create departmental budgets, arrange the course-schedule offerings, handle student concerns and issues, work to resolve a host of conflicts between faculty or between faculty and students, as well as participate in decision making and planning at the college or university level. Table 25.3 presents a summary of job duties of this particular type of academic administrator.

Research Looking at Academic Administrators

Job satisfaction, intent-to-leave positions, and role concerns of academic administrators were first reported in the early 1990s, with concerns over the scope of mid-manager positions, such as the department chair discussed earlier. The following three selected research studies looked at the concerns of the academic administrators in the 1990s. More recent studies will be reported in the next section of this chapter.

Chieffo (1991) explored factors related to organizational commitment and job satisfaction exhibited in leadership teams within community colleges in New Mexico. The *Survey of Organizations, General Satisfaction Scale* (Taylor & Bowers, 1972) measured job satisfaction, and the *Organizational Commitment Questionnaire (OCQ)* measured organizational commitment (Porter & Smith, as cited in Cook, Hepworth, Wall, & Warr, 1981). Scores on both scales indicated that administrators at these colleges were satisfied and committed to their colleges in their current roles. Role clarity was positively related to job satisfaction and organizational commitment. Being involved in decision-making meetings with the President was also deemed to be a significant factor in job satisfaction and overall commitment to the college.

Glick (1992) was one of the first researchers to look at job satisfaction across Presidents, Vice Presidents, and Deans of liberal arts universities. The revised *Job Descriptive Index (JDI)* was the instrument to assess job satisfaction across five scales (Paul, Kravitz, Balzer, & Smith, 1990). A key finding was that Vice Presidents and Deans reported dissatisfaction with the nature of their work. The Deans also demonstrated statistically significantly lowered scores on the Promotion and Supervision scales, as compared to Presidents. Not surprising, the median length of time in this position was reported to be less than 5 years. The author strongly encouraged that action be taken to improve job satisfaction in these critical management positions.

Murray and Murray (1998) explored job satisfaction of Department Chairs in 2-year colleges in relation to intent-to-leave. The authors adapted a number of scales that measured job satisfaction, predisposition to vacate a position, and role perception in creating their own tool. A major demographic finding of importance was that the majority of Department Chairs ($n=108$; 39.0%) were in these positions under 5 years, with 70% ($n=194$) in positions under 10 years. The majority of Department Chairs did report high levels of job satisfaction and a low desire to leave. However, high role ambiguity and medium levels of role conflict were reported. Of concern was that, if these role dilemmas increased, desire to leave the institution would increase as well. Additional research in these areas was encouraged by all investigators of these above seminal works.

More recently, in following up this line of investigation, Kuo (2009) explored the relationships between academic faculty (staff) and administrators at one US public research university (using a qualitative research approach). It was found that the most satisfying and productive environment for all is when both the faculty and administrators maintained a cohesive and positive relationship with similar views on goals and ideals. In opposition, a fragmented experience occurred when a lack of interaction and misunderstandings occurred, which increased frustration and resulted in an "us versus them" division that can be destructive if it continues for any length of time. The author concluded that both groups must work in tandem in order to understand their similarities and differences in dealing with situations and challenges, and then find a common ground for the most harmonious work environment.

Research Specific to Nursing Academic Administrators

Specific reference to the nursing academic administrators began in the 1980s. Not only do nursing academic administrators perform a host of typical Department Chair functions, but they also are responsible for a pre-licensure program to the state board of nursing and other credentialing agencies. This involves added responsibilities, such as negotiating with hospitals and clinical sites for student rotations; maintaining a skills lab with high fidelity simulation and technology; assuring that the curriculum meets current standard of practices; and the processing and admitting of students two

Table 25.4 Unique additional responsibilities of nursing academic administrators

Additional departmental	State of the art curriculum
	State of the art skills laboratory—financial and equipment
	Adhering to specific admission criteria and program progression per each student
	Additional meetings related to theory/clinical failures and processing of students
Liaison to hospitals/clinical sites	Securing sites/paperwork yearly/yearly renewal of contracts
	Resolving issues/conflict with faculty/with students/with nurses
Nursing state board/credentialing	Maintain program, faculty, and director approvals
	Write and oversee accreditation reports and visitations by approving boards
	Assist and process new nursing candidates for licensure; oversee preparation, paperwork, and submission of completed forms

or three times a year. As such, maintaining a "state of the art" nursing program, so that graduating students are well equipped to pass national boards and perform appropriately in a clinical setting, are additional critical elements. Table 25.4 presents a summary of these unique responsibilities for the nursing academic administrator. Early in the nursing education literature, concerns focused on the need to prepare and mentor those seeking nursing academic administrative positions (George, 1981; Hall, Mitsunaga, & de Tornay, 1981). Too often, faculty are promoted into academic administrative positions without the necessary prerequisites for learning this position. The second issue raised addressed stress, workload, and role responsibility concerns (Carpenter, 1989, George & Coudret, 1986). The following three studies review key findings specifically related to nursing academic administrators. The first study by Princeton and Gaspar (1991) reiterated these concerns, and reported findings of first-line academic administrators, representing 42 schools that offered Bachelor and graduate degree nursing programs. Telephone surveys were conducted using a demographic data instrument, nine created questions that assessed on administrative experiences, and an adapted competency assessment for nursing academic administrators. With respect to overall stress and strain, nursing administrators reported that excessive workload that extended beyond the normal work day was causing the greatest strain. The second area of strain was related to managing their faculty, and faculty needs and conflicts. At that time, only 37.5% (21/56) reported that they were planning on continuing in their current administrative positions. Over 20 years ago, the authors concluded that issues related to workload and stress had to be addressed, or continued difficulties recruiting and retaining nursing academic administrators would remain problematic. Unfortunately, to this day, these troublesome issues are still present.

Nursing academic administrators have once again been a population of interest over the last 5 years. High turnover, extended position announcements, and a lack of interest from potentially viable prospects was an increasing trend noted in the mid-2000s. Adams (2007) explored factors that could influence nursing faculty to investigate or plan for future academic administrative positions. The *Leadership Practice Inventory*, using both self and observer scales (Kouzes & Posner, 2001), and two investigator-created questionnaires that asked about response to recruitment into administration, along with career aspirations toward the future, were used. The faculty who participated in this study had a perception that academic administrative positions have high workloads, deal with increased conflict and working with conflicts, and are not granted a significantly different salary to offset the added workload. Only 18% of faculty participants shared that they might consider an academic administrative position in the future. Lack of training and/or preparation opportunities for advancement were also noted. Additionally, nursing academic administrators were asked if they would consider advancing into a higher administrative position. Workload, budget issues, and handling conflict were the three noted factors dissuading current administrators from pursuing another position in the future.

Mintz-Binder and Fitzpatrick (2009) explored social support (Weinert, 2003) and job satisfaction (Spector, 2005) across nursing program directors ($n=61$) at community colleges in California. A number of unusual trends were noted for the first time in this study. First, there were 14 different titles stated for the Program Director position, ranging from Dean, Assistant or Associate Dean, to Department Chair to Nursing Directors. Secondly, there were 31 different combinations of nursing and non-nursing programs under management, with responsibility ranging from 1 to 9 different programs. Third, 15 (24.6%) stated that they were in interim positions at the time of the survey. Lastly, the mean age of respondents was 55.3 years old and all were female. Social support was rated above average, but did not specifically address support exclusive to the college setting. Job satisfaction was rated as average, with low means in operations, pay, promotion, and reward dimensions. The operations subscale looked at paperwork processing and the overall functioning of the nursing program within a college structure, and it was rated the lowest. Additionally, directors rated their stress as 8.03/10 on an investigator-created rating scale.

National Work Environment Study

Noting the concerns expressed in the above studies, the National League for Nursing awarded a research grant in 2008 for a national study of nursing program directors within community colleges. The *Copenhagen Psychosocial Questionnaire II (COPSOQII) Middle Version* was selected as the instrument to assess 28 subscales of work environment variables (Pejtersen, Kristensen, Borg, & Bjorner, 2010). Survey monkey was used to email requests to 580 NLNAC-approved associate degree nursing (A.D.N.) programs. The response rate of useable surveys was 41.2% ($n=242$). Forty-two states were represented by respondents, as well as Washington, DC. The effect of work demand on the overall well-being of program directors was the first of three published studies (Mintz-Binder & Sanders, 2012). The *Work Demand Scale* was designed to include measures of quantitative demands (tasks and amount of time needed), work pace (expected time to complete a task), and emotional demands (intensity of the work). The *Health Well-Being Scale* was designed to include measures of one's general overall physical functioning, physical and emotional exhaustion, level of tension and irritability, and assessment of sleep behavior related to their job (Mintz-Binder & Sanders, 2012; Pejtersen et al., 2010). Values above 60, or below 40, are considered to be statistically different from the reported national average of 50. Possible median scores range from 0 to 100.

The *Work Demand Scale* was the highest of all scales, with a median of 63.5, indicating that the directors viewed their work demands as very high. The second highest calculated scale was the *Health Well-Being Scale* at 47.9. A positive statistical significance was found between these two scales with a Spearman's Rho correlation of 0.523 ($p<0.01$). The majority of the subscales within these two scales also correlated significantly. The highest correlation occurred between the stress and burnout subscales ($\rho=0.83$; $p<0.01$). Additionally, sleep-related concerns correlated highly with both stress and burnout ($\rho=0.67$; $p<0.01$). Thus, the perception by A.D.N. directors and their faculty of a high workload associated with this position was validated in this study. However, what is most troubling is that the effect of workload on overall physical health and well-being is not being addressed. These positions continue to expand and grow while departmental budgets are either stagnant or reduced. The subsequent stress and burnout that follows will either cause the director to resign or, worse yet, become physically ill.

The second manuscript from this study reported the relationships among job satisfaction, role issues, and supervisor support of A.D.N. program directors (Mintz-Binder, accepted for publication).

The two scales that addressed these issues were *The Work-Individual Interface Scale* that included job satisfaction and work/family balance subscales, and the *Interpersonal Relationships/Leadership Scale* that included role clarity, role conflict, social support, and recognition subscales. All six of these subscales correlated with each other, with a range of Spearman's ρ values of 0.24–0.68 ($p<0.01$). These findings confirm that A.D.N. directors are struggling with job satisfaction, role clarity issues, role conflicts, insufficient supervisory support, and difficulties managing a work/family balance. Given the stress and the workload inherent in a management level position, adding these other variables to the overall portrait of this position does validate why recruitment into these positions is troublesome. Also reported was an inconsistent presence and use of assistant nursing program directors. With a goal of "on the job training" and succession planning for the future, the training and use of assistant nursing program directors would seem to be a critical need that has not been fully recognized.

The third manuscript looked specifically at a surprise finding of the presence of bullying reported by A.D.N. directors in this study (Mintz-Binder & Calkins, accepted for publication). The definition of bullying was provided by the *COPSOQII* as "a person is repeatedly exposed to unpleasant or degrading treatment and that person finds it difficult to defend himself or herself against it" (Copenhagen Psychosocial Questionnaire, 2003). One-third of A.D.N. program directors reported bullying from students or faculty ($n=77$; 32.8%). Thirty-three of the 77 directors identified their nursing faculty as the primary offender, followed closely by 30 directors identifying students as the next largest group engaging in bullying. Seventy-four percent of directors who experience bullying reported it as occurring a few times over the last year ($n=57$). The highest percent of reported bullying was within their first year of their directorship ($n=10$; 13%), and the majority of bullying reported was by directors in their positions under 5 years ($n=40$; 51.9%). Also noteworthy was that none of the five male A.D.N. directors who responded to this survey reported any bullying behaviors toward them. When comparing subscale scores on the COPSOQII between directors reporting bullying to those who did not, those directors reporting bullying behaviors reported lowered self-rated health, higher stress, and increased sleep issues. The presence of bullying did appear to create a more difficult and more stressful work experience for these directors.

Pre-assessment of a Hardiness Study

In 1979, Kobasa introduced the concept of *hardiness* as a key variable in the assessment of stress and physical illness of male executives. Since that time, hardiness training programs have emerged to help offset high stress levels in administrators (Judkins & Furlow, 2003). Nurse managers in the hospitals responded positively to hardiness training programs and, as such, determined that nursing academic program directors could also benefit from training was proposed. Funded by the National Organization of Associate Degree Nursing (NOADN) in 2010, this study assessed three components of *hardiness* in current A.D.N. program directors in the USA. The 15-item *Dispositional Resilience Scale-Hardiness* (Bartone, 2007) was the instrument selected to send through email via survey monkey to NLNAC-accredited nursing program directors. This scale can be subdivided into (a) *Commitment* that assesses if they are committed to their position and their proactive nature; (b) *Challenge* that assesses how accepting one is with challenges presented and whether they react in a positive way; and (c) *Control* that assesses how they view their own personal control over events and their response to stress. Of the 487 directors with viable emails, the response rate was 38.0% ($n=184$). The mean of *hardiness* was 31.51, with 51.6% ($n=95$) of directors exhibiting high hardiness, and 48.4% ($n=89$) exhibiting low hardiness. The three subscales correlated with each other, as well as with the total score of the instrument ($p<0.05$). The amount of secretarial/clerical support correlated with the total hardiness scores and 2 of 3 subscales ($p<0.05$). *Control* was the one subscale that did not reach statistical significance with secretarial/clerical support. However, when looking at the use and significance of an assistant director in the program, results were unexpected. Sixty nine percent of directors reported that they did not have an assistant program director assigned to their program. Of the 31% that did use an assistant director, the use varied from availability of 1–2 hours week, to having one or more full-time directors assigned. However, measures of *hardiness* did not correlate with any use of assistant directors. Those program directors who were fortunate to have more than one assistant director assigned, however, did report highest levels of *hardiness* (Mintz-Binder, 2012).

Lindley and Mintz-Binder (2012) thematically analyzed 346 comments made by these directors in response to a question asking each to share their top two critical issues that they face in their position. Faculty-related issues ($n=99$) was the highest, with comments about staffing, motivation, conflict, performance, and work ethic concerns. Workload issues ($n=70$) was second, with comments about too much to do, "wearing too many hats," difficulty meeting administrative expectations, and no time for needed grant writing. Struggling with insufficient resources ($n=40$) was third, with comments about needing additional clerical support, clinical coordinators to assist with student clinical placements and program budgets and funding concerns. Dealing with student issues was fourth ($n=35$), with comments about their behaviors, lack of positive contact, processing course failures and subsequent grievances, and dealing with students' parents. Supervisory Hierarchical Issues ($n=18$) was fifth, with comments about system issues, feelings of powerlessness and overall experiencing a lack of understanding from the higher administration. Lastly, issues related to the curriculum ($n=14$) surfaced, with comments about the curriculum needing improvements, constantly needing to maintain currency, and concerns over producing a high-quality nursing graduate.

On the basis of the above results, hardiness training could be a very useful intervention for some of the nursing program directors as reflected by this study. Hardiness training involves a combination of lecture, discussion, role playing and group work with a cluster of participants. Topics range from assertiveness training, to negotiation skill development, to delegation and communication techniques. When in a discussion with nursing program directors, many reported that they did not have the financial support to attend because their departmental budgets had been cut due to financial issues. They also shared that they could not take the time to leave their workplace and attend a 2 or 3 day training such as this.

The lack of effective use of assistant directors was also a surprising finding. When considering the high workload of these program directors, an available well-trained, assistant director would be the key person to offer positive and strong assistance to them. An assistant director would be a faculty member who was interested in an administrative opportunity in the future and would be the ideal person to learn the nuances of this position in succession planning for the future. If properly and systematically taught components of program managing, the assistant director would offer the most assistance to the program director to offset the workload and manage portions of the job responsibilities. The absence and/or underutilization of assistant program directors need further exploration in the future.

The Next Steps: Nursing and Beyond

From the review of the prior studies, there is no question that nursing academic administrators are in need of significant intervention to offset their stress, decrease their workloads, and improve their overall health. What that intervention might be is currently being considered. It appears that an intervention needs to be brought to the directors rather than expecting them to attend a workshop or group meeting away from their college setting. Use of technology, such as podcasts, webinars, and/or conference calls, would be viable options. However, competing with the workload demands could provide a challenge too difficult to overcome. Academic nursing directors must see an intervention as meaningful and of value worthy of their attention to offset their work priorities at the scheduled time of an online activity. Nurses, and those in academia as well, are traditionally known to not always take care of themselves, or put themselves first, even if their health depends on it.

Additionally, appealing to the next generation of future nursing academic directors is critical for the success of the field of nursing and the developing profession. A focused approach to teaching the administrative role of academia to assistant directors is without question an essential need that is predominantly unrecognized and significantly underutilized. Exploring more about why this trend is occurring is a critical need for succession planning, as well as providing a hands-on learning opportunity for faculty who may be contemplating administrative careers in the future. Whether current directors feel that they are too overwhelmed to attempt to divert their energy to mentoring a novice assistant director, or they just do not have enough faculty to release someone a few hours a week to devote to learning the roles are major problems. The fact remains that not directly engaging a viable candidate is short-sighted and could have far-reaching consequences for the program should the director take ill or unexpectedly leave.

Although, at this time, the same level of studies has not been aimed at other non-nursing program directors or the administrative tier of universities, we can generalize that some, if not most, of these same findings may be occurring. A critical position in the university system that has received some attention, for example, is that of the University Research Administrator (URA). Katsapis (2010) reported that URAs are under high levels of occupational stress and strain. The types of occupational stressors most commonly reported were role ambiguity and role overload. The level of role ambiguity reported was at a level that suggested the possibility of maladaptive stress responses could occur. From this study, it is safe to generalize that some university-based academic administrative positions are, in fact, experiencing high levels of stress and strain as well.

Raines and Alberg (2003) made a poignant observation in stating that higher education apparently does not value the mid-level academic manager due to the lack of educational offerings for preparation of someone with this career objective. Without solid academic program offerings, academic administrators almost seem "set up" to fail. Rather, a prospective new leader has been quickly offered an interim chair or assistant dean for a short period of time and, hopefully, the work was mutually satisfying and appreciated by all involved parties. However, once in the actual permanent position, a high learning curve is expected. But preparation before assuming the position seems absent in academic environments, which truly is ironic. Why would programs that would successfully prepare future academic leaders be nonexistent or minimally available in institutions of higher learning? Certainly, the need is apparent. Without solid program offerings, a new administrator is left with "on the job training" which could be extremely valuable or unsatisfactory. Mentoring by a seasoned academic leader, either within or outside the institution, is critical. As part of the mentoring process, self-reflection, expanding listening and communicating skills with all levels of personnel, and committing to a process of continuous growth are essential recommended strategies. Hoppe (2003) underscored the need for nurturing new and novice academic leaders. Helping new leaders make positive and appropriate decisions takes the development of fortitude, a characteristic that is not always present, or may not come forth without high-quality support, encouragement, and role modeling. Knowing that the transition from a program perspective to an organization perspective takes time, effort, and self-reflection is worth sharing with the new academic leader in supportive conversations. Hoppe also makes an excellent point when stating that a faculty member willing to move into a leadership role does not necessarily mean that person will be effective or successful. Finding a good future leader and nurturing that person through a transition from faculty to academic leader over time is one of the best and most efficient strategies.

Summary and Future Directions

Although the focus of this chapter has been predominantly on the nursing academic director, it is fair to say that similar pressures, strains, and workloads are occurring throughout higher education. Faculty and administrators within community colleges, state colleges, universities, and the private colleges and universities are all feeling the effects of tighter budgets, less secretarial or clerical support, larger classes, increased online course offerings in distance education, as well as a shift toward older students who present with more complex personal, socioeconomic, and cultural challenges. The academic administrators at all levels must be poised, prepared, and ready to take on a host of challenges that continue to confront colleges and universities, from fluctuating budgets, to student athlete infractions, to the potential of terrorism or shootings on campus. Many of the issues reviewed in other chapters of this handbook (such as work-related strain and, its physiological/health consequences, occupational burnout, resiliency, social support, and bullying) were found to be active in the present "real world" of higher education. Thus, for example, doing what is necessary to prevent burnout is critical to maintain continuity and consistency in higher-education positions. Research and suggestions from Maslach et al. (2001) suggested that changing the organizational structure is a better solution than focusing solely on changing the individual. The job environment plays a major role in whether an administrator feels job satisfaction, work overload, stress and, ultimately, burnout. Being cognizant of mismatches of qualified applicants, yet perhaps not a good match for the institution or the administrative position, is critical. In this time of fewer available or qualified future administrators, placing someone rather than the "right one" is of great concern. As academic administrative positions continue to grow, change and expand, extremely qualified applicants with the proper training, personality characteristics, and vision should only be considered. No doubt, positions that are overwhelming and have grown beyond the capability of one person must be reassessed and divided accordingly.

Not only does offering courses or degrees specifically in higher education academic administration seem critical, but also nurturing and mentoring the careers of viable future administrators appears equally essential. When workload increases or budgets tighten, it seems to follow that extending mentoring opportunities or engaging in quality dialog about these roles simply vanishes. The risk to the academic institution is extremely high when a dedicated succession plan is either placed "on hold" or not initiated in a focused and dedicated way. The time may very well be now for top-tier administrators to take note of what these current studies reviewed in this chapter are displaying, and address concerns related to work demand, stress, burnout, job satisfaction, role confusion, potential for bullying, and the lack of succession planning occurring in some higher education organizations. Managing and feeling the financial effects of turnover can be extremely taxing when institutions are already feeling fiscal restraints. Presidents and Vice Presidents need to take the time to connect with stressed and overloaded mid-level administrators. Making that effort may bring forth extremely positive rewards and offset a prospective vacancy which would only strengthen that college, and be seen in a very positive light.

So why would someone consider a career as an Academic Administrator after reading this chapter? There is no question that this is a demanding role with a steep learning curve and is not a position that any seasoned faculty member can subsume. However, for those who have personality characteristics and ambition to succeed in academic administrative careers, the rewards are quite positive. Achieving a higher professional status, higher salary, and higher institutional recognition are a few of the extrinsic rewards attributed to administrative advancement (Murphy, 2003). One of the strongest intrinsic rewards of an Academic Administrator is the sense of making a difference or leaving behind a strong legacy. Meeting one's personal leadership goals or aspirations is another very strong intrinsic reward for some people. Ultimately, it appears to be a need or willingness to serve others that may in fact be the strongest motivation. Whatever the motivation might be, balancing all aspects and complexities of this role, along with handling the inherent stress and crises, are critical. Planning far ahead for a future in academic administration, and taking necessary steps to prepare including early mentoring, seems to be the best strategy for success. Taking the time to learn about the future position (the scope, the job description, the expectations as well as beginning the process of self-assessment) are critical steps at this preparatory stage. Improving one's communication skill-set, which includes critical listening as well as effective and transparent responses, would also be essential at this time. Finding a quality mentor and beginning the mentoring process before transitioning into a leadership role would also be extremely advantageous and useful. There is no question that there is a need for well-prepared future academic administrators in the near future. There also appears to be a great need to contain and control these positions at the organizational level if recruiting efforts are to be successful. High-stress positions with role ambiguity and extreme workloads are not currently appealing to this generation of new faculty, adding to the concern of expanding vacancies in academic administration. The process of increasing job descriptions beyond an appropriate workload of those in middle management positions cannot continue if recruiting the best and most competent person for the job remains the priority. Sadly, many with the qualities and proper preparation will not take on high-stress positions because they understand the effect of stress on one's physical health. At what point and with what number of vacancies need exist for serious reconstitution of these Academic Administrative positions to occur? In the midst of a lack of qualified Academic Administrator applicants, when will positions be brought back to reasonable levels? At what point will proper succession planning occur at the administrative levels in order to prepare the future academic leaders? And lastly, when will Academic Administrative leadership programs at the Masters level be created to support and offer the proper training for a future generation of prospective leaders? These are four major questions that must be answered to assure a positive, successful and well-developed pool of academic administrators with appropriate job responsibilities and roles. Hopefully, these elements are being put in motion before a catastrophic exodus occurs.

References

Adams, L. (2007). Nursing academic administration: Who will take on the challenge? *Journal of Professional Nursing, 23*(5), 309–315.

American Association of Community Colleges. (2005). *Competencies for community college leaders*. Retrieved March 23, 2012 from http://www.aacc.nche.edu/Resources/leadership/Pages/six_competencies.aspx

Bartone, P. T. (2007). Test re-test reliability of the Dispositional Resilience Scale-15, a brief hardiness scale. *Psychological Reports, 101*, 943–944.

Carpenter, K. D. (1989). Academic middle managers for baccalaureate nursing: Work, motivation and satisfaction. *Journal of Nursing Education, 28*, 256–264.

Chieffo, A. M. (1991). Factors contributing to job satisfaction and organizational commitment of community college leadership teams. *Community College Review, 19*(2), 15–24.

Cook, J. D., Hepworth, S. J., Wall, T. D., & Warr, P. B. (1981). *The experience of work: A compendium and review of 249 measures and their use*. Orlando, FL: Academic.

Copenhagen Psychosocial Questionnaire. (2003). Retrieved on August 27, 2007 from http://www.mentalhealthpromotion.net/resources/english_copsoq_2_ed_2003-pdf.pdf

Filan, G. L., & Seagren, A. T. (2003). Six critical issues for midlevel leadership in postsecondary settings. *New Directions for Higher Education, 124*(Winter), 21–31.

Foster, B. L. (2006). From faculty to administrator: Like going to a new planet. *New Directions for Higher Education, 134*(Summer), 49–57. doi:10.1002//he.216.

George, S. (1981). Associate and assistant deanships in schools of nursing. *Nursing Leadership, 4*, 25–30.

George, S., & Coudret, N. A. (1986). Dynamics and dilemmas of the associate and assistant dean roles. *Journal of Professional Nursing, 2*, 173–179.

Glick, N. L. (1992). Job satisfaction among academic administrators. *Research in Higher Education, 33*(5), 625–639.

Hall, B., Mitsunaga, B., & de Tornyay, R. (1981). Deans of nursing: Changing socialization patterns. *Nursing Outlook, 29*, 92–95.

Hoppe, S. L. (2003). Identifying and nurturing potential academic leaders. *New Directions for Higher Education, 124*(Winter), 3–12.

Judkins, S., & Furlow, L. (2003). Creating a hardy work environment: Can organizational policies help? *Texas Journal of Rural Health, 21*(4), 11–17.

Katsapis, C. A. (2010). The incidence and types of occupational role stress among university research administrators. *The Journal of Higher Education Management, 25*(1), 7–32.

Keim, M. C., & Murray, J. P. (2008). Chief academic officers' demographic and educational backgrounds. *Community College Review, 36*(2), 116–132.

Kobasa, S. C. (1979). Stressful life events, personality, and health: An inquiry into hardiness. *Journal of Personality and Social Psychology, 37*(1), 1–11.

Kouzes, J. M., & Posner, B. Z. (2001). *Leadership Practices Inventory (LPI) participant's workbook*. San Francisco, CA: Jossey-Bass.

Kuo, H. (2009). Understanding relationships between academic staff and administrators: An organizational culture perspective. *Journal of Higher Education Policy and Management, 31*(1), 43–54.

Lindley, M., & Mintz-Binder, R. D. (2012). *Exploring the challenges of the academic nurse leader role*. Southern Nursing Research Society Conference, New Orleans, LA (Poster session).

Locke, E. A. (1969). What is job satisfaction? *Organizational Behavior and Human Performance, 4*, 309–336.

Maslach, C. (1976). Burned-out. *Human Behavior, 5*, 16–22.

Maslach, C., & Jackson, S. E. (1981). The measurement of experienced burnout. *Journal of Occupational Behavior, 2*, 99–113.

Maslach, C., & Leiter, M. P. (1997). *The truth about burnout*. San Francisco, CA: Jossey-Bass.

Maslach, C., Schaufeli, W. B., & Leiter, M. P. (2001). Job burnout. *Annual Review of Psychology, 52*, 397–422.

McNair, D. E., Duree, C. A., & Ebbers, L. (2011). If I knew then what I know now: Using the leadership competencies developed by the American Association of Community Colleges to prepare community college presidents. *Community College Review, 39*(1), 3–25.

Mintz-Binder, R. D. (2012). *What are the critical factors affecting hardy (Poster session). functioning of academic program directors?* New Orleans, LA: Southern Nursing Research Society Conference.

Mintz-Binder, R. D. (accepted for publication). Exploring job satisfaction, role issues, and supervisor support of associate degree nursing program directors. *Nursing Education Perspectives*.

Mintz-Binder, R. D., & Calkins, R. D. (accepted for publication-proofs returned). Exposure to bullying at the associate degree nursing program director level. *Teaching and Learning in Nursing*.

Mintz-Binder, R. D., & Fitzpatrick, J. J. (2009). Exploring social support and job satisfaction among associate degree program directors in California. *Nursing Education Perspectives, 30*(5), 299–304.

Mintz-Binder, R. D., & Sanders, D. L. (2012). Workload demand: A significant factor in the overall well-being of directors of associate degree nursing programs. *Teaching and Learning in Nursing, 7*(1), 10–16.

Murphy, C. (2003). The rewards of academic leadership. *New Directions for Higher Education, 124*(Winter), 87–93.

Murray, J. R., & Murray, J. I. (1998). Job satisfaction and the propensity to leave an institution among two-year college division chairpersons. *Community College Review, 25*(4), 45–58.

Paul, K. B., Kravitz, D. A., Balzer, W. K., & Smith, P. C. (1990, August). *The original and Revised JDI: An initial comparison*. Paper presented at a meeting of the Academy of Management, San Francisco.

Pejtersen, J. H., Kristensen, T. S., Borg, V., & Bjorner, J. B. (2010). The second version of the Copenhagen Psychosocial Questionnaire. *The Scandinavian Journal of Public Health, 38*(Suppl. 3), 8–24.

Plater, W. M. (2006). The rise and fall of administrative careers. *New Direction in Higher Education, 134*(Summer), 15–24. doi:10.1002/he.213.

Princeton, J. C., & Gaspar, T. M. (1991). First-line nursing administrators in academe: How are they prepared, what do they do and will they stay in their jobs? *Journal of Professional Nursing, 7*(2), 79–87.

Raines, S. C., & Alberg, M. S. (2003). The role of professional development in preparing academic leaders. *New Directions for Higher Education, 124*(Winter), 33–39.

Reille, A., & Kezar, A. (2010). Balancing the pros and cons of community college "grow-your-own" leadership programs. *Community College Review, 38*(1), 59–81.

Spector, P. E. (2005). *Job satisfaction survey overview*. Retrieved May 1, 2006 from http://chuma.cas.usf.edu/~spector/scales/jssovr.html

Taylor, J. C., & Bowers, D. G. (1972). *Survey of organizations: A machine-scored standardized questionnaire instrument*. Ann Arbor, MI: University of Michigan, Center for Research on Utilization of Scientific Knowledge.

Weinert, C. (2003). Measuring social support: PRQ2000. In L. Strickland & C. Dilorio (Eds.), *Measurement of nursing outcomes: Vol. 3. Self care and coping* (2nd ed., pp. 161–172). New York, NY: Springer Publishing.

Occupational Health and Wellness: Current Status and Future Directions

26

Robert J. Gatchel

Overview

This Handbook has provided a comprehensive overview of the growing clinical research evidence related to the emerging transdisciplinary field of occupational health and wellness. This ever-expanding field has become especially more important today because of the growing costs, including socioeconomic as well as those associated with human suffering. In today's World of international business and finance, these costs are becoming even more significant because of the intertwining of world-wide economies. Indeed, a "hiccup" in one country will drastically affect others, as attested by recent economic "meltdowns" in various countries throughout the World. What makes these "meltdowns" even more troubling is the fact that there are so many disparities across countries in terms of economic and occupational variables, such as, working conditions and human rights, workers' compensation benefits, mental and physical health disorder rates, socialized vs. privatized health-care costs, retirement ages and related pension costs, etc. Thus, one major issue that needs to be addressed is whether there is any way that these variables can be standardized across countries in order to produce a "level playing field?" This has been tried by some countries, such as the establishment of the European Union (EU), but there are now also "cracks" occurring in the EU because of wide economic disparities that are emerging among the participating nations. Of course, solutions to such issues are beyond the scope of the current Handbook. We have addressed only those issues that we may be able to control/modify in the present zeitgeist. Of course, we must also introduce a word of caution concerning the material presented in this Handbook. A vast majority of it emanated from works translated into English and conducted in North America, Western Europe, and certain Nordic countries (e.g., Scandinavia and Finland). Thus, it would be unforgivable hubris to assume that such findings/suggestions would automatically generalize to all countries, especially the emerging industrial nations of the East and Pacific Rim. Actually, an important area of future research is to evaluate the generalizability of such issues and topics to these emerging industrial countries such as China, Taiwan, South Korea, and India.

R.J. Gatchel, Ph.D., A.B.P.P. (✉)
Department of Psychology, The University of Texas at Arlington,
Arlington, TX, USA
e-mail: gatchel@uta.edu

Of course, occupational health and wellness is still a relatively new emerging specialty within science and business. However, there is now an acceptance that the overall health of both organizations and individual workers need to be taken into account in order to yield the most efficient productivity while eliminating costly factors such as disabilities, impairments, and pain that may be caused by "unhealthy" occupational conditions. Throughout this Handbook, the various chapters provided a state-of-art discussion of important issues that are now recognized to be important in this field, and where there has been some significant progress made to date. These included the nature and causes of occupational stress, major symptoms and disorders often found in the workplace (e.g., musculoskeletal disorders, cardiovascular disease, cancer, mental health issues), the problem with absenteeism and presenteeism in the workplace, job-related burnout, self-medication and illicit drug use in the workplace/workforce, and the relatively new problem of bullying and violence in the workplace. A number of chapters were also dedicated to the evaluation of occupational causes and risks to workers' health, such as those related to healthy vs. non-healthy workplaces, safety issues and the problem of enforcement in the workplace, and the role of work schedules in occupational health and safety. Other issues, such as the fine balance between work–family issues and work–leave policies, as well as workers' compensation and other health-care policies for injured workers, were reviewed. These chapters provided a comprehensive evaluation of how these risks and causes of such occupational health threats are extremely important to consider. This series of chapters then segued into the now important area of prevention and intervention methods to apply in the workplace. Methods such as health and wellness promotion in the workplace, job-stress reduction programs for the workplace, primary and secondary prevention of illness in the workplace, organizational culture and workers' mental health, and employee-assistance programs were presented to the reader. Finally because it is a hallmark of scientific inquiry, the subsequent chapters were dedicated to documenting the prevalence and effectiveness of the occupational therapeutic impact that the aforementioned chapters provided. That is to say, it is one thing to provide clinical anecdotal comments about the presumed importance of the various issues discussed, and how to impact those areas; but it is another important scientific necessity to objectively document and quantify the seriousness of the noted issues, and then to objectively document and quantify their prevalence and any methods developed to modify their impact. Therefore, the review of epidemiological methods for documenting potential occupational health and illness issues, as well as program evaluation techniques to objectively quantify the efficacy/effectiveness of prevention and intervention programs, were presented. Finally the important issue of "can we decrease illness costs in the workplace?" was addressed. With this compendium of information now on hand, a major goal is to try to synthesize the current status of this information, as well as to comment on future important directions that need to be considered. These are the goals of the present chapter.

Revisiting/Updating Past Research Areas

In most areas of scientific inquiry, a common phenomenon that often occurs is that, after a great deal of research activity which subsequently appears to highlight or "answer" all the relevant empirical questions and integrates them in a well conceived and validated theoretical model, scientists then "move away" from that area and go on to the next research challenge. However, a decade or two later, this past research (which had been "shelved" or "archived") may be rediscovered because the dormant area again resurfaces as important to address; or, a new technology emerges, or a theoretical heuristic surfaces, that can lead to further advances. The older model is now "dusted off" and stimulates new research to expand/modify its basic theoretical/practical tenets. As a case in point, a book published in the early 1980s by McDonald and Doyle (1981) was about "… mental and physical health at work,

Table 26.1 Stresses, strains, and their long-term consequences (McDonald & Doyle, 1981)

Stresses	Strains
Poverty, insecurity of work and unemployment	*Physical reactions* Headaches, backache, muscle cramps, poor sleep, indigestion
Excessive overtime, shiftwork	
Pressure of work –excessive pace, mechanical pacing, production deadlines	*Psychological reactions* Fatigue, anxiety, tension, irritability, depression, boredom, inability to concentrate, feelings of unreality, low self-esteem
Work that is monotonous and requires little skill but demands constant attention	
Working in danger	*Behavioral effects* Heavy indulgence in smoking, alcohol and drugs; impulsive, emotional behavior; accidents
Interpersonal conflicts and tensions	
Uncertain responsibilities	*Social effects* Poor relationships with others at home and at work; inability to fulfill social and family roles; social isolation
Social isolation at work	
Poor physical environment at work (e.g., noise)	

Note: Factors outside work can also combine with the stresses of work to increase the strain on a worker, e.g., housing problems, domestic and family problems, bereavement, racial prejudice, etc.

and ways in which psychological and social aspects of working conditions can harm the health and well being of workers" (p. 1). In that book, they presented a table that summarized the various stressors at the workplace, and the consequences of such stressors on health (see Table 26.1). As can be seen, many of these issues/factors presented at that time are now (three decades later) again receiving increased attention.

As a further example of this current phenomenon, there are two such areas that will be considered here—the effects of unemployment/nonwork on mental and physical health, and the effects of environmental/occupational crowding on health and wellness.

Unemployment/Nonwork

The interest in this area has waxed and waned in unison with changes in unemployment rates. Jahoda and colleagues have been constant investigators in this area, from their earlier work on unemployment in Europe during the 1930s (Jahoda, Lazarsfeld, & Zeisel, 1933), and then throughout the rest of the century (Jahoda, 1982, 1988). This later research focused primarily on unemployment and economic recession factors that affected the psychosocial well-being of the unemployed. At the same time, Kasl and Cobb initiated their own research documenting changes in health status associated with job loss (e.g., Kasl & Cobb, 1970; Kasl, Gore, & Cobb, 1975), as had Feather and O'Brien (Feather, 1990; O'Brien & Feather, 1990). Most recently (2008–2012), with the Worldwide recession producing high rates of unemployment, there has been a dramatic increase in mental health problems (especially depression). For example, the Centers for Disease Control and Prevention (CDC) reported that the rate of depression in the USA in 2002 was 6.6%; it increased to 9% in 2010 (Seale, 2011). Moreover, the CDC has shown that suicide rates are also closely related to rises and falls in the economy. Suicide rates increased the most during the Great Depression from 1929 to 1933 (to an all-time increase of 22.1%), and has similarly gone up whenever the economy has fallen into a revision. This is also true worldwide, such as the 25% increase in the suicide rate in 2010 over the previous year, concomitant with the great unemployment rate in Greece (Kentikelenis et al., 2011).

Taking a slightly different approach to evaluating the detrimental effects of unemployment, Main, Phillips and Watson (2005) reviewed research that addressed the detrimental effects of unemployment due to musculoskeletal disorders such as low back pain. They highlighted the negative impact of such disorders on quality of life and the development of additional health problems of injured workers. These workers were also more likely to suffer from mental health problems, increased consultation rates for other physical complaints, and even lower life expectancy rates. Such data reveal the large public health concerns associated with unemployment due to the inability of returning individuals back to work because of musculoskeletal and other work-related injuries. Later in this chapter, the increases in vocational rehabilitation efforts to return workers back to the workplace as soon as possible will be discussed.

Environmental Psychology and Crowding Research

Environmental psychology is an area of study that evaluates the environment as a determinant or influence on human behavior and mood. Bell, Greene, Fisher, and Baum (1996) had earlier reviewed how high-density living environments/conditions, such as urban areas, crowded commuter trains, dormitory areas, prison settings, etc. can lead to:

> "… more negative affective states … and high levels of physiological arousal, as measured on a wide variety of indices. Further, there is evidence … that high density is associated with illness …" (p. 338).

McCoy (2002) has more recently reviewed the significant role that work environments play in performance and creativity, as well as the health, safety, and social behaviors of workers. One common concomitant of high-density work environments is increased noise. Such "noise pollution" has been shown to have detrimental physical and mental health consequences (Bronzaft, 2002). In fact, Raymond, Kerr, McCullagh, and Lusk (2011) have noted that noise is one of the most common occupational health hazards. They have reported that the prevalence of hearing loss among noise-exposed factory workers was 42% (based standards of the Occupational Safety and Health Administration). Another interesting finding of this study was that 76% of the workers reported that their hearing ability was good or excellent. This surprising finding suggests that, over time, the hearing loss was insidious in nature, with the workers accommodating to the gradually increasing levels of loss. Taken together, the findings of this investigation argue for the further development and implementation of surveillance methods and programs to address this important occupational health issue. Thus, the simple physical design of the workplace, which minimizes crowding and the noise levels that workers are exposed to, is an important factor to consider in occupational settings. Of course, as noted in the very first chapter of this Handbook, the economic pressures on companies to make money often trumps the immediate needs to make expensive workplace redesigns/renovations, unless political pressure can be brought to bear to make such changes. Of course, just as in the past, this will be a recurring problem/theme in the future that will need to be monitored and addressed throughout occupational settings.

Vocational Rehabilitation

"… where a man having an injury, has admittedly not recovered, returns to work … and then again breaks down, or who still has an obviously physical disability."
Sir John Collie, 1916

The above quote was taken from an article by Escorpizo, Gümunder, and Stucki (2011) which was the lead article for a Special Section of the *Journal of Occupational Rehabilitation* that focused on recent advances in better understanding and measuring vocational rehabilitation (VR) processes and outcomes. Indeed, a traditional bane of all employers and employees who were faced with occupational injury was how to return the injured worker back to the workplace as quickly as possible. As we just discussed earlier, Main et al. (2005) reported the detrimental effects of unemployment due to musculoskeletal disorders. They suggested the need to get these workers rehabilitated and back to work as soon as possible in order to avoid these effects. The field of VR has been at the forefront of developing methods to best facilitate work-return after injury. An important development in this field, which was a major topic of this Special Section [entitled, "Advancing the field of vocational rehabilitation with the International Classification of Functioning, Disability and Healths (ICF)"] was to "… provide stakeholders and advocates in VR a unifying perspective based on the ICF, a biopsychosocial model developed by the World Health Organization … and illustrate how the VR community can benefit from using the ICF" (Escorpizo et al., 2011). This represents an enlightened and important starting point for developing a common vernacular and measurement language that can be used when addressing work disability issues, and that can be utilized by multiple stakeholders (i.e., employers, employees, the social security and insurance system, health policy authorities, etc.), across different occupations, and across different countries.

Indeed, the above effort should be applauded because it provides an "anchor-based language" to address the often complex and non-isomorphic relationships among the various areas discussed throughout the present Handbook, such as different type of jobs, various work environments, occupational health issues, and specific Health-related conditions. This common language can now be used when communicating across the various disciplines and sciences involved in the complex field of occupational health and wellness.

Organizational Health: Integrating Physical Design Factors and Workers' Needs

Industrial research scientists such as Luczak (1992) have argued for the importance of a good work design environment which should be "anthropocentric" in nature (i.e., placing the individual worker at the center of the overall work design environment). This is in striking contrast to the traditional "technocentric" approach in which the work technology and economic considerations were at the center of the design process; the workers were expected to accommodate to the work environment characteristics. Of course, these do not have to be mutually exclusive approaches. For example, good ergonomic and work safety designs do not only benefit efficient production and cost-savings from management's perspective, but also protect workers from needless accidents and injuries. However, additional empirical studies are still needed to clearly delineate how to integrate these two apparently disparate approaches in a cost-effective and satisfactory manner for both the organization and its workers.

Of course, as Baum, Gatchel, and Krantz (1997) have reviewed, two important variables have been shown to significantly affect occupational stress in the work environment: job demands (i.e., job conditions that tax or interfere with the workers' performance abilities such as workload and work responsibilities); and level of job autonomy or control (i.e., the ability of the worker to control the speed, nature, and conditions of work). Low levels of control over one's job and excessive workloads seem to be a particularly important combination in heightening job-related stress. Much of this work was initially conducted by Mary Ann Frankenhauser (1979) in Sweden. Karasek and Theorell (1990) subsequently proposed that conditions of high demand and low control created *high strain* situations. Their "job-demand/control" hypothesis has been tested in several populations by applying a job characteristics scoring system based on responses to several national surveys of workers (a more thorough review of this work has been presented in earlier chapters by Dewe, O'Driscoll and Cooper, as well as Theorell in this Handbook). These job characteristics scores can then distinguish between occupations along the dimensions comprising job strain, and it has shown the ability to predict cardiovascular disease and mortality in studies of male Swedish workers and studies of men and women in the USA. Results such as these clearly indicate that work environments that are constructed to decrease "job strain" can have a significant impact on worker health and well-being. Thus, this "anthropocentric" factor would be an apparent and important one to consider in developing a good work design environment.

Occupational Injury Administrative and Legal Issues

We would be remiss if we did not introduce the reader to administrative issues that often emerge after an occupational injury or illness. Melhorn and colleagues have provided additional information on these important issues in their earlier chapter of this Handbook. Such information is quite important because many health care and human resources professionals are not well versed in these issues. As a starting point, it should be pointed out that it is now recognized that the most comprehensive and heuristic approach to the evaluation/management of medical conditions, especially those involving pain, is the biopsychosocial perspective (Gatchel, 2005; Gatchel, Robinson, Pulliam, & Maddrey, 2003; Turk & Monarch, 2002). This *biopsychosocial model* focuses on the complex interaction among biological, psychosocial, and medicolegal variables that patients encounter when dealing with persisting and, distressing medical conditions, such as chronic pain. Such an interaction may perpetuate, and even worsen, the clinical presentation. It also accounts for the likelihood that patients' lives are adversely affected in a variety of ways by their medical condition, thus requiring a more comprehensive assessment and treatment approach designed to address all aspects of required care, both biological and psychosocial. This approach is in striking contrast to the outdated, overly simplistic biomedical reductionist approach, which erroneously assumed that most medical illnesses could be broken down into distinct, independent physical and psychosocial components. As a case in point against this outdated approach, one study highlighted how individuals differed significantly in the frequency they report physical symptoms, and their tendency to visit physicians when experiencing identical symptoms, as well as in their responses to the same treatment (Gatchel, Kishino, & Strezak, 2006). Often, the nature of patients' responses to treatment has little to do with their objective physical conditions.

Another important aspect of the biopsychosocial model that deserves independent mention is in the area of *compensation injuries* (e.g., workers' compensation, short/long-term disability, and personal injury litigation). It has long been known that objective, societal outcomes, such as return-to-work, future healthcare utilization, and recurrent injury rates, are considerably lower than in the general population for similar injuries, independent of the severity of injury or treatment (e.g., Gatchel, 2005). For example, a large meta-analysis demonstrated that return-to-work rates for spinal fusion surgery to be as low as 16% in workers' compensation populations (Turner et al., 1992). It has become clear that financial secondary gain is closely related to patient behaviors when compensation is being provided

Fig. 26.1 The overlap between the construct of pain (a common symptom of illness), impairment, and disability

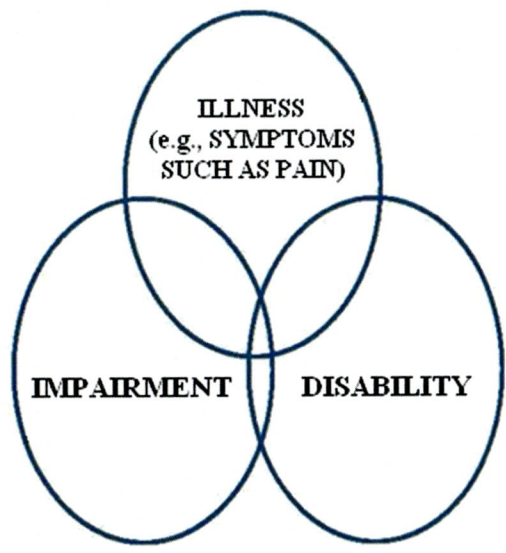

for illness. Secondary gain can be briefly defined as an individual's attempt to avoid certain activities (such as work), obtain monetary payment (through legal settlements), or to avoid certain activities in order to receive other support (e.g., sympathy or attention) from his or her environment that otherwise would not be forthcoming (Dersh, Polatin, Leeman, & Gatchel, 2004). Compensated illness is a frequent finding in almost all industrialized countries and is a significant financial strain on employers and the healthcare system.

As recently reiterated by Gatchel, Kishino, and Minotti (2010), in addition to the aforementioned fact that there are often complex interactions among the three biopsychosocial referents of illnesses such as pain, what makes this assessment area even more complicated is that there may also be complex interactions among the construct of *illness/pain* and the two related constructs of *disability* and *impairment*. These three constructs frequently do not display high concordance with one another, thus creating a second layer of complexity. Indeed, as previously highlighted by Gatchel (2005) and Gatchel and Kishino (in press), it is extremely important to be aware of the important administrative distinctions among the constructs of *pain*, *disability*, and *impairment*. This is again due to the fact that there is often discordance, or a low degree of correlation, among levels of chronic pain, impairment, and disability. For example, in an early influential report by Waddell (1987), the problem of discordance in the evaluation of chronic low back pain was noted (see Fig. 26.1). Although correlations were found among these three constructs, there was not perfect overlap among these phenomena. Although they are all logically and clinically related to one another, there is usually not a 1:1:1 relation among them. Waddell (1987) found correlations among them to be in the range of only about 0.6. Also, what makes these imperfect correlations even more complex is the wide range of differences in such concordance from one individual to the next (Turk & Melzack, 2001). Healthcare professionals, therefore, need to be cognizant of the varying relationships among these constructs during the evaluation of patients. For example, one patient may display very little medical impairment that can be objectively evaluated, although he/she may verbally report a great many symptoms of illness. Ratings of disability may perhaps fall somewhere in between the two in terms of severity. In stark contrast, another patient with a seemingly comparable injury may report very few symptoms (such as pain), but may display a great deal of impairment and disability. Obviously, clinicians need to be aware of the operational definitions of these above three constructs or phenomena because they are fundamentally different. Also, it is important to be aware of what construct you are being asked to assess in specific diagnostic situations, with the expectation that there may also be complex interactions among them that may differ from one patient to the next, as well as from one assessment time period to the next. These three constructs have been further discussed in the medical impairment and disability evaluation literature (e.g., Dembe, 2000; Gatchel, 1996, 2005). We will again briefly review them next.

Pain

We just discussed the construct of pain, which is a common symptom of occupational injuries and illness in general. Chronic pain (i.e., pain lasting for greater than three months) is a biopsychosocial concept based primarily on an experiential or subjective evaluation (Gatchel, 2004, 2005). The construct of pain is frequently used to infer the presence of some biopsychosocial mechanisms that prompts patients' complaints and inhibition of normal functioning and behavior. It is often difficult to quantify chronic pain in a totally objective and reliable manner. This is also frequently true for other illnesses, such as multiple sclerosis, chronic fatigue syndrome, whiplash injuries, PTSD, etc. Usually, simple patient self-report measures are used, which can often be too subjective and unreliable (Gatchel, 2005).

Impairment

Impairment has traditionally been a medical term which is used to refer to an alteration of an individual's usual health status (i.e., some anatomical or pathophysiological abnormality) that is evaluated by medical methods. The *American Medical Association's Guides to the Evaluation of Permanent Impairment (Sixth Edition)* defines impairment as "a significant deviation, loss, or loss of use of any body structure or body function in an individual with a health condition, disorder, or disease" (Rondinelli et al., 2008). The evaluation of impairment via an independent medical evaluation is conducted to determine some inferred pathophysiology or anatomical dysfunction that is assumed to have a negative impact on a patient's current health status or behavior (such as a significant loss, or loss of use, of a body structure or function). Unfortunately, however, such impairment evaluation relies upon methods that are often not totally reliable (physical examination findings tend to have a low inter-examiner reliability) and that are often subject to examiner bias, as well as patient effort. Nevertheless, its assessment is supposed to be standardized and should remain the same for any individual, regardless of differences in occupation. Thus, an injured worker who sustains a traumatic amputation of the dominant third finger will have the same impairment rating under a workers' compensation system claim, regardless of whether the worker was a truck driver who is still able to driver trucks or a data entry person who now has to change jobs. It is therefore important to inform patients that, if their case falls under an impairment-based system, then their monetary award will have little to do with their functional abilities and pain. Such monetary award differences may occur when determining disability. Finally, it should also be pointed out that progress towards recovery will often have no impact on the impairment evaluation or, conversely, a lack of recovery may not increase the impairment evaluation. This will be the case when a designated physician documents that Maximum Medical Improvement (MMI) has been reached by the patient. MMI is typically defined "… in part as the earliest date after which, based on reasonable medical probability, further material recovery from or lasting improvement to an injury can no longer be reasonably anticipated" [Texas Department of Insurance—Division of Worker's Compensation, 2008, 401.011 (30) (A)]. The "reasonable medical probability" part of this definition suggests that an MMI may often be quite subjective and may differ from one designated physician to the next. With this in mind, a healthcare professional should not prematurely insist on the documentation that MMI has been reached if there is any chance that progress in recovery is no longer a possibility (which may be manifested by improvement in physical findings such as range-of-motion and lifting capacity). This is because that once MMI has been documented as having been reached, then there is no longer the possibility of changing the patient's impairment rating.

Disability

Disability is more of an administrative term that refers to a diminished capacity or inability to perform certain activities of everyday living or occupational demands (or to meet statutory or regulatory requirements of a job) as a result of loss of function, due to impairment. Again, though, disability evaluations are not totally reliable and may also be subject to various examiner and patient response biases. Nevertheless, disability will vary depending on the "gap" between what the person can do and what the person needs or wants to do. Thus, under a system that uses a disability-based formula, such as Social Security Disability Insurance or personal injury litigation, the loss of the dominant third finger would have a much greater impact on the monetary award for the data entry person than the truck driver because the award would take into account future earning capacity. Under such systems, the clinician may be asked to render an opinion about work capacity, pain, and suffering, and other issues outside the immediate realm of medical opinion or the impairment rating. It should also be noted that the aforementioned "disability-based formula" will differ from one venue to the next. For example, each State has its own workers' compensation system, with different guidelines. As a healthcare professional, it is up to you to be well versed in such differences in medicolegal jurisdictions. These different jurisdictions, in turn, may have different levels of "secondary gain" issues associated with them.

How to Enhance Organization and Employee Health

Throughout this present Handbook, we have reviewed various health disorders, interventions and possible organizational programs to address health and wellness issues. At this point in time, the great deal of research and theory developed in this field has not yet been fully integrated in order to address important issues such as matching jobs and work design, related interventions to improve health issues that may arise, and how organizational structure can help employee health. In terms of the latter issue, it will be important to ensure that there is a healthy feedback system within the entire organization so that the needs of the "company" and those of the "workers" are constantly being appropriately monitored and addressed in an integrated manner. That is to say, the "left hand" needs to know what the "right hand" is doing at all times in order to avoid sudden increases in grievances and morale problems, health issues, productivity, economic problems, etc. This will be no easy task, and a great deal of coordinated effort is needed to accomplish the ultimate "healthy organizational hierarchical system." As an example of such a system, Fig. 26.2 presents the various components that need to be integrated and monitored into a meaningful whole in order to maximize worker productivity, safety, and health.

Public and Private Organizations/Agencies Included in the Field of Occupational Health and Wellness

It is not surprising that, with the emergent advances and recognized importance of the field of occupational health and wellness, there has been a concomitant growth of organizations and agencies specializing in various areas in this large field. In this section, we will provide a brief review of many of these to serve as a reference guide to readers.

ADMINISTRATION LEVEL

GOOD WORK ENVIRONMENTAL DESIGN

- Proper ergonomics and worker safety standards.
- Continuous feedback among administration, human resources, supervisors, occupational medical staff and workers concerning possible modification of the above.
- Monthly status reports concerning the financial health of the organization.
- Profit-sharing plan for employees?
- Encouragement of feedback from employees to increase productivity and safety improvement.

HUMAN RESOURCES LEVEL

AVAILABILITY OF PROGRAMS FOR ALL EMPLOYEES

- Employee-assistance programs for issues such as substance abuse, family problems, work issues, absenteeism, etc.
- Health-promotion programs, such as exercise, diet/weight loss, smoking cessation, stress management, anger/frustration control, etc.
- Recent information of interest to all.

OCCUPATIONAL MEDICINE RESOURCES

GOOD OCCUPATIONAL HEALTH CENTER

- Programs to prevent and provide early VR interventions for work-related injuries.
- Comprehensive interdisciplinary programs (such as functional restoration) to manage longer-term work disability issues.
- Wellness medical check-ups.
- Referral network for serious medical conditions.

HEALTH & ECONOMIC EVALUATION RESOURCES

PROGRAM/ORGANIZATION EVALUATION

- Effectiveness of Work Environmental Design, Human Resources, and Occupational Health Center in reducing prevalence of accidents, injuries, and health problems.
- Cost-savings of the above.
- Overall functioning and profitability of organization.

Fig. 26.2 Various components that need to be integrated and monitored into a meaningful whole in order to maximize worker productivity, safety, and health

- *National Institute for Occupational Safety and Health* (NIOSH). NIOSH has been mandated by federal law in the USA to stimulate/support research that addresses working conditions that may be hazardous to employees' mental or physical health and well-being. A further mandate is to disseminate the research and knowledge in order to prevent workplace injuries.
- *World Health Organization* (WHO). WHO helps to coordinate and sponsor a wide range of health-related research, from epidemiological to prevention and intervention studies that are designed to have a major impact on health and safety issues around the World.
- *World Bank*. The World Bank focuses on improving the well-being of individuals with disabilities living in developing countries.
- *The International Labour Organization* (ILO). The major goals of the ILO are the following: to enhance the social protection of workers as well as to strengthen the dialogue focused on work-related issues, to promote rights at work, and to encourage decent employment opportunities for those seeking work.
- *The International Classification of Functioning, Disability and Health* (ICF). The ICF seeks to develop a common reference and language for use with national and international organizations that seek to further vocational rehabilitation and health services for injured workers.
- *The European Academy of Occupational Health Psychology*. This academy was originally developed as a joint collaboration among scientists in the UK, Sweden, and Denmark. Its focus is on supporting regular conferences that promote research, clinical practice, and education in the field of occupational health psychology.

- *The International Commission on Occupational Health* (ICOH). The ICOH is an international scientific society dedicated to stimulate scientific progress, knowledge and development in the wide array of areas involved in occupational health and safety.
- *American College of Occupational and Environmental Medicine* (ACOEM). ACOEM's major goals are to promote and protect the health of workers through state-of-the-art clinical care, preventive services, interventions, etc.
- *Agency for Healthcare Research and Quality* (AHRQ). AHRQ is an arm of the Department of Health and Human Services in the USA developed to summarize the available medical evidence of appropriate treatments for various conditions, as well as developing practice guidelines. AHRQ replaced the earlier controversial AHCPR.
- *American Psychological Association* (APA). Besides having specific divisions dedicated to many issues of occupational health and wellness (e.g., Division 14, Industrial & Organizational Psychology; Division 38, Health Psychology), APA also often collaborates with other national and international organizations interested in promoting occupational- and health-related issues.
- *Society for Occupational Health Psychology* (SOHP). SOHP was the first organization founded in the USA that is devoted to occupational health psychology.
- *Workers' Education Association* (WEA). The WEA seeks to provide access to education and lifelong learning to workers throughout the World.
- *American Medical Association's Guides to the Evaluation of Permanent Impairment*. This edited compendium defines the latest innovative and new international standard for impairment assessment. It is now in its Sixth Edition.
- There have also been a number of scientific journals devoted to issues involved in occupational health and wellness: *Journal of Occupational Rehabilitation*; *Journal of Environmental and Occupational Medicine*; *Journal of Occupational Health Psychology*; *Health Psychology*.

Finally, in the USA, one specialty area within psychology is Industrial and Organizational Psychology. As noted by Briner and Rousseau (2011): "The founders of our field, including James McKeen Cattell and C.S. Myers, originated the application of systematic research to workplace issues ... Most of what we do in I-O psychology draws on or at least is informed by some type of evidence ..." (p. 3). However, in a special issue of the journal, *Industrial and Organizational Psychology* (2011, Volume 4, Issue 1), a plea for more evidence-based practice approaches is made. Indeed, this is one field that is greatly needed to help address many of the issues that we have addressed in this Handbook. However, to date, integration of new developments of work practice models with the evidence-based documentation of their validity/reliability has not been forthcoming. For the future advancement of this field, and the vital role it can play in occupational health and illness issues, further integration and growth is urgently needed.

Summary and Conclusions

As we have noted, occupational health and wellness is still a new emerging specialty within science and business. Nevertheless, there is now an acceptance of the fact that the overall health of both organizations and individual workers needs to be taken into account in order to yield the most efficient productivity while, simultaneously, eliminating costly factors such as disabilities, impairments, and pain that may be caused by "unhealthy" occupational conditions. Throughout this present Handbook, the various chapters provided a state-of-art discussion of important issues that are now recognized to be important in this field, and where there has been some significant progress made to date. A major goal of the current chapter was to attempt to synthesize the current status of this information presented, as well as to comment on future important directions that need to be considered. We initially addressed two areas that, although investigated widely two decades ago, are now being "rediscovered" as important in the field of occupational health and wellness: the effects of unemployment/nonwork on mental and physical health and the effects of environmental–occupational crowding on health and illness. It was revealed that there is a large public health concern associated with unemployment due to the inability of returning individuals back to work because of musculoskeletal and other work-related injuries. We also addressed the current increase in vocational rehabilitation efforts to return workers back to the workplace as soon as possible. We then introduced the reader to the important area of environmental psychology, with specific emphasis on how crowding research is of particular relevance to the field. Indeed, researchers are now reviewing the significant role that work environments play in performance and creativity, as well as the health, safety, and social behaviors of workers. One common concomitant of high-density work environments is increased "noise pollution," which has been shown to have detrimental physical and mental health consequences. Thus, the physical design of a workplace, which minimizes crowding and noise levels that workers are exposed to, is an important factor to consider in occupational settings.

Industrial research scientists have long argued for the importance of a good work design environment which should be "anthropocentric" in nature. This is in striking contrast to the traditional "technocentric" approach which emphasized that workers were expected to accommodate to the work environment characteristics. However, we pointed out that these two approaches do not have to be mutually exclusive. Good ergonomic and work safety designs do not only benefit efficient production and cost-savings from managements' perspective, but also protect workers from needless accidents and injuries. For example, two important variables that have been shown to significantly affect occupational stress in the work environment are job demands and level of job autonomy or control. Much of this research was initiated in Sweden by Frankenhauser and then expanded by Karasek and colleagues. These investigators proposed a "job-demand/control" hypothesis that created *high strain* job situations. *High strain* jobs were found to be associated with increased health problems in workers.

We also introduced the reader to administrative issues that often emerge after an occupational injury or illness. The biopsychosocial model was emphasized as important in better understanding the complex interactions among biological, psychological, and medicolegal variables that patients' encounter when dealing with persisting, distressing medical conditions. This biopsychosocial model is important to keep in mind when dealing with important occupational health areas such as compensation injuries. Constructs such as pain, disability, and impairment, and the fact that there is often a discordance or a low degree of correlation among the three, was also discussed. It is extremely important for professionals in the field of occupational health and wellness to become well-versed in the various administrative and legal issues associated with injuries and health issues. We then went on to discuss how to enhance organization and employee health in general. A model was proposed that took into account regular components that need to be integrated and monitored into a meaningful whole in order to maximize worker productivity, safety, and health. Finally, as was emphasized, with the emergent advances and recognized importance of the field of occupational health and wellness, there has been a concomitant growth of organizations and agencies specializing in various areas in this large field. We provided a brief review of many of these to serve as a reference guide to readers. A special call was also made for the field of Industrial and Organizational Psychology to increase its contributions of evidence-based approaches to work practice issues.

Other Future Directions

Each chapter in this Handbook concluded with a section with suggestions for future directions needed to further advance the key concepts/issues discussed. To those, some additional ones should be noted. These are delineated below.

- The actual understanding/definition of "work" as we now know it will be continuing to change in the future. Indeed, the earlier assembly line type of jobs are already being replaced by more automatic/robotic streamlined production. Where will a worker interface with this type of production? Also, new needs (such as drone aircraft controllers) may continue to expand, as will "virtual reality" methods of solving business issues and problems.
- Relatedly, what will happen to the traditional blue collar, unionized workers who manned the assembly lines? Can these "blue collar" workers be transitioned to more "white collar" jobs? This will undoubtedly create some political fall-out in terms of the "union vote" and politicians up for reelection. Indeed, with the recent trends in the "downsizing" by many companies, and their greater reliance on "outsourcing" to part-time or contingent workers, new issues are arising concerning how these workers will interface with traditional workers. Some of these issues were discussed in the chapter by Cole.
- Related to the above is the fact that we are already seeing a great outsourcing of jobs to countries with a workforce that is content with a minimum wage. How can this be better managed so that it can be a "win–win" situation for both the countries involved, as well as their workers? Can occupational health issues be carefully considered and managed by both the developed and underdeveloped countries involved?
- Superimposed on all of the above issues/questions is the great concern of decreasing natural resources to keep up with the industrial growth that is occurring across the globe. What type of international controls can be created to monitor this? This will create an entirely new international administration to help in this monitoring and coordination. No longer will negotiations between workers and employers be limited to individual countries, but it will have to expand across countries.
- How can we ensure that good work safety and health standards be incorporated around the globe?
- We are beginning to see a growth in the number of intervention strategies to increase occupational health and wellness. However, the traditional methods of documenting their efficacy/effectiveness will need to "change with the times." It is now not enough to simply empirically demonstrate that one approach is better than another. With the staggering and growing healthcare costs in the USA, the federal government is now moving towards finding the best ways to develop interventions that are both therapeutically efficacious and *cost-effective* (Lauer & Collins, 2010). This has stimulated the need for more comparative effectiveness research (CER; Manchikanti, Falco, Boswell, & Hirsch, 2010; Sox, 2010). One vital feature of CER is the use of cost-effectiveness analyses in order to help objectively document the most *cost-effective* intervention method. This has been sorely lacking in past intervention research in the field, and will need to be in the forefront of future efforts in the development/documentation of prevention and intervention methods in the workplace.
- There has been a definite increase in the number of workplace wellness programs being offered by employers, due to the research in this area demonstrating potential cost-savings and worker productivity. In their chapter, Shaw and colleagues highlighted the fact that the number of employers offering workplace wellness programs with financial incentives to employees in the USA has been steadily rising despite the recent recession-economic environment. That is the good news. However, some have voiced the concern that such wellness programs could actually be used as a means to discriminate against potentially sicker employees who cannot meet a given incentive (e.g., lose × number of pounds for a merit-pay increase or a decrease in your insurance deductible). As referenced by Kliff (2012) from a *Business Week* article:

> … Georgetown authors cite one wellness program that wields a stick. It suggests employers raise deductibles from, say, $500 to $2,500. Workers can then "earn credits" worth $500 each to lower the deductible if they meet certain targets for four factors: body-mass index, blood pressure, cholesterol, and tobacco use. A nonsmoking, normal-weight employee with healthy cholesterol and blood pressure winds up back at the $500 deductible. "If

you're on the wrong end of any of those four tests, your costs have gone up ..." The Georgetown authors say they want to make sure wellness incentives actually make people healthier and don't just shift costs onto sick workers. "There's really strong research showing that the higher the deductible, the greater the barrier to accessing care," ... "Someone may not be getting basic primary care or necessary care to treat a chronic condition."

Thus, one must always be concerned that a well-intentioned program can be "hijacked" for inappropriate purposes.

With the above areas in mind, it will be important to develop more comprehensive theoretical, economic, and prevention/intervention frameworks that take into account workers, worksites, employers, local and national administrations, as well as international cooperation, in order to address occupational health and wellness issues.

References

Baum, A., Gatchel, R. J., & Krantz, D. S. (Eds.). (1997). *An introduction to health psychology* (3rd ed.). New York, NY: McGraw-Hill.
Bell, P. A., Greene, T. C., Fisher, J. D., & Baum, A. (1996). *Environmental psychology* (4th ed.). New York, NY: Holt, Rinehart & Winston.
Briner, R. B., & Rousseau, D. M. (2011). Evidence-based I–O psychology: Not there yet. *Industrial and Organizational Psychology, 4*(1), 3–22. doi:10.1111/j.1754-9434.2010.01287.x.
Bronzaft, A. L. (2002). Noise pollution: A hazard to physical and mental well-being. In R. B. Bechtel & A. Churchman (Eds.), *Handbook of environmental psychology*. New York, NY: Wiley.
Dembe, A. E. (2000). Pain, function, impairment and disability: Implications for workers' compensation and other disability insurance systems. In T. G. Mayer, R. J. Gatchel, & P. B. Polatin (Eds.), *Occupational musculoskeletal disorders: Function, outcomes and evidence*. Philadelphia, PA: Lippincott Williams & Wilkins.
Dersh, J., Polatin, P. B., Leeman, G., & Gatchel, R. J. (2004). The management of secondary gain and loss in medicolegal settings: Strengths and weaknesses. *Journal of Occupational Rehabilitation, 14*(4), 267–279.
Escorpizo, R., Gmünder, H., & Stucki, G. (2011). Introduction to special section: Advancing the field of vocational rehabilitation with the International Classification of Functioning, Disability and Health (ICF). *Journal of Occupational Rehabilitation, 21*(2), 121–125. doi:10.1007/s10926-011-9309-1.
Feather, N. T. (1990). *The psychological impact of unemployment*. New York, NY: Springer.
Frankenhauser, M. (1979). Psychoendocrine approaches to the study of emotion as related to stress and coping. In H. E. How & R. A. D. Dienstbier (Eds.), *Nebraska symposium on motivation 1978* (pp. 123–161). Lincoln, OR: University of Nebraska Press.
Gatchel, R. J. (1996). Psychological disorders and chronic pain: Cause and effect relationships. In R. J. Gatchel & D. C. Turk (Eds.), *Psychological approaches to pain management: A practitioner's handbook* (pp. 33–52). New York, NY: Guilford.
Gatchel, R. J. (2004). Comorbidity of chronic mental and physical health disorders: The biopsychosocial perspective. *American Psychologist, 59*, 792–805.
Gatchel, R. J. (2005). *Clinical essentials of pain management*. Washington, DC: American Psychological Association.
Gatchel, R. J., & Kishino, N. D. (in press). Chronic pain, impairment and disability. In A. Rice, R. Howard, D. Justins, C. Miaskowski, & T. Newton-John (Eds.), *Textbook of clinical pain management* (2nd ed.). London: Hodder Arnold Publishers.
Gatchel, R. J., Kishino, N. D., & Minotti, D. E. (2010). The three major components of behavior used for assessing pain: Problems faced when there is discordance among the three. *Psychological Injury and Law, 3*, 212–219.
Gatchel, R. J., Kishino, N. D., & Strezak, A. (2006). The importance of outcome assessment in orthopaedics: An overview. In J. M. Spivak & P. J. Connolly (Eds.), *Orthopaedic knowledge update: Spine*. Chicago, IL: American Academy of Orthopaedic Surgeons.
Gatchel, R. J., Robinson, R. C., Pulliam, C., & Maddrey, A. M. (2003). Biofeedback with pain patients: Evidence for its effectiveness. *Seminars in Pain Management, 1*, 55–66.
Jahoda, M. (1982). *Employment and unemployment: A social psychological analysis*. Cambridge: Cambridge University Press.
Jahoda, M. (1988). Economic recession and mental health: Some conceptual issues. *Journal of Social Issues, 44*, 13–23.
Jahoda, M., Lazarsfeld, P. F., & Zeisel, H. (1933). *Marienthal: The sociography of an unemployed community*. London: Tavistock.

Karasek, R. A., & Theorell, T. G. (1990). *Healthy work*. New York, NY: Basic Books.

Kasl, S. V., & Cobb, S. (1970). Blood pressure changes in men undergoing job loss: A preliminary report. *Psychosomatic Medicine, 32*, 19–38.

Kasl, S. V., Gore, S., & Cobb, S. (1975). The experience of losing a job: Reported changes in health, symptoms and illness behavior. *Psychosomatic Medicine, 37*, 106–122.

Kentikelenis, A., Karanikolos, M., Papanicolas, I., Basu, S., McKee, M., & Stuckler, D. (2011). Health effects of financial crisis: Omens of a Greek tragedy. *The Lancet, 378*(9801), 1457–1458. doi:10.1016/s0140-6736(11)61556-0.

Kliff, S. (2012). *Will workplace wellness programs work?* Retrieved March 16, 2012 from http://www.washingtonpost.com/blogs/ezra-klein/post/will-workplace-wellness-programs-work/2012/03/13/gIQABWUU9R_blog.html

Lauer, M. S., & Collins, F. S. (2010). Using science to improve the nation's health system. *The Journal of the American Medical Association, 303*(21), 2182–2183. doi:10.1001/jama.2010.726.

Luczak, H. (1992). "Good work" design: An ergonomic, industrial engineering perspective. In J. C. Quick, L. R. Murphy, & J. J. Hurrell Jr. (Eds.), *Stress and well-being at work: Assessments and interventions for occupational mental health* (pp. 96–112). Washington, DC: American Psychological Association.

Main, C. J., Phillips, C. J., & Watson, P. J. (2005). Secondary prevention in health-care and occupational settings in musculoskeletal conditions focusin on low back pain. In I. Z. Schultz & R. J. Gatchel (Eds.), *Handbook of complex occupational disability claims: Early risk identification, intervention and prevention*. New York, NY: Springer.

Manchikanti, L., Falco, F. J., Boswell, M. V., & Hirsch, J. A. (2010). Facts, fallacies, and politics of comparative effectiveness research: Part I. Basic considerations. *Pain Physician, 13*(1), E23–E54.

McCoy, J. M. (2002). Work environments. In R. B. Bechtel & A. Churchman (Eds.), *Handbook of environmental psychology*. New York, NY: Wiley.

McDonald, N., & Doyle, D. (1981). *The stresses of work*. London: Nelson, Walton on Thames.

O'Brien, G. E., & Feather, N. T. (1990). The relative effects of unemployment and quality of employment on the affect, work values and personal control of adolescents. *Journal of Occupational Psychology, 63*, 151–165.

Raymond, D., Kerr, M., McCullagh, M., & Lusk, S. (2011). Prevalence of hearing loss and accuracy of self-report among factory workers. *Noise & Health, 13*(54), 340–347. doi:10.4103/1463-1741.85504.

Rondinelli, R., Genovese, E., Katz, R., Mayer, T., Mueller, K., Ranavaya, M., et al. (2008). *Guides to the evaluation of permanent impairment* (6th ed.). Chicago, IL: American Medical Association.

Seale, S. (2011). *The economy's depression epidemic*. Retrieved October 9, 2011 from http://www.dailyrx.com/feature-article/how-unemployment-and-foreclosures-are-creating-mental-health-crisis-america-15477.ht

Sox, H. C. (2010). Comparative effectiveness research: A progress report. *Annals of Internal Medicine, 153*, 469–472.

Texas Department of Insurance—Division of Worker's Compensation. (2008). *Quick reference guide for designated doctors*. C508-002A (5-08).

Turk, D. C., & Melzack, R. (2001). *Handbook of pain assessment* (2nd ed.). New York, NY: Guilford.

Turk, D. C., & Monarch, E. S. (2002). Biopsychosocial perspective on chronic pain. In D. C. Turk & R. J. Gatchel (Eds.), *Psychological approaches to pain management: A practitioner's handbook* (2nd ed.). New York, NY: Guilford.

Turner, J. A., Ersek, M., Herron, L., Haselkorn, J., Kent, D., & Ciol, M. A. (1992). Patient outcomes after lumbar spinal fusions. *Journal of the American Medical Association, 268*(7), 907–911.

Waddell, G. (1987). Clinical assessment of lumbar impairment. *Clinical Orthopedic Related Research, 221*, 110–120.

Index

A
ABCT. *See* Alcohol behavioral couple therapy (ABCT)
Absenteeism and presenteeism
   acute gastrointestinal illness, 160
   alcoholism/smoking, 164–165
   allergies, 158–159
   anxiety, 166
   arthritis, 162
   depression, 166
   fibromyalgia, 162–163
   health behaviors, 164
   health-care costs, 151
   influenza, 159–160
   intervention strategies
      depression, 171
      DM and LM program, 169–170
      obesity/physical activity, 172–173
      occupational injury prevention, 173–174
      Shell's Disability Management Program, 170
      smoking and alcohol cessation, 171–172
      stay at home, 168–169
      vaccinations, 169
   job satisfaction, 167–168
   job type, demand and schedules, 167
   migraine, 160–161
   multiple sclerosis, 163
   musculoskeletal injuries, 163–164
   obesity, 165
   occupational stress, 167
   osteoarthritis, 162
   physical activity, 165
   premenstrual disorders, 161
   pulmonary diseases, 161–162
   quantitative measurement approaches
      Absenteeism Screening Questionnaire, 157
      EWPS, 154
      FABQ, 157
      Friction Cost Method, 157–158
      HLQ, 154
      HPQ, 153–154
      Human Capital Approach, 157–158
      HWQ, 154
      MIDAS, 156
      MWPLQ, 156
      National Health Inventory Survey, 154–155
      PHQ-15, 157
      WLQ, 153
      WPAI, 153, 156
Absenteeism Screening Questionnaire, 157
ACC. *See* Anterior cingulate cortex (ACC)
ACOEM. *See* American College of Occupational and Environmental Medicine (ACOEM)
Acupuncture, 73
Adrenocorticotropic hormone (ACTH), 13
Adverse work schedules
   early start times, 299
   fatigue risk management
      caffeine and stimulant use, 308
      education programs, 307
      employer occupational health programs, 305
      healthful work schedules, 307
      modifying light conditions, 307–308
      occupational screening, sleep disorders, 306
      organizational interventions, 305
      pharmacotherapy, 309
      planned napping, 308
      shift work sleep disorder, 306
      sleep timing, 308–309
   governmental regulation and public policy
      EWTD, 310–311
      hours of service (HOS) regulations, 309
      organized labor, 311–312
      OSHA, 309–310
   health and safety risks of
      accidents and injuries, 300
      alcohol use, 302
      cancer, 304
      cardiovascular disease, 301
      drowsy driving, 300, 313–315
      exercise, 302
      gastrointestinal disorders, 303
      infectious disease, 304
      menstrual changes, 304–305
      metabolic and cardiovascular disease risk, 303
      musculoskeletal disorders, 300–301
      pregnancy loss, 305
      smoking, 301–302
      unplanned pregnancies, 305

Adverse work schedules (*cont.*)
 personal responsibility, 299
 rotating shift pattern, 298–299
 shift work, 298
 staffng, 299
Age
 cancer survivors, 139
 CTS, 75
 epicondylitis, 72
 low back pain, 77
Agency for Healthcare Research and Quality (AHRQ), 559
Agoraphobia, 107
Alcohol behavioral couple therapy (ABCT), 212
Alcoholics' Anonymous (AA), 213
Alcohol use
 absenteeism and presenteeism, 164–165
 adverse work schedules, 302
Allergies, 158–159
Allostatic load, 95
American Academy of Orthopedic Surgeons, 79
American College of Occupational and Environmental Medicine (ACOEM), 559
American Federation of Labor and Congress of Industrial Organizations (AFL-CIO), 311–312
American Psychological Association (APA), 42, 559
Americans with Disabilities Act (ADA), 306
Amoco Cadiz oil tanker, 267
Anterior cingulate cortex (ACC), 227
Antisocial personality disorder, 7
Anti-stressors, 384
Anxiety, 166
Arthritis, 162
Asthma, 161–162
Atherosclerosis, 87
Australian Human Rights Commission, 105

B
Berufsgenossenschaften, 342
Binge eating disorder, 223
BLS. *See* Bureau of Labor Statistics (BLS)
Boston Carpal Tunnel Questionnaire, 75
Breast cancer, 304
Bullying
 cognitive functioning, 227
 cyber bullying, 229–230
 definition, 220–221
 employee protections, 231–233
 history of, 221
 immune functioning, 227
 negative affect, 228
 neuroendocrine function, 226
 personality characteristics, 228
 physical and psychological health outcomes, 223–225
 sex differences, 225
 social support, 228–229
 styles and prevalence, 222
 theoretical model, 219–220
Bureau of Labor Statistics (BLS), 64–65, 267, 405, 476

Burnout. *See* Occupational burnout
Burnout Measure (BM), 188

C
California Family Leave Act, 326
California Industrial Accident Act, 4
Canadian Charter of Rights and Freedoms, 311
Canadian Community Health Survey, 423
Cancer survivors
 employer perspective, 143–144
 epidemiology, 132
 financial strain, 133
 return-to-work
  interventions, 146
  occupational health and recommendations, 144–145
 working population, age of, 132–133
 work model, 138
  age, 139
  cancer site, 140
  discrimination, 143
  education and income, 139
  flexibility, 142–143
  personal preferences, 141–142
  physical and psychological work demands, 142
  stage at diagnosis, 140
  support and environment, 143
  symptoms, 141
  treatment type, 140
  work ability, 142
 work patterns
  individual trajectories of work level, 136–138
  return-to-work, 134
  unemployment, 135
  work disability, 135
  workplace discrimination, 135–136
  work sustainability, 135
Cardiovascular disease (CVD), 415
 adverse work schedules, 301, 303
 direct and indirect cost of, 87
 effort–reward imbalance model
  evidence, 91–92
  vs. job strain model, 92
  measurement, 91
 health promotion programs, 96
 job strain model
  decision latitude, 88
  evidence, 89
  hypertension, 90–91
  iso-strain model, 90
  measurement, 89
  psychological demands, 88
  social support, 88–89
  subclinical indicators, 90
 job stress, 92
 organizational prevention strategies, 96–97
 overtime work, 93
 psychosocial risk factors, 87
 shift work, 93

Index

stress-management, 96
worksite intervention programs, 97
work stress
    and gender, 93–94
    health behaviors, 94
    negative emotions, 95
    psychobiological mechanisms, 95
Carpal tunnel syndrome (CTS)
    biomechanical risk factors, 74
    disease-specific self-report questionnaires, 75–76
    electrodiagnostic tests, 75
    individual risk factor, 75
    psychosocial risk factors, 74–75
    Tinel and Phalen tests, 75
    treatment approaches, 76
CATS. *See* Cognitive Activation Theory of Stress (CATS)
CBI. *See* Copenhagen Burnout Inventory (CBI)
Centers for Disease Control and Prevention (CDC), 552
Central nervous system (CNS), 12
Certified Employee Assistance Professional (CEAP) status, 446
Chernobyl nuclear power plant, 267
Chronic obstructive pulmonary disease (COPD), 161–162, 376
Clean Air Act, 6
Cocaine Anonymous (CA), 213
Code of Hammurabi, 342
Cognitive Activation Theory of Stress (CATS), 385
Cognitive appraisal model, 49–50
Communication, 253–254
Compensation neurosis, 344–345
Computerized tomography (CT), 70
Conservation of resources theory (CRT)
    occupational burnout, 187–188
    stress, 31–32
Contingency management (CM), 213
Copenhagen Burnout Inventory (CBI), 189
Copenhagen Psychosocial Questionnaire II (COPSOQII), 542
Coronary heart disease (CHD). *See also* Cardiovascular disease (CVD)
    diet, 484
    occupational stress, 11–12
    risk factors of, 165, 225
Corticosteroids
    CTS, 76
    epicondylitis, 73
Corticotrophin releasing hormone (CRH), 13, 226
Cost-benefit analysis (CBA), 505
Cost effectiveness analysis (CEA), 376, 505
Cost-Utility analysis (CUA), 376
Council on Accreditation (COA), 447
CTS. *See* Carpal tunnel syndrome (CTS)
Cultural values and behaviors
    collectivism–individualism dimension, 517
    cross-national differences, 517
    job choice, 519
    masculinity–femininity dimension, 517
    power distance, 517
    presenteeism, 519
    uncertainty avoidance, 518
    verbal abuse and bullying, 518
    workaholics, 519
CVD. *See* Cardiovascular disease (CVD)
Cyber bullying, 229–230

D

Dehydroepiandrosterone sulphate (DHEA-s), 386
Demand–Control Model, 51
Denmark cancer rehabilitation center, 133
Depression, 166, 171
Diabetes
    CTS, 75
    epicondylitis, 72
Dietary and physical activity interventions
    cardiovascular disease, 369
    employer-provided health insurance, 370
    environmental strategies, 367
    intensive and sustained interventions, 368
    non-randomized studies, 370
    overweight and obesity, 367
    primary prevention, 368
    secondary and tertiary prevention efforts, 369
    subgroup analysis, 370
Disease management (DM), 169–170
Drowsy driving
    motor vehicle crashes, 300
    US lawsuits, 314–315

E

EAPs. *See* Employee assistance programs (EAPs)
Effort–reward imbalance (ERI) model, 91–92, 249
Elbow pain. *See* Work-related musculoskeletal disorders (WRMDs)
Employee and Family Assistance Programs (EFAPs), 443
Employee Assistance Professional Association (EAPA), 447
Employee assistance programs (EAPs)
    brief history, 442
    business models and markets, 446
    Canada, 443
    clinical effectiveness, 449
    core technology
        alcohol and drug abuse, 445
        linkages and referral, 445
        manager training, 444–445
        work focus, 444
    cost benefit, 451
    definition of, 442
    Europe, 443
    evidence
        historical themes of, 448–449
        nature of, 448
    outcomes, 450
    overview, 441
    primary services, 443

Employee assistance programs (EAPs) (cont.)
   professional standards, 447
   promotion and use of, 446–447
   services, 443–444
   trends
      alcohol issues, 453–454
      disability, 454
      employee engagement, 456
      influences, 458–459
      proactive EAP, 457–458
      study methodology, 457
      study results, 457
      technology, 456–457
      wellness/prevention, 455–456
      work/life, 454–455
   United States, 442
   workplace outcomes
      absence, 452
      financial value, 453
      hourly compensation rate, 452
      outcomes data, 452
      productivity, 452
      ROI, 453
Employee Assistance Society of North America (EASNA), 442
Employee-involvement programs, 254
Employer occupational health programs, 305
Employer's Liability Act, 342
Endicott Work Productivity Scale (EWPS), 154
Energy mobilization and regeneration
   anti-stressors, 390–392
   cultural participation, 392–395
   factors, 387
   financial arguments, 388
   good emotional and instrumental support, 387–388
   manager education, 388–390
   participatory action research, 387–388
   reasonable challenges, 387
   well-planned reorganizations, 387
Engel's biopsychosocial model, 16
Environmental Protection Agency, 6
Epicondylitis
   acupuncture, 73
   assessment and diagnosis, 72
   biomechanical risk factors, 71–72
   classification of, 71
   corticosteroid injections, 73
   extracorporeal shock therapy, 73
   health-care costs, 71
   individual risk factors, 72
   NSAIDs, 73
   physical therapy, 73
   psychosocial risk factors, 72
   surgery, 73
   symptoms, 71
Epidemiology, occupational health and illness issues
   adverse medical conditions, 473
   aggravation, 473
   apportionment, 474, 487–489
   causal association, 486–487
   causation analysis, 417–472
   death, 473
   disability, 473
   evaluation, 491
   evidence, 475–476
   evidence-based medicine, 472
   exacerbation, 474
   exposure evidence, 487
   impairment, 473
   literature review
      accuracy and precision, 483
      bias, 483
      case–control study, 481–482
      chance, 482–483
      clinical epidemiology, 479
      cohort study, 481
      confounding, 483–484
      continuous variable, 485
      cross-sectional study, 482
      dependent variable, 485
      etiologic epidemiology, 479
      false negative, 486
      false positive, 486
      independent variable, 485
      internal validity, 479
      negative predictive value, 486
      odds ratio, 485
      parametric/nonparametric data, 485
      positive predictive value, 486
      questionnaires/reporting methods, 481
      relative risk, 485
      statistical hypothesis test, 484–485
      statistical tests, 481
      study design pyramid, 480
      true negatives, 486
      true positives, 486
   loss of consciousness, 473
   medical and legal causation, 490
   medical conditions, 473
   medical treatment, 473
   nonoccupational exposures, 473
   numerator data, 476
   occupational exposures and physical factors, 473
   OSHA, 476
   rates, 477–478
   recurrence, 474
   study design, 478–479
   survey's illness measures, 477
   testimony validity, 489–490
   work environment, 473
   workers' compensation compensability, 489
Equal Employment Opportunity Commission (EEOC), 517
European Working Time Directive (EWTD), 310–311
EWPS. *See* Endicott Work Productivity Scale (EWPS)
Exercise
   adverse work schedules, 302
   epicondylitis, 73
   low back pain, 78

Extracorporeal shock therapy, 73
Exxon Valdez oil tanker, 267

F
Fair Labor Standards Act, 45, 325
Family and Medical Leave Act (FMLA), 169, 325
Fatal Accident Act, 4
Fatality Assessment and Control Evaluation (FACE), 285
Fear-Avoidance Beliefs Questionnaire (FABQ), 157
Federal Coal Mine Safety Act, 268
Federal Employees Compensation Act, 4
Fellow-servant doctrine, 3–4
Fibromyalgia, 162–163
FMLA. See Family and Medical Leave Act (FMLA)
Friction Cost method, 157–158
Fukushima I nuclear plant, 267
Functional dyspepsia, 160

G
GAD. See Generalized anxiety disorder (GAD)
Gastroesophageal reflux disease (GERD), 160
Gastrointestinal disorders, 160, 303
Gender and cultural considerations
　changing workplace
　　employment projections, 513
　　globalization, 513
　　healthy work environment, 514
　　organizational benefits, 514
　context, 521–523
　CTS, 75
　discrimination and exclusion, 519–521
　diversity and health, 514–515
　diversity environments, 523–524
　EEOC, 517
　epicondylitis, 72
　equality, 525–526
　ethnicity and race, 515
　healthy organizational environment, 527–528
　legal mandate, 524–525
　low back pain, 77
　multiculturalism, 526–527
　sex and gender, 517
　subjective culture, 515
　values and behaviors
　　collectivism–individualism dimension, 517
　　cross-national differences, 517
　　job choice, 519
　　masculinity–femininity dimension, 517
　　power distance, 517
　　presenteeism, 519
　　uncertainty avoidance, 518
　　verbal abuse and bullying, 518
　　workaholics, 519
Generalized anxiety disorder (GAD), 107
GERD. See Gastroesophageal reflux disease (GERD)
Global Assessment of Functioning (GAF), 449
Globalization, 43

Ground fault interrupter (GFI), 278
Group motivational interviewing (GMI), 213

H
Handbook of Occupational Health and Wellness, 39
Hawthorne Effect, 41
Health and Labor Questionnaire (HLQ), 154
Health and Work Performance Questionnaire (HPQ), 153–154
Health behaviors
　Health Belief Model, 408–409
　Precaution Adoption Process Model, 410–411
　predictive ability, 413
　Theory of Reasoned Action and Planned Behavior, 409–410
　Transtheoretical Model, 411–412
Health insurance
　contingent workers, 283
　contract workers, 284
　in USA, 4
Health Management Organization (HMO) Act, 4
Health risk appraisal (HRA), 372–373, 455
Health Well-Being Scale, 542
Healthy Work, 42
Healthy workplace bill (HWB), 231–232
Heel pain
　assessment and diagnosis, 79
　biomechanical risk factors, 78
　individual risk factors, 78–79
　psychosocial risk factors, 78
　treatment approaches, 79
HLQ. See Health and Labor Questionnaire (HLQ)
Human Capital Approach, 157–158
Hypertension, 90–91
Hypothalamic Pituitary Adrenocortical (HPA) axis, 12–13, 226, 386
Hypothalamo Pituitary Gonadal (HPG) axis, 386

I
ICOH. See International Commission on Occupational Health (ICOH)
Illness and injuries
　BLS, 405
　health behaviors
　　Health Belief Model, 408–409
　　Precaution Adoption Process Model, 410–411
　　predictive ability, 413
　　Theory of Reasoned Action and Planned Behavior, 409–410
　　Transtheoretical Model, 411–412
　medical costs, 406
　mental health disorders, 406
　narcotic analgesics, 406
　prevention strategies
　　cancer, 416–418
　　CVD, 415–416
　　mental health disorders, 418
　　occupational injuries, 413–414

Illness and injuries (*cont.*)
    primary prevention, 407
    quaternary prevention, 408
    secondary prevention, 407
    tertiary prevention, 407–408
    tobacco, consumption of, 414–415
ILO. *See* International Labour Organization (ILO)
Immigrant workers, 286
Independent Medical Examinations (IMEs), 352
Individual Placement and Support (IPS) program, 117
Infectious disease, 304
Influenza, 159–160
Instant Messaging (IM), 253
Institute of Work, Health and Organisations (I-WHO), 42
International Classification of Functioning, Disability and Health (ICF), 553, 558
International Commission on Occupational Health (ICOH), 559
International Covenant on Economic, Social and Cultural Rights (ICESCR), 106
International Labour Organization (ILO), 558
International Workers of the World (IWW), 272
Iso-strain model, 90

J
Job content questionnaire (JCQ), 89
Job demands–control (JDC) model, 32–34
Job demands–resources (JD-R) model, 186–187
Job Descriptive Index (JDI), 540
Job–Person Fit Model, 185–186
Job-related stressors. *See also* Work stress
    ergonomics and occupational injuries, 46–47
    external stress-related factors, 48
    physical working conditions, 44–45
    preventative stress management, 53–54
    work-place psychosocial stressors, 47–48
    work schedules, 45–46
Job strain model
    decision latitude, 88
    evidence, 89
    hypertension, 90–91
    iso-strain model, 90
    measurement, 89
    psychological demands, 88
    social support, 88–89
    subclinical indicators, 90
Job stress. *See also* Work stress
    absenteeism and presenteeism, 167
    cardiovascular disease, 92
Justice salience hierarchy (JSH), 52

K
Karasek model, 245–246
Kentucky Employees Mutual Insurance Company (KEMI), 286

L
Labor unions, 311
Lazarus's transactional model, 26–28
Leadership, 249, 252
Lifestyle management (LM), 169–170
Low back pain
    acetaminophen, 78
    assessment and diagnosis, 77–78
    biomechanical risk factors, 77
    health-care costs, 77
    individual risk factors, 77
    lifetime prevalence rates of, 76–77
    non-pharmacologic therapy, 78
    psychosocial risk factors, 77
    self-care, 78

M
Macrosystem interventions, 427–428
Magnetic resonance imaging (MRI), 75
Malingering
    assessment of, 10–11
    occupational injuries, 7–8
    workers' compensation, 9–10
Maslach Burnout Inventory (MBI), 188
Maximum Medical Improvement (MMI), 556
Medicare, 4
Mental health
    bullying(*see* Bullying)
    burnout, 192–193
    framework, 243, 250–251
    job design
        choice and control, 245–246
        flexibility, 248–249
        job content/workload, 244–245
        physical work environment, 246–247
        reward systems, 249
        role ambiguity/conflict, 246
        work schedule, 247–248
    job future
        career development, 260–261
        job security, 259–260
    leadership, 249, 252
    organizational culture
        communication, 253–254
        employee participation/involvement, 254
        organizational justice and fairness, 254–255
        psychological health/safety climate, 257–258
        social support, 255–257
        work-life balance, 258–259
Mental Health Commission of Canada, 428
Mental health disorders
    best evidence-informed work accommodations, 432
    comorbidity, 107, 108
    disability management practices, 424
    incidence and prevalence of, 107
    interventions
        return-to-work process, 117–121
        unemployment, 115–116

Index 571

work disability, 117
occupational mental health
  employment outcomes, 426
  macrosystem interventions, 427–428
  mesosystem interventions, 429–432
  physical disorders, 107–108
  psychological symptoms, 423
  research gaps, 434–435
  social stigmatization, 424
  systemic solutions center, 433–434
  work accommodations
    inclusion and social process, 425
    occupational stress, 425
    person-environment conceptualization, 426
    recovery-oriented vision, 425
    stigma, 426
    unemployment, 426
  work disability, effects of
    decreased productivity at work, 109–110
    disability absence, cost of, 111–112
    short- and long-term disability, 111
    types of, 109
    unemployment, 108–109
    work loss days, 110–111
  work-related risk factors
    job characteristics, 113–114
    job security, 115
    targeting factors, 114
Mesosystem interventions
  employment outcomes
    disability management, 430–431
    job accommodation, targeting barriers, 431–432
    job matching, 431
    supported employment, 431
  primary prevention
    accommodations costs, budget, 429–430
    management, training of, 430
    restructuring organization, 429
    written policies, health and wellness, 429
Metabolic syndrome, 94
Migraine Disability Assessment (MIDAS), 156
Migraine Work and Productivity Loss Questionnaire (MWPLQ), 156
Minnesota Multiphasic Personality Inventory-2 (MMPI-2), 205
Missouri Workers' Compensation Law, 489
Mood disorders, 166
Motivational interviewing (MI), 212–213
MRI. *See* Magnetic resonance imaging (MRI)
Multiple sclerosis, 163
Musculoskeletal injuries, 163–164, 300–301
MWPLQ. *See* Migraine Work and Productivity Loss Questionnaire (MWPLQ)

N
Narcotics Anonymous (NA), 213
National Agricultural Safety Database, 276
National Cancer Institute, 133

National Health Inventory Survey, 154–155
National Institute for Occupational Safety and Health (NIOSH), 42, 285, 475, 558
National Organization of Associate Degree Nursing (NOADN), 543
National Research Council (NRC), 64
National Transportation Safety Board (NTSB), 307
Neck pain. *See* Work-related musculoskeletal disorders (WRMDs)
Night shift workers
  EWTD, 311
  fatigue risk management
    caffeine and stimulant use, 308
    modifying light conditions, 307–308
    planned napping, 308
    sleep timing, 308–309
  health and safety risks of
    alcohol use, 302
    cancer, 304
    drowsy driving, 300, 313
    gastrointestinal disorders, 303
    menstrual changes, 304–305
    occupational accidents and injuries, 298, 300
    pregnancy loss, 305
    smoking, 301–302
    SWSD, 306
    unplanned pregnancies, 305
  rotating shifts, 298
NOADN. *See* National Organization of Associate Degree Nursing (NOADN)
Nonsteroidal inflammatory medications (NSAIDs), 73
North American Industry Classification System (NAICS), 476
NRC. *See* National Research Council (NRC)
NTSB. *See* National Transportation Safety Board (NTSB)

O
Obesity
  absenteeism and presenteeism, 165
  CTS, 75
  epicondylitis, 72
  low back pain, 77
Occupational burnout
  CRT model, 187–188
  future research, 196
  history of, 182–184
  JD-R model, 186–187
  Job–Person Fit Model, 185–186
  Maslach's model, 183–185
  predictors of, 190–192
  prevention
    person-centered approaches, 195–196
    situation-centered approaches, 196
  psychosocial inventories
    Burnout Measure, 188
    Copenhagen Burnout Inventory, 189
    Maslach Burnout Inventory, 188

Occupational burnout (*cont.*)
    Oldenburg Burnout Inventory, 189
    Shirom-Melamed Burnout Questionnaire, 188–189
    Utrecht Work Engagement Scale, 189–190
    special populations
        health-care workers, 193
        law enforcement, 194
        mental health, 192–193
        teachers, 193–194
Occupational health and wellness
    behavioral pathogens, 14–15
    economic meltdowns, 549
    environmental psychology and crowding research, 552
    healthy organizational hierarchical system, 557
    medicolegal issues and occupational injuries
        compensation neurosis, 9
        litigation neurosis, 9
        losses and gains, 7
        malingering, 7–8
    occupational injury administrative and legal issues
        biopsychosocial model, 554
        compensation injuries, 554
        correlations, 555
        disability, 557
        impairment, 556–557
        pain, 555
    organizational health, 553–554
    public and private organizations/agencies, 557–559
    research activity, 550
    stress (*see* Stress)stresses, strains and long-term consequences, 551
    transdisciplinary model
        biopsychosocial model, 15–17, 19
        interdisciplinary approach, 17–18
    unemployment/nonwork, 551–552
    unhealthywork environments, 5–6
    vocational rehabilitation, 553
    workers' compensation (*see* Workers' compensation)
Occupational health psychology
    globalization, 43
    handbooks and journals, 39
    Hawthorne Effect, 41
    job-related stressors
        ergonomics and occupational injuries, 46–47
        external stress-related factors, 48
        physical working conditions, 44–45
        work-place psychosocial stressors, 47–48
        work schedules, 45–46
    occupational health researchers, 41–42
    organizations, 42
    preventative stress management, 53–54
    principles of scientific management, 40–41
    technology, 43
    work practices, 43–44
    work stress
        cognitive appraisal model, 49–50
        Demand–Control Model, 51
        Effort–Reward Model, 51–52
        organizational justice, 52–53
        P–E fit theory, 50–51
        theoretical models of, 49–50
Occupational injury prevention
    factor matrix, 275
    fatal roadway collision, 277
    injury prevention categories, 274
    safety training, 278–279
    unsafe work practices, 277
    young women and child workers, 276
Occupational mental health
    employment outcomes, 426
    macrosystem interventions, 427–428
    mesosystem interventions
        employment outcomes, 430–432
        primary prevention, 429–430
Occupational Safety and Health Act (OSHA), 45, 268, 309–310
Occupational workplace issues
    academic administrators, 539–540
    academic middle managers, 537
    administrative roles, 536
    American Association of Community Colleges competencies, 537
    faculty role, 536
    higher education, 535
    high job strain, 535
    nursing academic administrators
        hardiness study, pre-assessment of, 543–544
        Leadership Practice Inventory, 541
        National Work Environment Study, 542–543
        pre-licensure program, 540
        social support, 542
        telephone surveys, 541
        unique additional responsibilities, 541
        URAs, 545
        workload demands, 544–545
    organizational management concepts
        job burnout, 537–538
        job responsibilities, 539
        job satisfaction, 538
        stress, 539
Oldenburg Burnout Inventory (OLBI), 189
Organisation for Economic Co-operation and Development (OECD), 344–345
Organizational Commitment Questionnaire (OCQ), 540
Organizational culture
    communication, 253–254
    employee participation/involvement, 254
    organizational justice and fairness, 254–255
    psychological health/safety climate, 257–258
    social support, 255–257
    work-life balance, 258–259
Organized labor, 311–312
OSHA. *See* Occupational Safety and Health Act (OSHA)
Osteoarthritis, 162

P
Panic disorder, 107
Participatory action research (PAR), 388

Patient Health Questionnaire (PHQ), 157
Peer victimization. *See* Bullying
Personal protective equipment (PPE), 279
Personal time off (PTO), 326
Person–environment fit theory, 28–30, 50–51
Phalen test, 75
Pharmacotherapy, 309
PHQ. *See* Patient Health Questionnaire (PHQ)
Physical therapy, 73
Post-traumatic stress disorder (PTSD), 107, 223
Premenstrual disorders, 161
Presenteeism. *See* Absenteeism and presenteeism
Prevention and intervention methods
    assessments, 498
    barriers, 506
    cost-effectiveness, 505
    critical-emancipatory approach, 499
    formative evaluation
        black box evaluation, 501
        internet-based interventions, 500
        qualitative research, 500
        theoretical model, 501
    health promotion programs, 496
    interpretive approach, 499
    intervention mapping
        adoption and implementation plan, 507–508
        monitoring and evaluation plan, 508
        production and integration, 507
        proximal program objectives, 507
        theory-based intervention methods and practical strategies, 507
    interventions, 495
    positivist approach, 498
    process evaluation
        fidelity, 502
        formal and informal process factors, 503
        social and political realities, 502
    research methods/concepts
        effectiveness, 497
        external and internal validity, 497
        Federal agencies, 496
        generalizability, 497
        inherent barriers and limitations, 496
        multiple theories and techniques, 496
        scientific method, 496
        study validity, 497
    statistics, 497–498
    summative evaluation, 504–505
Prevention strategies
    cancer, 416–418
    CVD, 415–416
    mental health disorders, 418
    occupational injuries, 413–414
    primary prevention, 15, 407
    quaternary prevention, 408
    secondary prevention, 15, 407
    tertiary prevention, 15, 407–408
    tobacco, consumption of, 414–415
Productive Rehabilitation Institute of Dallas for Ergonomics (PRIDE), 352

Psychological health and safety (PH&S), 257–258
Psychological Injury and Law, 10
Psychological job strain questionnaire (PSJSQ), 89
Psychological stress. *See* Stress
PTSD. *See* Post-traumatic stress disorder (PTSD)
Pulmonary diseases, 161–162

Q
Quality Adjusted Life Years (QALYs), 376
Québec Charter of Human Rights and Freedoms, 311
Quick Inventory for Depressive Symptoms Self-Report (QIDS-SR), 171

R
Randomized control trial (RCT), 457
Receiving operator characteristic (ROC) analysis, 157
Return-on-Investment (ROI), 451
Return-to-Work (RTW), 454
Revenue Capacity Factor (RCF), 452
Role ambiguity, 246
Rotating shift pattern, 298–299

S
Screening, brief intervention, and referral to treatment (SBIRT), 172, 453
Self-medication and illicit drug use
    behaviorist model, 203
    empirical evidence, 205–206
    integrated model, 203–204
    interventions
        alcohol behavioral couple therapy, 212
        behavioral couple therapy, 212
        contingency management, 213
        group motivational interviewing, 213
        inpatient treatment programs, 214
        motivational interviewing, 212–213
        outpatient treatment programs, 214
        psychosocial treatment, 211–212
        screening, 209–210
        self-help groups, 213
        stress reduction, 210–211
        therapeutic communities, 214
    psychodynamic model, 202–203
    work-stress paradigm, 209
        coping deficits model, 207
        cultural model, 207
        empirical evidence, 208–209
        meditation model, 206
        moderated meditation model, 207
        moderation model, 206–207
        physical availability, 208
        simple cause–effect model, 206
        social availability, 208
        spillover/generalization model, 207
        work stress model, 207
Service Employees International Union (SEIU), 311
Shell's Disability Management Program, 170

Sherbrooke Model, 118–119
Shift work. *See also* Adverse work schedules
  cardiovascular disease, 93
  job-related stress, 45–46
Shift work sleep disorder (SWSD), 306
Shirom-Melamed Burnout Questionnaire (SMBQ), 188–189
Shoulder pain. *See* Work-related musculoskeletal disorders (WRMDs)
Sick Leave Ordinance, 169
Sleep disorders
  drowsy driving, 300
  occupational screening, 306
Smoking
  absenteeism and presenteeism, 164–165
  adverse work schedules, 301–302
  cardiovascular disease, 87
  CTS, 75
  epicondylitis, 72
  low back pain, 77
SNS. *See* Sympathetic nervous system (SNS)
Social Security Disability Act, 4
Society for Occupational Health Psychology (SOHP), 559
State Disability Insurance (SDI), 326
Stress
  conservation of resources theory, 31–32
  coronary heart disease, 11–12
  definitions of, 24–26
  and health, 13–14
  job demands–job control model, 32–34
  Lazarus's transactional model, 26–28
  nature of, 12–13
  P–E fit theory, 28–30
  savouring the positive, 35–36
  work and happiness, 35
Stress reduction programmes
  anti-stress health promotion programmes, 383
  employee health change organization
    assembly-line workers, 398
    counter clock-wise schedule, 395
    HPG activity, 396
    PAR, 396
    psychosocial work environment, 397
    quasi-experimental design, 397
    shift work schedule, 395
    urinary catecholamine excretion, 398
  energy mobilization and regeneration
    anti-stressors, 390–392
    cultural participation, 392–395
    factors, 387
    financial arguments, 388
    good emotional and instrumental support, 387–388
    manager education, 388–390
    participatory action research, 387–388
    reasonable challenges, 387
    well-planned reorganizations, 387
  individual stress management, 398–400
  individual *vs.* organizational stress reduction approaches

  individual stress management level, 384–385
  intervention efforts, 384
  stress reaction and regeneration, 386–387
  structural and individual factors, 384
Structured Interview of Reported Symptoms (SIRS), 10
Substance abuse professional (SAP) services, 445
Supported employment (SE) program model, 116–117
Survivorship Care Plan, 145
Swedish Insurance Company, 388–390
SWSD. *See* Shift work sleep disorder (SWSD)
Sympathetic nervous system (SNS), 12–13, 226

T
TBI. *See* Traumatic brain injury (TBI)
Temporary Disability Insurance (TDI), 169
Tennis elbow, 71
TENS. *See* Transcutaneous electrical nerve stimulation (TENS)
Tetraethyl lead, 5
The Handbook of Occupational Health Psychology, 39
The Journal of Occupational Health Psychology, 39
The Principles of Scientific Management, 40–41
Therapeutic Return-to-Work (TRW) program, 119
Three Mile Island nuclear energy plant, 267
Tinel test, 75
Total Permanent Disability (TPD), 350
Transcutaneous electrical nerve stimulation (TENS), 71
Traumatic brain injury (TBI), 353
Triangle Shirtwaist factory, 269–271
Trust and Betrayal in the Workplace, 253
Type II diabetes, 72

U
Unemployment
  cancer survivors, 135
  mental disorders, 115–116
Universal Declaration of Human Rights, 106
University Research Administrator (URA), 545
Utrecht Work Engagement Scale (UWES), 189–190

V
Vaccination, 169
Vocational rehabilitation (VR), 553
Voucher-based reinforcement therapy (VBRT), 213

W
Washington Administrative Codes (WACs), 352
WEA. *See* Workers' Education Association (WEA)
WFHN. *See* Work Family and Health Network (WFHN)
WHO. *See* World Health Organization (WHO)
Work Demand Scale, 542
Work Disability Diagnostic Interview for Common Mental Disorders (WoDDI-CMD), 119
Workers' compensation
  California Industrial Accident Act, 4
  case studies

Index

behavioral medicine evaluation, 353
chronic opioid therapy, 352
insurer's obstructionist policies, 354
L&I Claim manager, 353
psychopharmacological intervention, 354
return-to-work rates, 352
secondary gain, 353
vocational reactivation, 352
compromise and release, 343
employer negligence, 342
Fatal Accident Act, 4
Federal Employees Compensation Act, 4
fellow-servant doctrine, 3–4
health insurance, 4
Health Management Organization Act, 4
indemnity and disability
    Canadian qualitative study, 347
    caregiver role, 346
    claim managers' errors, 348
    compensation neurosis, 344
    disability management, 347
    employment status, 344
    financial support, 343
    medical bills, 346
    Medicare fee schedule, 349
    negative progression, 347
    neutral phenomenon, 346
    pain specialists, 349
    return-to-work process, 345
    rigidity and unresponsiveness, 348
    secondary gain, 345
    tertiary gain, 345
lump-sum payment, 343
malingering, 9–10
monetary compensation, 341
national health expenditures, 5
negligent accidental injuries, 3–4
private insurance carriers, 342
US health-care expenditures, 6
vocational retraining, 341
Washington, 350–351
work-related injuries, 342
Workers' Education Association (WEA), 559
Work Family and Health Network (WFHN)
    employee health, 331
    family outcomes, 331–332
    moderating factors, 332
    workplace intervention, 329–330
    workplace outcomes, 330–331
Work–family balance issues
    biopsychosocial model, 327–328
    care demands, 325
    demographic behaviors, 325
    nonmarital childbearing, 324
    paid market labor, 324
    role incompatibility, 324
    schedule consistency, 323
    work-family conflict
        employee health, 331
        family outcomes, 331–332
        moderating factors, 332
        workplace intervention, 329–330
        workplace outcomes, 330–331
Work–leave policies
    employee usage, 327
    Fair Labor Standards Act, 325
    federal government, 325
    FMLA, 326
    sick leave, 326
    telework, 327
Work Limitations Questionnaire (WLQ), 153, 212
Workplace bullying. *See* Bullying
Workplace disasters
    alternative/contingent workers, 283
    attitudes, 289–290
    capital and social relations, 280–282
    congressional action, 269
    contract workers and injury risk, 284
    dynamic work environments, 287–288
    economics and injury consequences, 285–286
    environmental toll, 267
    examples of, 268
    government sources, 267
    Heinrich injury pyramid, 279–280
    immigrant workers, 286
    Lawrence Woolen Textile Mill Strike, 271–273
    methane, 268
    narrative guides and directs behavior, 289
    outsourcing and subcontracting, 283–284
    safety climate, 273
    safety practices, 288–289
    social activity, 282–283
    Triangle Shirtwaist factory, 269–271
    US Underground Coal Mining Disasters, 269
    William Haddon Jr.
        factor matrix, 275
        fatal roadway collision, 277
        injury prevention categories, 274
        safety training, 278–279
        unsafe work practices, 277
        young women and child workers, 276
    Workers' Compensation insurance premiums, 268
Work Productivity and Activity Impairment Questionnaire (WPAI), 153
Work-related musculoskeletal disorders (WRMDs)
    conceptual model, 66–68
    distribution of, 66
    economic burden of, 65–66
    elbow
        acupuncture, 73
        assessment and diagnosis, 72
        biomechanical risk factors, 71–72
        corticosteroid injections, 73
        epicondylitis, 71
        extracorporeal shock therapy, 73
        individual risk factors, 72
        NSAIDs, 73
        physical therapy, 73
        psychosocial risk factors, 72
        surgery, 73

Work-related musculoskeletal disorders (WRMDs) (*cont.*)
  future research, 80
  hand and wrist
    assessment and diagnosis, 75–76
    biomechanical risk factors, 74
    individual risk factor, 75
    psychosocial risk factors, 74–75
    treatment approaches, 76
  incidence and prevalence rates, 64–65
  knee, foot, and ankle
    assessment and diagnosis, 79
    biomechanical risk factors, 78
    individual risk factors, 78–79
    psychosocial risk factors, 78
    treatment approaches, 79
  low back pain
    acetaminophen, 78
    assessment and diagnosis, 77–78
    biomechanical risk factors, 77
    health-care costs, 77
    individual risk factors, 77
    lifetime prevalence rates of, 76–77
    non-pharmacologic therapy, 78
    psychosocial risk factors, 77
    self-care, 78
  neck and/or shoulder
    assessment and diagnosis, 70
    cognitive-behavioral intervention, 70–71
    ergonomic interventions, 70
    improper static postures, 68–69
    individual risk factors, 69–70
    prevalence of, 68
    psychosocial risk factors, 69
    repetitive work activities, 68
    symptoms, 68
    TENS, 71
  types of, 68
Work schedules. *See also* Adverse work schedules
  absenteeism and presenteeism, 167
  job-related stress, 45–46
  workplace mental health, 247–248
Worksite health and wellness promotion
  business case, 375–377
  comprehensive worksite health promotion programs, 373–375
  development of, 366
  dietary and physical activity interventions
    cardiovascular disease, 369
    employer-provided health insurance, 370
    environmental strategies, 367
    intensive and sustained interventions, 368
    non-randomized studies, 370
    overweight and obesity, 367
    primary prevention, 368
    secondary and tertiary prevention efforts, 369
    subgroup analysis, 370
  evolution of
    chronic health conditions, 365
    economic and organizational benefits, 366
    financial incentive, 367
    historical timeline, 366
    physical and psychosocial well-being, 365
  HRA and tailored health advice, 372–373
  integration of, 377–378
  smoking cessation, 370–372
Work stress
  cardiovascular disease
    ERI model, 91–92
    gender, 93–94
    health behaviors, 95
    job strain model (*see* Job strain model)
    negative emotions, 95–96
    psychobiological mechanisms, 95
  cognitive appraisal model, 49–50
  conservation of resources theory, 31–32
  definitions of, 24–26
  Demand–Control Model, 51
  Effort–Reward Model, 51–52
  job demands–job control model, 32–34
  Lazarus's transactional model, 26–28
  organizational justice, 52–53
  P–E fit theory, 28–30, 50–51
  savouring the positive, 35–36
  self-medication and illicit drug use
    coping deficits model, 207
    cultural model, 207
    empirical evidence, 208–209
    meditation model, 206
    moderated meditation model, 207
    moderation model, 206–207
    physical availability, 208
    simple cause–effect model, 206
    social availability, 208
    spillover/generalization model, 207
    work stress model, 207
  theoretical models of, 49–50
  work and happiness, 35
World Bank, 558
World Health Organization (WHO), 153, 423, 553, 558

Printed in the United States
By Bookmasters